W9-DCN-841

PEDIATRIC
SURGERY *volume 1*

PEDIATRIC SURGERY *third edition*

Volume 1

edited by

ORVAR SWENSON, M.D.

Surgeon-in-Chief
The Children's Memorial Hospital
Chicago, Illinois
Professor of Surgery
Northwestern University Medical School

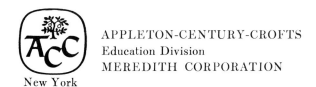

APPLETON-CENTURY-CROFTS
Education Division
MEREDITH CORPORATION

New York

Copyright © 1969 by
MEREDITH CORPORATION

All rights reserved. This book, or parts thereof, must not be used or reproduced in any manner without written permission. For information address the publisher, Appleton-Century-Crofts, Division of Meredith Corporation, 440 Park Avenue South, New York, New York 10016

629-1

Library of Congress Card Number: 68-10853

Copyright © 1962 by Meredith Publishing Company

Copyright © 1958 by Appleton-Century-Crofts, Inc.

PRINTED IN THE UNITED STATES OF AMERICA

M-85913

CONTRIBUTORS

JOSEPH E. ALFANO, M.D.
Head, Division of Ophthalmology
The Children's Memorial Hospital
Assistant Professor of Ophthalmology
Northwestern University Medical School

DAVID ALLAN, M.D.
Head, Division of Anesthesia
The Children's Memorial Hospital
Assistant Professor of Anesthesia
Northwestern University Medical School

LUIS V. AMADOR, M.D.
Head, Division of Neurosurgery
The Children's Memorial Hospital
Clinical Associate Professor
The University of Illinois College of Medicine

LESLIE B. AREY, Ph.D., Sc.D.
Robert Laughlin Rea
Professor of Anatomy, Emeritus
Northwestern University Medical School

THOMAS G. BAFFES, M.D.
Associate Attending Surgeon
The Children's Memorial Hospital
Associate, Department of Surgery
Northwestern University Medical School

JOHN M. BEAL, M.D.
Professor of Surgery and Chairman
Department of Surgery
Northwestern University Medical School

ARTHUR DE BOER, M.D.
Associate Attending Surgeon
The Children's Memorial Hospital
Assistant Professor of Surgery
Northwestern University Medical School

WILLIAM L. DONNELLAN, M.D.
Associate Attending Surgeon
The Children's Memorial Hospital
Associate in Surgery
Northwestern University Medical School

THOMAS J. EGAN, M.D.
Attending Physician and Director
Clinical Study Center
The Children's Memorial Hospital
Associate Professor of Pediatrics
Northwestern University Medical School

JOHN ELSEN, M.D.
Head, Division of Otolaryngology
Assistant Professor of Otolaryngology
Northwestern University Medical School

JEANNE M. FOLEY, Ph.D.
Research Psychologist

ORVILLE C. GREEN, M.D.
Head, Division of Endocrinology
The Children's Memorial Hospital
Associate Professor of Pediatrics
Northwestern University Medical School

PAUL H. HOLINGER, M.S., M.D.
Head, Division of Bronchology
The Children's Memorial Hospital
Professor of Bronchoesophagology
The University of Illinois College of Medicine

FAROUK S. IDRISS, M.D.
Head, Division of Cardiac Surgery
The Children's Memorial Hospital
Assistant Professor of Surgery
Northwestern University Medical School

JAMES M. KIDD, M.D.
Associate Pathologist
The Children's Memorial Hospital

LOWELL R. KING, M.D.
Head, Division of Urology
The Children's Memorial Hospital
Assistant Professor
Northwestern University Medical School

HUGH L. MOFFET, M.D.
Head, Division of Infectious Diseases
The Children's Memorial Hospital
Assistant Professor of Pediatrics
Northwestern University Medical School

CLARENCE W. MONROE, M.D.
Head, Division of Plastic Surgery
The Children's Memorial Hospital
Associate Clinical Professor of Surgery
The University of Illinois College of Medicine

HENRY L. NADLER, M.D.
Assistant Attending Physician
The Children's Memorial Hospital
Assistant Professor of Pediatrics
Northwestern University Medical School

WILLIAM L. RIKER, M.D.
Associate Surgeon-in-Chief
The Children's Memorial Hospital
Associate Professor of Surgery
Northwestern University Medical School

JOYCE A. SCHILD, M.D.
Associate Attending Bronchologist
The Children's Memorial Hospital
Clinical Associate in Otolaryngology
The University of Illinois College of Medicine

JEROME L. SCHULMAN, M.D.
Head, Division of Psychiatry
The Children's Memorial Hospital
Professor of Pediatrics and
Professor of Psychiatry and Neurology
Northwestern University Medical School

ORVAR SWENSON, M.D.
Surgeon-in-Chief
The Children's Memorial Hospital
Professor of Surgery
Northwestern University Medical School

MIHRAN O. TACHDJIAN, M.D.
Head, Division of Orthopedic Surgery
The Children's Memorial Hospital
Associate Professor of Surgery
Northwestern University Medical School

DAVID T. A. VERNON, Ph.D.
Research Psychologist

PREFACE

When the time came to plan a third edition of our textbook on pediatric surgery, so many advances had occurred that a single individual could not adequately deal with all the surgical conditions of infancy and childhood. To be useful to students, house officers, physicians, and surgeons, the text had necessarily to include the whole spectrum of pediatric surgery, and so a number of individuals skilled in the various specialties of pediatric surgery were asked to contribute their experience to the work. The advantages of having several contributors are obvious. There are also certain disadvantages, among them the lack of continuity and style which is inherent in multiple authorship. It was decided, therefore, to limit the contributors to members of The Children's Memorial Hospital and the Northwestern University School of Medicine surgical staff. The book thus includes detailed considerations of the pediatric surgical specialties: Orthopedics, Urology, Otolaryngology, Bronchology, Neurosurgery, Cardiac Surgery, Ophthalmology, and Plastic Surgery, as well as chapters concerning the conditions now treated in general Pediatric Surgery. It has been our constant effort to avoid needless repetition and to bring a reasonably consistent form to the finished work in order to assist more ready comprehension by our readers.

It is becoming evident that as clinical problems become more and more complex the surgeon must work in close relationship with various pediatric medical specialists. We have therefore requested men in certain of the pediatric disciplines to contribute their experience to the book. In this way the reader is presented with information regarding fields of medicine which are important to the management of surgical patients. The sections on teratology, fluid and electrolyte balance, bleeding disorders, and genetics have been directed to subjects which are of particular value to the surgeon who becomes involved in the care of infants and children.

The book is an attempt to present well-tried diagnostic and therapeutic methods in a manner that readers can follow from work-up through treatment of patients in an orderly and comprehensive way. We believe that the principles outlined here will continue to be relevant for some time to come, and that their correct application can result in excellence of surgical care for patients in the pediatric age group.

Attention to the endless details required in the preparation of this manuscript has fallen to the secretaries of our department, Miss Viola Muffler and Mrs. Anna Tyas. Mrs. Tyas kept track of the large number of illustrations, legends, bibliographies, as well as preparing the manuscript. To both, our sincere thanks and appreciation. Appreciation to Elsa Swenson who has compiled the index (and does not think it is for the birds).

The majority of photographs were taken by our hospital photographer, Miss Helen Silver. We are proud of her work. The illustrations were started by Miss Sally Stengel. Matrimony drew her away from our projects. She was ably replaced by Miss Diane Nelson.

This book would have been impossible without the counsel and direct help of the publisher, especially Mr. David Stires, Editor-in-Chief of Medical Books, and two of his able assistants, Miss Judith Schwartz and Miss Adele Spiegler.

CONTENTS

Volume 1

section four   THE ABDOMEN

xi

Volume 2

section five   **THE SKIN**

section six   **PEDIATRIC UROLOGY**
Lowell R. King

COLOR PLATES

Selected pictures illustrating
Orvar Swenson's treatment of Hirschsprung's disease
(Chapter 45)
(From Swenson. Surgical Procedures, 4:1, 1967.
Courtesy of Warner-Chilcott Laboratories.)

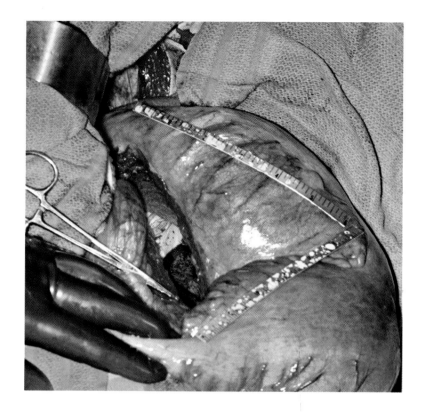

Looking into the pelvis, the change in diameter of the colon from sigmoid to rectosigmoid is apparent. In this large child, the proximal line of resection was determined by measuring 12 inches proximally from the narrow segment into the dilated segment. Absence of ganglion cells usually extends 3 to 8 inches into the dilated colon above the funnel lesion. The patient's age and size determines this distance. For instance, in a 1-year-old child this length is 3 to 4 inches.

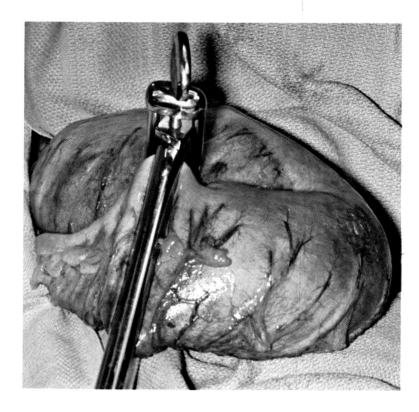

The Von Petz stapling clamp has been placed across the colon at the predetermined point of proximal resection. Note that the proximal bowel in the left side of the photograph has been decompressed by manually forcing the intestinal contents into the bowel that is to be resected. Small impactions can be dealt with in this manner. The blood supply proximal to the clamp is ample.

The rectosigmoid is being held up to provide a view into the pelvis. Note that freeing of the rectosigmoid and rectum has been accomplished by keeping the dissection on the bowel wall, leaving the pelvic structures undisturbed.

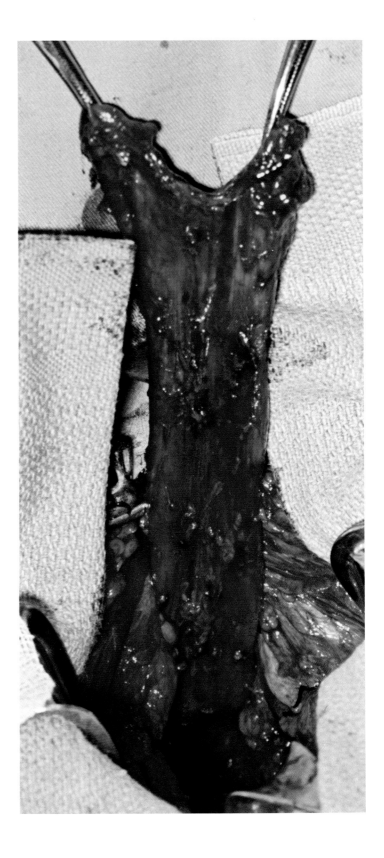

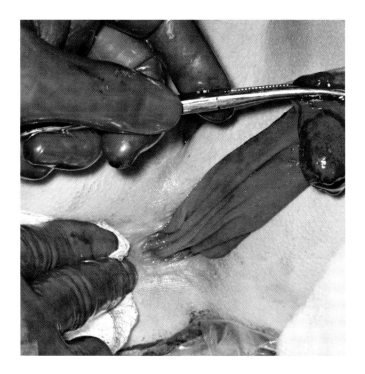

The rectosigmoid and rectum have been prolapsed through the anal canal. By traction on the prolapsed colon and counter traction on the perianal skin, the cutaneous mucosal junction can be clearly identified. Unless this is possible, the distal segment has not been sufficiently freed.

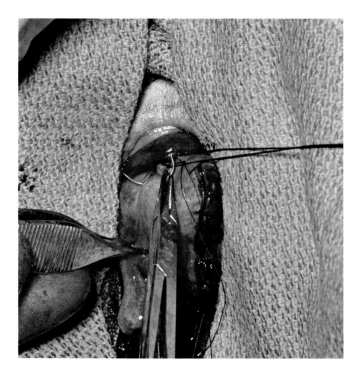

The prolapsed rectum has been divided about 2 cm from the mucocutaneous margin anteriorly. The cut will be continued diagonally backward so the rectum is transected almost at the cutaneous margin posteriorly. The proximal colon has been pulled through the incision. It is imperative to have adequate length particularly at the mesenteric side of the bowel. The first suture line is being placed. It consists of 5-0 silk sutures which include the muscular coats but do not perforate the mucosa.

The first layer of interrupted silk sutures has been placed completely around the bowel except for a short space posteriorly. This is the most difficult area to close. The surgeon must be sure that these last few sutures are carefully placed to assure a watertight anastomosis.

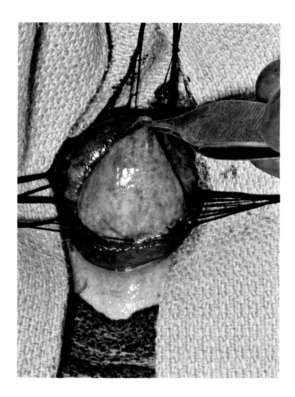

The stapled end of the prolapsed segment has been partially divided and the mucosa of the two segments united with interrupted 5-0 chromic catgut sutures. When the sutures are cut the anastomosis recedes into the pelvic cavity.

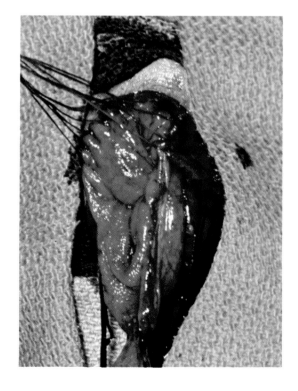

1

Orientation—The Surgical Team

Pediatric surgeons are primarily concerned with malformations in the neonate. In order to treat them most effectively they must be trained to recognize and deal intelligently with the various pathological entities that commonly occur in this age group. It is a serious mistake for the surgeon to consider that the pathology he is so familiar with in adults will be completely useful in dealing with infants—for the spectrum of pathological entities in the neonatal and infant period is entirely different from what one has to deal with in the adult. For example, a partial duodenal obstruction caused by malrotation with an associated volvulus of the midgut is an entity practically never encountered in adults. Unless the surgeon is cognizant of the condition, its signs, symptoms, roentgen diagnosis, and surgical treatment, he may either overlook it or fail to correct it adequately.

An additional problem with infants is that the history of the illness must be obtained from the parents or other observers, and this often introduces mistakes unless a determined effort is made to secure an accurate report. Many times the diagnosis can be reached more quickly and will be more accurate when based upon a concise detailed description of the progression of events of the illness than upon the physical findings or the laboratory data. This is particularly true because there is no cooperation from the infant during physical examination. The performance of a meaningful examination on infants requires special skill and, more important, experience. A surgeon treating infants has to cope with a set of postoperative problems different from that of adults under similar circumstances. Abnormalities of the whole metabolic process in infants, particularly dehydration and electrolyte imbalance, occur with greater speed and require more precise treatment for correction and maintenance than in large patients. Intelligent care for the postoperative patient requires an understanding of caloric requirements and special information on formula composition, intervals of feeding, and dietary progression to the inclusion of solids. To be sure, he has the help of pediatric consultants; nevertheless, an appreciation of these problems improves his ability to work intelligently with the pediatrician.

Precision in surgical technique is extremely important in pediatric surgery. The newborn is approximately one-thirtieth the size of an adult, and this miniaturization requires technical precision. Suturing with 3–0 silk and catgut sutures is comparable to using heavy cord to suture adults. It is amazing how the human body can withstand the invasion of

1

various organ systems and body cavities with profound alterations in the internal structure and still survive. As more extensive operations for the correction of malformations in the neonate are performed a precise, gentle surgical technique becomes more important. To ensure high survival rates, to reduce morbidity in the hospital, and to achieve better functional results, there is no substitute for the use of fine instruments, minute sutures, and a technique that appreciates that tissue damage should be reduced to a minimum during the operative procedure. These facts are reviewed here to emphasize that the pediatric surgeon requires special knowledge, skills, and techniques in addition to a broad basic training in general adult surgery if he is to provide optimum care for the surgical pediatric patient.

The skill of the pediatric surgeon can be nullified without adequate ancillary professional services. A pediatrician, with his knowledge of the normal physiology of the newborn and his skill and experience in the diagnosis and treatment of the sick baby, is an important member of the team, essential both for the diagnosis and later in the postoperative management of the patient. This is particularly true when serious postoperative complications arise that have unexpected far-reaching effects on various organ systems of the body outside the immediate area subjected to operative manipulation.

Of equal importance is the presence of a pediatric radiologist to conduct the numerous examinations that are required for accurate diagnosis of surgical conditions in infancy. Special training and exquisite patience are important in his search for lesions that are unknown in adult radiology and must be sought for in an uncooperative, squirming, noisy infant. Special equipment, such as for image intensification at the fluoroscopic screen, with equipment to make cinegraphic studies is necessary so that, in addition to static roentgen films, dynamic studies of function can be recorded on movie film.

A third essential person on the team that provides optimum surgical care for the infant is a pathologist. The tumors, the congenital malformations, and the metabolic disorders in the pediatric age group are entirely different from those in adults. Consequently the best and most experienced adult pathologist proves of very little value in the diagnosis of surgical conditions in the neonate. Frequently the surgeon is dependent upon the skills, as in making frozen sections, and upon the judgment of the pediatric pathologist to guide him in surgical therapy. The peculiar tumors and the many small deviations from normal that the pathologist must detect on frozen section while the surgeon in the operating room is waiting for a decision can only be successfully performed by one specially trained in this area of pathology. Unless such a person is available, operative procedures can be wasted as far as therapy for the patient is concerned. Wrong operative procedures can be undertaken, and multiple operations are often required in order to achieve the desired result because a trained pediatric pathologist was not available initially to help guide surgical therapy.

The fourth person, who is probably the most important of all on the team treating the surgical problems of infancy, is the anesthesiologist. A man can have the most profound knowledge and extensive experience in dealing with adult anesthesia and be unable to cope safely with the problems of infant anesthesia. Because of the small tidal air volume and the miniature size of the airways, special instruments and equipment are required in pediatric anesthesia. In addition to the administration of the anesthetic agent, the anesthesiologist has assumed the responsibilities of checking the volume of blood loss and administering fluids, blood, and special medication during the course of the operation. This permits the surgeon to concentrate his efforts completely on the operative procedure. The pediatric anesthesiologist offers an important service in appraising the patient preoperatively, helping to reach a sound judgment on what can be accomplished, particularly in determining when an extremely ill patient is ready for surgery and what magnitude of surgical procedure can be tolerated. Today, operations are performed on patients who were considered prohibitive operative risks two decades ago. The anesthesiologist has also become an important member of the team responsible for the postoperative care of the patient. The pediatric anesthesiologist is vitally interested in the maintenance of stable postoperative environmental factors, encompassing what is generally referred to as inhalation therapy. He is interested in the airway and the pulmonary function in the immediate postoperative period, and because of these interests and skills he becomes an extremely valuable person on the team that must band together for optimum care of the postoperative patient.

Another fact about an infant's condition that the pediatric surgeon must take into account is that it can deteriorate with appalling rapidity, and the baby's survival depends on the prompt detection and treatment of the changes that have occurred. This is particularly true with respect to the airway and pulmonary function. Consequently the surgical team must visit the infant patient frequently, and to accomplish this over a 24-hour period a competent house staff of pediatric surgical interns and residents must be available. Unless such a group of trained surgeons can be in attendance 24 hours a day, many of the more complicated procedures now performed quite routinely on neonates should not be undertaken. Because of the rapid deterioration and change, particularly in relation to the airway, there must be a house staff available on call so that the patient can be attended immediately when trouble arises.

Often the nurses' role in the care of surgical pediatric patients is unappreciated. Their special skills and experience provide for the child's comfort and for the prompt, effective administration of postoperative orders. In addition their close observation of the patient in the postoperative period enables them to call attention to complications in the incipient stages when prompt remedial measures will prevent disaster. The need for an intensive care unit staffed by nurses who have had long experience in caring for pediatric postoperative patients is essential if major complicated surgery is to be undertaken. These devoted people are keen observers and will detect variations from normal early in the development of postoperative complications. Such skills require long training and experience, and the services gained from a well-trained nurse in the intensive care unit cannot be expected from a staff nurse who sees pediatric postoperative patients only on rare occasions.

Of equal importance in the care of the patient postoperatively is the availability of laboratories and personnel to supply promptly and accurately the results of various tests that may be required in the areas of bacteriology, blood typing, and biochemistry. Of particular importance is the ability of the chemistry laboratory to perform microdeterminations so that electrolyte concentrations can be checked on small quantities of blood secured from heel pricks. The 10 ml of blood necessary for standard macro techniques, especially when daily determinations are required, may be difficult or impossible to obtain postoperatively from a small, sick infant.

It is possible to perform simple, straightforward operations without elaborate facilities and still secure acceptable results. However, the outcome of complicated operations, such as the correction of esophageal atresia and tracheoesophageal fistula, is dependent to a large extent on all the skilled personnel and the complete laboratory facilities that have been discussed.

The surgical team has a grave responsibility in caring for infants and children with anomalies because in many instances the anomalies are being repaired for a lifetime of 70 years or more. Children with malformations often have mechanical problems whose correction will permit them to lead normal, useful lives. The surgeon who makes the first effort to correct the deformity has the opportunity to produce the most acceptable and enduring result. If he fails, the next procedure in most instances will be less successful than a properly conceived and adequately performed initial operation.

ORVAR SWENSON

REFERENCES

POTTS, W. J. Pediatric surgery is growing up. J.A.M.A., 166: 462, 1958.

2

Neonatal Physiology

A knowledge of neonatal physiology is imperative for the surgeon who embarks upon the operative treatment of the newborn. Such knowledge improves diagnostic skill by providing a background of normal function against which to compare abnormalities observed in the patient; it also improves postoperative care by giving insight into metabolism and providing the specific normal data that make the results of laboratory tests on patients meaningful.

RESPIRATORY SYSTEM

At times the newborn has variations in respirations that are alarming to the attending physician because of their irregularity. The types of respiratory patterns that the newborn exhibit have been studied by Deming and Washburn (1935), who classified the movements into three major groups:

(1) A regular pattern in which expiration and inspiration are equal and there is no appreciable pause after expiration. It is the most common configuration observed in the newborn.

(2) A cog-wheel type in which the movements may be slightly jerky and a prolonged expiratory phase is followed by a pause. This form is uncommon.

(3) A periodic form with periods of regular respirations interrupted by pauses such as are observed in Cheyne-Stokes respirations of the elderly patient. There may be complete irregularity without distinct pauses.

As would be anticipated these abnormalities, particularly the periodic type, are more common in the premature and postoperative patients. The significance of the periodic type of respiration is not clear. Studies have been conducted by Miller (1937) and others, who found that the administration of higher concentrations of oxygen than are found in the normal atmosphere eliminated the periodicity and transformed the irregular form into a regular pattern. This should not be interpreted as indicating that one pattern provides more effective ventilation than another. Unless the attending physician, surgeon, and nurse appreciate that these variations of the respiratory pattern are normal there will be unnecessary concern about the postoperative patient who exhibits such variations. Although the irregularities are apt to disappear in the first week or so of life, in some infants they may persist for a month or more. Consequently, the possibilities of these types of respiratory patterns being seen postoperatively, even in four- to six-week-old infants, must be borne in mind. In some neonates, there are periodic deep respiratory efforts; the cause of this is debated. It may be that it serves a useful function in the newborn by opening up atelectatic areas that may be present during the first 12 to 24 hours after birth. The average respiratory rate of the newborn varies from 25 to 35 per minute. Rates beyond this may be observed in normal infants. However, when the rate exceeds or is below these limits investigations should be undertaken to rule out pathology as the cause of the change from the average rate.

The infant's chest is relatively small in volume compared to the abdominal cavity. As the child grows into adulthood, the proportion of volume increases in favor of the thoracic cavity until it approaches unity. The most effective air exchange in the infant's chest is achieved with diaphragmatic breathing. The contribution to respiration of rib cage movement by the intercostal muscles is far less in the infant than in the adult. The infant's type of respiratory movement should be taken into account by the surgeon. Diaphragmatic respiratory movements may be disturbing during abdominal operations, and it may be dangerous in such situations for the surgeon to urge the anesthesiologist to achieve a deeper level of anesthesia. A wiser course is to have the patient intubated and to assist respirations by mechanical or manual means, thus providing a tranquil field for the surgeon and ensuring that the patient's respiratory requirements are met.

In observing newborns, particularly prematures, some suprasternal retraction may be noted, and this may be normal. Such retraction is caused by the thinness of the thoracic cage and the power of the diaphragmatic musculature in producing negative pressure in the thoracic cavity. Hasty conclusions based on a slight retraction that a mechanical airway obstruction exists are unwarranted. However, the appearance of retraction in a patient who previously exhibited none is a cause for concern.

The vital capacity is difficult to determine in the newborn. It has been measured on the basis of deep inspiratory efforts, and it is judged to be about 180 ml in the average newborn. The tidal air has been computed to be between 12 and 20 ml.

For many decades it has been suspected that the fetus and newborn have resistance to anoxemia beyond that of an adult. Experiments have been performed in animals, and these indicate that their newborn have a re-markable resistance to anoxemia. In some adult animals, survival after removal of the midbrain, thus abolishing respiratory efforts, will be on the average of 3 to 4 minutes. In their newborn the survival after this type of experiment may be 30 to 45 minutes. It has been repeatedly observed in caring for newborns with lungs consolidated to an extent to render them incapable of serving as oxygen-absorbing mechanisms that the patient has survived for as long as half an hour. The explanation of this is difficult. It may be that the resuscitating efforts made or the gasping movements of these infants fill the upper gastrointestinal tract with air, and this may be an avenue of oxygen supply to the infant. Although it is impossible to give any definite figures, since one can only infer from animal experimentation and clinical observations, it is safe to say that many newborns will tolerate a period as long as 15 minutes of severe anoxemia without permanent damage to vital structures.

A peculiarity of newborns, especially prematures, is that they show some ill effects from being immersed in high concentrations of oxygen in tents or incubators. The appearance of retrolental fibroplasia in premature infants was found to coincide with the therapeutic use of oxygen. There seems to be a susceptibility of the small arterioles of the retina to develop spasm and be functionally occluded when the infant breathes a high oxygen concentration. This is followed by swelling and edema with fibrosis, progressing to such an extent that vision becomes severely impaired. Studies now indicate that there is relative safety in administering oxygen providing the concentration does not exceed 40 percent. It would seem inadvisable to deny the premature infant oxygen when needed. Fortunately in most situations a concentration in the incubator below 40 percent is effective with the prematures requiring oxygen therapy. Generally, there is a tendency to misuse oxygen therapy. Oftentimes the patient who is not doing well will be given oxygen in the hope that some benefit will be derived. Such procedure robs the patient of the benefits of a thoughtful analysis of the situation and of the direct help available from carefully selected roentgenographic studies and laboratory tests that may indicate specific therapy that makes oxygen administration unnecessary.

One of the peculiarities of the newborn is his unwillingness or inability to breathe through the mouth. This is not a universal behavior, for occasionally the newborn will breathe perfectly well through the mouth, as has been demonstrated by rare and unusual cases of choanal atresia with untroubled mouth respirations. Usually the baby with this disease will have respiratory obstruction until an airway is provided. Furthermore it is not unusual to see postoperative patients who are either unwilling or unable to respire through the mouth. For this reason, nasogastric tubes may disturb respiratory function more than anticipated because one channel, which is a needed respiratory passage, is being obstructed. Such patients must be closely observed to ensure that an adequate respiratory exchange is maintained.

In association with the peculiarity of nasal breathing, the absence of the cough, gag, or swallowing reflex is common in the newborn. Anesthesiologists have taken advantage of this and performed intratracheal intubations without anesthesia. Although this can be accomplished in the newborn, in the two- or three-month-old infant it may be a difficult and traumatic procedure. The absence of the cough reflex and gag reflex, particularly the former, may have serious implications postoperatively. It has been reported that unattended postoperative infants have been found dead in their cribs, and postmortem examinations have revealed mucous plugs in the larynx or trachea accounting for the asphyxia. For these reasons, it is mandatory in the postoperative care of infants to provide constant nursing care so that by vigilance the airway is maintained unobstructed. Physicians and surgeons should impress upon the intensive care nursing personnel the peculiar absence of the cough or gag reflex in some infants and thus alert them to the necessity of careful observation and assiduous care in the cleaning of the oropharynx so that mucus and saliva will not be inhaled and produce a partial or complete block in the respiratory system.

HEMATOLOGY

There are differences in the hematology of the newborn and the adult. The most striking is that the newborn retains fetal hemoglobin for a period after birth. Extensive studies have been made on the difference between fetal hemoglobin and adult hemoglobin with regard to the oxygen-carrying capacity and its disassociation curve, and, although there have been differences established, these appear to be of no real significance as far as the newborn's capacity to maintain adequate oxygenation is concerned. In general, this statement is agreed to by most workers. Recently, Klaus and Meyer (1966) stated that "the ability of fetal hemoglobin to carry more oxygen at any partial Pa_{O_2} is a distinct advantage to the infant, but makes clinical recognition of hypoxia more difficult since cyanosis will be observed at a lower oxygen tension."

Fetal hemoglobin does provide a means of determining whether the blood a newborn vomits is his own or swallowed maternal blood, for by a simple bedside test based on the resistance of the fetal hemoglobin to ammonium hydroxide fetal hemoglobin can be identified. It is not unusual for a patient who has vomited blood in the first 24 hours of life to undergo radiographic studies to detect a bleeding point in the gastrointestinal system. Such examinations may be avoided by the test for fetal hemoglobin in the vomited blood.

The red blood count of the newborn varies from 5.5 million to 6 million, and there are usually 10 nucleated red blood cells per 100 white blood cells. The values are somewhat different depending on whether the blood is capillary or venous, as is demonstrated by the finding of 20 g per 100 ml of blood in capillary blood, whereas venous blood contains 17 g per 100 ml. The erythrocyte of the newborn is larger than that of adults, the difference being about 20 percent. These high values tend to fall in the first two weeks of life. The hematocrit of the newborn or of the baby during the first few days of life varies between 45 and 55 percent. The white blood cells may be as high as 45,000 on the first day, but during the first week the number will fall to about half this value. There is considerable variation in the white blood count, and occasionally in postoperative patients who have been operated upon in the first day or two of life blood counts may be obtained in the range of 30,000 to 40,000. In view of the normal range observed in infants who have not undergone any surgical procedure, these figures can be viewed without concern providing that there are no indications of infection. There is also a change in the type of white cells during the first week, there being an increase in lymphocytes and some increase in monocytes during this period. Studies of the fibrinogin content of the newborn compared to that of the mother indicates that they are almost equal. The sedimentation rate of the newborn is extremely slow, which is hard to explain in view of the normal fibrinogin levels.

COAGULATION OF BLOOD

As the infant gets older there is an increase in the platelet count, which at three months reaches a somewhat elevated level. The maximum is usually given as under 500,000, with a minimum of 200,000. At birth the capillary values range from a low of 160,000 to a high of 320,000. It is important to keep these values in mind, particularly in dealing with patients with large hemangiomas. It is possible at times to make important decisions in a patient with a hemangioma and a decrease in the platelet count and a fall of hemoglobin. In such situations, the trapping of platelets in the hemangioma may be of such severity that serious coagulation defects result unless the hemangioma is promptly removed. The various substances involved in coagulation are essentially at normal levels at birth. For instance, the accelerator globulin (AcG) is usually within normal. The proconvertin or SPCA, like prothrombin, has been shown to be normally reduced at birth, to fall somewhat during the ensuing day, and subsequently to reach adult level. For these reasons the administration of vitamin K is important and should be a routine procedure. However, the surgeon should be warned against considering vitamin K administration capable of correcting all types of bleeding in the newborn. When a hemorrhagic disease of the newborn is encountered—and this is not too common—the cause of the situation may be extremely complicated and require a complicated laboratory study to be completely understood. From a practical standpoint, the use of fresh blood will be effective in correcting most such problems.

CIRCULATORY SYSTEM

During a brief period following birth the circulatory system undergoes profound changes, for in the fetus the pulmonary system has been bypassed by a series of shunts and a large flow provided for the placenta; these shunts must close in order for the postnatal circulation to be established. The ductus arteriosus is one of these shunts, and, although it is anatomically open, functional closure takes place in the first few days of life. The closure is achieved by fibers in the wall of the structure itself and is governed by complex factors. Anatomical closure does not occur until about the second month. For a brief period after birth the aortic and pulmonary artery pressures remain equal, and for this reason there is probably no blood shunted through the ductus arteriosus during this period. After birth the blood oxygen saturation rises rapidly to 90 percent or more, and this is evidence that a significant right to left shunt is not present.

The blood volume at birth is given as about 300 ml. The normal resting pulse ranges from 110 to 140. When the infant is crying his pulse rate may go to 180 or 190. Such parameters of normal pulse rates are important to remember, particularly in evaluating the postoperative patient. A pulse rate of 160 postoperatively is satisfactory, and, immediately following operation, transient rates as high as 180 and 190 are not alarming. Slow rates, however, are more ominous and may precede cardiac arrest. It is entirely satisfactory for the postoperative patient in the third or fourth day to exhibit a pulse rate of 140. The blood volume is usually calculated to be 85 ml per kg of weight. The cardiac output is estimated to be from 500 to 600 ml per minute. This output is two times greater in proportion to the weight than in adults. The stroke volume corrected for weight is about the same in infants and adults; the difference in cardiac output is therefore attributable to the increased neonatal heart rate.

Blood pressures reported by various observers have not shown absolute agreement, and this is probably related to the differences in the techniques used in making the measurements. There is a gradual rise in pressure during the first week and an even slower rise thereafter, until adult levels are reached. When a cuff $2\frac{1}{2}$ cm in width with a pneumatic pad completely encircling the arm is used, some observers find that the systolic pressure at birth varies between 65 and 75 mm of mercury. These values climb to 70 to 80 mm at one week of age. There has been a reluctance in the past to make use of blood pressure measurements taken on infants. This attitude probably stems from noting the variety of values that have been published and from a failure to appreciate the need for a standardized cuff. It is important to realize that an observer using a single technique can obtain reproducible blood pressure values, and this technique can then be useful in following the postoperative infant.

There is a central pooling of blood in the newborn with peripheral constriction. The clinical importance of this is that in the newborn there is often a persistence of cyanosis in the hands and feet because of sluggish peripheral circulation. This is a physiological phenomenon and should be taken into account in evaluating cyanosis in the preoperative and postoperative infant.

Heart size is important in evaluating the newborn, particularly when surgery is anticipated, for it is an accurate and simple method of detecting congenital cardiac lesions. When chest films are taken with the tube at a standard distance from the patient so that distortion is minimized, it is generally stated that the normal heart diameter is 50 percent of the thoracic width. Some workers follow the rule that newborn cardiac silhouettes of more than 5.7 cm in width are abnormal and warrant further investigation for the presence of a cause for the cardiomegaly. In auscultation of the heart in the first week of life, murmurs may be detected. It is stated by some observers that less than one in ten of such murmurs persists and proves to be caused by an organic lesion. There are differences in the ECG tracing of the neonate compared to that of a baby several months of age. These differences consist of a right ventricular predominance and alterations in the T-waves.

METABOLISM

In comparing newborns with adults the difference in their surface areas is extremely important. For example, if one compares an adult with a newborn on the basis of weight, heat production is twice as great in the newborn. Actually, when surface area is the basis of comparison, heat production is either the same in the two age groups or slightly less in the neonate. At first heat production utilizes predominantly carbohydrates. Subsequently the respiratory quotient indicates that fat is used when feedings are withheld. Generally, it is considered that prematures depend on carbohydrates rather than on fats or protein. Heat regulation is unstable, and most dramatically so in the premature. Temperatures tend to be low and usually stabilize in the first 24 hours or less at 98° to 99° F. Premature infants are notoriously more unstable, their homeostatic temperature mechanisms being even more undeveloped than those of full-term newborns. It is interesting that various preliminary studies have indicated that to maintain a premature at a low temperature is probably detrimental despite the fact that theoretically this should reduce metabolic processes while the premature reaches full development.

Clinical experience has led to the conclusion that normothermic infants do better postoperatively than when the temperature is depressed. Often during operations, before the days of careful monitoring, a considerable drop in temperature was observed near the end of the procedure. The general condition of such babies was always precarious until rewarming was accomplished. Careful monitoring of temperature and, in most situations, maintenance of normothermic levels during the operation and postoperatively is preferable.

LIVER FUNCTION

Concern is occasionally expressed by surgeons regarding the adequacy of neonatal liver function. Actually, by known methods of quantifying liver function, it is normal in the neonate except that Bromsulphalein is cleared somewhat more slowly from the blood during the first week of life than thereafter. This is particularly true of the premature infant. In approximately 50 percent of newborns there is visible jaundice, labeled as icterus neonatorum or physiological jaundice. It usually appears on the second day and reaches a peak at six days and then rapidly subsides; there are no known deleterious long-term effects. There is considerable debate whether the level of bilirubin can reach a point where kernicterus can be associated with physiological jaundice, and the possibility has not been excluded. The complete explanation of the so-called physiological jaundice is not available. Certainly the hemolysis of blood during the period of jaundice is not excessive. The defect seems to be that the enzyme system which conjugates the bilirubin is taxed beyond its ca-

pacity, and this is a function the liver had to assume rather abruptly, since the maternal circulation performed this clearance during fetal life.

DIGESTIVE TRACT

During the first 24 hours the intestine's activity consists of clearing itself and preparing for a very active function, for by two weeks of age the infant's digestive system must handle one half liter of formula per day. On the basis of body weight, this is equivalent to 10 to 12 quarts in the adult. This indicates the greater need of the infant for fluids than that of the full-grown individual. There has long been a clinical impression that fetal distress results in meconium being evacuated into the amniotic sac. It is a common observation in the experimental laboratory and in the operating room that when the blood supply is diminished to a segment of intestine and there is beginning ischemia, the first reaction is contraction of the intestine, so that the passage of meconium during fetal distress would not be a surprising phenomenon. It has generally been estimated that the gastrointestinal tract of an infant is proportionally longer than that of adults. Certainly the activity of the intestinal tract is somewhat different from the pattern observed in adults. Gastric peristalses are less frequent, and consequently there may be some delay in emptying the stomach. The pattern is variable in that there may be quite prompt partial emptying with a small retention that may last for as long as 24 hours. Hunger contractions are observed in infants and may occur 1 to 2 hours after feeding; these can be recorded as periods of peristaltic activity with a progression in intensity.

The small intestine shows some activity, but there is a tendency for barium to be segmented into isolated masses, similar to the configuration observed in the so-called celiac disease syndrome. It may be generalized that there is a deficient tonus in all of the gastrointestinal tract except the lower intestine and colon. This is demonstrated by transit times determined after the ingestion of radiopaque material by the newborn and its subsequent appearance in the cecum. In the newborn this varies from 3 to 6 hours, as compared to $2\frac{1}{2}$ hours in the adult. The transit time from ingestion to elimination in the adult is taken to be about 24 hours. This function is much more rapid in infants, where the average is about 8 hours. This is evidence of increased colonic activity. The colon is somewhat elongated and haustrations are shallow if present at all. This is important from a radiologic standpoint, for it is now well-known that the identification in plain roentgenograms of the colon in the newborn and the distinguishing of it from the small intestine is not possible because of the absence of haustral depressions. The colon is rather small, and studies have demonstrated radiographically that 60 to 75 ml of opaque material completely fills the neonatal colon. It is interesting that observations made on premature infants usually establish that there is a somewhat more rapid transit time in this group than in full-term infants.

The passage of air into the intestinal tract is dramatic, for the stomach partially fills with air with the first breath. Precise investigations indicate that this may not be invariably true, but it certainly takes place in the first 5 or 10 minutes after birth. The progression of air through the intestinal tract is phenomenally rapid; it reaches the cecum in 2 hours and may be expelled quite shortly after this, since the transit time through the colon is rapid. This speedy filling of the gastrointestinal tract with air is taken advantage of since air is an excellent contrast medium for radiographic examinations. In many instances, particularly in the upper gastrointestinal tract, the air, with its speed of descent, establishes a readily available contrast material that can be studied by radiographic means, and patency of the intestinal tract can be established by this simple technique.

The mucosa of the gastrointestinal tract is highly developed without any serious deficiency. The glands of the stomach are known to develop in the fourth and fifth months of life, and presumably hydrochloric acid, pepsin, and renin are present shortly after this.

Enzymes are present in the intestinal tract from the fourth month on. Pancreatic lipase and trypsinogen are present at the fourth or fifth month and are not deficient at birth. One of the exceptions to this is amylase, which may not have appeared at the time of birth and may remain at a rather low level, for as long as the first year of life.

There has been considerable interest in the pH of the gastric contents of the newborn, and it is found that initially this is essentially neutral. The pH varies from 3.15 to 8.33, the majority being between 6.5 and 8. At four to five hours it has fallen to an average of from 3 to 1. This trend progresses and by 24 hours is usually in the vicinity of 1 or 2, which is equal to about one-tenth normal hydrochloric acid. The volume of the gastric contents remains quite small, being about $2\frac{1}{2}$ ml per 24 hours. While these are average figures it is well to keep in mind that there is considerable variation, with a number of neonates being achlorhydric. Most of the acid is in the fundus, with a lesser concentrate in the pyloric area. The high levels subside in a matter of weeks and become somewhat lower than in adults for the first year.

Meconium has always been of interest to physicians, and in the past extensive investigation of its composition has been made. The volume is between 50 and 200 g, and it is made up of vernix caseosa, hair, and cells from the skin and gastrointestinal tract, as well as bilirubin. The consistency of the meconium has clinical implications, for meconium ileus is caused by an increased viscosity of the material. In the infant with meconium plug syndrome, Clatworthy (1956) studied the composition of the plug and found no tryptic activity in nine cases, despite the fact that these babies eventually developed normal enzyme activity. Normally, 50 percent of newborns pass meconium within 12 hours, and practically all have passed meconium within 24 hours. Following this, there are transition stools that tend to be greenish, curdled, and watery, followed by yellow soft stool. In normal infants bowel movements vary from one to six per day.

Newborn infants, both premature and full-term, have excellent digestive powers; their management of carbohydrates and proteins is essentially that of an older child or adult. The efficiency of the glucose mechanism is exemplified by the fact that dextrose appears in the blood with equal rapidity when monosaccharides or disaccharides are ingested. Fat-splitting enzymes, by measurement, seem to be adequate. However, when diets are given which tend to be high in fat, they are not handled as well as formulas containing normal amounts of fat. It is probably for this reason that diets excessive in fats are less well tolerated than the ones containing a moderate amount of fat. In dealing with surgical patients, particularly those who have through some accident sustained an extensive loss of small intestine, the need for limiting fat is more noticeable than in normal infants. That proteins are well handled is demonstrated by the fact that as protein ingestion is started a positive nitrogen balance ensues quite promptly. The NPN rises in the blood during the first week to levels not greatly above normal, averaging from 50 to 60 mg. The serum protein in the newborn is somewhat lower than in adults. There is a slight deficiency in globulin and a more noticeable one in the albumin, and, as would be expected, these changes in the serum protein are more pronounced in the premature. The relation of this to the edema encountered in the premature infant from time to time is not fully elucidated. Blood sugar levels fall postnatally and vary from 40 to 100 mg during the first ten days of life. Glysuria is a finding that parallels the situation in older children, there being no remarkable feature about this in the newborn.

MINERALS AND VITAMINS

The newborn has a reserve of minerals and vitamins to rely upon, their exact level being directly related to the maternal state. The infants who have not been able to acquire any substantial reserve of these substances from the mother may not show depletion for several days to a week or so after birth. Therefore, the administration of these substances in the first few days after delivery is not essential. The administration of vitamins becomes necessary after the second or third week of life, and at such time the administration of vitamins is a preventive measure rather than a corrective one. Calcium and inorganic phosphorus in the blood are generally normal, although there may be some transient rise in the inorganic phosphorus level and a fall in calcium probably representing a temporary physiologic hypoparathyroidism. Most diets given to infants have adequate amounts of calcium. It must be recalled that absorption of calcium from the intestine requires vitamin D, and after two or three weeks this substance should be administered in order to prevent rickets. The amount given is 400 international units per day. The neonate has a marginal supply of iron, and here again it is somewhat related to the state of the maternal blood levels of iron. It is well to remember that cow's milk is poor in iron. The question often arises whether the physiological anemia seen at two or three months of age can be prevented by the administration of iron. Although the severity of this phenomenon might be ameliorated, it is doubtful that it can be entirely prevented by administering iron. The ascorbic acid level is maintained above that of the mother, and falls from 1.5 mg per 100 ml in the plasma to about 0.7 mg within the first 24 hours of life. Since the boiling of formulas, which is common today, destroys vitamin C, it is important that 25 to 50 mg of ascorbic acid or orange juice be included in the diet after three weeks of age. Vitamin A, riboflavin, and thiamine are well supplied by the average diet and need not be supplemented.

REGULATION OF WATER AND ELECTROLYTES

It is generally agreed that the kidneys begin to function after the fourth month of fetal life. That this function is not essential to the well-being of the fetus is demonstrated by the fact that babies born without renal tissue of any significance are normal in every respect, demonstrating the adequacy of the placental mechanism in caring for renal function. It has been suggested by Rosa (1951) that the fetus swallows about 500 ml of amniotic fluid in 24 hours and that the kidneys excrete 40 ml and retain 25 ml for metabolism. The remainder appears to be transported across the placental circulation.

The progressive hypotonicity of the amniotic fluid is thought to be caused by the addition of fetal urine. This has been proposed by Zangemeister and Meissels. Further evidence of intrauterine renal function is that any mechanical obstruction will cause dilatation of the ureter or renal pelvis proximal to the block. At birth the fetal bladder is not empty but contains a small amount of dilute urine. The infant's kidney is definitely inferior in performance to the kidneys seen in older children. The differences cannot be reconciled by the consideration of differences in surface area, metabolic rate, or weight alone. Taking all of these factors into consideration, there is a definite depression of urea clearance per unit of surface area to a value that does not become adult until the child reaches two years of age or more.

McCance and Widdowson (1947) have shown that if one compares function to the total volume of water rather than to the surface area, the discrepancy between neonatal and adult renal function becomes less pronounced. However, even with this mode of calculation, there is a relative reduced clearance in the first two months or so. Glomerular filtration measured by inulin clearance or creatinine clearance indicates that the newborn has some lag in function when compared with adults, whether one makes the comparison on the basis of units of body water or on the basis of surface area. By the body water method of comparison, the filtration rate becomes quite adequate at adult levels at about six weeks, whereas the surface area method of computation does not indicate that the glomerular filtration rates reach the adult level of function until the second

year after birth. The determination of renal plasma flow in infants is not well documented. There are questions particularly regarding the PAH as a method of determining this flow. Should these tests be eventually substantiated as effective measures of renal plasma flow it will then have been shown that there is a greater reduction in this function than in the glomerular filtration rate. Tubular reabsorption when measured by standard techniques is again somewhat depressed in the neonate. The ability of the infant kidney to conserve water and to excrete urine with a high osmolarity value is important to the clinician. There seems to be a definite lack in this regard, for adults may exhibit a urine of 1,200 to 1,400 osmolarity, whereas infants under stressful situations cannot achieve more than about 600 milliosmoles. It is interesting that the premature infant has about the same power in this regard as the full-term infant. There are many factors to be considered in any explanation of this reduced function; it would appear that the main depression is in the tubular resorption. This phenomenon of the newborn period is important because dehydration might not be accompanied by a urine of high osmolarity, particularly when one expects the same levels to be reached as those seen in adults. The ability of the newborn kidney to excrete large quantities of dilute urine is a problem. There is some indication that for the first few weeks of life there is a definite limitation in this regard. This would have considerable importance to the surgeon, since overhydration during the immediate postoperative period in the newborn might have deleterious effects.

Of universal importance to clinicians is the level of the blood urea nitrogen in the newborn. It is found to range from 10 to 25 mg per 100 ml of blood, and occasionally higher. Consequently, high levels of this type in the newborn for a period of a week or so should be interpreted with caution as an indication of renal disease. It is incorrect to assume that proteinuria or albuminuria in the newborn's urine is normal. This assumption is based on earlier concepts, which were formed with data collected with faulty techniques. More precise techniques have proved that proteinuria and albuminuria are uncommon in the newborn. The newborn infant has a greater component of water in his general makeup than the average adult; this is largely extracellular water. Weight loss is definite and occurs during the first 72 hours after birth and is caused by the loss of meconium and water, and the insensible loss of water from the lungs and skin and of some vernix from the body surface. The impression formerly held that the weight loss was primarily the result of a diuresis is erroneous. The volume of urine that the average baby passes on the first day is about 20 ml, and it gradually rises by the end of the first week to about 150 ml per day. In view of the average weight loss of about 7 percent of the total weight in the first 72 hours it is obvious that the urine output cannot account for this. The time of the first voiding is of interest in examining newborns; studies have shown that in 12 hours approximately half of the babies have voided, and only a very small percentage goes beyond 24 hours without having passed urine. However, it is handy to keep in mind that voiding may not occur for as long as 48 hours and still be consistent with a normal urinary tract. The loss of water from the skin and the lung surfaces has been studied and found to average about 1 g of water per kg per hour.

There is some evidence that the newborn tends to be a little acidotic, with a low PCO_2. The variation from normal is not great, being given at about 34 mm of mercury. This picture is somewhat more pronounced in prematures, and the fact that the PCO_2 is depressed indicates that this is a metabolic acidosis. Studies of sodium concentration in the serum of the neonate reveal that it is not significantly at variance with the range found in adults. In contrast, potassium appears to be somewhat elevated in the neonatal period. Magnesium may be somewhat elevated for the first week of life, after which it assumes a level not far from the normal in adults. There is a slight hyperchloremia, with a concentration as high as 110 mEq per liter of plasma. These findings are usual in premature infants. It should be summed up that abnormal losses of water and solutes through either vomiting or diarrhea may be more significant in neonates because of some immaturity of their systems and may rapidly become clinically significant.

It would appear that the endocrine system is as ready as any of the mechanisms of the newborn to cope with extrauterine life. Certainly this system as a whole probably exhibits more maturity and a more normal function than other systems, and it is certainly adequate to the degree that substitu-

TABLE 1.   ANTIBODIES PASSIVELY ACQUIRED BY THE FETUS*

ANTIBODIES IN CORD BLOOD EQUAL TO OR HIGHER THAN THOSE IN MATERNAL BLOOD	ANTIBODIES IN CORD BLOOD LESS THAN THOSE IN MATERNAL BLOOD, AT TIMES ABSENT
Tetanus antitoxin	Streptococcus agglutinins
Diphtheria antitoxin	*Hemophilus influenzae* antibodies
Smallpox hemagglutinins	Blood group isoagglutinins
Antistreptolysins	Shigella antibodies
Antistaphylolysins	Poliomyelitis antibodies
Bacillus pertussis antibodies	Salmonella somatic (O) antibodies
Toxoplasma (complement-fixing and neutralizing)	*Escherichia coli* (H and O) antibodies
Salmonella flagellar (H) antibodies	Rh complete antibodies
Rh-blocking antibodies	Heterophilic antibodies

* From Schaffer. Diseases of the Newborn, 2nd Ed. Courtesy of W. B. Saunders Co.

tion therapy of any kind is not a practical necessity. That the infant may have some physiological endocrine disturbances caused by maternal influences is well established. Changes in the genital organs of the female, in the prostate gland in the male, and in the breasts in both sexes are evidence of such maternal influence. The common disease of diabetes in mothers probably has more serious effects on the newborn than any other condition. There may be increased weight, both total and of individual organs, and the disease may be reflected in the metabolism as an elevation of blood glucose. It would appear that the correction of hypoglycemia could affect the high mortality rate of diabetic neonates. This has not been completely proved to be the case. The syndrome of the diabetic mother's child is a complicated one and has been only partially elucidated. Hyperthyroidism may be transmitted to the fetus. It can occur even with a mother who has been effectively treated by surgery.

IMMUNITY
IN THE NEWBORN

The newborn infant receives immunities from the mother (see Table 1) depending on the level of the mother's titer against specific infectious diseases. There is good immunity against diphtheria and tetanus, as well as against measles, mumps, smallpox, vaccinia, poliomyelitis, ordinary respiratory viruses, the Coxsackie virus, and the virus of herpes simplex. The exact levels of immunity in the newborn infant cannot be predicted. The general rule is that for the infec-

tions listed above there is immunity for at least six months. It is well to keep in mind that chicken pox is not among the infections against which there is immunity, and thus it is possible for small babies to contract this disease.

The main defense against bacterial infection is I_gG or 7S gamma globulin, which has a molecular weight of 165,000 and is transferred through the placenta. Its concentration in the neonate varies directly with the duration of the gestation period. In the adult it comprises 75 to 80 percent of the total gamma globulin. However, the high molecular weight immunoglobin (I_gM or 19S) gamma globulin, which seems specific in protection against gram-negative infections, fails to cross the placental barrier. This may partially explain the infant's notorious inability at times to resist gram-negative bacterial infections.

A persistent notion in pediatric thinking that the neonate is immunologically incapable is now challenged by a number of studies. These studies, less than a year old, indicate that the fetus, the premature infant, and the newborn are to a degree capable of producing the two immunoglobulins of major protective importance, I_gG and I_gM.

Another cause of the premature infant's susceptibility to infection is proposed by Gluck and Silverman (1957), who have demonstrated that the leukocyte's ability to phagocytize particulate matter is deficient in the premature. This function increases with the maturation of the infant, and at full term there is an adult level of activity.

ORVAR SWENSON

REFERENCES

ADAMS, F. H., and LIND, J. Physiologic studies on the cardiovascular status of normal newborn infants. Pediatrics, 19: 431, 1957. (With special reference to ductus arteriosus.)

AMES, R. G. Urinary water excretion and neurophysial function in full term and premature infants shortly after birth. Pediatrics, 12: 272, 1953.
ANDERSEN, B., and ORTMANN, G. On number

of erythrocytes and content of haemoglobin in blood of newborn children. Acta Med. Scand., 93: 410, 1937.

AVERY, M. E. The Lung and Its Disorders in the Newborn Infant. Philadelphia, W. B. Saunders Company, 1964.

BARNETT, H. L. Renal physiology in infants and children. I. A method for estimation of glomerular filtration rate. Proc. Soc. Exp. Biol. Med., 44: 654 1940.

———— VESTERDAL, J. The physiologic and clinical significance of immaturity of kidney function in young infants. J. Pediat., 42: 99, 1953.

BRAMBELL, F. W. R., HALLIDAY, R., BRIERLEY, J., and HEMMINGS, W. A. Transference of passive immunity from mother to young. Lancet, 1: 964, 1954.

BRANNING, W. S. Acid-base balance of premature infants. J. Clin. Invest., 21: 101, 1942.

BRINES, J. K., GIBSON, J. G., Jr., and KUNKEL, P. Blood volume in normal infants and children. J. Pediat., 18: 447, 1941.

BUCHANAN, D. J., and RAPOPORT, S. Chemical comparison of normal meconium from a patient with meconium ileus. Pediatrics, 9: 304, 1952.

BYRN, J. N., and EASTMAN, N. J. Vitamin A levels in maternal and fetal blood plasma. Bull. Hopkins Hosp., 73: 132, 1943.

CALCAGNO, P. L., RUBIN, M. I., WEINTRAUB, D. H., KELLEHER, M. K., and STUBBINS, M. H. Studies on the renal concentrating and diluting mechanisms in the premature infant. J. Clin. Invest., 33: 91, 1954.

CLATWORTHY, H. W., HOWARD, W. H. R., and LLOYD, J. The meconium plug syndrome. Surgery, 39: 131, 1956.

COOK, C. D., CHERRY, R. B., O'BRIEN, D., KARLBERG, P., and SMITH, C. A. Studies of respiratory physiology in the newborn infant. I. Observations on normal premature and full-term infants. J. Clin. Invest., 34: 975, 1955.

CUTTER, R. D. Normal gastric secretion of infants and small children following stimulation with histamine. J. Pediat., 12: 1, 1938.

DEMING, J., and WASHBURN, A. H. Respiration in infancy; method of studying rates, volume and character of respiration. Amer. J. Dis. Child., 49: 108, 1935.

DILLON, J. G. Respiratory function of digestive tract as basis of roentgenographic life test. Amer. J. Roentgen., 48: 613, 1942.

DUBS, E. Osmolarity of urine in the infant. Amer. J. Dis. Child., 77: 114, 1949.

EBERS, D. W., SMITH, D. I., and GIBBS, G. E. Gastric acidity on the first day of life. Pediatrics, 18: 800, 1956.

ELDRIDGE, F. L., HULTGREN, H. N., and WIGMORE, M. E. The physiologic closure of the ductus arteriosus in the newborn infant. J. Clin. Invest., 34: 987, 1955.

FASHENA, G. J. Experimental demonstration of functional hepatic immaturity. Amer. J. Dis. Child., 76: 196, 1948.

FEINSTEIN, M. S., and SMITH, C. A. Digestion of protein by premature infants. Pediatrics, 7: 19, 1951.

FELDMAN, W. M. The Principles of Ante-natal and Post-natal Child Physiology, Pure and Applied. London, Longmans, Green & Co., Ltd., 1920.

FRIIS-HANSEN, B., HOLLIDAY, M., STAPLETON, T., and WALLACE, W. M. Total body water in children. Pediatrics, 7: 321, 1951.

FRIMANN-DAHL, J., LIND, J., and WEGELIUS, C. Roentgen investigations of the neo-natal gaseous content of the intestinal tract. Acta Radiol., 41: 256, 1954.

GAMBLE, J. L. Chemical Anatomy, Physiology and Pathology of Extracellular Fluid. Cambridge, Mass., Harvard University Press, 1954.

GLUCK, L., and SILVERMAN, W. A. Phagocytosis in premature infants. Pediatrics, 20: 951, 1957.

———— WOOD, H. F., and FOUSEK, M. D. Septicemia of the newborn. Pediat. Clin. N. Amer., 13: 1131, 1966.

GORDON, H. H., HARRISON, H. E., and McNAMARA, H. Urea clearance of young premature and full-term infants. J. Clin. Invest., 21: 499, 1942.

GREENWALD, H. M., and PENNELL, S. Carbohydrate metabolism of the normal newborn infant. Amer. J. Dis. Child., 39: 281, 1930.

HENDERSON, S. G., and BRIANT, W. W., Jr. The colon in the healthy newborn infant. Radiology, 39: 261, 1942.

HOFFMAN, W. S., PARMELEE, A. H., and GROSSMAN, A. Electrolyte balance studies on premature infants. Amer. J. Dis. Child., 77: 49, 1949.

HOWARD, P. J., and BAUER, A. R. Irregularities of breathing in the newborn period. Amer. J. Dis. Child., 77: 592, 1949.

HSIA, D. Y., ALLEN, F. H., Jr., DIAMOND, L. K., and GELLIS, S. S. Serum bilirubin levels in the newborn infant. J. Pediat., 42: 277, 1953.

KATO, K. Leukocytes in infancy and childhood. J. Pediat., 7: 7, 1935.

KLAUS, M., and MEYER, B. P. Oxygen Therapy for the Newborn. Pediat. Clin. N. Amer., 13: 3, 1966.

MAKEPEACE, A. W., FREMENT-SMITH, F., DAILEY, M. E., and CARROLL, M. P. Nature of amniotic fluid: Comparative study of human amniotic fluid and maternal serum. Surg. Gynec. Obstet., 53: 635, 1931.

McCANCE, R. A., and WIDDOWSON, E. M. Blood-urea in the first nine days of life. Lancet, 1: 787, 1947.

———— YOUND, W. F. Secretion of urine by newborn infants. J. Physiol., 99: 265, 1941.

MILLER, H. C., and BEHRLE, F. C. Changing patterns of respiration in newborn infants. Pediatrics, 12: 141, 1953.

PAINE, J. R., and NESSA, C. B. Observations on the distribution and transport of gas in the gastrointestinal tract of infants and young children. Surgery, 11: 281, 1942.

ROSA, P. Study of the circulation of the amniotic fluid in man. Gynec. Obstet. (Paris), 60: 463, 1951.

RUSSELL, S. J. M. Blood volume studies in

healthy children. Arch. Dis. Child., 24: 88, 1949.

SALMON, G. W., and RICHMAN, E. E. Liver function in the newborn infant. J. Pediat., 23: 522, 1943.

SCHAEFFER, A. J. Diseases of the Newborn, 2nd ed. Philadelphia, W. B. Saunders Co., 1965.

SELLE, W. A., and WITTEN, T. A. Survival of respiratory (gasping) mechanism in young animals subjected to anoxia. Proc. Soc. Exp. Biol. Med., 47: 495, 1941. *Also* Amer. J. Physiol., 133: 441, 1941.

SHERRY, S. N., and KRAMER, I. The time of passage of the first stool and first urine by the newborn infant. J. Pediat., 46: 158, 1955.

SMITH, C. A. The Physiology of the Newborn Infant. Springfield, Ill., Charles C Thomas, Publisher, 1959.

TALBOT, N. B., SOBEL, E. H., McARTHUR, J. W., and CRAWFORD, J. D. Functional Endocrinology from Birth Through Adolescence. Cambridge, Mass., Harvard University Press, 1952.

WALLER, H. K., and MORRIS, D. Resuscitation of the newborn with intragastric oxygen. Lancet, 2: 951, 1953.

WASCH, M., and MARCK, A. The radiographic appearance of the gastrointestinal tract during the first day of life. J. Pediat., 32: 479, 1948.

WASHBURN, A. H. Blood cells in healthy young infants: Study of 608 different leukocyte counts with final report on 908 total leukocyte counts. Amer. J. Dis. Child., 50: 413, 1935.

WIDDOWSON, E. M., and SPRAY, C. M. Chemical development in utero. Arch. Dis. Child., 26: 205, 1951.

WILSON, J. L., et al. Anaerobic metabolism in the newborn infant. I. On the resistance of the fetus and newborn to oxygen lack. Pediatrics, 1: 581, 1948.

3

Teratology

The incidence of malformations in infants surviving the neonatal period is about 7 percent. Nearly half of that number show more than one anomaly, and 1 child in 40 is born with a structural defect that demands treatment. The percentage of total malformations involving each of the various organ systems has been given as follows: musculoskeletal, 38 percent; integumentary, 20 percent; central nervous, 14 percent; cardiovascular, 9 percent; gastrointestinal, 9 percent; and respiratory, 2 percent.

TERATOGENESIS

The ways in which malformations arise are related to hereditary mechanisms, to environmental influences, and to cooperative action between the two. It has been suggested that 20 percent of all congenital anomalies are genetic in origin, 10 percent are caused by abnormal distributions of chromosomes, 10 percent may spring from viral infections, whereas the remaining 60 percent are without known antecedents at the present time. The basic causes of abnormal development fall into two categories: environmental and genetic.

ENVIRONMENTAL FACTORS

A considerable number of different agencies constitute environmental factors in teratogenesis.

EXTERNAL MECHANICAL TRAUMA

External mechanical trauma is an improbable source of malformations in mammalian embryos. Even amniotic adhesions or bands, once widely advocated as a direct cause, are now known to be secondary sequelae of focal dysplasia in fetal tissues. It is conceivable, however, that too little amniotic fluid in the later months of pregnancy may lead to the distortion of the so-called compression baby.

TEMPERATURE

Thermal changes, applied to vertebrate embryos other than mammals, readily induce abnormal development. By contrast, the constancy of temperature in the mammalian uterus renders it unlikely that thermal changes play any significant role in mammalian teratogenesis. Experiments, as well as observations on pregnancies complicated by pyrexical infections, support this conclusion.

IRRADIATION

The efficacy of x-rays, applied at different stages of pregnancy, as a teratogenic agent on embryos has been amply demonstrated in rodents. Supporting, but less precise, evidence has been gained from pregnant women; notable are the sequelae of the atomic bombings of Japan. The ability of radiation to damage effectively the gonadal germ cells has also been proved in small rodents. Similar evidence is lacking in the human female, although the potency of even weak radiation (including cosmic rays) in producing such effects as mutations is credited by some authorities.

OXYGEN LACK

Either oxygen deficiency or carbon dioxide excess (by direct experiment) is an effective cause of maldevelopment in lower vertebrates, and even in some birds and rodents. Information concerning the human embryo is less direct.

CHEMICAL POISONS

Among other chemical agents the salts of certain heavy metals and a toxic dye, trypan blue, have been used extensively as teratogens on rodent embryos, and with marked success. The efficacy of the drug thalidomide as a teratogenic agent on the human embryo is common knowledge.

METABOLIC AGENTS

The absence or excess of certain vitamins in the maternal diet produces a nutritional imbalance that may result in abnormalities. Certain chemicals, such as urethane and nitrogen mustard, acting as inhibitors, interfere with the growth processes, thereby inducing malformations.

HORMONES

Endocrine products, administered in excess, act variously as teratogenic agents. Disturbances of the embryo's own endocrine glands can produce alterations in target organs. Examples of such alterations are pseudohermaphroditism (gonad; suprarenal cortex), anencephaly and cyclopia (adenohypophysis, ACTH), cretinism (thyroid), and dwarfism and gigantism (adenohypophysis, growth hormone).

INFECTIONS

In man the virus of rubella is the only virus known to be a competent teratogen, although in some other mammals additional viruses have been reliably proved to be teratogens. Certain other microorganisms are able to pass the human placental barrier, invade the embryo, and produce disease there. Congenital syphilis, toxoplasmosis, and fetal malaria are among this group. For the most part such disturbances are purely pathological, but some sequelae are teratological, such as tooth anomalies (syphilis) and hydrocephalus (toxoplasmosis).

DEFECTIVE CIRCULATION

Vascular deficiencies owing to an abnormal heart, the lack of a heart (acardiac twin), or poor vascular communications with the placenta are related to various major and minor malformations.

IMMUNITY AGENTS

The Rh factor provides the basis for a natural experiment in which maternal antigen passing the placental barrier interferes with the successful termination of the erythropoietic process in the embryo.

GENETIC FACTORS

One fifth of all malformations are estimated to result from mutations and one tenth from other chromosomal mishaps. Mutational changes operate according to the laws of genetics. Nevertheless, there are many complications, involving some environmental factors, that alter the incidence, intensity, and expression of a given mutant, and these may make the actual mode of transmission uncertain in any specific case. Whatever biological mechanisms the genes control, be they unitary enzymic creations or not, these mechanisms are disrupted by the abnormal genes in some way. Moreover, the environmental agents, already mentioned, that induce malformations are not free from suspicion of an involvement based on genetic instability. Indeed, some authorities even hold that the majority of congenital defects arise from combinations of such factors. Syndactyly is an example of a dominant mutation, albinism of a recessive mutation, and hemophilia of a mutation carried by an X chromosome.

Chromosomal aberrations result from the abnormal behavior of chromosomes during meiotic divisions of sex cells (and, to a degree, during the later somatic mitoses as well). They include nondisjunction, translocation, and deletion. Syndromes such as Down's, Turner's, and Klinefelter's result from such mishaps in chromosome distribution during meiotic divisions.

MECHANISMS

The idea that specifc malformations are produced by specific teratogenic agents holds true only for rare exceptions. Thalidomide medication is a notable illustration of a particular drug producing marked and conspicuous dysgenesis of the limbs, but its effect is not limited to this particular regional malformation. In general, the same teratogenic agent induces different kinds of abnormalities when acting at different phases in embryonic differentiation. Contrariwise, the same abnormality may be induced by different kinds of agents acting at a time characterized by a particular phase of differentiation. In some instances different chemical agents produce unlike results when applied at the same developmental moment. This is presumably because they interfere with different chemical processes in the differentiating organism.

The former identification of a properly timed retardation or arrest in development as the sole or prime environmental factor in producing abnormalities has lost favor with the years. Nevertheless, the general concept of the differential susceptibility of an embryonic part at a particular critical moment in the schedule of organ advances remains as an important basic principle. Other parts may or may not be so scheduled as to be sensitive, at that specific moment, to competent disruptive influences. A part that is sensitive (and susceptible to producing a specific defect) at one particular time is immune to the same influence at an earlier or later period of development.

Experiments imply that there are several ways in which teratogenic agents can affect susceptible embryonic cells: (1) Mitosis may be inhibited. (2) Enzymes may be blocked or destroyed, with a consequent crippling or destruction of cells. (3) Synthesis may proceed in such a manner that certain uncustomary chemicals substitute for the usual participants in a chain of reactions within cells, but these substitutes are then incompetent to act so as to meet the metabolic needs of those cells. (4) Other chemicals act by altering certain radicals of the nucleoproteins in the chromosomes of cell nuclei; this especially damages cells with high mitotic rates. Whatever the manner of interference may be, the final result is probably either cell impairment or death, or a changed rate of growth. In the first instance a cellular deficiency occurs in the definitive organ or part. As to growth, this type of activity can be affected by halting it for a time, by slowing it, or by accelerating it. Any one of these measures puts local growth out of step with adjoining parts and upsets the coordinated schedule of development. Continued, unrestrained growth is a condition leading to the development of congenital tumors.

CLASSIFICATION OF MALFORMATIONS

One scheme of classification can be based on the abnormal developmental functionings that result from the operation of the following factors: (1) effective stimulus, (2) tissue responsiveness, (3) growth capacity, (4) degenerative tendency, (5) enzyme function, and (6) hormone function. Another method is to classify malformations according to the different ways in which imperfect development departs from normality. The following account is presented in categories that come under the latter scheme, that of departures from normality. In many instances special explanations, deemed to be helpful, are added as supplementary comments.

At times a practical problem in classification arises—for example, should cleft palate be assigned to the category of growth failures or to that of failures to fuse? In all such instances the decision has hinged on what seems to be the primary faulty factor.

TOTAL DEVELOPMENTAL FAILURE

In total developmental failure—agenesis or aplasia—a specific developmental product fails to differentiate. As a practical matter, atypical results are not included in this category if they are present but so small as to be without practical significance.

EXTERNAL FORM

EXAMPLE: *fetus amorphus.*

Such nonviable specimens are somewhat globular in shape and are virtually lacking in recognizable external modeling.

ORGANS OR PARTS

EXAMPLES: *cranial vault (acrania), combined with virtual lack of a brain (anencephalia); eyes (anophthalmia); lens (aphakia); lower jaw (agnathia); teeth (anodontia); total limb (amelia); individual bones (e.g., radius, vertebra, phalanx); nails (anonychia); spinal cord (amelus); breast (amastia); nipple (athelia); hair (atrichia); cardiac valves; other organs (e.g., kidney, gallbladder, heart (acardia), diaphragm, vertebra, ribs, muscles).*

In agnathia a tiny rudiment representing the lower jaw can usually be found by careful dissection in the suprahyoid midline. In this condition the ears lie forward on the neck and sometimes are joined (synotia).

Some limb defects are strongly heritable. Perhaps the clearest example of muscle lack is absence of the pectoralis major.

PARTIAL DEVELOPMENTAL FAILURE

Incomplete development may affect many organs or parts and may derive from different kinds of arresting factors.

EXTERNAL FORM

EXAMPLES: *acardia; hemicardia; aprosopia.*

There are many gradations between amorphic fetuses and less severe examples of faulty modeling.

An acardiac fetus is a free twin not only lacking a heart but also deficient in the general features of the external body.

Hemicardius designates a free twin possessing only half a heart but whose external form is recognizable.

An example of local, but essentially complete, developmental failure is a featureless face (aprosopia).

HISTOGENESIS

EXAMPLES: *hemicrania; hemivertebra; incomplete clavicle; virtual absence of limb, except for hand or foot (phocomelia); absence of part or all of distal half of limb (hemimelia); absence of hand (achiria), foot (apodia), or phalanx (aphalangia); shallow acetabulum; local hypoplasias (e.g., nonelastic skin, some stenoses and atresias, incomplete cardiac valve).*

These defects are primarily owing to an inability of cells to proliferate and undergo tissue differentiation. The deficiency may involve a total unit in a larger complex (e.g., absence of the arm in phocomelia), or it may be a failure to complete a unit (e.g., hemivertebra). The lack of a complete row of phalanges produces one form of brachydactyly.

GROWTH

GENERAL

EXAMPLE: *dwarfism (microsomia)*.

Congenital dwarfism is of different types and causes. The midget is small, even at birth. Growth proceeds slowly and ceases at the usual times, thus making a miniature adult; the condition is of genetic origin. Another genetic type slows in growth after birth because of a secondary deficiency of the growth-promoting hormone. Such an adult has the skeleton of a child of about seven years.

A cretin is a dwarf whose incomplete differentiation is due to a congenital lack of thyroid tissue.

Achondroplasia denotes a dwarf condition characterized by a cessation of growth at the base of the skull and in the long bones; it is apparently due to a genetic mutation.

LOCAL

EXAMPLES: *head (microcephalia); lower jaw (micrognathia); cleft lip (cheiloschisis); cleft mandible (dignathia); bifid tongue (diglossia); bicornuate uterus; limb (micromelia); premature synostosis; incomplete pericardium or diaphragm; short esophagus; stunted organs (e.g., brain, ear, spleen, uterus, penis); persistent interventricular foramen; persistent foramen primum of septum primum.*

An undersized mandible (micrognathia) is at times a component of the Pierre Robin syndrome, which is also characterized by a posterior displacement of the tongue and often by a cleft soft palate.

Lateral cleft lip is not produced by a failure of the maxillary and median nasal processes to unite, as was formerly held. Rather, it results from a faulty growth and spread of mesenchyme into the wholly continuous epithelial forerunners of those so-called processes. Absence of mesenchyme at the lines of junction between the ridges, thus formed, can lead to a secondary separation of the basic epithelial components of the lip. The rare median cleft lip represents a similar failure with respect to the paired medial nasal processes. It may be associated with duplication of the nose. Likewise, cleft mandible and bifid tongue result from failures of mesenchymal masses to spread and merge.

A bicornuate, or two-horned, uterus results when the medial, facing walls of the two unfused müllerian ducts at this level do not elevate and create a domed fundus.

Premature closure of the cranial bones produces a deformed skull. Most commonly the sagittal suture is at fault, resulting in a keel-shaped cranium (scaphocephaly). Next in frequency is the obliteration of all sutures over the vault, resulting in a tall cranium (oxycephaly). Third in order is the premature closure of the coronal suture, producing a broadened skull (brachycephaly).

The rare open pericardium derives from an incomplete pleuropericardial membrane. The more common unclosed diaphragm results from an incomplete pleuroperitoneal membrane. Both conditions strongly favor the left side.

Growth failures of the septum primum of the primitive atrium and of the interventricular septum of the common ventricle are responsible for permanent communications between the two sides of the heart.

UNION

EXAMPLES: *cleft palate (uranoschisis); cleft sternum; bifid spine (rachischisis); eyecup fissure (coloboma); unmerged ear components; unfused septum primum and septum secundum of atrium; notched spleen; unanchored mesentery; uterovaginal septation or doubling; polycystic kidney; and thoracoabdominal fissure (thoracogastroschisis).*

Cleft palate, cleft sternum, and bifid spine represent failures of bilateral halves to meet and fuse.

Coloboma results from a disturbance in the closure of the normal fissure in the embryonic optic cup. The common term, "choroid fissure," is inappropriate, since the primary defect is in the optic cup. The gap may affect the iris, ciliary body, retina, or choroid tunic. Coloboma could also be classified as a partial embryonic survival.

Elevations on the branchial arches normally merge and produce an auricle. They may fail to fuse properly.

The postnatal fusion of the septum primum and septum secundum in the region of the foramen ovale fails in about 23 percent of hearts. In most instances, however, the defect is only a probe-patent communication between the two atria.

The spleen arises as several hillocks on the greater omentum. Failure of these to merge completely results in incisures.

Failure of the mesentery of the total intestine to make its normal partial attachment and obliteration predisposes to a twisting (volvulus) about the mesenterial root.

The several degrees of doubling of the uterus and vagina can be traced to varying failures of fusion between the two primitive müllerian ducts.

Polycystic kidney has been traditionally explained as the failure of the secretory tubules and excretory ducts to unite. Other possible explanations have been advanced, but probably no single explanation accounts satisfactorily for all conditions encountered.

Ventral midline fissures in the thorax or abdomen or both lead to protrusion of the heart (ectocardia) or of the abdominal viscera (eventration). Both conditions result from a failure of the paired primitive body folds to join.

SEPARATION

EXAMPLES: *merged eyes (cyclopia); tracheoesophageal fistula; exstrophy of the bladder; and conjoined parathyroid and thymus.*

Cyclopia follows the failure of a wedge of neural plate and head mesenchyme to develop in the region where primitive optic centers organize in a primitive common eye field. Normal separation of the eye primordia then fails.

Tracheoesophageal fistula is perhaps best interpreted as an incomplete separation of the laryngotracheal groove from the early foregut. It is almost always accompanied by atresia of the esophagus, at or below the level of the fistulous connection between the two tubes.

At one stage of development the bladder region of the common cloaca is separated from the exterior by the cloacal membrane only. Failure of mesoderm to invade this infra-umbilical region, followed by rupture of the combined ectoentodermal membrane, apparently produces the exposed, exstrophic condition. Severe eversion of the bladder tends to be accompanied by spread pubic bones and either a grooved (epispadiac) or a bifid penis or clitoris.

The superior parathyroids and the thymus take origin from the third pair of pharyngeal pouches. Failure of these glands to separate results in the burial of a parathyroid in the thymus.

SUBDIVISION

EXAMPLES: *unpartitioned body cavity; unpartitioned heart chambers; some stenosis of aorta or pulmonary artery; persistent cloaca; reduced lobation of lung or liver.*

Compartmentalizing of the coelom fails when a pleuropericardial membrane does not completely separate the pericardial cavity from a pleural cavity or when a pleuroperitoneal membrane does not complete the separation of a pleural cavity from the peritoneal cavity.

Septation of the primitive cardiac chambers is imperfect when the interventricular septum or the atrial septa fail to complete their normal development. In the case of the septum primum of the atria the defect may result from a persistent foramen primum or from a foramen secundum that fails to overlap completely the foramen ovale in the septum secundum.

Some stenoses of the aorta or pulmonary artery derive from an unequal longitudinal division of the truncus.

Incomplete subdivision of the cloaca usually produces a rectovestibular fistula in the female and a rectovesical or rectourethral fistula in the male.

MIGRATION

ORGANS

EXAMPLES: *thoracic stomach; undescended testis (cryptorchism); pelvic kidney; cervical thymus; ears beneath mandible (synotia); lack of abdominal musculature.*

Thoracic stomach is correlated with a short esophagus that fails to lengthen typically. As a result, normal descent cannot occur.

The reason for failure of testicular descent is unclear because the factors responsible for normal descent are obscure. Traction by the gubernaculum can no longer be credited, since it is not attached at its scrotal end and it converts into soft, jellylike tissue before descent begins.

The kidneys arise in the pelvis and normally ascend the distance of four vertebral segments. On arrival they normally rotate 90 degrees about their longitudinal axis.

The thymus may retain the approximate level of its pharyngeal pouch origin. This corresponds to the region of the future neck.

The ears arise in the branchial arch region and normally shift position as the mandible develops. As an accompaniment of agenesis of the mandible, the ears remain in the low, more or less horizontal (and sometimes fused) state.

A notable deficiency is the lack of the abdominal musculature, leaving a flaccid, loose, and wrinkled wall. This condition follows when the primitive myotomes of the dorsolateral trunk fail to send extensions ventrad.

CELLS

EXAMPLES: *megacolon; nonmedullary suprarenal gland; agenesis of branchial arch skeleton; sterile gonad; and virtual agenesis of spleen.*

This group, as a whole, is characterized by migratory failure on the part of distinctive cells. Megacolon results from a lack of autonomic ganglion cells in the lower colon, and especially in the rectum. The precursors of these cells arise in the primitive spinal ganglia. With normal migratory activity they become, in serial order, the ganglionated sympathetic trunks, the collateral ganglia, and the terminal ganglia of such visceral organs as the colon.

The medullary rather than the cortical component of accessory suprarenal glands especially tends to be lacking. The medullary cells arise in the primitive spinal ganglia, migrate, normally invade the cortical component of the suprarenal, and aggregate centrally within it.

Experimental evidence from embryos of amphibians and birds indicates that the branchial arch skeleton normally derives from migratory cells that originate in the primitive craniospinal ganglia. Hence, deficiencies in mammals and man may have their origins in a similar migratory failure.

The primitive germ cells arise caudal to the embryonic disk. Normally they migrate craniad in the early lining and mesenchyme of the gut and invade the genital ridge. Failure to do this produces a sterile gonad.

Congenital lack of a significant spleen is thought by some to be related to the failure of migratory thymic cells to immigrate into the spleen, proliferate, and populate it.

SYNTHETIC PROCESSES

EXAMPLES: *proteins (alkaptonuria, sickle cell anemia), carbohydrates (galactosemia), lipids (Gaucher's disease), or pigments (albinism, congenital porphyria).*

This group of defects comprises those "inborn errors of metabolism" in which enzyme deficiency blocks the course of intermediary metabolism and results in abnormal chemical functioning. The abnormal products may be stored or excreted.

Alkaptonuria represents an incomplete oxidation resulting in the excretion of homogentisic acid in the urine.

In sickle cell anemia, resulting from mutation, a single incorrect amino acid is substituted for one of the 557 amino acids that make up the peptide chains of the hemoglobin molecule. This renders the hemoglobin incompetent to function normally.

Galactosemia results from an enzyme deficiency that fails to convert galactose to glucose. Galactose is then stored in the liver and spleen and also excreted in the urine.

Gaucher's disease involves an abnormal storage and retention of cerebrosides in the reticuloendothelial cells.

General pigmentation is lacking when tyrosinase fails to act on tyrosine.

Through an error in porphyrin synthesis the precursors of porphyrin may be found in the plasma, urine, and feces.

DEVELOPMENTAL EXCESS

The category of developmental excess comprises results originating from processes that exceed normality or from the occurrence of events at a site at which they do not normally occur.

GENERAL OVERGROWTH

TOTAL GIGANTISM

EXAMPLE: *macrosomia.*

Historically giants are those who exceed 79 inches in height, but because of modern increases in stature this measure should probably be revised upward. Usually the condition starts before birth and the oversized newborn continues to grow at an accelerated rate. Another type of giant, one with a hereditary predisposition, does not begin excessive growing until some time in childhood. The basic cause of general gigantism is overproduction of the growth-promoting hormone, and a contributing factor is a delay in the closure of the epiphysis.

REGIONAL GIGANTISM

EXAMPLES: *cranium (macrocephalia); hydrocephalus; enlarged jaw (macrognathia); limb (macromelia); digit (macrodactylia); cervical or lumbar rib; male breasts (gynecomastia); female virginal breasts; male genital precocity; hypertrophy of clitoris.*

Hydrocephaly has a mechanical basis. Distension by cerebrospinal fluid accompanies impaired drainage, caused by stenosis of the aqueduct or by obstruction of the outlet of the fourth ventricle.

Local gigantism, as of a digit, seemingly represents an exaggerated tissue reaction to the same factors that elsewhere elicit a more moderate response.

A prominent rib at the lowest cervical (or highest lumbar) level is an exaggeration of the rudimentary rib, normally present and fused with the vertebra.

Gynecomastia in the male child and abnormal hypertrophy of the female breast at puberty are consequences of endocrine dysfunction. Such male breasts usually persist, and the corresponding female breasts never revert to their normal size.

Precocity of the male external genitalia and hypertrophy of the clitoris are further illustrations of endocrine dysfunction.

LOCAL HYPERPLASIA

EXAMPLES: *stenosis (some); exostosis; fibroma; hemangioma; lymphangioma (cystic hygroma); nevi (pigmented, sebaceous); polyposis; lipoma; rhabdomyoma; ichthyosis; and neurofibromatosis.*

Stenoses vary as to the hyperplastic tissue concerned. In the pylorus the muscle sphincter is at fault. In the gallbladder, bile ducts, and intestine, stenosis represents a retention of the normally temporary occlusion resulting from massive proliferation by the intestinal lining. Some intestinal types are attributed to rapid elongation and to an interference with the blood supply.

All but the first item in the preceding list are designated as *hamartomas.* They represent tissue excesses either prenatal or appearing during postnatal tissue maturation. Often called tumors, they are not neoplastic.

INCREASED NUMBERS

TOTAL REPETITION

EXAMPLES: *true twins; triplets; and so forth.*

Monozygotic, separate twins are the product of abnormal development (subdivision of an embryonic mass or duplication of an embryonic axis). The abnormal quality of this kind of twinning is made obvious when conjoining occurs. Such union varies in degree, and the twins may be equal or unequal in size.

SUPERNUMERARY PARTS

EXAMPLES: *vertebra; digit (polydactylia); phalanx (hyperphalangia); hand (dichiria); foot (dipodia); nipple (hyperthelia); double ureter.*

Except for the cervical region, vertebrae at other levels may vary above (or below) the normal number.

An extra digit, added as a *postminimus* in the hand or foot series, produces the ordinary polydactyly.

Hyperphalangia denotes the addition of one or more phalanges in the regular finger or toe series.

Dichiria or dipodia designates a more or less successful doubling of the hand or foot.

Hyperthelia occurs in at least 1 percent of individuals and along the course of the embryonic mammary ridge between the axilla and groin.

Duplication of the ureter depends upon the development of separate ureteric buds from the same mesonephric duct. They induce the formation of a single kidney from the metanephrogenic tissue into which they grow; only rarely are wholly duplicate kidneys produced.

SEPARATE (ACCESSORY) ORGANS

EXAMPLES: *pancreas; tooth (hyperdontia); breast (hypermastia); thyroid; parathyroid; suprarenal; spleen; placenta.*

An accessory pancreas derives from a supernumerary, separate primordium or perhaps from displacement of the early, diffuse formative tissue.

An accessory tooth, breast, or thyroid originates only along the course of the dental lamina, mammary ridge, or thyroglossal strand, respectively.

Accessory parathyroids originate from the four pharyngeal pouches that normally produce only one each.

An accessory suprarenal is often located in close relation to the kidney or gonad. This reflects propinquity in the sites of origin of these organs.

The spleen normally arises from the fusion of separate primordial hillocks on the greater omentum. A supernumerary spleen originates from one or more extra hillocks.

An accessory placenta arises from a separate, persisting patch of chorionic villi.

SUBDIVISION

EXAMPLES: *gallbladder and duct; Y-shaped ureter; accessory lobes of lung or liver; bifid digits; cleft hand or foot; bifid rib; local duplication of digestive tube; or supernumerary cusps of cardiac valves.*

Bifurcation and duplication of the gallbladder (and sometimes the cystic duct) is a product of branching, imitating that which produced the cystic and hepatic ducts from the common stem duct.

A double renal pelvis and calyx in relation to a branched ureter results from the bifurcation of the so-called ureteric diverticulum (which buds off the mesonephric duct).

Accessory lobes of the lung or liver sometimes occur; they correspond to lobes normal for lower mammals.

A bifid digit, cleft hand or foot, and a bifid rib are examples of duplication by branching.

Local parallel duplication of the digestive tube sometimes occurs, and at all levels. This condition would seem to be intimately related to blind diverticula that reach a maximum length of some three feet. The method of formation of either type, although postulated, is uncertain.

DEVELOPMENTAL MERGER

The category of developmental merger comprises organs that combine because of the proximity of their primordia, their subsequent growth, and often the failure of other factors that normally act to insure their separate state.

ABNORMAL UNION

EXAMPLES: *kidneys (horseshoe or cake); digits (syndactylia); lower limbs (sympodia); ears (synotia); annular pancreas; teeth; placenta.*

The permanent kidney primordia arise in close relation to each other, and sometimes fuse—usually by their caudal ends. Rarely the two kidneys lie on the same side and then are usually fused.

Syndactylia favors the fusion of the middle and third digits but may involve others.

Fusion of the lower limbs results from the developmental failure of a median, wedge-shaped mass of trunk mesenchyme, which ordinarily keeps them apart.

Union of the ears depends on a retention of their original location in a nearly ventral position on the future neck and on their subsequent fusion. This result follows the failure of the mandible to develop significantly and its consequent failure to force the ears apart.

An annular pancreas is perhaps caused by the development of the normally suppressed member of the paired ventral pancreatic buds. This outgrowth possibly joins the regular ventral and dorsal buds and so completes the encirclement of the duodenum.

Tooth fusion is a result of developmental proximity on the dental lamina.

Through growth the placentas of ordinary twins may unite when the implantation sites are fairly close together. In this instance a seam of junctional tissue prevents a vascular union.

EMBRYONIC SURVIVALS

The category of embryonic survival comprises permanent conditions that represent arrested states along the course of normal progressive or regressive development.

TOTAL SURVIVAL

EXAMPLES: *cervical (branchiogenic) fistula; umbilical (yolk stalk) fistula; intestinal herniation into stump of umbilical cord (omphalocele); umbilical (urachal) fistula; persistent tail; clubfoot (perhaps); persistent truncus; persistent ductus arteriosus; imperforate anus; imperforate hymen; coarctation of aorta (some); misshapen placenta.*

A complete cervical fistula represents the rare retention of a complete but temporary, "gill slit" condition occurring in embryos of early weeks. Those from the first slits open, externally, high on the ventrolateral surface of the neck and internally into the external auditory meatus. The more common fistulas are from the second slits; these open externally on the ventral border of the sternohyoid muscle and internally into the tonsillar fossa.

A fecal fistula results when that segment of the yolk stalk located between the navel and ileum is retained as a hollow tube.

An omphalocele represents a failure of the intestine to return from its temporary herniation into the umbilical cord. Its hernial sac is, therefore, covered by the thin amniotic reflection surfacing the cord.

A urinary fistula results when the urachus remains patent between the navel and bladder. The urachus is an attenuated portion of the bladder, and not the allantoic duct as was formerly thought.

The embryonic tail, maximally developed at five weeks, is then one sixth of the body length. During the next four weeks it normally disappears from external view. Specimens 3 inches long have occurred in the newborn. Most specimens are soft and fleshy, but a few have contained skeletal elements.

The origin of clubfoot has not yet been fully resolved. Some consider it to be a retention of a normal condition, transitory in the human fetus but permanent for apes.

The single truncus arteriosus normally undergoes longitudinal division into the aorta and pulmonary artery, but this process may fail to occur.

The ductus arteriosus is that part of the left sixth aortic arch located distal to the pulmonary artery. Its homologue on the right side regresses early, whereas the ductus normally remains patent only until shortly after birth.

The anal membrane is that portion of the primitive cloacal membrane that comes to separate the anal canal (proctodeum) from the rectum. Normally this membrane has a transitory existence.

The hymen is originally a complete membrane, located at the junction of the combined müllerian ducts with the urogenital sinus. Normally this membrane becomes variably perforate.

Coarctation of the aorta, just proximal to the attachment of the ligamentum arteriosum, may represent a persistence of the narrowing occurring there as long as the ductus is functional. Constriction opposite the ligamentum arteriosum is usually attributed to the pull of that cord.

A noncircular patch of chorionic villi giving rise to the placenta is responsible for a variously subdivided organ and for other irregularities of shape.

PARTIAL SURVIVAL

EXAMPLES: *pupillary membrane; broad oral opening (macrostomia); Meckel's diverticulum of ileum; kidney lobation; eyecup fissure (coloboma); urethral groove (hypospadias); pilonidal sinus; paradental cyst; thyroglossal cyst; preauricular or cervical (branchiogenic) cyst or sinus; yolk stalk cyst; urachal cyst or sinus; stenosis or atresia of the intestine, bile ducts, or gallbladder; accessory renal arteries; right or double aortic arch; left or double superior vena cava; left or double inferior vena cava; and double thoracic duct.*

Strands that partially obstruct the pupil are remnants of the pupillary membrane, or vascular covering over the front of the fetal lens.

A broad orifice to the mouth cavity is a partial retention of the relatively wider oral opening characteristic of the embryonic and early fetal period.

Meckel's diverticulum is most commonly a short proximal segment of the embryonic yolk stalk that remains patent and opens into the ileum. It may extend even to the umbilicus, and in some instances a more distal portion persists as a fibrous cord.

The fetal kidney shows external elevated areas, separated by grooves, outlining the bases of pyramids. In the human these grooves normally fill in, but such external lobation may persist (as it does in some mammals).

The so-called choroid fissure is really a defect based on the imperfect closure of the normally temporary fissure in the early optic cup. This anomaly can also be classified as a failure of union (Ch. 3).

Hypospadias results from the failure of the paired urethral folds of the fetus to meet and complete the urethral tube locally.

A pilonidal sinus is commonly interpreted as an enlarged and infected coccygeal fovea, which overlies the ending of the fetal neural tube in the integument. Nevertheless, similar dimples also occur at higher levels.

Cysts arise from remnants of embryonic epithelial structures that are usually obliterated. Among them are the following: paradental cysts, from the dental lamina or enamel organ; thyroglossal cysts, from the strand originally extending from thyroid to tongue; cervical cysts, from the first or second gill slit tissue (cervical sinuses are similar remnants that usually open externally, and rarely into the pharynx); yolk stalk cysts, from remnants of the embryonic duct between ileum and navel; and urachal cysts, from remnants of the urachus between bladder and navel.

Stenosis or atresia of the intestine and bile ducts is referable to a retention of the normally temporary occlusion of the lumen by epithelial proliferation.

The embryonic renal arteries are more numerous than those that ordinarily persist. The final number and pattern are quite variable.

Anomalies of the aortic arch, superior vena cava, inferior vena cava, and thoracic duct reflect the choice of unusual paths in the bilateral pattern of early vessels.

MISPLACEMENT

The category of misplacement is often designated as *heterotopia* or *ectopia*.

SITE OF ORIGIN

EXAMPLES: *tooth; thyroid; accessory parathyroid; pancreas; spleen; suprarenal; ectopic hair; and so forth.*

An ectopic tooth, thyroid, or parathyroid can only originate from an unusual portion of the primitive dental lamina, thyroglossal strand, or pharyngeal pouch, respectively.

An ectopic pancreas, spleen, kidney, or suprarenal arises by an additional primordium, separate from the normal one.

Long, coarse hair may develop in regions ordinarily covered by the downy type. Examples of a general body coat are known, but more common are local tufts ("tails" or "manes") in the midline of the back.

TRANSPOSITION

EXAMPLES: *aortic arch; aorta and pulmonary artery; heart (dextrocardia); total thoracic viscera; total abdominal viscera; or total thoracoabdominal viscera.*

The right fourth aortic arch of the embryo may be the one that develops (rather than the left one), as is characteristic of birds.

The aorta and pulmonary artery presumably become transposed and connected to the wrong ventricles when the spiral septum subdivides the truncus in such a way that the usual crossed relation does not result.

In dextrocardia that is not a part of general visceral inversion, the heart lies on the right of the midplane. Its chambers may be transposed or not.

The cause of mirror imaging of the viscera is not known. It is a part of the larger problem of the determination of asymmetry and bilateral symmetry in the embryo.

ABNORMAL TRANSPORT

EXAMPLES: *ectopic organs (testis, heart, parathyroid); ectopic endings (ureter); "undescended cecum"; nonrotation of intestine; volvulus; reversed rotation of intestine.*

The testis may descend but come to lie outside the scrotum.

The heart is displaced to the right in dextrocardia.

The parathyroids may become located away from the thyroid, and may even follow the thymus into the thorax.

The ureter may open into the urethra or the genital duct of the male and into the urethra, vagina, or vestibule of the female. The urethral sites are the results of atypical absorptions of the common stem of the future ureter and male duct. The proximity of the mesonephric duct and its ureteric bud to the müllerian ducts predisposes to a communication between the two.

A ureter may cross to the opposite side and connect with an ectopic kidney that it induces there.

When the intestine withdraws from the umbilical cord and rotation occurs, the cecum is normally located at the iliac crest. So-called undescended cecum is actually a cecum that rises secondarily, following the cranially retreating liver.

On its return from temporary herniation into the umbilical cord the intestine may fail to rotate, whereupon the typical pattern is not established. An accompanying failure of the mesenteries to become obliterated in part (and so anchor the intestines) predisposes to the twisting characteristic of volvulus.

A reversed rotation of the returning intestine results in a mirror image of the normal pattern.

HERNIATION

EXAMPLES: *diaphragmatic hernia; indirect inguinal hernia; umbilical hernia (exomphalos); omphalocele; meningocele; meningoencephalocele; meningomyelocele; ectocardia; eventration.*

Some two thirds of all diaphragmatic hernias are made possible by the failure of a particular component (pleuroperitoneal membrane) of the diaphragm to fill in its allotted area. This leaves a defect (foramen of Bochdalek) through which abdominal viscera can push into the pleural cavity. In some cases the membrane is intact but thin. It may then yield to pressure and produce a hernial sac. This apparently results from mechanical weakness because of the failure of muscle to reinforce the original membrane.

The foundation for a herniation of abdominal viscera through an overly large esophageal hiatus in the diaphragm may be laid when the descent of the stomach into the abdomen, occurring during the time of the development of the diaphragm, is delayed by tardy elongation of the esophagus. In some instances the esophagus remains short, so that the upper part of the stomach lies in the lower mediastinum. This is really a failure of descent of the stomach rather than a secondary herniation.

Herniation through the ventral aspect of the diaphragm (so-called foramen of Morgagni) is least common. The ectopic viscera are contained within the bulging membranous sac. This condition probably arises through a failure of muscular reinforcement of the early, membranous septum transversum.

Indirect inguinal hernia is made possible when the tubular segment of the processus vaginalis remains open, or partly open, even into adult life.

An umbilical hernia is conditioned by the incomplete closure of the fusion of the umbilical ring, following the return of the intestine to the abdomen. A loop of small intestine can then push past this defect and come to occupy a sac covered by skin.

The herniated intestinal loops may fail to return to the abdomen from their normal, temporary location in the umbilical cord. This condition (omphalocele) is characterized by the distinctive composition of the containing sac; it consists of a thin membrane composed solely of the transparent amniotic covering of the cord and a peritoneal lining.

Meningocele is herniation of the meninges accompanying an imperfect closure of the spine or cranium. This defect permits the protrusion of a sac, filled with cerebrospinal fluid and covered with skin.

When a meningeal herniation in the cranial region also contains cerebral tissue, it becomes a meningoencephalocele. When the spinal cord herniates locally into the meningeal sac, the condition is called meningomyelocele.

External protrusion and free exposure of the heart (ectocardia) or abdominal viscera occurs when the folds that form the body wall fail to meet in the midventral line.

ACTIVATOR LACK

Evidence of activator lack is based largely on experiments performed on amphibians and birds, since the mammalian embryo is virtually inaccessible to experimental procedures.

INDUCTIVE INADEQUACY

Accumulating experimental evidence demonstrates increasing numbers of developmental dependencies between embryonic parts. These are related sequentially as cause and effect. One part in contact with another imparts to it a chemical substance that educes a particular type of developmental response. This sequence of stimulus and response constitutes an induction. Much, at least, of agenesis and partial development is related to inductive inadequacies.

Examples of normal ectodermal inductions are the lens (by the optic cup); the cornea (by the lens); and the membranous labyrinth, adenohypophysis, and cartilaginous body axis (by the neural tube).

Examples of normal mesodermal inductions are the neural tube and myotomes (by the notochord); the müllerian duct (by the mesonephric duct); and the kidney (by the ureteric bud growing out from the mesonephric duct).

Examples of normal entodermal inductions are those acting in part on the heart and on the optic vesicle.

HORMONAL INADEQUACY

EXAMPLES: *cretin dwarfism; male pseudo-hermaphroditism; sexual infantilism.*

True hormones, produced by endocrine glands, are not primary, creative factors in development. Yet they do play a role in development, and especially in its later phases. When certain parts have arrived at a given state of differentiation (including hormone sensitivity) they react to the chemical stimulation supplied by the hormone substances appropriate for those particular parts.

Thyroid deficiency is notably responsible for cretinism.

The hormone of the fetal testis normally suppresses the female duct system and permits the male ducts and external genitalia to dominate; an inadequate influence of this kind leads to the indecisive or mixed conditions of these auxiliary genital organs.

Inadequacy of the hypophysis-gonad endocrine sequence results in a stunted female tract and a rudimentary prostate and seminal vesicles in the male.

ATYPICAL DIFFERENTIATION

TISSUE SUBSTITUTION

EXAMPLE: *heteroplasia.*

In tissue substitution, or heteroplasia, a tissue differentiates in a location that is nor-mally foreign to it. Such abnormal location constitutes an incongruity.

An ectodermal example is hairy skin as a patch in the moist stratified epithelium of the conjunctiva. Mesodermal examples are skeletal muscle in the thyroid or lung and cartilage in a tonsil or kidney. An entodermal example is a patch of gastric (fundic) epithelium in the upper esophagus. Other substitutions in development are ligaments for precartilage and testicular tissue for ovarian medulla in an ovotestis.

INCORRECT HISTOGENESIS

EXAMPLES: *achondroplasia; osteogenesis imperfecta; local melanism; albinism; congenital cataract; erythroblastosis.*

In this type of aberration an attempt is made to produce the normally expected tissue, but the histogenetic differentiation is faulty.

RETROPLASIA

EXAMPLE: *retrograde displasias.*

Striking are the retrograde processes in fetal parts that lead secondarily to adhesions to nearby portions of the amnion. Such localized necroses also are responsible for fetal amputations.

Quite different, and wholly normal, is dedifferentiation. In this process the steps of differentiation are reversed and a return is made to the simpler forerunner tissue. An example is the cartilage of the fetal internal ear, which reverts first to precartilage and then to a mesenchymal reticulum in order to make room for the developing perilymph spaces.

EMBRYONIC NEOPLASMS

EXAMPLES: *neuroblastoma; embryoma (Wilms' tumor); retinoblastoma; hepatoblastoma; rhabdomyoblastoma; teratoma.*

These tumors arise in prenatal or early postnatal development. Their sources are particular organ primordia or tissue, that are still in an immature state. Such tumors differ causally from acquired tumors of mature tissues because they result from intrinsic disturbances of normal developments. They differ in structure because they continue to differentiate at an embryonic level, thereby producing masses of immature tissue. They rate both as neoplasms and as malformations.

The peculiar growths known as teratomas occur most frequently in the ovary and sacrococcygeal region. They are not "included twins" but are tumors containing tissues foreign to the region where found. An immature type, with poorly differentiated tissue, is an *embryoma,* which is highly proliferative and usually malignant. The simplest type with mature tissue is commonly called a *dermoid cyst,* yet such specimens usually possess representatives of all three germ layers. Conspicuous in every teratomatous specimen is the lack of an orderly arrangement of tissues and parts. All types probably represent responses to induction at an abnormal time and place. The chief deficiency is an inability to organize as a whole.

HERMAPHRODITISM

TRUE TYPE

The true variety of hermaphroditism (*h. verus*) is a condition in which representatives of male and female gonads occur in the same individual. Of the numerous cases described, in some there are a separate ovary and testis; in others there is an ovary or a testis paired with an ovotestis; and in still others there is a pair of ovotestes. The sex chromosome pair has been reported both as XX and as a mosaic (XY/XO); hence, a generalization is at present impossible. The internal genitalia are faulty bisexual, and sometimes representatives of the internal genital organs of both sexes occur on one or both sides. External genitalia may be intermediate in structure, and secondary sexual characteristics are usually mixed. The two kinds of gonads presumably derive from the primitive indifferent gonad, which has bisexual potentialities. The dual activity of the cortical (female) and medullary (male) components seems to depend on an abnormal genic balance controlling these parts.

FALSE TYPE

In the false variety of hermaphroditism (*h. falsus*), or *pseudohermaphroditism,* an individual has the gonads of one sex, but the external genitalia and secondary sexual characteristics tend to be intermediate or to approximate those of the opposite sex. The internal sexual tract can be that of either sex. Also, it may be double or mixed; commonly it is atrophic in part.

In the common masculine pseudohermaphroditism the individual possesses testes, inferior in quality and often undescended, but the external genitalia (by retarded development and severe hypospadias) and secondary sexual characteristics resemble those of the female. The internal sexual tract may be that of either sex, or it may be double or mixed. This feminization results from an inadequate suppressive influence exerted by the testicular hormone during the fetal period. The fetal ovaries are ineffective in influencing either duct system of the external genitalia. By contrast, it is the testes that normally stimulate the external genitalia and male ducts while suppressing the female ducts.

In the rare *feminine pseudohermaphroditism* recognizable ovaries may be present, and even descended, but the other sexual characteristics, sometimes even including an enlarged clitoris and fused labias, tend to simulate the male. This masculine trend can be produced by the excessive androgenic action of an enlarged suprarenal cortex or by a tumor with masculine structure that develops in the medulla of the ovary. The second method depends on the significant fact that the embryonic ovary, like the testis, has inherent bisexual potencies.

CHROMOSOME ABERRATION SEQUELAE

Unusual assortments of chromosomes in the somatic cells of the embryo result from mishaps, usually during meiotic divisions in the germ cells. Such abnormal behavior includes nondisjunction, translocation, and deletion.

AUTOSOMES

EXAMPLES: *trisomy; triploidy; mosaicism.*

Trisomy denotes the presence in somatic cells of three chromosomes of one kind instead of the usual pair. This condition is produced during gametogenesis when the chromosomes of a given pair fail to separate and both pass into one daughter cell. Mongolism is related to trisomy of chromosomes number 21 in the human series.

Triploidy denotes the presence of three sets of chromosomes in somatic cells instead of the customary two sets. This can be brought about by the union at fertilization of a diploid and a haploid gamete. Examples are known in amphibians and mammals.

Aberrations occurring in the divisions of somatic cells can also produce abnormal assortments of chromosomes. When such an aberration takes place relatively early in embryonic development the cellular progeny is so distributed that normal and abnormal regions of the body compose a mosaic pattern. The mosaic state is known to be responsible for some discrepant blood groups and for circumscribed regions showing neurofibromatosis.

SEX CHROMOSOMES

EXAMPLES: *Turner's syndrome; Klinefelter's syndrome; superfemales; mosaics.*

Turner's syndrome designates a genetic female whose sex chromosome assortment is XO. Accompaniments are infantilism, sterility, and mental deficiency.

Klinefelter's syndrome designates a genetic male whose sex chromosome complex is XXY, XXXY, or XXXXY. It was this condition (and the XO combination, above) that proved that sex determination is related to the presence or absence of Y and not to the presence of X alone (male) and XX (female), as formerly believed. Accompaniments are enlarged breasts, lack of beard, and sterility.

Superfemales, so called, have sex chromosome complexes of XXX or XXXX. This condition is associated with impaired mentality. Otherwise such individuals are nearly normal and may even be fertile.

Mosaics of sex chromosomes (XY/XO) have been reported in true hermaphrodites.

SYNDROMES

Among syndromes are those named for the following persons: Down; Eisenmenger; Fallot; Kast; Klippel-Feil; Laurence-Moon-Biedl; Marfan; Peutz; Sturge.

In general, syndromes do not arise in sequence through a chain of direct dependencies. On the other hand, and this clearest when the malformed parts are well separated spatially, they may occur because different parts become susceptible at the same time and respond atypically to a common teratogenic influence. Other results may reflect the influence of defective genes, since the same gene may participate in syntheses related to different parts.

LESLIE B. AREY

4

Genetics in Surgery

Human genetics has primarily been concerned with individual differences in man and has made its major contribution to medicine predominantly in the area of the classification of human disease. The clinician and the human geneticist attempt to divide groups of diseases with similar symptoms into specific entities of which the particular pathogenesis, therapeutics, and prognosis may be utilized in the practice of medicine.

GENERAL PRINCIPLES

The individual is made up of numerous hereditary factors, or genes. These genes are present in duplicate and are located on pairs of chromosomes in all somatic cells. Each individual has inherited one member of each pair of genes from his father and one from his mother. During the formation of germ cells only one chromosome of each pair—

TABLE 1.   PAIR OF GENES DETERMINING THE MN BLOOD GROUP IN MAN. OUTCOME OF VARIOUS MATINGS OF HOMOZYGOUS AND HETEROZYGOUS INDIVIDUALS

MATING OF A HETEROZYGOUS MOTHER (MN BLOOD GROUP) AND A HOMOZYGOUS FATHER (MM BLOOD GROUP).

		Mother *Genotype* *MN*			
	Germ cells	M			N
Father			Zygotes		
Genotype	M	MM			MN
MM	M	MM			MN

MATING OF A HETEROZYGOUS MOTHER AND A HETEROZYGOUS FATHER (MN BLOOD GROUP).

		Mother *Genotype* *MN*			
	Germ cells	M			N
Father			Zygotes		
Genotype	M	MM			MN
MN	N	MN			NN

34

and hence one gene of each pair—reaches the mature germ cell. When fertilization takes place, the diploid, or paired, number of chromosomes is restored, and pairs of genes are then present in the zygote, or fetus. If the genes present at a specific location on a pair of homologous chromosomes are similar, the individual is said to be homozygous with respect to that gene. If the genes are different, the individual is called heterozygous, and the genes are called alleles. Homozygous individuals can produce only one type of gamete with respect to this gene, whereas heterozygous individuals will produce equal numbers of gametes with each type of gene (see Table 1).

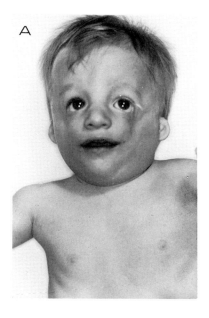

COMMON PATTERNS OF INHERITANCE

AUTOSOMAL DOMINANT

Autosomal dominant inheritance in man may be recognized by the following features: (1) The dominant trait is also present in one parent of the affected child (mutation presents an exception); (2) the trait is transmitted by an affected person to one half of his children, regardless of their sex; and (3) unaffected family members do not transmit the trait to their children. (Figure 1 shows a patient with Treacher-Collins syndrome and his pedigree, illustrating autosomal dominant

Fig. 1. A. Patient with mandibulofacial dysostosis. B. His family pedigree demonstrating an autosomal dominant mode of inheritance.

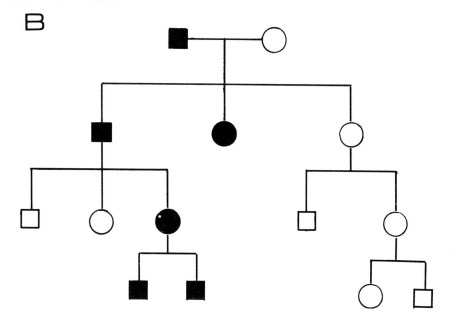

inheritance.) Some examples of conditions inherited in this fashion are (1) Marfan's syndrome—long, slender limbs, luxation of the lens, hernias, aneurysm of the aorta; (2) Ehlers-Danlos syndrome—excessive elasticity of the skin, hyperextensibility of joints, poor wound healing, bleeding tendency; (3) Osler's telangiectasia hemorrhagica—multiple telangiectases, nosebleeds, arteriovenous aneurysms in the lungs, occasionally multiple hemangioendotheliomas of all organs; (4) multiple sebaceous cysts of the skin; (5) osteogenesis imperfecta—blue sclera and multiple fractures with resultant limb deformities; (6) Treacher-Collins syndrome—deformity of the ears, maxillary and mandibular hypoplasia, hearing deficit; and (7) familial polyposes of the colon, multiple polyps, benign and malignant.

AUTOSOMAL RECESSIVE

Autosomal recessive inheritance in man may be recognized by the following features: (1) The trait characteristically appears only in siblings; (2) on the average, one fourth of the siblings of an affected individual, regardless of sex, are affected; (3) the children of affected persons are rarely affected; and (4) the parents of the affected child may be related. (Figure 2 shows the pedigree of a family with galactosemia.) Some examples of conditions inherited as autosomal recessive disorders are (1) galactosemia—mental retardation, cataracts, and liver disease; (2) cystic fibrosis of the pancreas—meconium ileus of the newborn, repeated pulmonary infection, cirrhosis of the liver, absence of pancreatic enzymes; (3) xeroderma pigmentosum—photophobia, telangiectasis, wartlike hyperkeratoses, superficial ulcers with malignant transformation, severe scarring of face and hands; and (4) Hurler's syndrome—progressive mental retardation, hepatosplenomegaly, spinal deformity, inguinal and umbilical hernias.

X-LINKED RECESSIVE

X-linked recessive inheritance may be recognized by the following features: (1) The trait is transmitted by carrier females to one half their sons; (2) males are affected predominantly; and (3) an affected male never transmits the disease to his sons, but all his daughters will be carriers. Classic examples

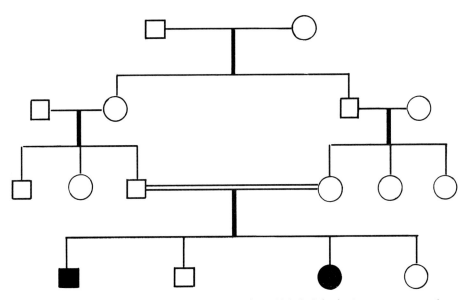

Fig. 2. Classical pedigree of a family with galactosemia, which is inherited as an autosomal recessive disorder.

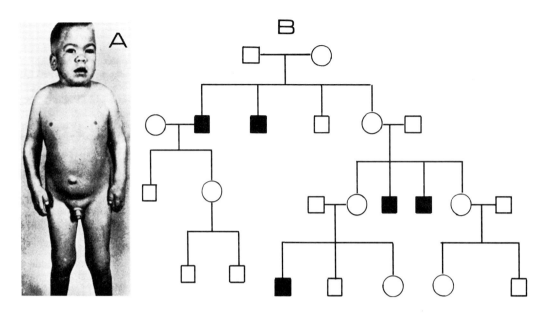

Fig. 3. A. Patient with Hunter's syndrome. B. Pedigree showing it as inherited as an X-linked recessive disorder.

of this disorder are red-green color blindness, hemophilia A and B, anhidrotic ectodermal dysplasia, and Fabry's disease. (Figure 3 shows a patient with Hunter's syndrome and his pedigree.)

CHROMOSOMAL ABERRATIONS

CHROMOSOME ANALYSIS TECHNIQUES

In the past decade, since the technique of study of human chromosomes has been simplified and standardized, the clinician has gained some understanding of the etiology of a number of the common congenital malformation syndromes. The technique of chromosome analysis performed utilizing peripheral blood is as follows: Heparinized blood is collected in a sterile tube and allowed to sediment. The plasma containing lymphocytes is removed and suspended in a culture medium containing phytohemagglutinin, which stimulates the lymphocytes to divide. After three days, colchicine is added

to the culture to arrest cell division at a stage where the chromosomes are easily studied. The cells are then exposed to a hypotonic solution in order to disperse the chromosomes, and slides are prepared. (Figure 4 is a photograph of human chromosome preparation.) The chromosomes are photographed, counted, and arranged in an order dependent on both the size and the position of the centromere. These characteristics determine the karyotype. (Figure 5 shows types of human chromosomes; Figure 6 shows the karyotype of a normal female; Figure 7 shows the karyotype of a normal male.) The normal chromosome complement in the female consists of 22 pairs of autosomal chromosomes and one pair of sex (X) chromosomes, a total of 46 (Fig. 6). The normal chromosome complement of a male consists of 22 pairs of autosomal chromosomes and 2 sex chromosomes (X and Y), a total of 46 (Fig. 7).

The sex chromatin body, or Barr body, is different from the sex chromosome. It is a darkly staining body located along the nuclear membrane in most of the cells of the normal female (Fig. 8). It is absent in the

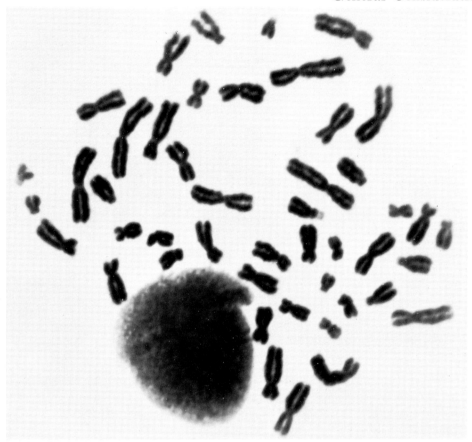

Fig. 4. Human chromosomes during mitosis after exposure to colchicine and hypotonic solution.

normal male. A constant relationship exists between the X chromosomes and the sex chromatin bodies: there is one less sex chromatin body than the number of X chromosomes. Epithelial cells from the buccal mucosa are studied by analyzing 100 to 200

METACENTRIC SUBMETACENTRIC ACROCENTRIC

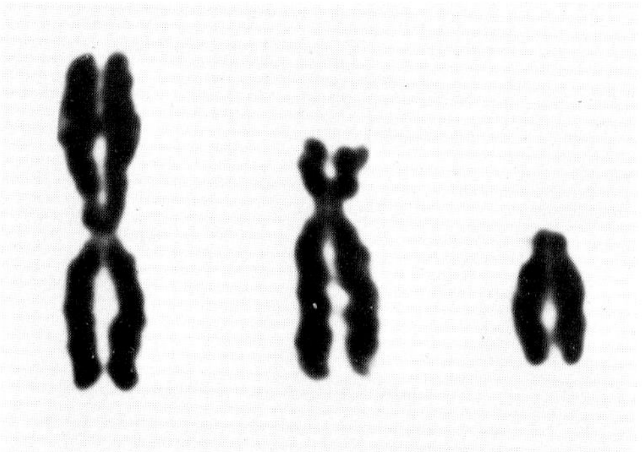

Fig. 5. Types of human chromosomes named relative to the position of the centromere.

cells and the number of sex chromatin bodies counted.

ABNORMALITIES OF AUTOSOMAL CHROMOSOMES

AUTOSOMAL TRISOMY SYNDROMES

DOWN'S SYNDROME

Down's syndrome (mongolism) is characterized by mental retardation, hypotonia, a brachycephalic head with flat occiput, epicanthic folds, Brushfield spots, a low nasal bridge, protruding tongue, short and broad hands, a horizontal palmar crease (simian line), a curved fifth finger, abnormal dermatoglyphics, a wide gap between first and second toes, congenital heart disease, and an abnormal pelvis. There is an increased inci-

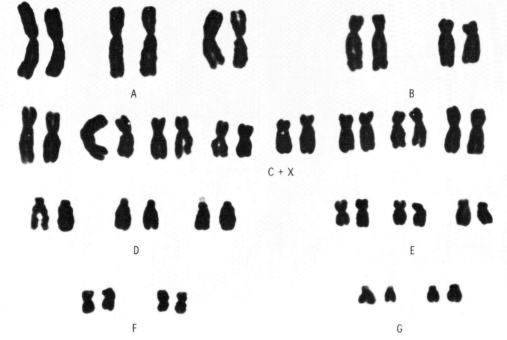

Fig. 6. Karyotype of a normal female.

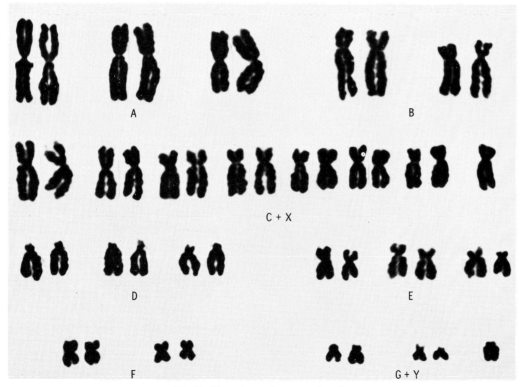

Fig. 7. Karyotype of a normal male.

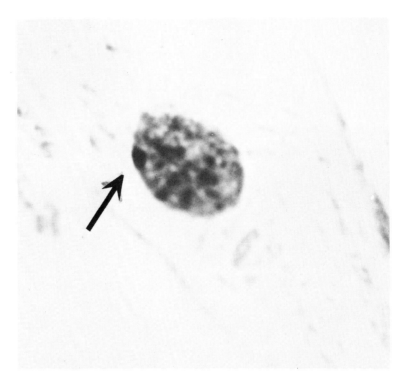

Fig. 8. Buccal smear obtained from a normal female demonstrating a sex chromatin mass located at the periphery of the nucleus. (Courtesy of Wayne Borges.)

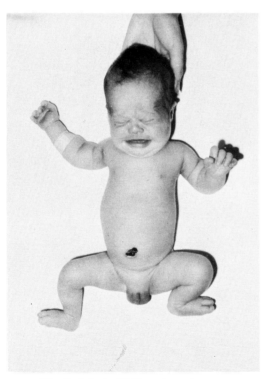

Fig. 9. Infant with Down's syndrome.

dence of both duodenal atresia and congenital aganglionosis in this condition. (Figure 9 shows an infant with Down's syndrome.) The majority—about 95 percent—of children with Down's syndrome have 47 chromosomes. The extra chromosome is a small, acrocentric chromosome of the G group, usually referred to as chromosome 21 (Fig. 10). The incidence of Down's syndrome is approximately 1 in 700 births. The risk of a mother less than 29 years of age having a child with Down's syndrome is about 1 in 2,000. The chance increases to 1 in 50 for mothers over the age of 40 years. A small number of children with Down's syndrome are found to have only 46 chromosomes. Close examination of the chromosome preparation demonstrates two chromosomes attached to one another (translocation—see Figure 11). In some of these cases the translocated chromosomes may be inherited from either parent, and usually from the mother. The importance of this finding is that parents carrying translocated chromosomes may

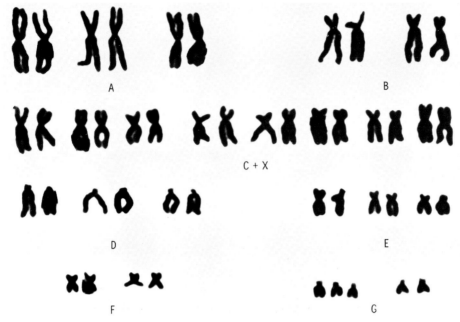

Fig. 10. Karyotype from infant with trisomic Down's syndrome. Note extra G group chromosome.

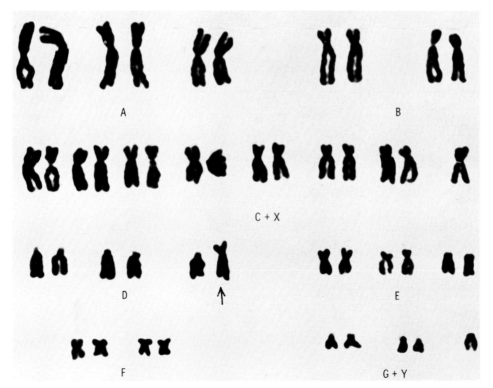

Fig. 11. Karyotype from infant with Down's syndrome. Note the presence of the translocation of a G group chromosome to one of the D group chromosomes (D/G translocation).

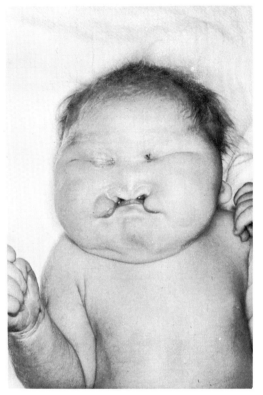

Fig. 12. Infant with D_1 trisomy syndrome.

have a risk as high as 100 percent of having children with Down's syndrome. Although the incidence of translocations is about 2 percent of all patients with Down's syndrome, the incidence in mothers below age 30 may be 5 to 10 percent. It is the usual procedure to refer every mother below 30 years of age who has had a child with Down's syndrome, every mother with more than one affected child, and all families with histories of Down's syndrome for chromosomal analysis.

D_1 TRISOMY SYNDROME

The D_1 trisomy syndrome is characterized by mental retardation, cleft lip and palate, microphthalmia, cataracts or coloboma, polydactyly, congenital heart disease (CHD), abnormal dermatoglyphics, ·prominent heels, and death in early infancy. This disorder is associated with the finding of 47 chromosomes, the extra one belonging to the D group of chromosomes (Fig. 12).

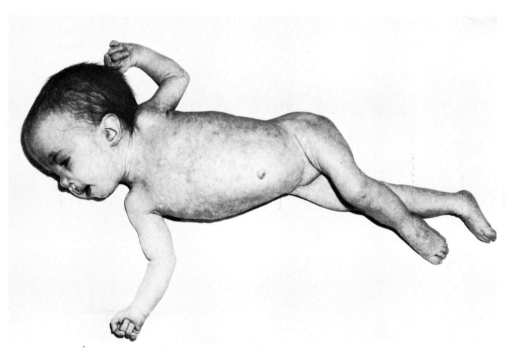

Fig. 13. Infant with 18 trisomy syndrome.

18 TRISOMY SYNDROME

The 18 trisomy syndrome (E trisomy syndrome) comprises mental retardation, failure to thrive, low-set malformed ears, flexion deformity of the hands with the second finger overlapping the third and the fifth overlapping the fourth, abnormal dermatoglyphics, CHD, and rocker-bottom feet. This condition is associated with 47 chromosomes, the extra one being a number 18 chromosome (Fig. 13).

AUTOSOMAL DELETION SYNDROMES

A number of autosomal deletion syndromes in man are known. The cri du chat (cat-cry syndrome) results from the deletion of the short arm of a B group chromosome, and the syndrome involving the deletion of the short arm of chromosome 18 are discrete congenital malformation syndromes.

SEX CHROMOSOME ABNORMALITIES

TURNER'S SYNDROME

Girls with Turner's syndrome (gonadal dysgenesis) have the following abnormalities (Fig. 14): short stature; lymphedema of the hands and feet in the newborn period; a low hairline and webbing of the neck; congenital heart disease; coarctation of the aorta (25 percent); increased lateral carrying angle at the elbow; renal malformations; telangiectasia of the bowel, producing unexplained melena; and amenorrhea. Chromosome analysis reveals the presence of 45 chromosomes with a missing X chromosome, and examination of a buccal smear reveals the absence of the sex chromatin body.

KLINEFELTER'S SYNDROME

Males with Klinefelter's syndrome are usually detected during adolescence. The principal findings are small testes, azospermia, gynecomastia (with carcinoma of the breast

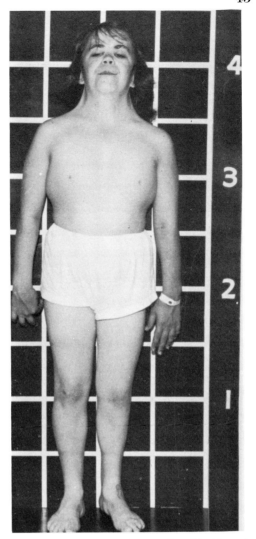

Fig. 14. Thirteen-year-old female with Turner's syndrome (XO).

recorded in a number of cases), eunuchoid features, and either behavioral difficulties or mental retardation (25 percent). Examination of buccal smears demonstrates the presence of a sex chromatin body, and chromosome analysis reveals the presence of 47 chromosomes with an extra X chromosome.

REFERRING PATIENTS FOR ANALYSIS

The physician is faced with the problem of determining which children should be referred for chromosomal analysis. The following guide is one that I use in selecting cases for such analysis: (1) children with any of the specific syndromes known to be associated with a chromosomal abnormality, such as Down's syndrome, and D_1 trisomy syndrome, (2) children with three or more congenital malformations although without specific syndrome complexes—the likelihood of finding a chromosome aberration among them is approximately 10 percent, and (3) children with congenital malformations from families with histories of similar malformations or numerous abortions. The child with an isolated congenital malformation involving any system is unlikely to have a chromosome aberration. This does not preclude the possibility that this entity is familial. The physician must obtain a family history if he is to recognize and counsel those families in which the entity is genetically determined.

HENRY L. NADLER

REFERENCES

STERN, C. Human Genetics. San Francisco, W. H. Freeman and Company, 1960.

LENZ, W. Medical Genetics. Chicago, University of Chicago Press, 1963.

ROBERTS, J. A. F. An Introduction to Medical Genetics. New York, Oxford University Press, 1963.

CLARKE, C. A. Genetics and the Clinician. Philadelphia, F. A. Davis Company, 1964.

KNUDSON, A. G. Genetics and Disease. New York, McGraw-Hill Book Company, Inc., 1965.

McKUSICK, V. A. Human Genetics. Englewood Cliffs, N.J., Prentice-Hall, Inc., 1964.

EGGEN, R. R. Chromosome Diagnostics in Clinical Medicine. Springfield, Ill., Charles C Thomas, Publisher, 1965.

VALENTINE, G. H. The Chromosome Disorder. Philadelphia, J. B. Lippincott Company, 1966.

THOMPSON, J. S., and THOMPSON, M. W. Genetics in Medicine. Philadelphia, W. B. Saunders Company, 1966.

5

The History and the Physical Examination

It is understandable that as medical knowledge increases and diagnosis becomes more dependent upon radiographic and laboratory examinations there is a tendency to pay less attention to the history of a patient's illness. Such a change of emphasis is not in the best interest of the patient. The value of laboratory and radiographic tests is not here being denied, for they are and will continue to be of increasing importance. However, as an aid in clearly delineating the patient's problem and in selectively ordering x-ray examinations and laboratory tests, there is no substitute for a carefully obtained history. At times a problem that has failed to be resolved despite many complicated laboratory investigations has been elucidated by a careful reconstruction of the development of the illness. This is particularly true in the case of small children and infants, who are uncooperative and on whom the physical examination is difficult to perform.

Obtaining a history and performing a physical examination of an infant or a child present problems not encountered in caring for adult patients. The history of a child's illness must be secured from parents or relatives or other adults rather than from the patient, and in appraising such a history it is important to evaluate the reliability and accuracy of the narrator's information. Generally, mothers are careful observers; having cared for their children in good health they are quick to perceive deviations from normal behavior. The tendency to disregard some seemingly irrelevant information which the mother supplies should be resisted, for these observations often help in making a diagnosis.

It is normal for parents to be disturbed when their child is ill, and it is wise for the doctor to alleviate their anxiety by permitting them, without interruption, to describe their child's illness. In this way, without having to ask leading questions, the examiner is given an unbiased account of the child's troubles. He can then ask questions that will fill in gaps in the progression of the illness and secure a full system, prenatal, past, and family history. It is helpful for the doctor, by appropriate questions and observations, to gain some insight into the family's economic and emotional situation, for this information is valuable in appraising the child during his hospital stay and in planning followup care.

During the history taking, especially if it is conducted in the physician's office or in the hospital, the child will have an opportunity to become accustomed to his new surroundings and acquainted with the physician. It is a mistake for the examiner to deny the child this period of accommodation and to proceed brusquely with the examination. Haste may provoke the child into being uncooperative and may make the examination difficult to perform and the findings hard to evaluate.

Patience and a sincere effort to gain the child's confidence will help prevent such unfortunate episodes. Often during the conversation with the parents the child will, of his own accord, approach the physician, and this is a sure indication that the child has gained confidence in the doctor and will be cooperative during the examination. When children have been informed by their parents of what the visit to the doctor entails, they will usually approach him without fear. Children enjoy being the center of attention, and the examiner will be successful if he keeps this fact in mind. In coping with timid or uncooperative children, he should try various approaches—for example, offering the child a toy or, better still, suggesting to the child that he come over and show the examiner some toy he has or some part of his clothing which is obviously new. Children are proud of such items and will often forget their shyness and insecurity in their eagerness to show off a new dress or jacket. When the child has made a voluntary approach to the doctor, the situation can be made more secure by the doctor's conversing with him about his brothers, sisters, or pets or about school and other activities. After a few minutes of such conversation, permission to perform an examination is often obtained from the child. Once the child has given his consent, the doctor rarely fails to conduct a satisfactory examination.

Occasionally, regardless of how assiduously the child's confidence is courted, it becomes necessary to use force to examine the child. In such situations it is advisable to ask the parents to leave the room to permit the doctor and nurse to proceed with the examination. Having the parents leave the room will often quiet the child, and in some instances permitting the parents to return to the examining room will ensure a cooperative attitude on the child's part.

In examining infants, a feeding during the procedure is helpful, for it quiets the baby so that chest auscultation and abdominal palpation can be performed satisfactorily. When it is inadvisable for the infant to have fluids orally, a nipple containing cotton with sweetened water can be offered to him.

The first step in conducting the examination is to remove all clothing so that the whole body can be inspected. Often a rash that is the key to the diagnosis will be overlooked if the child remains partially dressed during the examination. It is important to turn the patient over and look for rashes on the back and extremities as well as on the neck, chest, and abdomen. At the same time the color of the skin can be noted, and cyanosis, icterus, or pigmentation can be detected without disturbing the child. Observations of the child's posture and movements are important, for they may give clues to the nature of the illness. In acute appendicitis the child's posture will be stooped and his gait deliberate; when he lies down he will often recline on his right side with his legs flexed.

A surgeon is primarily concerned with pathology in a localized area; nevertheless, it is important that he perform a complete examination. Abdominal pain may be related to an upper respiratory infection, and unless the signs of inflammation are sought in the ears, nose, and throat the possibility of mesenteric adenitis will be overlooked and an incorrect diagnosis of appendicitis made. Abdominal pain may also be related to pneumonia, so that examination of the chest is imperative.

The simple manipulations that are not uncomfortable to the patient should be performed first. It is a good idea to begin with percussion and auscultation of the chest. Permitting the child to become familiar with the stethoscope will divert his attention during this part of the examination. The heart sounds are then elicited, and percussion for determination of heart size and position is performed. Blood pressure should be taken to determine whether hypertension exists or whether arm and leg blood pressure differ, so that coarctation of the aorta will not be overlooked in the asymptomatic stage.

After the chest has been examined it is well to proceed to the abdomen. In evaluating a child's reaction to abdominal palpation the doctor must be careful not to ask repeatedly if palpation of the abdomen, particularly of localized points, produces pain. The examiner will often obtain false positive findings by persistent questioning concerning abdominal tenderness. It is better to divert the child's attention during the abdominal examination by conversation concerning unrelated situations. Simple questions about the child's associates and activities are useful. The child readily becomes an active participant in a conversation about school, games, and pets, and his attention is diverted from the examination so that the doctor can determine the areas of true tenderness by observing the child's facial expression. When the examination is conducted in this manner, voluntary spasm is not usually encountered. If the patient does exhibit abdominal muscle spasm, constant gentle pressure will often overcome it and thus allow its differentiation from true spasm. Talking to the child about things other than abdominal tenderness and observing his face for signs of discomfort are also of value in examining the occasional child who is stoic and who will not indicate when abdominal palpation produces pain.

Sometimes it is impossible to gain a child's confidence and conduct a satisfactory abdominal examination. This is particularly true of the two- and three-year-olds. In such a situation Nembutal may be given to provide conditions for an adequate examination. A child who will not permit a satisfactory abdominal examination is probably hyperactive, and a moderate dose of Nembutal will quiet him or produce light sleep. Under such circumstances true tenderness or spasm can be detected. (An average dose is 2 mg of Nembutal per pound of body weight, up to 30 pounds. For heavier children a proportionate part of the adult dose, computed by weight, is suitable. The medication is given in a capsule which has been perforated in several places by a needle and is administered by inserting the capsule into the rectum.) It is possible by observing his face to detect areas of localized abdominal tenderness upon palpation; certainly the spasm occurring under these conditions can be relied on. Under no

circumstances should medication be administered to a child with abdominal pain until the attending surgeon has had an opportunity to see the patient and to make a preliminary examination.

Often the patient with an acute retrocecal appendix has a normal abdomen on examination, and it is not until palpation is directed to the flank above the iliac crest that tenderness and spasm are elicited. This maneuver is frequently omitted by surgeons because of haste or a failure to appreciate the value of such tenderness in making the diagnosis of an acutely inflamed appendix. Flank tenderness must be clearly differentiated from costovertebral angle tenderness, which is elicited by pressure at the costal phrenic angle and which is a sign of renal or perirenal inflammation.

Testing for rebound tenderness in children under 10 or 12 years of age is of no value, for often a false positive response is observed which is probably the child's normal reflex reaction to the sudden release of pressure on the abdominal wall and not due to peritoneal irritation. In older children, cough tenderness should always be used as a check on rebound tenderness. It is impossible to elicit cough tenderness in young children because it is difficult to induce small children to cough. Auscultation of the child's abdomen is extremely important in order to determine the absence or presence of peristalsis. A series of high-pitched sounds occurring at frequent intervals is a physical sign that can be relied on and is indicative of intestinal obstruction.

Considerable information can be gained from rectal examination, which can be performed without upsetting the child, provided that a few precautions are taken. First, the child must be given a notion of what the examination involves, and this can be conveyed by explaining that rectal examination is similar to the administration of an enema or to taking a rectal temperature, experiences which most children have had. Second, one should explain to the child that he must bear down to relax the anal sphincter and to permit the examiner's finger to be inserted, which can then be accomplished with a minimum of discomfort to the child. If his cooperation is obtained, the child will not be disturbed by the examination, and the examiner can make a reliable appraisal of conditions within the pelvic cavity.

In about 10 percent of children with appendicitis, the appendix is pelvic in position, and examination of the child's abdomen may be negative. Rectal examination, when there is a simple appendicitis, reveals right-sided pelvic tenderness. The abscess which forms after perforation of the appendix may be detected as a pelvic mass.

The extremities should be observed, the reflexes tested, and an attempt made to elicit Kernig's sign; the neck should be carefully examined for rigidity. It is then well to proceed with examination of the eyes, ears, nose, and throat. Frequently, examination of the eyegrounds is omitted, an omission that should be condemned, for crucial information may be overlooked. In patients with acute abdominal complaints it is extremely important to be sure of the status of the eardrums to exclude otitis media. Pharyngeal and tonsillar infection must be excluded by careful inspection of the mouth and throat. It is wise to leave to the end of the examination those maneuvers which are definitely uncomfortable to the patient, and undoubtedly those involved in examining the ears and throat present more difficulties than any others. During the course of the examination some idea of the patient's emotional status is gained. In dealing with an extremely apprehensive child the surgeon must realize that many of the positive findings are probably not accurate. On the other hand, an extremely stoic child may lead the examiner to underestimate the reactions to various parts of the physical examination unless he is alert to the child's emotional status.

ORVAR SWENSON

6

The Psychological Effects of Hospitalization

Marked concern about the adverse psychological effects of hospitalization and illness is evident in the hundreds of articles that have appeared in professional journals and in popular literature. Research findings suggest that these concerns are warranted. With few exceptions (Cassell, 1965; Ylppo et al., 1956), studies of children's posthospital behavior support the idea that the experience is psychologically upsetting to many children, if not to most, particularly in the absence of special ameliorative programs (Fagin, 1964; Jessner et al., 1952; Prugh et al., 1953; Schaffer and Callender, 1959; Weinick, 1958; Woodward, 1959; Stott, 1956). Vernon et al. (1965) review the literature on children's psychological responses to hospitalization and illness and provide additional data and discussion on this point as well as on the factors that contribute to upset.

Discussions of these effects suggest that there is considerable agreement about the aspects of hospitalization that contribute to psychological upset. These include, most commonly, the child's separation from his parents and, to a lesser extent, the unfamiliarity of the hospital setting, parental anxiety, lack of adequate relationships with the staff, reduced opportunities for activity and play, and the child's own misconceptions. Individual differences in vulnerability to upset are often considered to be related to the child's age, his adjustment prior to hospitalization, and his life situation.

As the size of this list of potential determinants suggests, the situation is complex. The number of published recommendations for helping the hospitalized child is correspondingly formidable, ranging from the use of candy-coated tongue depressors to major programs involving the mother's staying in the hospital with her child.

Unfortunately, proposals for improving hospitalization have far exceeded investigations of their effectiveness, and, in addition, the findings of existing studies are often difficult to interpret. Although it is apparent that there is no simple formula for making hospitalization a wholly positive experience, it seems worthwhile to consider several major areas in which the physician has a unique opportunity to aid his patients through his relationships with them, their parents, and the hospital staff. The focus of this discussion is on ways in which he can enhance the child's capacity to cope with the experience and on ways in which adaptation can be facilitated by the reduction or elimination of potential sources of upset.

The first area involves the provision of psychological preparation. There is considerable evidence that preparation is helpful in alleviating upset and in promoting psychological benefit (Cassell, 1965; Prugh et al., 1953; Weinick, 1958; Jackson et al., 1953; Vaughan, 1957). Discussions of preparation usually suggest that its value lies, in part, in reducing the unfamiliarity of the situation by imparting information to the child. It is assumed that vague, partially understood threats are especially anxiety arousing and that the unexpected is more stressful than that which is anticipated. In the absence of accurate information, or with the aid of misinformation, children are likely to develop fantastic and distorted ideas about what will happen to them in the hospital. In addition to the importance of accurate information, preparation is often considered important in encouraging children to express their emotions and in having them form relationships of trust and confidence in the person concerned with their care.

Despite considerable agreement on the importance of psychological preparation, it appears that it is frequently neglected. It seems likely that this is partly because preparation requires time. The pressures of a busy schedule may lead the physician to feel that preparation is relatively expendable or to the hope that someone else—the parents or perhaps the nurses—will assume the responsibility. Psychological preparation may also be neglected because of uncertainty about effective approaches in terms of content, timing, age limitations, and the informant.

With respect to content, the particular information to be imparted is likely to vary with such factors as the age of the child, the informant, the time available, and the reason for hospitalization. It has often been suggested, however, that the child be told what will happen, why it will happen, and what he will experience (see, feel, smell, etc.) and that this be told simply, reassuringly, and at a level appropriate to the child's development. This leaves considerable latitude, and it is well to remember that too much information, such as an overly graphic description of surgical procedures, may be as bad as too little.

The second question involves the timing of preparation. Virtually all who have considered this apparently feel that there is an optimal time for preparation to begin. This point was stated in general terms by Anna Freud (1952): If preparation begins too soon it allows too much time for the spreading of id fantasies, and if it begins too late

the ego has insufficient time for preparing defenses. Differences of opinion exist with respect to its translation into practice, however, with recommended times ranging from several weeks to a day or two before admission. Although there are no studies that provide comparisons of the effectiveness of preparation done at different times, several studies indicated that children were aided by preparation performed even after they were admitted to the hospital (Cassell, 1965; Weinick, 1958; Vaughan, 1957).

The third question involves the extent to which effective preparation is possible in terms of the child's age. Although it is apparent that the child's capacity to understand and to communicate increases with age, the lower limits at which preparation may be of some value is a subject for debate. For example, Robertson (1957) stated that the child of two and one half or three may seem to understand that mother is going to leave him, but this is in fact a concept the real nature of which he is incapable of appreciating. In contrast, Sexton (1960) stated: To a child under two years of age, words may mean little; but if these words are directed to the child rather than to the parents and are said in an honest and sincere way, the child will get an idea that something is going to happen that may not be pleasant, but has to happen, and that everything will be done to make it as easy as possible. . . . I believe as early as two years, or even earlier, they can get a feeling of reassurance from the way they are handled and talked to."

A study by Gofman and her associates (1957) presented data relevant to these issues. While their findings suggested a positive relationship between age and adequacy of preparation, they concluded that children as young as three or four can gain some understanding of their illness, provided the explanations are made in simple terms.

The possibility of preparing young children through play techniques has been little investigated, but parents frequently report that children respond well to potentially frightening experiences when they can become familiar with them through games. For example, one mother prepared her young child for the bandages following correction for strabismus through games of blindman's bluff. A home camera may dramatize the taking of x-rays.

Differences of opinion are evident with respect to who should provide preparation. Robertson (1958) proposed that preparation is likely to be most effective when the informant is the child's mother, presumably because the child trusts her and because she is well acquainted with means of communicating with her child and with his particular needs. Others have pointed out, however, that the parents may not have enough information to provide proper preparation or that the parents' anxiety about the situation may distort or weaken preparation. It is interesting to note that the one study that failed to show that preparation reduced upset relied on parents to provide the information (Jessner, et al., 1952). In addition, it may be argued that the value of psychological preparation in providing an opportunity for the child to establish trust and confidence in the persons who will be in charge of his treatment is lost if the parents are the sole informants.

Plank (1962) advocated an approach to the problem which combines the efforts of a variety of people. In essence, she suggested that preparation for surgery begin with parents and the family doctor prior to admission, that it continue with the surgeon and the anesthetist, and that it conclude with the hospital staff (i.e., nurses, play workers, etc.), who have more contact with the child and who see more of the apprehension and anxiety that children experience prior to surgery. We may note, however, that the effectiveness of preparation in Vaughan's (1957) and Cassell's (1965) studies raises questions about the necessity, but not necessarily about the desirability, of an elaborate program of this type. In each of these studies, preparation was done by one person (a psychiatrist and a psychologist, respectively) after the child had entered the hospital.

While existing research suggests that the person who provides the preparation need not be involved in the child's treatment, it is our feeling that the physician who plans the child's admission should assume a major share of the responsibility for preparation. This need not mean that he alone prepares the child but that he at least begins the process and enlists the aid of the parents and members of the hospital staff in following through.

In addition to psychological preparation as a means in helping the child to cope with the unfamiliarity of the hospital setting, his experience may be made less strange or threatening through the modification of the hospital environment. Recommendations with respect to such modification include making the hospital more homelike, encouraging the child to bring personal possessions such as a favorite toy or blanket, serving foods that he likes, and using his nickname. Recommendations involving preoperative medication and anesthetizing the surgery patient before he leaves his room suggest that such procedures may serve a similar function. Örsten and Mattsson (1955) noted (p. 90) that this approach relieves the child of the "unpleasant experience of passing through long corridors, seeing the instruments and the staff in their mouth masks."

Medical rounds have received considerable attention as a source of fright because the child tends to misunderstand and misinterpret what he hears. It has frequently been urged that discussion of the child's case not take place in his hearing and that all remarks concerning his illness be carefully phrased to avoid stimulating anxiety.

A second area of concern involves children's separation from their parents during hospitalization. The adverse effects of separation have, of course, been mentioned very frequently. A great deal has already been written on the value of frequent visiting in alleviating upset, and it scarcely seems necessary to labor this point. Although a survey of current hospital policies on visiting is not available, it appears that considerable progress is being made and that restricted visiting is the exception.

The literature suggests that the major issues may involve the amount and timing of parent-child contacts. Whereas liberal visiting is generally assumed to be sufficient for older children, it is recommended by many authors that the mother be permitted to stay with the young child of about six months to four years of age for whom the trauma of separation is likely to be greatest. Although there has been little investigation of the contribution of living-in, one study (Fagin, 1964) indicated that children one to three years of age tended to be better adjusted following hospitalization when they were accompanied by their mothers, while those who were permitted only visiting showed upset. Obviously, the evidence is not overwhelming, but a growing number of reports of positive experiences with living-in suggest that more thought should be given to providing facilities for mothers. While many hospitals have not been planned for living-in, the program described by Hunt (1956–1957) suggests that relatively simple arrangements (a ready supply of cots for mothers) may be workable and may eliminate the problem of providing a private room for each mother and child. That such arrangements may also be satisfactory to the parent is suggested by one mother's report of her experience (Hemmendinger, 1956–1957).

The second issue, the timing of parent-child contacts, involves the desirability of the parents' presence at times of particular stress for the child. Although there is considerable agreement that the parents should remain with the child during admission procedures and until he becomes familiar with the ward, marked differences in opinion are apparent about the parents' presence before and immediately after surgery and during examinations and treatments. Those who favor the parents' presence whenever possible suggest that it provides needed support. They point out that even though a child may cry less when his mother is excluded, this does not mean he is less upset but simply that he is too frightened to cry. In contrast, some authors argue that the child actually is better off without his mother and note that the doctor finds it easier to establish rapport when he is alone with the child. Others recommend that the parent be excluded because of her own distress (a factor which may further upset the child) and because the nurse or physician may find her presence disturbing, particularly when a difficult or potentially dangerous procedure is being performed.

At present there is no research that helps one in weighing the advantages and disadvantages of the parents' presence. It seems worthwhile, however, for the physician to examine existing policies that lead to the exclusion of parents. In some cases the reason for parents' presence or absence may be based largely on expediency or established routines—the mother of the outpatient may accompany him during many tests because she is needed to help hold the child; the mother of the inpatient may be excluded from the same tests because it is customary for an aide or nurse to accompany the child. Clearly, each situation requires evaluation not only in terms of possible reduction of upset for the child but in terms of the feelings of the parent and the persons performing the procedure. Our own ongoing research has provided some observations on the mother's presence during anesthesia induction for tonsillectomy. Although the data on children's responses are not ready for analysis, it is clear that the mothers who are present greatly favor this approach.

A third major concern for the physician involves the parents. It is well recognized that parents whose child is entering the hospital are likely to be anxious and may, therefore, be less able to provide the emotional support their child needs. In addition, the parent's anxiety may be transmitted to the child. While the focus here is on the importance of allaying parental anxiety in terms of children's reactions, it may be noted that helping the parents to weather this difficult experience is in itself a worthwhile objective. Furthermore, reducing their anxiety may make them substantially easier to get along with and thus contribute to more satisfactory relationships between the parents and the physician as well as other members of the hospital staff. To pursue this sequence one step further, good relationships between the staff and the parents may also affect the staff's relationships with the child.

One comprehensive list of suggestions for reducing parents' anxiety, their sense of confusion, and their unfamiliarity with the situation is provided by Gofman and her associates (1957). They include (1) adequate preparation of both parent and child prior to admission, (2) admission procedures that allow gradual separation of parent and child, (3) staff concern about the child's emotional and physical needs and understanding of and respect for the parents' concerns about the child, (4) continued preparation and support of both parent and child during hospitalization, and (5) providing parents with as complete an understanding as possible of findings and written instructions for home care.

Although the possibility of helping the child through providing emotional support for the parents has been little investigated, Mahaffy's study (1965) suggests that this approach is valuable. He reported that when the parents of children undergoing tonsillectomy had repeated contact and discussion with a nurse, the children showed significantly less upset both during and after hospitalization than those whose parents did not have this contact. The involvement of the social worker, the psychiatrist, or psychologist in helping parents with especially difficult problems may also be helpful. Woodward and Jackson's study (1961) of children hospitalized for severe burns provides support for the role of the social worker in alleviating long-term upset.

It is realistic to suppose, however, that regardless of the importance one attributes to aiding the parent, the time available for such activities is limited. The possibility of supplementing one-to-one approaches with group techniques merits consideration. Glaser (1960) suggests that parents benefit from having the opportunity to discuss concerns about their children's reactions with other parents and a member of the hospital staff. Others have suggested that a hospital service which provides information and the opportunity for group discussions of the care of particular types of illnesses and handicaps is of value. A movie concerning hospital facilities, personnel, and services might also be used in imparting information (a procedure now in operation at The Children's Memorial Hospital in Chicago).

The fourth area of concern involves the staff's relationships with the child. The literature contains many suggestions to the effect that friendly, reassuring relationships with staff members who understand the needs, feelings, and the problems of the child are beneficial.

Unfortunately, the means of achieving this are not simple. The high degree of specialization in modern hospitals contributes to situations in which, for example, one person gives the child his bath and another gives him his penicillin injection on one day, with different nurses performing these functions on successive days. The absence of a stable contact with a single individual may contribute to the child's sense of bewilderment and the feeling that no one really cares.

The problem is usually one of balancing the child's needs against a number of practical considerations. In this, the physician must play a strong leadership role; he should encourage inservice training for staff that emphasizes this problem, and he should attempt to provide for staffing that will furnish individual attention. When nurses' time is limited, it may be necessary to concentrate on children who appear most vulnerable to upset. Other professional groups (such as nursery school teachers and occupational therapists), child care workers, and volunteers may also make substantial contributions. A variety of approaches has been described in which nonmedically trained personnel play an active role in meeting children's emotional needs (Plank, 1962; Shore et al., 1965; Tisza and Angoff, 1961). A "mother bank" of mature women whose own children no longer require their attention has proved extremely useful in our hospital in the care of infants whose problems require intensive short-term contact.

These points are applicable to hospitalized children in general, but, as suggested previously, some children may be considered high-risk cases in that they are especially vulnerable to psychological upset. It is important for the physician to plan hospitalization in terms of the needs and problems of the individual child.

Differences in vulnerability to upset are linked to the child's age. The young child, from about the age of six months to four years, is thought to be more prone to upset than younger infants or older children because of his strong emotional and physical dependency on his parents and because of his limited ability to understand and cope with hospitalization. The idea of a differential susceptibility to upset for different age groups has received considerable support from research on children's reactions during hospitalization. This has led numerous authors to recommend that elective surgery either be done during the relatively safe period of early infancy or be postponed until the child is four or five years of age. It appears important, however, to consider the pros and cons of this approach for the particular child. For example, the psychological advantages associated with the repair of disfiguring congenital defects at an early age may far outweigh the possible upset arising from hospitalization.

A different but relevant point has been suggested by Solnit (1960). He stated that both the potential for psychological damage and the potential for psychological benefit are relatively high for the hospitalized child of preschool age. He reasoned that developmental problems centered on the child's relationship with his mother (i.e., separation anxiety, ambivalent feelings, and self-control of bodily functions) are most common in children under five years of age. Solnit proposed that such problems might be resolved

during hospitalization which was carefully planned for this purpose.

Emotional problems, such as neurotic personality, excessive dependency, shyness, aggressiveness, anxiety, and obsessional states, may also interfere with the child's adaptive capacities. Although the available research is suggestive at best, it seems reasonable to suppose that the child who finds it difficult to adjust to everyday situations may have difficulty in coping with the stresses associated with hospitalization and illness. The surgeon should move cautiously with the child who displays emotional problems. At times it is well to request an emotional evaluation prior to surgery. With elective procedures that may be postponed, the pediatrician may advise the parents to seek professional help for the child's problem before planning hospitalization. Special precautions may also be instituted for high-risk children. The mother might be encouraged to stay with the extremely dependent child, especially careful preparation might be provided for the anxious child, and the nurses might provide extra attention and emotional support when difficulty is anticipated.

In contrast to the idea that hospitalization is most likely to be psychologically detrimental to these children, a few authors have mentioned that hospitalization may contribute to adjustment. When the parents' relationship with their child is a source of difficulty, as frequently appears to be the case, the hospital may provide an opportunity for reeducating the parents. As the mother sees her child improve she is likely to question her own approaches, to learn by example, and to be willing to accept assistance, either from the staff or from other psychiatric services. The timid or insecure child who is helped to cope with the experience through the support of his parents and others may show positive gains in self-confidence and improvement in his relationships with others. The parents, in turn, may benefit from a newfound sense of adequacy.

Finally, the child who is encountering a difficult period in his life situation that makes special demands on his adaptive capacity may find hospitalization the one stress or problem too many. The birth of a sibling, death or illness in the family, difficulties between the parents, and a change in residence may all be danger signals of which the physician should be aware. At times it may seem advisable to delay surgery until the child has adjusted to the situation or, if immediate treatment is necessary, to provide special measures to alleviate upset.

Perhaps as physicians we encounter tragedy and drama so often that we erect a barrier against seeing or feeling it. This is quite sensible and desirable because if we should experience any significant percentage of the anxiety that our patients and their parents do, we should soon be in fairly serious difficulty. The physician whose own child is having a herniorrhaphy may recognize the routine nature of this surgery, but somehow it seems much more routine when the child is not his own. Much as it is risky to experience all that a patient experiences, it is also risky, even for the physician, to move too far in the other direction. The danger is that of converting the practice of medicine into a mechanical operation devoid of human values and satisfactions. At this extreme, the child is seen as a bothersome appendage to a hernial sac; surgery is an assembly-line procedure.

Physicians are given a rare opportunity. They are permitted, even encouraged, to participate in the drama of human life and death. They are automatically respected, their advice sought. For most people the greatest satisfactions in life come from contact with other human beings. This may be true of one's practice as it is of one's personal life. And, of course, if physicians manage to make this contact, the patients are certain to benefit.

JEANNE M. FOLEY
JEROME L. SCHULMAN
DAVID T. A. VERNON

REFERENCES

CASSELL, S. E. The effect of brief puppet therapy upon the emotional responses of children undergoing cardiac catheterization. J. Consult. Psychol., 29: 1, 1965.

FAGIN, C. M. The case for rooming in when young children are hospitalized. Nurs. Sci., 2: 324, 1964.

FREUD, A. The role of bodily illness in the normal life of children. In EISSLER, R. S., et al., eds. The Psychoanalytic Study of the Child. New York, International Universities Press, 1952, pp. 69–81.

GLASER, K. Group discussions with mothers of hospitalized children. Pediatrics, 26: 132, 1960.

GOFMAN, H., BUCKMAN, W., and SCHADE, G. H. Parent's emotional response to child's hospitalization. Amer. J. Dis. Child., 93: 629, 1957.

HEMMENDINGER, M. Rx: "admit parents at all times." Child Stud., 34: 3, 1956–1957.

HUNT, A. D., Jr. An experiment in team work. Child Stud., 34: 10, 1956–1957.

JACKSON, K., WINKLEY, R., FAUST, O. A., CERMAK, E. G., and BURTT, M. M. Behavior changes indicating emotional trauma in tonsillectomized children. Pediatrics, 12: 23, 1953.

JESSNER, L., BLOM, G. E., and WALDFOGEL, S. Emotional implications of tonsillectomy and adenoidectomy on children. In EISSLER, R. S., et al., eds. The Psychoanalytic Study of the Child. New York, International Universities Press, 1952, pp. 126–169.

MAHAFFY, P. R. The effects of hospitalization on children admitted for tonsillectomy and adenoidectomy. Nurs. Res., 14 (1): 12, 1965.

ÖRSTEN, P., and MATTSSON, A. Hospitalization symptoms in children. Acta Paediat., 44: 79, 1955.

PLANK, E. N. Working with Children in Hospitals. Cleveland, Western Reserve University Press, 1962.

PRUGH, D. G., STAUB, E., SANDS, H. H., KIRSCHBAUM, R. M., and LENIHAN, E. A. A study of the emotional reactions of children and families to hospitalization and illness. Amer. J. Orthopsychiat., 23: 70, 1953.

ROBERTSON, J. A mother's observations on the tonsillectomy of her four-year-old daughter. Nurs. Times, 53: 1395, 1957.

ROBERTSON, J. Young Children in Hospitals. New York, Basic Books, 1958.

SCHAFFER, H. R., and CALLENDER, W. W. Psychologic effects of hospitalization in infancy. Pediatrics, 24: 528, 1959.

SEXTON, H. M. Emotional preparation for hospitalization. Amer. Surg., 26: 422, 1960.

SHORE, M. F., GEISER, R. L., and WOLMAN, H. M. Constructive uses of a hospital experience. Children, 12 (1), 3, 1965.

SOLNIT, A. J. Hospitalization. An aid to physical and psychological health in childhood. Amer. J. Dis. Child., 99: 155, 1960.

STOTT, D. H. Infantile illness and subsequent mental and emotional development. J. Genet. Psychol., 94: 233, 1956.

TISZA, V. B., and ANGOFF, K. A play program for hospitalized children: The role of the playroom teacher. Pediatrics, 28: 841, 1961.

VAUGHAN, G. F. Children in hospital. Lancet, 272: 1117, 1957.

VERNON, D. T. A., FOLEY, J. M., SIPOWICZ, R. R., and SCHULMAN, J. L. The Psychological Responses of Children to Hospitalization and Illness: A Review of the Literature. Springfield, Ill., Charles C Thomas, Publisher, 1965.

WEINICK, H. M. Psychological Study of Emotional Reactions of Children to Tonsillectomy. Unpublished doctoral dissertation, New York University, 1958.

WOODWARD, J. Emotional disturbances of burned children. Brit. Med. J., 2 (No. 5128): 1009, 1959.

WOODWARD, J., and JACKSON, D. Emotional reactions in burned children and their mothers. Brit. J. Plast. Surg., 13: 316, 1961.

YLPPO, A., HALLMAN, N., LANDTMAN, B., and PIIPARI, R. Effect of short time hospitalization on the behavior and on some somatic functions of children. Ann. Paediat. Fenn., 2: 1, 1956.

7

Anesthesiology

Pediatric anesthesiology is attended by some misconceptions and fallacies that should be eliminated. If a surgical procedure is necessary and there is a reasonable hope of survival, a pediatric anesthesiologist should be able to administer an anesthetic without appreciably diminishing the chances of a successful result. Only on rare occasions is a child unacceptable for surgery because of a contraindication to anesthesia. The patient should be in as good a condition as possible, and the timing of the procedure should be optimum; this optimal time is a compromise between the requirements for surgery and those for anesthesia.

There has been a tendency on the part of the anesthesiologists in nonpediatric hospitals to manage children like little adults. There is as much difference anatomically, physiologically, and pathologically between an adult and a child as there is between a child and an infant, an infant and a neonate, and a neonate and a premature baby. Pediatric anesthesiology requires specialized knowledge and specialized equipment. Advances in pediatric anesthesiology have been brought about by increased knowledge of the physiology of the child and infant and by the use of more sophisticated apparatus. Whether a hospital does ten pediatric surgical procedures a year or ten thousand there are three basic requirements for success: (1) knowledgeable anesthesiology, (2) constant experience, and (3) proper equipment.

Hospitals are apt to spend large sums of money on operating room equipment, such as elaborate tables and complicated lights, but to be reluctant to spend like amounts on, for example, a ventilator suitable for infants. It is not uncommon for a hospital to invest ten thousand dollars a year in special cardiac sutures but insist on the reuse of endotracheal tubes beyond the point of safety. A hospital will not question the expense involved in providing sterile bronchology apparatus but may fail to appreciate that anesthesiology apparatus used in the same airways should be sterile. Any hospital that undertakes the surgical treatment of children must be prepared to supply the minimum amount of pediatric anesthesiology apparatus and to maintain it in a proper condition.

The statement that the best anesthetic agent is the one the anesthesiologist is most familiar with is not generally true. The anesthetic agent of choice is the one that is the best pharmacologically for a specific child in a particular situation. The anesthetic technique of choice is the one that disturbs least the physiology of the child.

The most significant advance in anesthesiology in the past decade has been the shift from qualitative to quantitative methods. Formerly such agents as diethyl ether were dripped on a cone and the depth of anesthesia was estimated in a variety of ways. Today anesthetic agents such as halothane are precisely metered, so that a known amount of agent is supplied to the patient.

Respirations are not assisted; rather, ventilation is totally supplied by apparatus which provides an accurate stroke volume at a fixed rate for the patient's calculated surface area. Humidification is supplied so that the patient is not dehydrated by a dry gas mixture.

PREPARATION OF THE PATIENT

There are controversial data on the effects of hospitalization on a child and on the aftereffects of the administration of an anesthetic. Nevertheless, there are two factors important in preventing undesirable aftereffects: the love for children and respect for their inherent intelligence. The ability to project one's love to a child is more effective than a sedative in gaining the child's confidence and reducing his anxiety. A preoperative visit should always be made.

The anesthesiologist should be thoroughly familiar with the condition of the patient and should aid the surgeon and pediatrician in bringing the patient into optimal condition for surgery. He should pay particular attention to anything that might have a bearing on the anesthetic management (e.g., preoperative and prior medication with cortisone, chlorpromazine, or reserpine). If he neglects to perform fully his part of the preoperative preparation, he may encounter insurmountable obstacles during the administration of the anesthesia. Since pediatric surgery is technically demanding because of the small, delicate bodily structures involved, the surgeon should be allowed to concentrate fully on the operation. The anesthesiologist should take over the responsibility of total environmental control and care of the patient during the operation. He must also be familiar with the surgical procedure, so that he will be successful in providing optimal working conditions for the surgeon.

PREOPERATIVE MEDICATION

Premedication is administered to prevent tracheal and bronchial secretions, to decrease vagal activity, and to produce sedation.

TABLE 1.   PREMEDICATION SCHEDULE*

WEIGHT OF CHILD (lbs)	WEIGHT OF CHILD (kg)	ATROPINE (mg)	MEPERIDINE (mg)	MORPHINE (mg)
4–8	1.8–3.6	0.1		
8–10	3.6–4.5	0.15		
10–20	4.5–9.0	0.2		
20–30	9.0–13.6	0.3	15	
30–40	13.6–18.1	0.4	25	
40–50	18.1–22.6	0.6	30	
50–60	22.6–27.2	0.6	40	
60–70	27.2–31.7	0.6		6
70–80	31.7–36.2	0.6		7
80–90	36.2–40.8	0.6		8
90–100	40.8–45.3	0.6		9
100–150	45.3–68.0	0.6		11

* A premedication schedule should be used only as a guide. No sedatives are necessary in infants. Morphine sulfate is used in older children because it is superior to meperidine in allaying anxiety.

Another objective may be to decrease peripheral oxygen consumption by lowering metabolism. As a rule premedication is mandatory for children, but there are exceptions; for example, the anticholinergic drying agents should be avoided if possible in patients with cystic fibrosis, for they will increase the retention of tenacious secretions in the bronchial tree and thus cause obstruction.

ANTICHOLINERGIC AGENTS

No premedication schedule had proved to be altogether successful, for such schedules assume that all children are of a standard type and make no provisions for individual variations. An anticholinergic agent, atropine sulfate, is recommended in all cases. The dose is calculated on the basis of mg/lb body weight, as shown in Table 1. It should be administered intramuscularly one half to one hour before the operation. Should the operating room schedule be delayed past one hour the drug should be repeated. In situations where an anticholinergic agent is to be avoided if possible, as in cystic fibrosis, access to a vein must be available. In infants so sick that vagal stimulation and subsequent bradycardia could lead to cardiac arrest, it is best that the atropine sulfate be administered intravenously by the anesthesiologist as soon as there is any indication of this train of events. Atropine sulfate is the anticholinergic drug of choice because of its vagolyte action. Its relative inadequacy as a drying agent is unimportant when halothane is used. The most common complication following the use of atropine is a blotchy generalized rash having no medical significance.

It should be emphasized that bradycardia is the greatest danger in pediatric anesthesia, since the oxygenation process has little reserve capacity. Bradycardia is avoided by adequate atropinization and oxygenation. With the use of a quantitative anesthetic delivery system and an adequate maintenance dosage of an anesthetic agent, bradycardia secondary to overdosage should not occur.

SEDATIVES

The amount of sedation that a child will require preoperatively depends on the psychic makeup of the individual and also on the external stimuli from the environment. Unfortunately, it is impossible to classify the various types of psychic makeups of children so that they can be managed in an individualistic manner; consequently, we are still treating children in standard groups.

The amount of sedation needed in a pediatric hospital is less than that necessary in a pediatric unit attached to a general hospital. This is because of the difference in the environment surrounding the child. It is always better to err on the light side than to oversedate children and face the risk of respiratory depression.

To lessen the danger of mistakes in calculating the ordered dose of sedation, a simplified technique for measuring the prescribed sedative is recommended. Meperidine and morphine are supplied in liquid form, and the multiple-dose vials are clearly marked to indicate milligrams per milliliter of solution. Fine tuberculin-like syringes whose barrels are divided into 100 increments are used to draw up the requisite dose. A simple calculation is necessary to measure out the prescribed dose of the sedative. This technique has lessened but not eliminated the instance of oversedation, which is usually caused by the misreading of the prescribed order in relation to decimal points. For this reason it is wise to place a "0" before the decimal point to emphasize that tenths of milligrams are ordered.

Since mistakes may be reduced but not eliminated, it is wise for each nursing unit to be supplied with equipment and drugs to provide immediate respiratory assistance when overdoses of such drugs as morphine sulfate occur (Fig. 1).

The inhalation therapy department should be responsible for supplying each nursing unit with a sealed box containing the necessary sterile equipment and drugs along with a self-inflating bag. Should the seal be broken

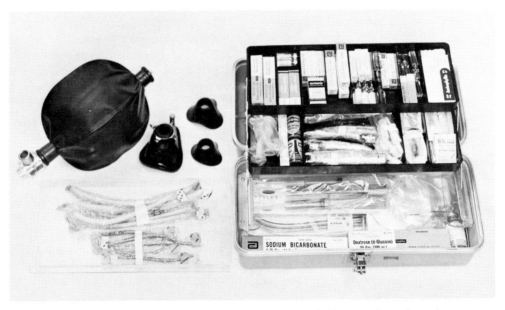

Fig. 1. Resuscitation equipment should be readily available on each nursing unit.

through use or from any other cause, the inhalation therapy department should replace the unit immediately, thus ensuring that at all times equipment is available and in functional condition.

RESTRICTION OF ORAL INTAKE

It is important that children, especially infants, do not go into surgery dehydrated. Children and infants are acceptable for anesthesia induction if they have not been fed for four hours preceding the operative procedure. Infants should be listed first on the schedule so that if there is a delay there will be minimal dehydration. A sick infant should be provided with an intravenous drip to eliminate dehydration during the period of no oral feedings in preparation for surgery. It should be remembered that restriction of oral intake for a four-hour period does not guarantee an empty stomach.

ACCEPTANCE OF A CHILD
WITH A FEVER

Beware of accepting for a routine procedure a child who has a low grade fever,

$100°$ F–$101°$ F (rectally). Should a bacteremia or viremia develop during anesthesia, it is difficult to prevent a serious complication.

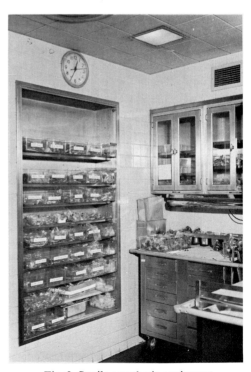

Fig. 2. Sterile anesthesia equipment.

PREOPERATIVE LABORATORY DETERMINATIONS

To decide on a hemoglobin level for a child of a specific age, one must know the normal hemoglobin value for his age group. However, the hemoglobin level is only significant if it is considered as part of his overall condition. As a guide, a child should not be accepted for surgery for a routine procedure whose hemoglobin is 10 percent under the normal for his age group. Thus, a three-month-old infant whose hemoglobin level is at the low ebb normally should not be accepted for routine surgery if it is under 9 g%. A second preoperative prerequisite is a urine analysis. If there is any possibility that a patient will require blood during an operation, the blood should be available in the operating room before the anesthetic is started.

EQUIPMENT

PREPARATION

Although it is true that anesthesia equipment should be as sterile as the surgical pack, it is not generally appreciated. The sterility is accomplished by a combination of steam and gas sterilizing. If the equipment is purchased with sterilizability in mind, it is possible to autoclave the bulk of equipment and gas sterilize the rest. With a view to cost, it is important to employ as much disposable apparatus as possible to reduce the number of personnel needed, which is the costliest expense in any hospital budget. When the equipment is sterilized it should be laid out in such fashion that it is easily accessible, as shown in the illustration (Fig. 2). The more commonly used apparatus is separated from the less commonly used material. There should be an inventory control, so that reordering can be accomplished with a minimum of effort. This will also facilitate the evaluation of a projected budget. A daily work schedule should be prepared for the technician, and this technician should be supervised by the anesthesiologist, employing such aids as culture control.

SELECTION OF APPARATUS

Pediatric anesthesia apparatus must (1) have a minimum of dead space, (2) be of low resistance, (3) be atraumatic, (4) be sterilizable, and (5) be light in weight.

Besides the child equipment there should be available specialized equipment for the management of infants. In regard to equipment an infant can be defined as a child weighing less than 12 kg.

A nonrebreathing technique is used exclusively because it provides minimum dead space, minimum resistance, minimum turbulence, easy assistance or control of ventilation, and easy quantitation of anesthesia, ventilation, and humidification. There are now adequate humidification methods along

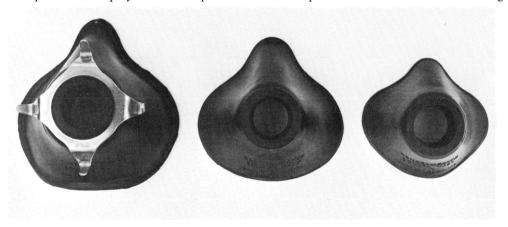

Fig. 3. Rendell-Baker Soucek infant masks.

with good temperature control apparatus which have overcome the dehydrating effects and reduction in temperature, which were not provided for in the early nonrebreathing systems.

MASKS

INFANT

Rendell-Baker and Soucek devised a series of three masks with very small dead space for use in infants (Fig. 3). These can be cold sterilized or, better yet, gas sterilized and individually packaged.

CHILD

The small trimar mask or medium Mc-Kesson mask fits the majority of children. The medium trimar is suitable for the larger child. These, too, are cold sterilized or gas sterilized and individually packaged.

ELBOWS AND CHIMNEY PIECES

INFANT

The Rendell-Baker infant chimney piece is the most physiological available (Fig. 4). Not quite so sophisticated is the MIE chimney piece with a pop-off valve (Fig. 5). The Rendell-Baker chimney piece (Fig. 6) has

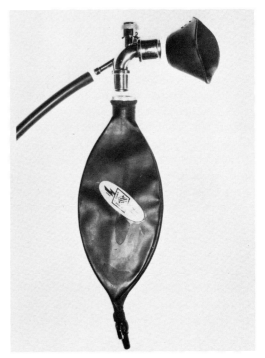

Fig. 5. The MIE chimney piece is not as sophisticated as the Rendell-Baker one and is heavier. It has the advantage of being autoclavable.

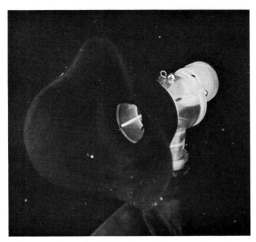

Fig. 4. The Rendell-Baker chimney piece has a dividing septum preventing the mixing of the inspired and expired gases.

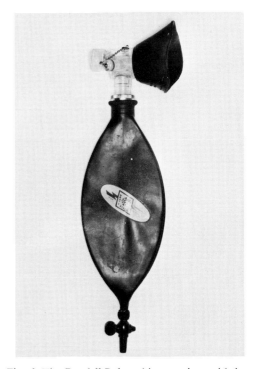

Fig. 6. The Rendell-Baker chimney piece with bag and mask.

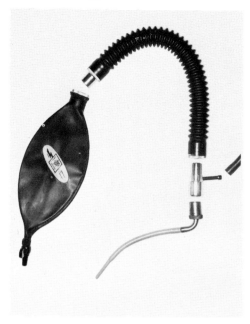

Fig. 7. No valves are used on infants. Instead, an Ayre's T piece is employed. The illustration demonstrates how the T piece is attached to the endotracheal tube connector and breathing bag. The gases are exhausted through the stopcock at the end of the bag.

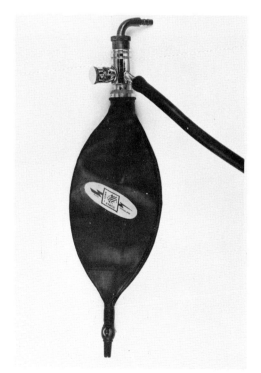

Fig. 8. An Ingliss valve may be incorporated on the Ayre's T piece.

to be cold sterilized or gas sterilized, whereas the MIE can be autoclaved.

CHILD

The Ohio elbow can be autoclaved.

NONREBREATHING VALVE

INFANT

No valves are used on infants. Instead, an Ayers T piece is employed (Fig. 7). This T piece may or may not have an Ingliss pop-off valve (Fig. 8). These can be autoclaved.

CHILD

The Sierra nonrebreathing valve is superior to any other available (Fig. 9). It is lightweight, being made of aluminum, and has a dead space of only 2 ml, and since its flapper disks are of silicone the whole assembly can be autoclaved and packaged. This valve has been demonstrated to be quite reliable, and maintenance is relatively simple. The incorporation of a pop-off valve on the assembly takes care of excess gas from too large a minute gas flow. The resistance also is minimal.

OROPHARYNGEAL AIRWAYS

There should be a full range of sizes of plastic sterile disposable airways. Bite blocks made of covered cork are very useful in safeguarding the lumen of the endotracheal tubes.

ENDOTRACHEAL TUBES

INFANT

The Cole tube is extremely satisfactory for infants. When nasal intubation is required, the Portland plastic tube is acceptable. Cuffed tubes are used only for large children. Armored tubes may be necessary when the head is extremely flexed. No en-

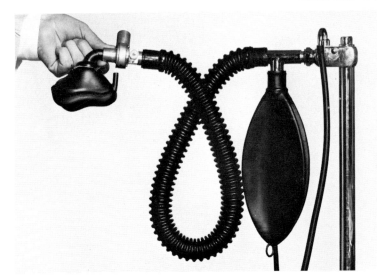

Fig. 9. The Sierra nonrebreathing valve is lightweight and has a dead space of only 2 ml. It can be auto-claved and its maintenance is simple. The incorporation of a pop-off valve takes care of excess gas from too large a minute gas flow.

dotracheal tube should be autoclaved more than three times because the surface becomes abraded and may cause irritation to the mucosa. It is preferable to gas sterilize endotracheal tubes. A guide or wire is inserted to ensure that the appropriate curves are retained, and the tube is packaged and sterilized.

CHILD

Portland plastic endotracheal tubes, uncuffed, are the most desirable. Rubber tubes

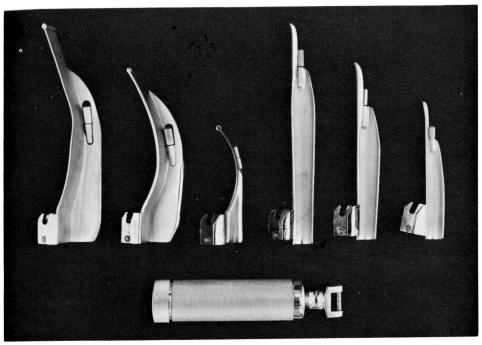

Fig. 10. A full range of laryngoscope blades should be available for both infant and child. Since the neonate has little or no neck, a Guedel #H670 premature blade is preferred.

may be employed. These are sterilized as before, packaged, and stored.

LARYNGOSCOPES

INFANT

There should be a full range of laryngoscope blades available for both the infant and the child (Fig. 10). Since the neonate has little or no neck, a Guedel # H670 premature blade is preferred. The alternative is an infant MacIntosh blade. For the larger infant, an infant-size Guedel blade may be used.

CHILD

There should be available a # 3 MacIntosh blade, a # 4 MacIntosh blade, and child and adult straight blades. Laryngoscope blades can be autoclaved, but there is a high incidence of nonfunctioning of the light, and therefore laryngoscope blades should be gas

sterilized. Battery handles should be of one standard size. Extra batteries and light bulbs should be available. For special situations, such as that created by a child Pierre Robin syndrome, a Holinger laryngoscope may be necessary. This blade prevents the large tongue from flopping over and obstructing the view.

GAS MACHINE

For nonrebreathing systems high flows are necessary so that both the nitrous oxide and oxygen flow meters should provide up to 10 per minute. The gas machine should be as simple as possible (Fig. 11), for the important part of a gas machine is the accuracy of the flow meters. To deliver a known amount of anesthetic agent, direct reading or non-direct reading systems are available.

The Vernitrol is the most common indirect reading system, and the Fluotec or Pentec is the most common direct reading system for achieving quantitative anesthesia. Either a ventilator can be mounted on the gas ma-

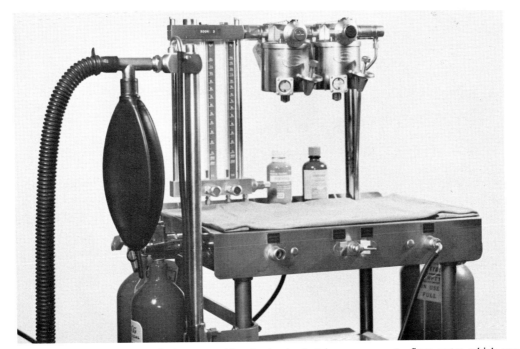

Fig. 11. The Canadian Heidbrinck gas machine is simple, but has an accurate flow meter which can provide a flow up to at least 10 liters per minute for use with the nonrebreathing systems.

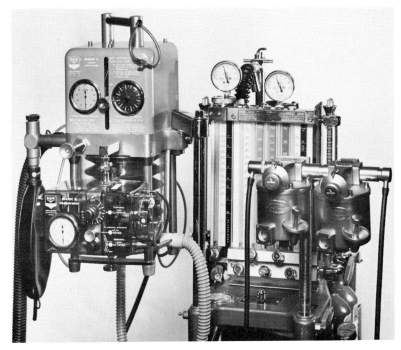

Fig. 12. The Ohio B333 has been modified to have a direct reading sidearm vernitrol for halothane. The Bird Mark IV + 8 combination can be adjusted to any height and an intermittent humidification system has been incorporated using the Bird main line micronebulizer.

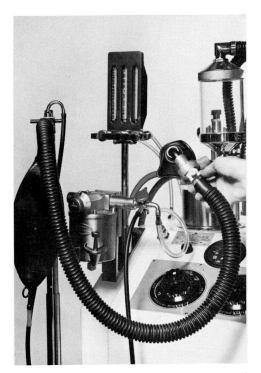

Fig. 13. An induction circuit has been added to the Engström model 200 respirator.

chine (Fig. 12), or the gas machine can be mounted on the ventilator (Fig. 13).

VENTILATORS

The Engström respirator model 200 is the most satisfactory respirator, especially for supplying infants with quantitative ventilation and humidification. The respirator is described in detail in the chapter on inhalation therapy. To achieve quantitative anesthesia along with quantitative ventilation and humidification a separate circuit was designed (Figs. 14 and 15). A high flow of gas can thus be provided over a Fluotec or Pentec to keep these instruments linear. The mixture is collected in a free-hanging bag. The respirator then draws from this mixture a calculated volume, which is introduced into the patient along with the desired humidification. For older children a Bird Mark IV plus 8 can be employed, provided that it is appreciated that the anesthesia is quantitative and the ventilation is qualitative. In

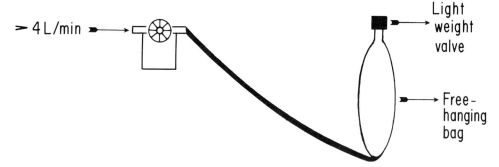

Fig. 14. To keep the Fluotec linear it is necessary to have a flow of at least 4 liters per minute. The anesthetic mixture is collected in a free-hanging bag fitted with a light weight valve for overflow. Thus no back pressure can be applied to the Fluotec.

addition, unless an ultrasonic nebulizer is placed in the circuit, the humidification system has to be used intermittently; otherwise the anesthesia becomes qualitative.

HUMIDIFICATION APPARATUS

Humidification apparatus is dealt with in detail in the chapter on inhalation therapy. Basically there are three types: (1) the Venturi mechanical nebulizer, (2) the heated humidifier, and (3) the ultrasonic nebulizer. It is vitally important to humidify when using a nonrebreathing circuit, particularly when the operation extends much beyond thirty minutes.

SUCTION APPARATUS

Miniaturized suction apparatus should be used when working with infants so that blood loss collected by suction can be measured in 2-ml increments. A standard apparatus has its lowest calibration at 400 ml. Suction catheters should be of the sterile disposable type and should be available in a full range of sizes.

STETHOSCOPE

A monaural or binaural stethoscope with a series of chest pieces of various sizes

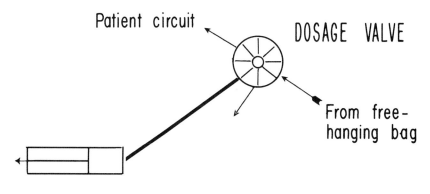

Fig. 15. A new dosage valve was designed to give accuracy at small minute volumes in particular. This valve is calibrated at 3 liters per minute instead of the usual 10 when used for infants. When the control of the valve is set at rebreathing, the back stroke of the cylinder will enable the placing of a known volume of a known concentration of anesthetic mixture from the free-hanging exposed bag into the free-hanging bag in the glass cylinder.

should be available, along with a range of sizes of esophageal stethoscopes.

SYRINGES

Syringes and needles of all sizes should be of the sterile disposable type.

MONITORING DEVICES

Besides the stethoscope, which is by far the most important monitoring device, the items discussed in the following sections should also be at hand.

BLOOD PRESSURE EQUIPMENT

Blood pressure cuffs suitable for all ages are necessary. The following sizes are recommended:

(1) Newborn infant's size, inflatable cuff, $5\frac{1}{4} \times 1\frac{1}{4}$ in.

(2) Large infant's size, inflatable cuff, $6 \times 2\frac{1}{4}$ in.

(3) Child's size, inflatable cuff, 6×3 in.

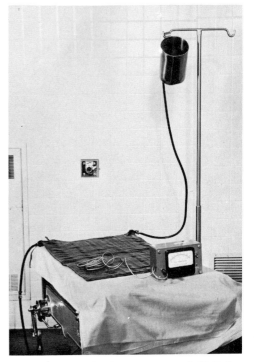

Fig. 16. An electric thermometer and McQuiston water mattress is used to control the temperature of the infant manually.

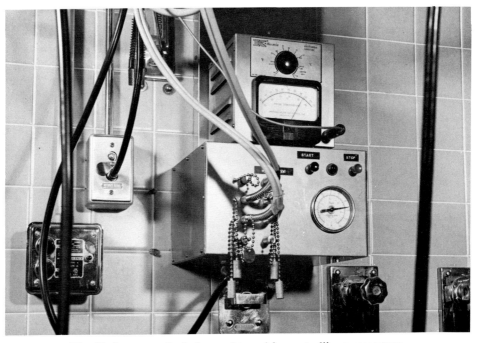

Fig. 17. An automatic device can be used for controlling temperature.

(4) Small adult's size, inflatable cuff, 9 × 4 inches.

Either a tycos with the bulb mounted beside the manometer or an oscillometer is then employed.

THERMOMETER AND TEMPERATURE CONTROL MATTRESSES

A continuous temperature indicator with rectal and esophageal probes is necessary for every patient. The temperature may be controlled manually (Fig. 16) or, preferably, automatically (Fig. 17).

PULSOMETERS

The Keating-Cottel pulsometer (Fig. 18) is a useful aid in monitoring the pulse, since it gives some information concerning diffusion at the tissue level and thus provides an

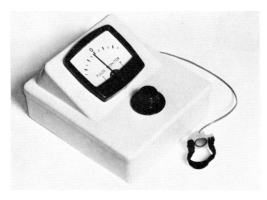

Fig. 18. The Keating-Cottel pulsometer.

index of the depth of the anesthesia. It is also useful as an aid in recording the blood pressure, especially under hypothermic conditions, although direct pressure manometric recordings are more accurate and dependable.

SPIROMETERS

A Wright spirometer is used with pressure constant, volume variable respirators. The Engström respirator has an excellent spirometer built into the expiratory line.

ECG MONITORS

An ECG monitor is extremely useful. The impulse from the R wave can activate a flashing light and sound signal.

DEFIBRILLATORS

It is mandatory that a DC defibrillator be readily available.

AIDS IN MONITORING CIRCULATING BLOOD VOLUME

Besides the stethoscope, blood pressure apparatus, and direct manometric recordings from arterial catheters, additional aids should be available to give some indication of blood loss and the adequacy of blood replacement. Total body weight can be measured by various types of scales. Provided dry sponges of constant weight are used, weighing sponges is an objective method of determining blood loss.

Miniaturized suction apparatus that provides measurement of 1-ml to 5-ml increments of blood is valuable in infant surgery. Total body preoperative and postoperative weight has a place in open heart surgery and in any procedure in which blood loss and replacement has been large. The recording of central venous pressure is extremely valuable, especially when large volumes of blood in relation to total volume must be replaced.

Facilities for measuring pH, PCO_2, and PO_2 are extraordinarily helpful during the ventilation of sick children. Samples can be taken during the operation and at the termination of anesthesia so that corrections can be made when there are variations from normal.

CHOICE OF AGENT

Halothane (Fluothane) is the anesthetic agent of choice in pediatric anesthesia. Its advantages are that it is pleasant and non-irritating, does not produce secretions, has a rapid action, is nonemetic, and, most important, is nonexplosive. Being neither parasympathomimetic nor sympathomimetic, it does not produce bradycardia through a parasympathomimetic action as does cyclopropane, but it may produce bradycardia because of its intense action when the concentration is increased too rapidly. In high concentrations it will act as a myocardial depressant, and like all anesthetic agents, with the possible exception of a light plane of diethyl ether or trichloroethylene, it is a respiratory depressant. Halothane is a poor relaxant, but children, especially infants, who have poorly developed musculature, do not require a great deal of relaxation. There has not been any direct proof that halothane is a hepatotoxic agent. One of the great auxiliary benefits of the introduction of halothane has been the development of quantitative, direct reading, temperature compensated vaporizers. It was the introduction of halothane that gave the impetus to the change from qualitative to quantitative anesthesia. Halothane should not be used routinely in the presence of epinephrine because it sensitizes the myocardium to epinephrine, and if the dose of epinephrine circulating in the bloodstream is high enough, ventricular extrasystoles or even fibrillation will supervene.

Methoxyflurane (Penthrane) is another satisfactory nonexplosive anesthetic agent. Its advantage is that it is fluorinated ether and is thus very stable. It has a great margin of safety and is a good relaxant; however, its deficits of prolonged induction and recovery times are difficult to overcome. It can be used in the presence of epinephrine, but there is a higher incidence of emesis than there is in the recovery from halothane. The prolonged recovery time can be put to good advantage in bronchography.

Nitrous oxide is a pleasant, nonexplosive anesthetic agent with good analgesia. Used in conjunction with relaxants it has proved to be of great value.

With the present choice of nonexplosive anesthetic agents, the use of an explosive agent in pediatric surgery is unjustified in most instances.

CHOICE OF TECHNIQUE

Nonrebreathing systems are the most physiological for use with children. They have minimal dead space and low resistance, and the anesthetic agent can be quantitated along with ventilation and humidification. With no other technique can this be readily accomplished. Former criticisms of the nonrebreathing technique no longer apply, since there are now excellent humidifying systems and the temperature of the patient can be easily controlled.

An arbitrary weight limit, 12 kg, is set for infants. Below this a nonvalvular modified Ayre's technique is employed. Above 12 kg a valve system using the Sierra nonrebreathing valve is recommended.

During difficult, complicated surgical procedures the Engström ventilator model 200 with the Allan anesthesia circuit is used, along with an ultrasonic nebulizer or a heated humidifier. This combination allows accurate control of anesthesia, ventilation, and humidification in a quantitative manner.

PREPARATION
FOR INDUCTION

The objective in anesthesia is to prevent complications rather than to overcome mistakes once they have been made. Diligent preparation for induction of anesthesia has many dividends. The anesthetic machine must be checked for leaks in the system and for a satisfactory supply of oxygen and nitrous oxide. The temperature and humidity of the room is noted. The suction apparatus for the anesthesiologist's use is checked for leaks. Monitoring aids are checked systematically. To ensure that enough resuscitation apparatus would be available to meet any exigency, an anesthetic cart (Fig. 19) was designed that is large enough to accommodate a full range of resuscitation apparatus and drugs. At The

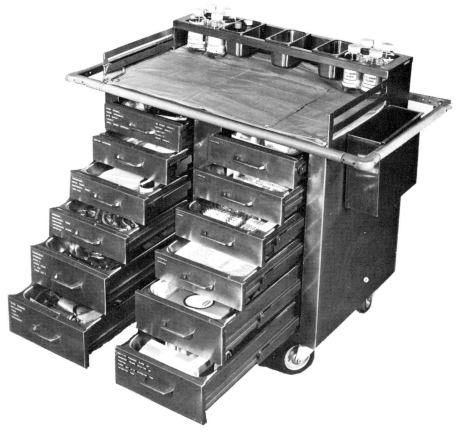

Fig. 19. The design of the cart was oriented towards maintaining a sterile aseptic technique. The contents of the drawers are clearly indicated. A considerable amount of apparatus and drugs are necessary to take care of any exigency.

Children's Memorial Hospital (Chicago) the administration of drugs, fluids, electrolytes, and blood is in the domain of the anesthesiologist in the operating room area. The design of this cart was also oriented toward the maintenance of a sterile aseptic technique. The contents of the drawers are clearly indicated. As is clear from the illustration, a considerable amount of apparatus and drugs is necessary to take care of any exigency. For every anesthetic there should be displayed a stethoscope, blood pressure apparatus with a cuff of suitable size, a laryngoscope with an appropriate blade in working condition, at least three endotracheal tubes of appropriate sizes with connectors of suitable size, oropharyngeal airways, a bite block, tape, a mask with

valvular or nonvalvular systems, large oral suction catheters and endotracheal suction catheters of appropriate sizes, syringes and needles, a tongue depressor, a head rest, sterile gauze, atropine, and succinylcholine. For more specialized procedures, additional equipment, such as esophageal stethoscopes, electrodes, pulsometers, and oscillometers, must be available on the anesthesiologist's cart. The temperature control mechanism should be checked for the accuracy of the thermometer and for the flow through the mattresses, with particular attention paid to the maximum mattress temperature. The intravenous solutions and set should be set up and the availability of blood investigated. When the nursing service is ready and the surgeon is present, the child is brought into the operating room. The circulating nurse must be free to assist the anesthesiologist during anesthesia induction.

INDUCTION OF ANESTHESIA

It is again emphasized that a smooth, safe induction of anesthesia in a child depends on the anesthesiologist's ability to project his love and respect for that child. Three agents are used for induction. They are nitrous oxide–oxygen, nitrous oxide–oxygen–halothane, oxygen–halothane, and short-acting barbiturates, such as sodium thiopental and methohexital. Under such circumstances, a short-acting relaxant prior to anesthesia has a distinct advantage once good ventilation has been established.

In infants under six months of age the neuronal cells are poorly developed. On this premise these infants are paralyzed with succinylcholine and intubated, and then anesthesia is commenced. Older children should be allowed to choose between a gaseous induction and the intravenous induction of a short acting barbiturate.

TECHNIQUE

CHILD

The precordial stethoscope is placed in such a position that both cardiac and breath sounds are audible. A blood pressure cuff of appropriate size is placed on the arm and the blood pressure checked. If sodium thiopental has been chosen, it should be administered slowly until the eyelash reflex is lost. The dose is 2–4 mg/kg. The child is oxygenated, and the nitrous oxide, oxygen, halothane, or methoxyflurane is administered.

Should intubation be decided upon, a short acting relaxant, such as succinylcholine, is administered immediately after the thiopental. The child is oxygenated with a bag and face mask and then intubated. Gaseous induction is done by gradually lowering the mask, which is fitted by an elbow to a Sierra nonrebreathing valve, over the patient's face (Fig. 20). Fifty percent nitrous oxide in oxygen is begun, followed by a gradual increase of the percentage of halothane. The top percentage of halothane necessary is usually 2.5 percent, and induc-

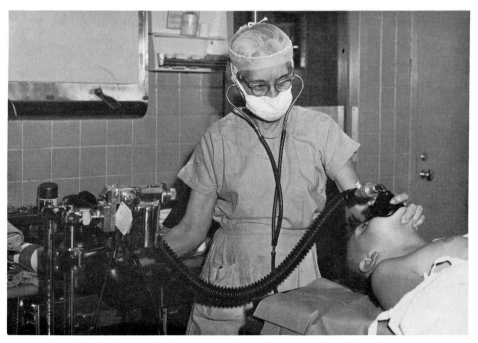

Fig. 20. Gaseous induction employing a Sierra nonrebreathing valve.

tion is accomplished in three or four minutes. Halothane maintained in the region of 1 percent is then employed. The gas flow necessary with a nonrebreathing valvular system is that which is necessary to keep the bag three quarters full. If the gas flow is too high for the patient's minute volume, the pop-off valve is used. The use of mask harnesses is actively discouraged because pressure syndromes can arise. At all times vigilance should be maintained for bradycardia. The two most common causes of bradycardia are overdosage with the anesthetic agent and inadequate atropinization. The remedy is obvious: lighten anesthesia, oxygenate with positive pressure, and repeat the atropine dosage. Unnecessary touching of the patient during induction should be actively discouraged so as to avoid detrimental reflex reaction, such as laryngeal spasm. Immediately after induction the thermometer probes are put in place.

INFANTS

If a shorter acting barbiturate is used for induction it is employed as for children. A gaseous induction with halothane, using a Rendell-Baker mask and MIE chimney piece (Fig. 21), is performed in the same manner as for the child, taking the safety precautions of having the precordial stethoscope and blood pressure cuff in place. It should always be remembered that a normal respiration pattern for a neonate is cyclical and that short periods of apnea may arise. Infants are nasal breathers, so the masks have to be properly placed on the infant's face. When a valveless system is used, the gas flow must be twice the minute volume, which is calculated from a nomogram. A rule of thumb is that the minute volume equals the rate times the tidal air, and the tidal air equals the dead space, i.e., 1 ml/lb $\times$ 3. Either an open ended tube, with which respiration can be assisted or controlled by closing the open end, or a miniature bag can be used. A good aid in measuring the depth of anesthesia in an infant is the tone of his fingers. Airway obstruction will first become evident by slight subcostal retraction, which will be followed by retraction of the sternum and supraclavicular area and by de-

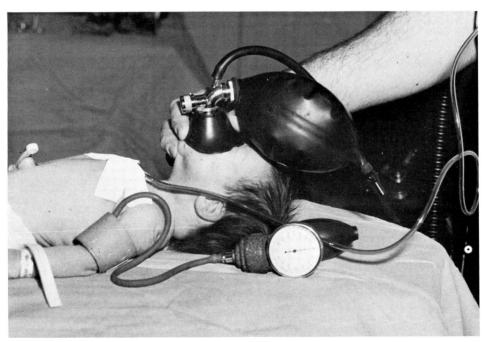

Fig. 21. Induction of the infant is accomplished using a valveless system with high flows. Note the erect position; the neck is not extended.

creased exchanges. Should this occur, the head should be repositioned; if obstruction is not thereby remedied, an oropharyngeal airway is inserted. If laryngospasm occurs, it generally can be overcome by positive pressure with oxygen supplied by means of a face mask and bag. On extremely rare occasions, succinylcholine may be necessary to overcome the spasm.

THE UNMANAGEABLE CHILD

Occasionally a child arrives for surgery in an unmanageable condition exhibiting great excitement. Sodium thiopental, 5 to 10 mg/lb given rectally, or methohexital, 8 to 10 mg/lb, may be used to calm the child. Should this fail, intravenous induction using either sodium thiopental or methohexital is resorted to. The child's hand can always be held securely for a few seconds and a # 25 needle inserted into a vein and the agent injected.

ENDOTRACHEAL INTUBATION

Endotracheal intubation is used to maintain an airway or to prevent interference with the surgical field.

ADVANTAGES

Some of the advantages of endotracheal intubation are the following:

(1) It prevents aspiration of blood and tissue from the mouth and pharynx. This is especially important in oral, dental, and nasal surgery.

(2) It prevents aspiration of vomitus. Endotracheal intubation is essential for patients with full stomachs or those who have upper intestinal obstruction.

(3) It is mandatory in open chest surgery, and it is common in apneic techniques of anesthesia and resuscitation.

(4) It can be used when the patient is sitting or prone.

(5) It can be used when the anesthesiologist is remote from the head because of the surgical field.

COMPLICATIONS

Some points should be remembered in preventing complications of endotracheal intubation.

(1) The size of the tracheal lumen is critical in children, especially in infants. To prevent damage to the tracheal mucosa and obstruction to respiration, thin walled tubes should be fitted in place gently. Cuffed tubes are not employed in small children and infants.

(2) Apparatus associated with endotracheal intubation should be carefully checked before it is used, to avoid equipment failure. Complications do arise at the time of intubation, such as respiratory depression and apnea, which can be controlled by positive pressure oxygenation. Any loose teeth should be removed before intubation, but on occasion teeth are dislodged.

(3) Nasal intubation is associated with a high incidence of hemorrhage caused by tearing of the mucosa and adenoid tissue. Often this occurs because of the operator's ignorance of the normal anatomy of the nasal passages. The tube should be gently passed under the inferior turbinate.

(4) If the proper endotracheal tube is used and the head position is maintained, no kinking will occur. The tube should be fixed firmly in place so that accidental extubation is prevented.

(5) Extubation spasm, which occurs frequently when cyclopropane is used, rarely occurs when halothane is used.

(6) Postintubation hoarseness and obstruction to the airway still occur. Such a complication can usually be traced to a rough intubation or roughing of the tracheal tube surface by repeated reuse and sterilization. Adequate humidification systems have diminished the incidence of endotracheal irritation.

INDICATIONS FOR USE

Mandatory indications for endotracheal intubations are:

TABLE 2. LARYNGOSCOPE BLADES AND TUBE SIZES
RECOMMENDED ACCORDING TO CHILD'S WEIGHT

WEIGHT OF CHILD	WEIGHT OF CHILD	SIZE OF TUBE INTERNAL DIAMETER	LARYNGOSCOPE SIZE	CONNECTOR SIZE	LENGTH OF TUBE*
(lbs)	(kg)	(mm)		(mm)	(cm)
0–10	0.45–4.5	3.0	Premature	4	13
10–20	4.5–9.0	3.5		4	14
20–30	9.0–13.6	5.0	Infant	4–4.5–5	15
30–40	13.6–18.1	5.5		4.5–5	17
40–50	18.1–22.6	6.5		5.5–6	19
50–60	22.6–27.2	7.0		5.5–6	20
60–70	27.2–31.7	7.5	Child	6–6.5	20
70–80	31.7–36.2	8.0		6.5–7	22
80–90	36.2–40.8	8.5		7–7.5	22
90–100	40.8–45.3	9.0		7.5–8	22

WEIGHT OF CHILD		COLE TUBES SIZE	INTERNAL DIAMETER	LARYNGOSCOPE SIZE	CONNECTOR SIZE	LENGTH OF TUBE*
(lbs)	(kg)		(mm)		(mm)	(cm)
3–4	1.36–1.81	12	2.5	Premature	4	12
4–6	1.81–2.72	14	3.0	Premature	4	12
6–8	2.72–3.62	16	3.5	Premature	4	13
8–10	3.62–4.50	18	4.0	Premature	4	13

* All tubes are cut to the greater length.

(1) Patients with full stomachs or upper intestinal obstructions, including pyloric stenosis.

(2) Intrathoracic procedures.

(3) Operations in the prone position.

(4) Intracranial operations.

(5) Major operations about the mouth, face, and neck. Operations in compromising positions, such as kidney or lateral jackknife positions.

(6) Arteriograms, pneumoencephalograms, and ventriculograms.

(7) All tonsillectomies.

Table 2 indicates laryngoscope blades and tube sizes recommended according to the patient's age and weight. The tube of indicated size along with the next larger and next smaller sizes should be selected as a group. Table 3 shows the average lengths of

TABLE 3. AVERAGE LENGTH OF TUBES

WEIGHT OF CHILD	WEIGHT OF CHILD	LENGTH OF TUBE
(lbs)	(kg)	(cm)
0–10	0.45–4.5	13
10–20	4.5–9.0	14
20–30	9.0–13.6	15
30–40	13.6–18.1	17
40–50	18.1–22.6	19
50–60	22.6–27.2	20
60–70	27.2–31.7	20
70–80	31.7–36.2	22
80–90	36.2–40.8	22
90–100	40.8–45.3	22

tubes. Although the table method is the most accurate, the lumen of the external nares is a useful index to the size of the glottis, particularly in infants.

SELECTION OF TIME TO INTUBATE

The incidence of trauma following awake intubation is much higher than that occurring when anesthesia plus relaxant or relaxant alone is employed. Before any attempt at intubation is made, the child should be well oxygenated.

INTUBATION UNDER RELAXANT ALONE

In infants under six months, when their neuronal cells are poorly developed, a useful method of intubation is to oxygenate, administer succinylcholine, 0.5 mg/lb intravenously or, less preferably, 0.75 mg/lb intramuscularly. Oxygenation is then repeated and intubation is accomplished under tranquil conditions.

INTUBATION UNDER ANESTHESIA ALONE

Induction is accomplished by the routine method using nitrous oxide–halothane or sodium thiopental. After five minutes of halothane administration the jaw is examined for relaxation. When the jaw is relaxed intubation must be accomplished swiftly, for in a space of three to five breaths cord movement will again make intubation impossible.

INTUBATION UNDER ANESTHESIA PLUS A RELAXANT

Either nitrous oxide–halothane or sodium thiopental is followed with intravenous succinylcholine, 0.5 mg/lb. After oxygenation the patient is readily intubated. Should another relaxant, such as gallamine or tubocurarine, be contemplated, it is preferable not to mix polarizing and depolarizing relaxants. If a longer acting relaxant is to be used, adequate muscular contractility should be reestablished before the second agent is given. A blockade monitor is a useful aid. Adequate atropinization is essential during intubation to prevent bradycardia.

Position is all-important for easy intubation (Fig. 22). The head and neck should be in the bronchoscopic position—that is, the head is slightly off the table and parallel to it, as shown in the illustration. After the head is positioned, the teeth are checked for looseness or fragmentation. The laryngoscope is then held between the thumb and forefinger and the blade inserted slightly to the right of the midline, displacing the tongue to the left. As the blade is carefully advanced, first the oropharynx and then the hypopharynx are exposed, and the epiglottis then comes into view. Using a straight blade, the epiglottis is usually lifted. Should there be difficulty in bringing the glottis into view, the larynx should be gently pressed with the little finger of the left hand. If the MacIntosh blade is used, it is inserted in the midline. The epiglottis comes into view, and the blade is placed behind the epiglottis. The difference between the management of the handle of the straight laryngoscope and that of the MacIntosh is that with the MacIntosh the handle is pushed straight ahead toward the feet and the epiglottis is lifted by anterior pressure and the glottis comes into view, while with the straight blade the handle is rotated and the epiglottis is picked up. The glottis should always be in view before the anesthetist tries to proceed with intubation.

The tube of appropriate size is selected and put into place. The distance between the glottis and the carina is estimated on the basis of standard figures, and the endotracheal tube is inserted one third of the distance between the glottis and the carina. The patient is immediately oxygenated, and then the tube is taped into place. Care should be taken that the tube itself is taped and not the connector, since the tube may become dislodged into the trachea.

It is vitally important that after every endotracheal intubation the breath sounds on

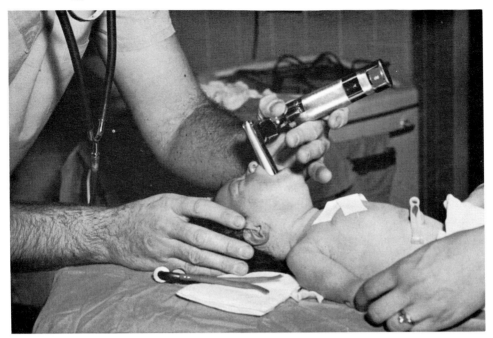

Fig. 22. Position is all-important for easy intubation of the infant. The larynx is located quite cephalad.

both sides of the chest are listened to, to make absolutely certain that the tube is not endobronchial. Either a bite block or an oropharyngeal airway is inserted to prevent occlusion of the tube by the teeth.

Should a tube less than 4 mm in diameter be employed of the non-Cole type, it is best that the connector be inserted over the tube or that another piece of tubing be inserted over the tube and then the connector inserted into the larger piece of tubing, so that the lumen of the tube is not diminished.

MAINTENANCE
OF ANESTHESIA

OBJECTIVES

The main objectives of the anesthesiologist during the operative procedure are (1) providing intensive care for the patient and (2) supplying the best possible working conditions for the surgeon.

The surgeon requires that the patient be immobile, that the area in which he is op-

erating be exposed, and, on occasion, that the patient be relaxed. There will be times when the surgeon's requirements cannot be met because of the unacceptable risk they pose to the patient. On these occasions the anesthesiologist and surgeon make a compromise. It is the anesthesiologist's duty to keep the surgeon fully informed of anything that pertains to the patient's care. Problems between anesthesiologists and surgeons usually result from lack of adequate communication.

GENERAL RULES

Constant observation is the most important factor in maintenance methodology. The anesthesiologist must use most of his senses for constant observation, and therefore the following rules should be observed during anesthesia.

(1) Unnecessary sound and movement is discouraged in the operating room.

(2) Everything possible should be organized before induction (i.e., infusions and transfusions should be ready to be hooked

to the patient, and all necessary drugs should be drawn up into syringes in the appropriate dosages and labeled). The aim is that extraneous movement and effort on the part of the anesthesiologist be reduced to a minimum. Nothing should be allowed to distract the anesthesiologist's attention from observation of the patient. He must not serve as surgical assistant, as is sometimes done in tonsillectomies. The anesthesiologist must at all times remain in contact with the patient and should move from the head of the table

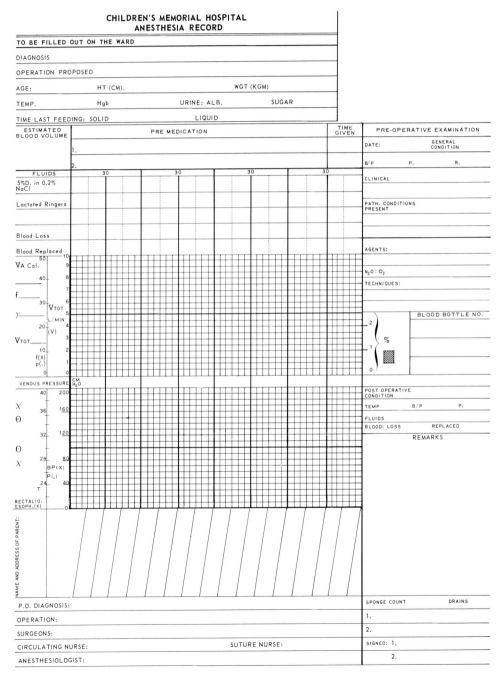

Fig. 23. Anesthesia record form. Front side.

only when there is some definite objective, such as observing the blood loss on the patient's perineum; but even then there should be monitoring parameters that he can observe from the foot of the table. Accidents in pediatric anesthesia may occur when the anesthesiologist is distracted by trying to help either the surgeon or the operating room nurses. Fatigue is a great hazard in pediatric anesthesiology, a fact that surgeons do not appreciate. It is extremely difficult to maintain maximum vigilance for more than four

RECOVERY ROOM AND POST ANESTHETIC RECORD

HOUR	T.P.R.	MEDICINE, TREATMENT ETC.	REMARKS	URINE	DEF'N.

POST ANESTHESIA SUMMARY:

SIGNATURE

ANESTHESIOLOGIST (OR) ANESTHETIST

Fig. 23 (cont.). Anesthesia record form. Reverse side.

hours at a time, and relief after four hours is advantageous.

(3) The anesthesiologist must constantly monitor the patient's heart sounds and respirations by means of a stethoscope. It is also very useful for him to keep a finger on a palpable pulse—usually the temporal artery or dorsalis pedia, depending on the position of the patient—as a direct check on the patient's circulation.

(4) Some part of the patient should be exposed, either the face or the foot, so that skin color can be observed. No obstructing apparatus that would prevent the application of suction to the patient's airway can be tolerated. The drapes should never be in a position which prevents the anesthesiologist from seeing the progress of the operation and thus changing his technique to best suit the changing surgical requirements. Inspecting the field of operation is again an additional aid in estimating the condition of the patient. The classical example is during heart operations. The best way to monitor the heart action is to observe it directly.

(5) An accurate anesthesia record should be prepared and maintained for each case (Fig. 23). The preoperative diagnosis and the condition of the patient should be noted; it is helpful to have the patient's height and weight recorded as well, so that the surface area can be calculated. The temperature, hemoglobin, and urinalysis must be recorded along with the time of the last feeding of both solids and liquids—the premedication should not be administered unless these data are available and recorded on the chart. Therefore, the chart should be begun on the wards. It is extremely useful to chart the fluid intake of both infusions and transfusions continuously in detail and at the same time to record the blood loss. Monitoring the classical data, such as blood pressure, pulse, and respiratory rate, is insufficient. The temperature should be continuously monitored in all cases, along with detailed respiratory parameters. Additional aids, such as the recording of central venous pressure, should be charted diligently. Since optimum anesthesia techniques are quantitative, the concentration of the anesthetic mixture should also be charted. Any drug that is administered is noted in detail, and all data are associated with time. At the end of the surgical procedure the total amount of fluid and blood given is recorded along with the estimated blood loss. A final check on the patient's condition is made and recorded. The value of an anesthesia record is directly related to the diligence with which it has been kept and to the detailed information it contains.

CHECKING THE PATIENT

Every anesthesiologist should work out a system by which he routinely checks a number of points indicating the patient's condition. This check procedure will depend on the type of case being managed, but a routine should always be followed. The anesthesia record should be designed so that the check procedure can be charted readily. The following sections outline a procedure that can be used as a guide.

ADEQUACY OF VENTILATION

The most important parameter to measure in pediatric anesthesiology is respiration. The patient should be continuously checked for any sign of obstruction. The stethoscope is extremely valuable in measuring respiration and diagnosing signs of obstruction. At all times one must watch for the characteristic sounds and signs of kinked tubes and stuck valves. If a breathing bag with a one-way valve system is used, one can estimate the adequacy of ventilation by momentarily shutting off the gas inflow and measuring the uptake from the bag. In major surgery when a constant volume ventilator is being used, continuous measurement of the volume exhaled is measured by a spirometer. The pressure in a nondistensible system can be measured, giving a good indication of changes in the compliance. In pressure-limited ventilators, a Wright spirometer should be used if the patient is in a position that makes the clinical assessment of the adequacy of respiration extremely difficult. In the more difficult cases the pH, PCO_2, and PO_2 should be monitored. The greatest danger in pediatric anesthesiology is hypoventilation. Changes in the patient's color and in the so-called vital signs are relatively late indications of hypoxia.

With the exception of a light plane of diethyl ether and trichloroethylene, all anesthetic agents are respiratory depressants. Therefore, respiration should always be assisted or controlled. Because it is extremely difficult to accurately assist respiration manually in the infant, it is more physiological to control respiration in the infant by mechanical means.

SIGNS OF ANESTHETIC LEVEL

Since the advent of halothane and methoxyflurane the classical signs of depth of anesthesia have had to be reassessed. The signs that are useful when these agents are used are signs of relaxation. One can achieve surgical planes of anesthesia with halothane by estimating the degree of relaxation of the hand, especially in an infant; the hand should be relaxed but not flaccid. The only eye sign of use is the loss of the eyelash reflex in light anesthesia and fixation of the pupils in surgical anesthesia. Halothane is a poor relaxant, and no effort should be made to attain complete abdominal relaxation with this agent. Overdosage is diagnosed by a fall in blood pressure and bradycardia. As with all pharmacological agents, there is a specificity between each patient and the drug being used. Small concentrations of halothane may give sudden hypotension for no apparent reason; thus, the amount of halothane necessary varies from patient to patient.

In the infant, respiratory signs of the depth of anesthesia may be difficult to assess. Usually the respiratory cycle will become quiet and more regular, but in the infant the cyclical type of respiration is common. If a child is sobbing before anesthesia, he is liable to

sob throughout the anesthetic. Laryngeal stridor occurs if the anesthesia is too light and is best managed by deepening the anesthesia while maintaining full oxygenation.

Methoxyflurane is similar to halothane in regard to clinical signs, but its action is slower and thus the signs change more gradually. Full abdominal relaxation can be obtained with this agent.

When training residents it is proper to teach them that if the patient is not inclined to move, he is too deeply anesthetized. When there is any doubt in regard to the depth of anesthesia, it should be lightened until movement occurs. It is no disgrace under these circumstances to have the patient move, provided the surgeon is forewarned.

CIRCULATION AND BLOOD PRESSURE

The cardiovascular system is checked by palpation for the pulse rate, rhythm, and quality. Blood pressure, stethoscopic heart sounds, and central venous pressure are monitored. Color, degree of warmth, and dryness of the palms of the hands are also useful clinical signs.

FLUID THERAPY

In the infant, the compressibility of the fontanel is a useful sign in relation to the fluid balance. Unexpected distension of the neck veins may indicate overhydration. Volume-controlled infusion apparatus with microdrips should be used along with increment blood transfusion apparatus. Blood should be warmed before administration. The blood loss in relation to sponges and suction should be continuously monitored. Central venous pressure recording is extremely useful in estimating blood loss.

BODY TEMPERATURE

The temperature of the patient should be monitored and charted continuously, and variation in temperature should be discussed with the surgeon. Recently an appreciable number of cases have been reported in which sudden, violent hyperthermia occurred, and extremely drastic action was necessary to save the patients. This hyperthermia has not been explained as yet, but speed in cooling is an absolute necessity in saving these patients. The surgeon should be made aware of the possibility of hyperthermia and of the urgency of combating it.

POSITION

The anesthesiologist may continue to check the patient's position, to avoid unnecessary trauma, especially to peripheral nerves.

GASTRIC DISTENSION

In the infant the stomach may be distended during controlled ventilation if an endotracheal tube is not being used. Stomach distension is prevented with the nasogastric tube. A distended stomach will splint the diaphragm and cause hypoventilation and may cause acute cardiovascular changes.

MACHINE OBSERVATION

During the procedure the anesthesiologist should routinely check the gas flow, the availability of continuing gas supply, the hookup of the apparatus, the position of the endotracheal connection or the mask position, and such monitoring aids as the spirometer and pressure gauge. If a water mattress is being used, its temperature must be monitored continuously so that it does not exceed 105° F. An effort is made to keep the mattress temperature at 100° F, especially if the underdrape becomes wet.

THE PATIENT'S RECOVERY

EXTUBATION OF THE TRACHEA

Care must be taken when extubating the patient. Before extubating, the patency of the suction apparatus should be checked. A Yankauer suction apparatus should be available for removing large volumes from the mouth and pharynx. DeLee type of catheters of suitable sizes should be made ready for sucking out the endotracheal tubes. The endotracheal tubes should be suctioned when indicated, with care being taken that the patient is not deoxygenated. The patient is always ventilated after suctioning. Apparatus for reintubation should be kept ready and a bag and mask kept available. The same care that is taken with the induction and intubation of a patient is taken with extubation. To avoid laryngospasm and hypoxia, the patient should always be oxygenated before being extubated. The best time for removal of the endotracheal tube is when the patient has recovered the swallowing reflex. When the reflex returns, the endotracheal tube is removed in stages during expiration. At all times the patient should be kept oxygenated. If there is any doubt whatsoever about whether there is an accumulation around the tube, suction should be performed under direct vision using a laryngoscope. A bite block should be left in place during extubation to prevent the patient from suddenly biting down on the tube. Routinely, a mask is placed on the face, and the adequacy of respiration is checked. The patient should be allowed to become fully awake before extubation when there are special circumstances, such as bowel obstruction, and then buckling of the tube should be avoided. Other such special circumstances occur when the patient has a full stomach and when it would be extremely difficult to reintubate the patient. During extubation the heart sounds are continuously monitored. It is not uncommon in the infant that following extubation there is a period of apnea. The patient should be ventilated manually. Should laryngospasm occur, it is usually possible to break the spasm with positive pressure. Succinylcholine should be readily available for the rare case in which positive pressure is ineffective. The abdomen should be inspected and the contents removed to prevent splinting of the diaphragm. In pediatric anesthesiology the patient should always be awake before being removed from the operating room. A final check on the stability of the various systems of the child should be done in the postanesthesia room.

If any complications are going to arise, they should occur in the operating room. The nursing staff and surgeons should be available for the awakening process and for the transit of the patient. The surgeon should always accompany the patient to the postanesthesia room, for the postanesthetic period is the most dangerous for the patient. During transportation, suctioning equipment should be readily available, along with a means of providing positive pressure respiration.

In the postanesthesia room the patient is better nursed with the head to the center of the room where observation can be accomplished more readily. Pulse, blood pressure, and respiration are again monitored continuously. The anesthesiologist should go over the anesthesia record with the postanesthesia room nurse with special reference to his final observations on the condition of the child and the fluid and electrolyte balance.

Both the postanesthesia area and the intensive care area should be fully equipped for resuscitation (Fig. 24).

THE ANESTHESIOLOGIST'S POSTOPERATIVE RESPONSIBILITIES

The anesthesiologist should work closely with the surgeon and pediatrician in the postoperative management of the patient. Although division of responsibility will vary from hospital to hospital, good liaison is absolutely essential. The anesthesiologist is usually responsible for the ventilatory requirements of the patient but should assist the surgeon in such matters as determining fluid and electrolyte requirements in the changeover period. The anesthesiologist is much more aware of the condition of the patient in the postanesthesia period than the sur-

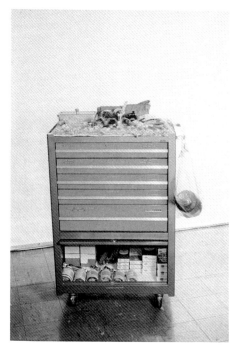

Fig. 24. The recovery areas should be fully equipped with a resuscitation cart.

geon is, and it is his responsibility to assist the surgeon in evaluating the postoperative condition of the patient.

LOCAL AND REGIONAL ANESTHESIA

In pediatric anesthesia there are a few indications for local and regional anesthesia. The statement that morbidity and mortality from local and regional anesthesia in children is less than that for general anesthesia has not been substantiated.

TOPICAL ANESTHESIA

As a topical agent, lidocaine (Xylocaine) 4 percent appears to provoke the fewest side reactions. If topical anesthesia is used, the dose should be measured (Figs. 25 and 26). In many operations in pediatrics the depth of anesthesia required for the actual operation is less than that required for obtunding the laryngeal reflexes. A good illustration of this type of operation is dental cavity repair.

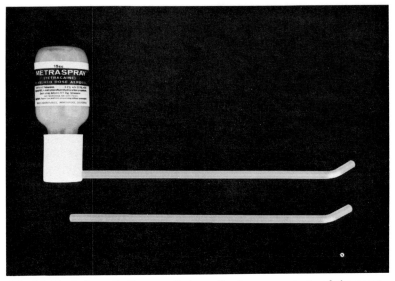

Fig. 25. Topical anesthetic spray that supplies known amounts of the agent.

The length of operation should be taken into account, for the topical anesthetic should be worn off before the end of the operation, thus preventing reflux and aspiration from the obtunded larynx. In bronchology a useful technique is to saturate the patient with methoxyflurane and liberally spray a topical anesthetic on the larynx and trachea.

LOCAL INFILTRATION

Local infiltration is used extensively in the emergency reception areas. It is preferable to settle on one agent and to have a schedule in relation to age and weight to serve as a guide for the residents. Lidocaine has proven to be excellent as a local anesthetic for infiltration. It should be emphasized that there is a different dose-weight relationship for each concentration of the drug.

REGIONAL BLOCK

Although block procedures have been used extensively on children, in a pediatric hospital the need for nerve blocks is small. In such an institution an occasional epidural anesthetic is used for extensive abdominal procedures in the presence of liver failure. An

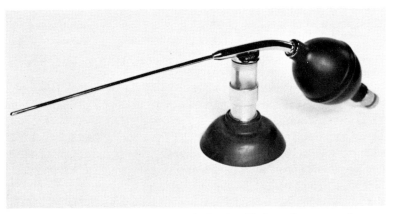

Fig. 26. The dose of topical anesthetics should always be measured.

indication for brachial block is the creation of an A-V dialysis shunt in the patient with renal failure.

A therapeutic block, such as a lumbar sympathetic, an epidural, or a caudal, has been employed on occasion as a means of controlling vasospasm.

Pudendal blocks have been used in conjunction with some urological procedures.

INTRAVENOUS BARBITURATES

Intravenous anesthesia can be employed in all age groups. With practice it is possible to perform an induction using short acting intravenous barbiturates in infants. Children vary in their acceptance of needle injections. It is a good practice to give them the choice of an inhalation or an intravenous induction. The retarded child is best managed with intravenous barbiturate induction. The most common barbiturate used in this fashion is sodium thiopental, and the dose range is 2 to 4 mg/lb in a 2.5 percent solution. The solution is administered slowly and is stopped when the eyelash reflex is lost.

The barbiturates are hypnotics and should not be used as anesthetics. They are useful in the treatment of convulsive disorders. A slow injection of a 2.5 percent solution of sodium thiopental is maintained until the convulsions cease.

Sodium thiopental is excreted at the rate of 10 percent per hour. Respiratory depression from an excessive rate of infusion is managed by positive pressure ventilation. If sodium thiopental is used in a concentration greater than 2.5 percent, there is an increased risk of laryngospasm, which is managed by positive pressure ventilation and, if necessary, by the administration of a short acting relaxant such as succinylcholine.

RELAXANTS

There is wide variation in the use of relaxants in children. The Liverpool school of Jackson-Rees uses nitrous oxide, curare, and hyperventilation routinely. In institutions relaxants are rarely used. It is safer to use an inhalation technique, which permits rapid pulmonary elimination, than an intravenously administered drug, which requires additional time and a biochemical degradation for elimination.

INDICATIONS FOR USE OF RELAXANTS IN PEDIATRIC ANESTHESIA

Intubation is aided by the use of a short acting relaxant, such as succinylcholine. This is administered intravenously, 0.5 mg/lb, after making sure that atropine sulfate in the appropriate dose has been given. Succinylcholine can also be administered intramuscularly; however, by this route the absorption rate is unknown, and therefore this method of administration should be discouraged. A short acting relaxant requires rapid intubation and consequently is not a satisfactory drug for the inexperienced person to administer. To intubate awake or under an inhalation anesthetic is advantageous for the inexperienced person.

In infants under six months of age an induction technique that is often employed is to oxygenate the infant, administer succinylcholine, intubate, and then begin administration of the anesthesia.

In very poor-risk infants, many of them with "cardiac" lesions, it may be dangerous to administer any anesthetic agent. Such patients may be made immobile by the intermittent administration of succinylcholine. For a 20-pound infant the dilution will be 2 mg/ml; for a 30-pound infant, 3 mg/ml; for a 40-pound infant, 4 mg/ml; and so on. To avoid excessive fluid infusion the dilution should not exceed 2 mg/ml. After each dose, respirations are allowed to become reestablished before another dose is given.

The longer acting relaxant of choice in pediatrics is gallamine chloride. The tachycardia following its use makes it the relaxant of choice in patients with relatively slow pulses. It is shorter acting than curarine and is also reversible. The dose of gallamine is initially 1 mg/kg and subsequently 0.5 mg/kg.

CONTRAINDICATIONS

There are definite contraindications to the use of relaxants in children. The most important of these are the genetic deficiencies such as that of pseudocholinesterase, a condition often associated with congenital glaucoma.

Unless one is extremely adept technically, relaxants are contraindicated if the patient has a distended full stomach, since there may be a rush of gastric contents through the relaxed cardiac sphincter that may flood the pharynx.

Should there be any doubt about the adequacy of the excretory renal or hepatic mechanism for any specific relaxant, the relaxant should not be used.

HYPOTENSIVE TECHNIQUES

On rare occasions a hypotensive technique is justified in pediatric anesthesia. In coarctation of the aorta and some urological procedures, a hypertension occurs which can be controlled by a ganglionic blocking agent, such as trimethaphan.

In infants there are certain procedures that entail considerable blood loss. If it is anticipated that this blood loss will be unmanageable using standard methods of control, a hypotensive technique is employed. Hypothermia, which is in itself a hypotensive technique, may be sufficient to achieve adequate control of the blood loss. If this is inadequate, the deeper planes of halothane anesthesia are used to produce additional hypotension.

HYPOTHERMIA

Hypothermia is now rarely used alone in pediatric anesthesia. It may be used in association with extracorporeal circulation when the surgeon is confronted with an un-

usual problem. The most common use of the hypothermia technique is in the management of hyperthermia associated with infection. Appendectomy is not delayed until there is a spontaneous fall of a high fever; rather, the patient is placed on a hypothermic blanket and rapidly brought to normothermia under anesthesia.

The value of maintaining the patient at a subnormal temperature following cardiac arrest is unknown.

SPECIAL PROBLEMS

ANESTHESIA FOR INFANTS

A common surgical mistake in dealing with the neonate is to be too vigorous in the preparation of the operative site, causing the towel that the infant is lying on to become wet, so that the infant rapidly cools. Again, if the infant is lying on a heating mattress and the covering towel becomes wet, there is a possibility that the infant will be burned even though the circulating fluid is maintained at or below 105° F.

OMPHALOCELE

When managing a case of omphalocele the wound should be closed without the use of relaxants, or diaphragmatic movement may be impaired postoperatively.

DIAPHRAGMATIC HERNIA

Relaxants should not be used during the abdominal closure of diaphragmatic hernia, or the diaphragmatic movement will be impeded. If there is any doubt whatsoever about the adequacy of respiration, it should be measured and, if found to be deficient, an automatic mechanical ventilator should be employed and monitored with pH, PCO_2, and PO_2 determinations. No attempt should be made to inflate the atelectatic lung.

TRACHEOESOPHAGEAL FISTULA AND ESOPHAGEAL ATRESIA

The main duty that the anesthesiologist has in the management of the patient with a tracheoesophageal fistula or esophageal atresia is the preoperative, operative, and postoperative tracheobronchial toilet. This should be accomplished under direct vision, great care being taken to be extremely gentle. If the trachea and bronchi are kept free of secretions, these cases, whether they are surgically managed extrapleurally or intrapleurally, should present no problem to the anesthesiologist.

ANOPLASTY AND ABDOMINOPERINEAL PULL THROUGH

Combined abdominoperineal procedures in infants are becoming more common in the treatment of imperforate anus and Hirschsprung's disease. Colitis is the great hazard in these patients. If there is any doubt about whether the child has colitis, it will soon be resolved during and immediately after induction of anesthesia. It is very difficult to achieve control of respiration and temperature in these patients in the presence of severe colitis. If it becomes evident, a short procedure is indicated. If these patients are operated on soon enough after birth—that is, before colitis has occurred—they present no anesthesia problem.

Small prematures do not tolerate long procedures. Infants weighing 4 to 8 pounds do not appear to be excessively disturbed by procedures requiring four to six hours. Gentleness in handling tissue is the most important factor in management of the neonate.

PYLORIC STENOSIS

Pyloric stenosis is an upper intestinal obstruction; consequently, before induction or intubation the stomach should be emptied with a Levin tube that should be left in

place during the operation and then discarded. Intubation is mandatory.

HERNIORRHAPHY

Patients undergoing herniorrhaphy are not intubated unless it is impossible to maintain an airway. The Ayre's technique is employed. Adequate depth of anesthesia should be reached before the peritoneum is pulled and the transfixing suture inserted; otherwise, laryngospasm may occur. Two percent halothane with 50 percent nitrous oxide and oxygen is usually adequate to achieve the desired level of anesthesia.

THORACIC SURGERY

The patient about to undergo thoracic surgery should be made familiar with the postoperative and intensive care management in relation to both the inhalation and respiratory physical therapy. The apparatus to be used should be demonstrated, and if postoperative ventilation by mechanical ventilator is contemplated, it should be explained to the child before he is operated on. In bringing the child into the best possible condition for surgery, respiratory physical therapy and inhalation therapy may be necessary.

Beware of the lesion of the lung that appears to be a tumor or a cyst because it may be an abscess whose contents may flood the tracheobronchial tree. A bronchoscopy setup should always be readily available when undertaking the anesthesiology management of such a lesion.

Anesthesiology management for operations on the heart and great vessels entails a detailed knowledge of the actual defects and their effects on the physiopathology of the patient. It is impossible to give a satisfactory anesthetic and to manage the patient well without this knowledge.

In a vast majority of these patients an inhalation anesthetic is administered quantitatively along with quantitative ventilation and humidification using the Engström model 200 with the Allan anesthesia circuit. This method leaves the anesthesiologist relatively free to monitor the patient continuously, attend to blood loss and replacement, and manage drug therapy.

As a routine, 1 to 1.5 percent halothane is used in a 50 percent nitrous oxide–oxygen mixture for maintenance in all open heart cases and those closed heart procedures in which the transsternal approach is employed. In these cases of closed heart and shunt procedures with a transpleural approach, one lung is compressed by retraction to provide exposure for the surgeon. This will add intrapulmonary shunting to the existing cardiac shunt and dangerously lower the arterial PO_2. Here nitrous oxide is not used, and halothane is administered in 100 percent oxygen. However, the lack of nitrous oxide in the gas mixture will necessitate an increase in halothane concentration to provide adequate anesthesia unless muscle relaxants are given. Our objection to muscle relaxants is that after their use we have noticed deleterious effects in the immediate postoperative period, consisting of diminished inspiratory and expiratory activity and low tidal volumes and arterial PO_2 values. These

values improve significantly after the administration of Tensilon or Prostigmin, indicating residual myoneural blockade. These anticholinesterase drugs have a profound effect of their own on the heart, along with the atropine sulfate that has to be given preceding them. Instead of imposing further burdens on the heart, which is at peak capacity and may have to cope with hypoxemia, we prefer the simple alternative of increasing the halothane concentration. This can be safely accomplished, provided that there is constant vigilance aided by various monitors. On the other hand, in cases in which extremely high concentrations of halothane would be required to avoid this, the careful intermittent administration of succinylcholine is justified. This applies to small babies with high metabolic rates and very high compensatory outputs as well as to those patients with extremely poor cardiac status.

In open heart surgery with the transsternal approach, muscle relaxants are usually not indicated, and there is no advantage in employing any inhalational agent other than halothane.

Ventilation is accomplished by the Eng-

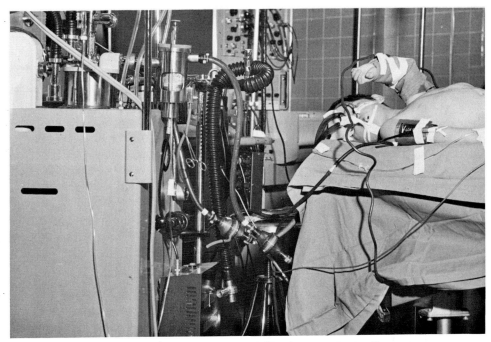

Fig. 27. Ventilation is accomplished by the Engström ventilator.

ström ventilator (Fig. 27). A nomogram serves as a baseline for calculating the required minute volumes and rates. The adequacy of these estimated settings is checked against the arterial PO_2 and PCO_2 determined from blood samples taken by means of an arterial catheter. Our experience has been that in most cases we have had to use slightly higher settings than those indicated by the nomogram. Of course, this may be a result of the need for slight hyperventilation that arises because of our reluctance to paralyze the patients.

Although the Engström respirator is a versatile and effective machine that has achieved clinical success, there is one instance where this respirator cannot replace the anesthesiologist's hands. In some procedures in which the situation is worsened by the addition of an artificial intrapulmonary shunt in the retracted lung, the so-called diaphragmatic flap is bothersome to the surgeon. The fast rhythmic actions of the diaphragm are due to oxygen hunger and are different in rate from the heart rate. It is difficult for the surgeon to cope with two uncoordinated rhythms while performing a delicate anastomosis. Since the arterial PO_2 cannot be elevated significantly in the presence of intracardiac or intrapulmonary shunts because of venous admixtures, it is impossible to overcome the patient's oxygen hunger by administering 100 percent oxygen alone. It has been proposed that the alveoli be moderately distended during expiration, and thus oxygen hunger will be alleviated by pressure being put on the stretch receptors. This has the disadvantage of increasing the physiological dead space in the lungs. To deliver as much oxygen as possible, there are two additional contributory measures:

(1) Increase the volume of effective alveolar ventilation. There is a certain limit imposed on this measure by both the thorax and the lungs. The lungs are inefficient ventilating organs in infants, with a respiratory surface per unit weight one fifth that of adults. In the presence of increased physiological dead space the relative augmentation of alveolar ventilation achieved by this measure alone is not sufficient to meet peripheral oxygen need.

(2) Increase the rate of ventilation up to 45 to 50 respirations per minute. The Eng-

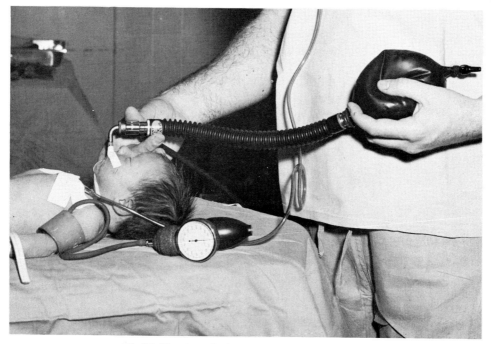

Fig. 28. Hand ventilation using the Ayre's T piece.

ström respirator can readily increase the tidal volume, the physiological dead space, or both. The rate cannot be increased over 35 per minute, which is well below the required 45 to 50 per minute. This rate can be maintained with hand ventilation (Fig. 28), obviating the need for a dangerous level of anesthesia or the use of muscle relaxants.

One of the most efficient ways to evaluate the patient's circulatory system during surgery and in the postoperative period is to measure the central venous pressure. This measurement will be an indication of the competence of the heart and of its ability to cope with the venous return. It must be emphasized that the venous pressure does not accurately reflect blood volume in the patient at any one time; it is only a useful aid in making an estimation of that volume. With a normal cardiovascular system the value should be between 7 and 12 cm of water pressure.

VASCULAR RING

In the patient with a vascular ring the trachea or the esophagus, or both, is compressed. Also, the trachea may be poorly developed and may collapse after the obstruction is removed. If the surgical attempt to prop up the trachea is inadequate, a supporting tube may have to be left in place. During the actual procedure all the effort is directed toward maintaining oxygenation, so the surgeon may have to work intermittently between periods when the lungs are fully inflated.

TETRALOGY OF FALLOT

In the tetralogy of Fallot the circulation time is prolonged. If an intravenous induction is used the sodium thiopental should be injected slowly, and great care must be taken to allow sufficient time for it to act.

GENERAL SURGERY

In cases with temperature elevations the patient is hydrated and taken to the operating room. The child is placed on a cooling mattress, and induction of anesthesia is accomplished using a high-oxygen technique. If the patient is prevented from becoming hypoxic, no complications from the hyperthermia will ensue. The temperature is brought to normal before the operation commences. Convulsions have not occurred when this procedure has been followed.

OPERATIONS INVOLVING THE LIVER

Blood loss can be massive in operations involving the liver. Should a partial hepatectomy be contemplated hypothermia may be indicated, since it is an excellent technique for preventing uncontrolled blood loss. Care should be taken that the inferior vena cava is not obstructed by a retractor. In patients with liver disease, care is taken to keep the PO_2 and PCO_2 within normal range. Drugs degraded in the liver should obviously be avoided.

OPERATIONS AROUND THE NECK, FACE, AND MOUTH

THYROGLOSSAL DUCT CYST

In operations for the removal of a thyroglossal duct cyst, an armored tube is used, and a Jensen gag is inserted into the mouth. Surgery is facilitated by the anesthesiologist's backing completely out of the field. When the surgeon wishes to know the depth of his dissection the Jensen gag is opened, and the anesthesiologist uses his finger to aid the surgeon in determining it.

ORTHOPEDIC SURGERY

The orthopedic patient most difficult to manage is the one undergoing extensive spinal fusion. Controlled respiration is essential because spontaneous ventilation is adversely affected by the operative procedure.

Position is extremely important in orthopedic procedures. It should be checked and rechecked throughout the operation.

PEDIATRIC NEUROSURGERY

The important facts to remember in pediatric neurosurgery are the following. The airway must be maintained under difficult circumstances. Armored tubes are of help, especially when the head is in extreme flexion, and they must be well secured. A means for mucus escape from the mouth and nose should be provided. The eyes must be protected, both by an ointment and by a hard protective covering. If the patient is to be in the sitting position, his legs are wrapped to prevent pooling of the blood. The alcohol-water circulating mattresses for temperature control are applied to a sufficient surface to ensure control of the temperature. All neurosurgical patients should be under controlled ventilation by an automatic ventilator, preferably one of the volume constant type. The ventilatory cycle is set in such a manner that within 30 to 60 seconds spontaneous respiration will occur when the machine is shut off. Thus, the respiratory cycle can still be used as a guide for the surgeon. Use of the ventilator precludes a buildup of carbon dioxide and the resulting congestion in the vessels of the brain. The danger of air embolism is minimized.

For premedication the standard table is followed. The narcotic is omitted in the comatose child. If the surgeon uses wet sponges an additional problem arises in estimating blood loss. He may also use large quantities of saline for irrigation. Measuring the hemoglobin content in the suction bottle aids in estimating the actual blood loss.

EYE, EAR, NOSE, AND THROAT OPERATIONS

All patients undergoing tonsillectomies should be intubated without exception. In ear operations, since epinephrine is used to control bleeding, methoxyfluorane is the anesthetic of choice.

In ophthalmic procedures adequate doses of atropine should be administered preoperatively and may even have to be repeated during the operation to prevent bradycardia from the ocular reflex.

LARYNGOSCOPY AND BRONCHOSCOPY

When laryngoscopy or bronchoscopy is performed the operator prefers to have unlimited access to the patient and an opportunity to view the larynx without any obstruction such as an endotracheal tube or catheters. This necessitates either undepressed spontaneous respiration or controlled respiration using a cuirass type of ventilator. The latter method is, on the whole, unsatisfactory in children. The anesthesiologist cannot control obstruction in the airway satisfactorily. Ventilation may be inadequate but not obviously so with the continued action of the respirator. The surgical requirements are further complicated when biopsy or such therapeutic procedures as the removal of papillomas are to be performed which require a considerable time for completion. The explosion hazards of electrical connections, light bulbs, and cautery or diathermy are considerable.

A technique was developed at The Children's Memorial Hospital which provides the surgeon with a patient who is breathing adequately and quietly during lengthy procedures on the larynx and trachea. There is no danger of explosion. It consists of local and general anesthesia with long acting methoxyflurane (Penthrane). Lengthy endoscopic procedures can be carried out during recovery from a prolonged methoxyfluorane induction. Premedication is usually confined to atropine sulfate to avoid respiratory depression. Induction is initiated either by a sleep dose of sodium thiopental or by halothane. The nitrous oxide and halothane are withdrawn after a few minutes and oxygen and methoxyflurane given until the jaw is relaxed; 4 percent lidocaine in a dose of 5 mg/kg of body weight is sprayed over the base of the tongue, the upper surface of the epiglottis, the piriform fossae, the larynx generally and each vocal cord separately, the posterior and anterior commissures, the lower surface of epiglottis, and the trachea. This is accomplished in two or three stages with intervals of a few minutes. Usually 20 minutes of satisfactory conditions will require a total induction time of 20 minutes using 1.5 percent methoxyflurane.

When there is considerable obstruction to the airway, as may be found in multiple papillomatosis of the larynx, one should be cognizant of the fact that the patient is hypoxic and that even slight respiratory depression by the anesthetic agent will tend to increase dead space. Therefore, the respirations should be assisted until respiratory exchange after relaxation is adequate. Vigilance is necessary to prevent respiratory depression.

BRONCHOGRAPHY

Anesthesia given in the x-ray department can be associated with several problems. These problems are minimal in a department that is close to a surgical suite which is completely equipped with anesthetic apparatus and in which anesthesia is frequently given; however, in a department that is not near the surgical suite, the following points must be remembered:

(1) Anesthetic equipment must be checked and fully maintained.

(2) An adequate supply of drugs must be on hand.

(3) Suction apparatus must be in the room.

(4) Skilled help in the management of such problems as massive blood loss and cardiovascular collapse is lacking and compounds the seriousness of this situation if it arises.

(5) Inordinately long, drawn-out procedures, particularly in premature babies and infants in air-conditioned departments, result in considerable heat loss, which must be monitored and then treated with portable thermal control mattresses, warm blankets, or the careful use of hot-water bottles.

(6) The postoperative journey through corridors and elevators to the recovery room or ward can be hazardous. A small portable foot pump suction apparatus is a necessity.

At all times there must be sufficient light available so that the patient can be observed. The danger in bronchography is that of flooding too much of the lung fields at any one time, which immediately causes hypoxia. This is prevented by careful placement of the contrast media. The introduction of the image intensification systems with television monitors has greatly facilitated bronchography and has been a great aid to the anesthesiologist in monitoring the procedure and the patient.

Any procedure in an x-ray department can be fraught with hazards. For example, following a carotid arteriogram a hematoma may compress the trachea. For the ventriculogram the patient is in the sitting position, and hypotensive episodes may arise which must be diagnosed and treated immediately.

DENTISTRY

Dental procedures that are related to anesthesiology management should be divided into two groups, pain-producing and non-pain-producing. In the former group are extractions and reconstruction of the alveolar ridges. In the latter group are repair and reconstruction of the teeth themselves. Surgical anesthesia is required for the painful operations, whereas very light anesthesia is called for in the others.

Nasal intubation is helpful in dental anesthesia, for it ensures an unobstructed operative field. A well-lubricated tube is placed inferior to the lower turbinate, and in this position hemorrhage is rare. Magill forceps are used to place the tube, under direct vision, into the larynx and trachea. The nasal tube should always be inspected carefully for foreign bodies after it has passed through the nares. An amazing collection of objects can be found in children's noses. In procedures that do not produce healing postoperatively an anesthetic local spray or anesthetic jelly can be used to obtund the laryngeal reflex. This allows the anesthesiologist to maintain a very light plane of anesthesia. At the end of any procedure the mouth and pharynx should be carefully inspected for foreign bodies. Only in extremely short procedures lasting only two or three minutes is intubation not used. Pharyngeal packs are frequently used to prevent blood and mucus from running down the edges of the nasal endotracheal tube. They should be kept reasonably clean and should be replaced at frequent intervals. The end of the pack should always be left outside the mouth and should have some means of identification, such as a metal ring, so that the pack is removed at the end of the procedure. All dental patients should be inspected by the anesthesiologist for foreign matter in the mouth and pharynx at the end of the procedure.

EMERGENCY AND UNSCHEDULED OPERATIONS

There are few conditions that demand emergency surgery. Uncontrolled hemorrhage and acute head injury may deserve immediate treatment, but in most types of acute pathology time must be taken to examine the child thoroughly for other illnesses or injuries, to treat shock or fluid imbalance, to administer sedatives and antibiotics, and to take any measures necessary to bring the child into suitable condition for anesthesia and operation.

It is extremely rare that a tracheostomy has to be done in an emergency. Usually an endotracheal tube can be put in position, thus terminating the emergency. It is only when one has failed to insert an endotracheal tube that a tracheostomy has to be done with alacrity.

THE FULL STOMACH

There are two factors to be considered in judging the most appropriate time to operate on a child who has eaten recently. One is the actual time of the meal, and the other is the time the accident occurred or the pain began. Digestion is apt to cease in the presence of pain, and gastric emptying may occur for four to six hours. A satisfactory routine is a four-hour interval between the last meal and the administration of anesthesia, but it does not guarantee an empty stomach. Gastric lavage is not of much help in the management of the child with the full stomach. Adequate large volume suction apparatus should be made available, and induction is begun either intravenously or by inhalation. The movement of the abdomen is carefully watched. The mask is frequently lifted from the patient's face to inspect for vomitus. If possible, intubation is carried out under the gaseous agent alone, but some anesthesiologists prefer to use a short acting relaxant and to intubate the patient very rapidly. Both these techniques are very dangerous, and the dexterity of the anesthesiologist is important. If aspiration occurs, a bronchoscopy is performed to clear the air passages.

Just as important as the insertion of the endotracheal tube is its removal. The child should be completely awake before the tube is removed, and again the large volume suction apparatus should be instantly available. The anesthesiologist should remain with the patient until the danger of aspiration has passed.

ACUTE OR CHRONIC RESPIRATORY DISEASE

There are occasions when surgery has to be performed in the presence of acute or chronic respiratory disease. These cases can be managed adequately if the basic rules of respiratory therapy are followed during the anesthetic management. Bronchial spasm can be controlled by the administration of intravenous hydrocortisone succinate sodium. Another useful method of treatment is the inhalation of an isopropylnorepinephrine (Isuprel) mist. This is accomplished either by introducing a Bird mainstream micronebulizer in the circuit or by incorporating an ultrasonic nebulizer.

MIST THERAPY DURING THE COURSE
OF AN ANESTHETIC

The most effective local therapy for obstructive lung disease is mist therapy. One third normal saline is nebulized in an ultrasonic nebulizer that is incorporated in the anesthetic circuit. The ultrasonic nebulizer is superior to the mechanical nebulizer because a gas flow is not necessary to generate the mist. Rather, ultrasonic energy is used to generate the mist, and no dilution of the anesthesia mixture by extraneous gas occurs. A good illustration of an obstructive lung disease is cystic fibrosis. In children with this disease it is best to try to avoid the use of atropine sulfate, but entrance to veins should be readily accessible and atropine sulfate administered intravenously at the first signs of bradycardia from reflex action. It is well to use ultrasonically produced mist therapy during long procedures on these children.

BLOOD DYSCRASIAS AND
LEUKEMIA

It is best to avoid intubation where there is a possibility of a bleeding tendency. A patient with such a defect has to be assessed on an individual basis in relation to the surgery to be performed.

DIABETES

The anesthesiologic management of diabetic children is similar to that of diabetic adults. Usually the patient is established on NPH insulin prior to the operation. Should this be accomplished on the day of the operation, the patient receives half of his daily dose of NPH insulin one hour prior to operation, and 5 percent glucose in water is administered through the procedure at an appropriate rate of 5 ml/kg. Following the operation the second half of the insulin is administered.

CONCLUSION

Pediatric anesthesiology can be successfully accomplished if enough attention is paid to detail. Constant vigilance is necessary for good patient care.

DAVID ALLAN

8

Inhalation Therapy

Inhalation therapy is an old science, the first institute of pneumotaxics having been formed in Bristol, England, in the nineteenth century. Interest in inhalation therapy waned, but in the last few years it has undergone a revival. In the practice of pediatric inhalation therapy there have been some important advances, particularly in the methods of humidification, nebulization, continuous and intermittent positive pressure respiration, hyperbaric oxygenation, and sterilization of equipment. Inhalation therapy is mainly achieved by quantitative alteration of the respired atmosphere. Its aim is to provide adequate cellular oxygenation and carbon dioxide elimination. The atmosphere is modified mainly by the percentage of oxygen being altered, water content being changed, therapeutic agents being introduced as mists, and the pressure of the atmosphere being increased.

OXYGEN

Soon after Joseph Priestley's discovery of oxygen in 1772 and Antoine Lavoisier's elucidation of respiration, oxygen therapy was introduced in England by James Beddoes. James Watt, engineer and inventor of the steam engine, was Beddoes' collaborator, and they were assisted by Sir Humphrey Davy. Their publication in 1794 in Bristol of "Considerations of the Medicinal Use and Production of Facetious Airs" can be regarded as the beginning of inhalation therapy. Exces-

sive enthusiasm and indiscriminate therapeutic applications led to many failures, and it was not until scientific investigations were made by such men as J. S. Haldane, A. V. Hill, and Sir Joseph Barcroft that oxygen therapy was placed on a sound physiological groundwork.

Hypoxia is a broad term indicating deprivation of oxygen regardless of etiology or site. It can arise from a variety of causes. Since methods of treatment are closely allied to etiology, the administration of oxygen infrequently corrects the basic defect. Rather, oxygen is applied as a stopgap until more fundamental measures can be instituted or can become effective or because specific therapy for the underlying disease is unavailable. In this capacity, administration of oxygen can be lifesaving. To facilitate the better application of oxygen therapy, Comroe and Dripps classified hypoxia into five categories: (1) delivery of an inadequate amount of oxygen to normal lung tissue, (2) inadequate pulmonary function, (3) venous-arterial shunts, (4) inadequate transport of oxygen by the circulation, and (5) inadequate tissue oxygenation. Using such a classification, the identification of disease entities producing hypoxia and their treatment with oxygen therapy is not difficult.

The diagnosis of hypoxia is problematic because the signs and symptoms are nonspecific and variable. Changes can occur in the respiratory, cardiovascular, and central nervous systems, as well as in other tissues and in metabolism. Blood oxygen transfer may be altered, with cyanosis sometimes being produced. Cyanosis is an unreliable guide to the arterial oxygen saturation, since it only signifies 5 g percent of reduced hemoglobin in the arterial blood. This represents an oxygen saturation of 67 percent when a normal hemoglobin level, 15 g percent in the adult, is present. However, when anemia lowers the hemoglobin to 10 g percent in the adult, then cyanosis is not apparent until the arterial blood circulation has decreased to 50 percent. The ability to recognize mild cyanosis varies from observer to observer.

Oxygen saturation and content of blood is related to the oxygen tension (PO_2), as illustrated by the oxygen dissociation curve (Fig. 1). A shifting of the curve either to the right or to the left by changes in the patient's partial pressure of carbon dioxide or by changes in his temperature and acid-base status should be noted. Infants particularly can become hypoxic from the oxygen dissociation curve's being moved to the left by

falls in temperature. The oxygen tension of the blood is reduced when (1) the partial pressure of oxygen in the inspired air is lowered, (2) the amount of oxygen delivered to the alveoli per minute is below physiological requirements, (3) the exchange of oxygen across the alveolar membrane is inadequate because of a mechanical block or a deficiency of surfactant-like substances, or (4) there is a venous-arterial (right-to-left) shunt. There are other conditions in which the blood PO_2 is normal, but either the oxygen content is low or the rate of oxygen delivery to the tissues is inadequate.

Hypoxia stimulates both the rate and the depth of respiration through the carotid and aortic bodies. This hyperpnea produces a fall in arterial carbon dioxide tension, which may in turn produce changes of its own. Hypoxia and dyspnea are not necessarily associated. Dyspnea usually occurs when the respiratory minute volume reaches approximately 50 percent of the maximal breathing capacity. There are many causes of dyspnea

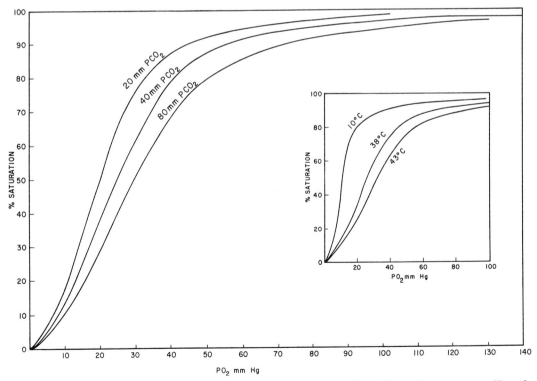

Fig. 1. Oxygen dissociation curve, interrelated with oxygen tension. The effects of temperature, pH, and carbon dioxide pressures are included.

other than hypoxia, and thus the indication for oxygen therapy is not dyspnea but hypoxia. When oxygen is given to a patient who has both hypoxia and dyspnea, therapy should not be stopped if oxygen fails to relieve the dyspnea.

Acute hypoxia results in an increase in heart rate, but in the infant this tachycardia is transient and consequently often undetected. Therefore, bradycardia is used as an index for hypoxia in the infant. The sign of hypoxia which is most often overlooked involves the central nervous system and is expressed as irritability. The use of sedatives under these circumstances is unwise.

Normally, inspired air contains 21 percent oxygen. At a barometric pressure of 760 mm Hg, this represents a partial pressure or tension of 159 mm Hg of oxygen in the inspired air. However, oxygen uptake and dilution with water vapor and carbon dioxide reduce the PO_2 in the alveoli to about 100 mm Hg. There is a small tension differential between alveolar gas and arterial blood, resulting in a normal arterial PO_2 of about 90 mm Hg (96 percent saturation). The inhalation of oxygen at one or more atmospheres of pressure raises the arterial PO_2 many times beyond its normal value and may lead to functional disturbances of tissues so exposed. Oxygen is carried by the circulating blood, mainly as oxyhemoglobin, with a small amount dissolved in physical solution. The effects of the inhalation of a high concentration of oxygen on the nitrogen concentration and carbon dioxide transport are important. Alveolar air contains 80 percent nitrogen. Since gases in the alveoli are in equilibrium with the blood, many liters of nitrogen are in solution in the body fluids and cavities. The partial pressure of nitrogen in the alveoli falls rapidly if oxygen is inhaled. Nitrogen diffuses from the body tissues into the blood and is eliminated by the lungs, a process by which almost the total nitrogen content of the body can be washed out if the oxygen therapy is administered for a sufficient period of time. Carbon dioxide is carried by the blood mostly in the form of bicarbonate. The transfer occurs readily when a hydrogen ion acceptor is available, as happens in the capillaries when oxyhemoglobin is converted to reduced hemoglobin, which is a stronger base and therefore a superior hydrogen ion acceptor. When a large amount of oxygen is carried in simple solution, as in hydrogen ion acceptor. When a large amount ically dissolved oxygen alone may be sufficient to satisfy tissue oxygen uptake requirements (e.g., 3 atmospheres of pressure), but because little or no oxygen is extracted from oxyhemoglobin the necessary quantity of reduced hemoglobin required for efficient carbon dioxide transport in the bloodstream is not available. When 100 percent oxygen is administered there is also a loss of sensitivity in the chemoreceptors. This is not usually significant unless the situation is magnified, as in hyperbaric oxygenation. Cardiac output can be reduced 15 percent by the administration of 100 percent oxygen.

THERAPEUTIC USES

Indications for oxygen therapy can be discussed in relation to the five categories previously given for the classification of hypoxia.

(1) Delivery of inadequate amount of oxygen to normal lungs: When there is an obstruction to breathing, and consequently inadequate oxygenation of the lungs (e.g., bronchial constriction), oxygen therapy can be of great value.

(2) Inadequate oxygenation because of abnormal pulmonary function: The chief indications for oxygen therapy are those associated with inadequate oxygenation of the blood resulting from abnormal pulmonary function. This is especially true when hypoxia is the result of poor diffusion of oxygen across the alveolar capillary membrane. Diffusion of gases through this membrane depends largely on water solubility, which is 20 times as great for carbon dioxide as it is for oxygen. Pulmonary edema and pulmonary fibrosis change the rate of diffusion of oxygen, which is proportional to the partial pressure differences of oxygen existing across

the alveolar capillary membrane. Therefore, oxygen inhalation can, within limits, overcome a diffusion defect.

(3) Venous-arterial shunts: Shunting of blood on the whole results in arterial desaturation. This is defined as a ventilation perfusion defect. Hypoxia can be corrected under these circumstances by oxygen inhalation only if the amount of shunting is very small owing to the constant dilution of arterial blood with desaturated venous blood. Hyperbaric oxygenation, of course, can improve the situation to some extent.

(4) Inadequate arterial transport of oxygen: Oxygen therapy is a valuable adjunct to the treatment of certain types of circulatory disorders. The oxygen therapy for carbon monoxide poisoning accelerates the conversion of carboxyhemoglobin to oxyhemoglobin. Hyperbaric oxygenation leads to increased transport of the gas in physical solution. This additional oxygen carried in the plasma in physical solution under normal or elevated pressures could be extremely valuable as an adjunct in the treatment of anemia and shock.

(5) Inadequate tissue oxygenation: Oxygen administration can help to satisfy abnormally high tissue demands, such as in thyrotoxicosis. Perhaps surgeons could make use of oxygen therapy in the treatment of intestinal obstruction, paralytic ileus, and postoperative distension. The gas that accumulates in the bowel is largely composed of nitrogen. The blood can retrieve little of this nitrogen, for it has already been exposed in the lungs to an atmosphere containing 80 percent nitrogen under normal circumstances. If, however, 100 percent oxygen is breathed, the partial pressure of nitrogen in the alveoli falls, and nitrogen will diffuse from the blood into the inhaled gases. As the nitrogen content of the blood decreases, the gas in the intestine diffuses into the circulation and is eliminated through the lungs. The same reasoning can be applied to the patient who is having difficulty after a pneumoencephalogram. Air can be largely eliminated by the inhalation of 100 percent oxygen. Subcutaneous emphysema may also be reduced by the same technique.

HYPERBARIC OXYGENATION

Professor Charles Illingworth of the University of Glasgow, a student of hyperbaric oxygenation, believes that more research is needed to assess the place of hyperbaric oxygenation in therapy. The effects of 1 to 4 atmospheres of oxygen on patients have been investigated in Scotland, Holland, and the United States. Hyperbaric oxygenation at 1 to 2 atmospheres is the treatment of choice in carbon monoxide poisoning. The patients are placed in mobile chambers, and in 20 minutes many are awake and well. Its use in circulatory disturbances, respiratory difficulties, and anaerobic and aerobic infections is still being evaluated.

ADEQUATE OXYGEN THERAPY

In the sick child increased physiological shunting is frequently present, in varying degrees. The shunting may be one of three types: either a portion of the cardiac output bypasses a certain area of the pulmonary capillaries, or a portion of the cardiac output perfuses nonventilating alveoli (atelectasis), or a combination of both occurs. It is thus impossible to predict the arterial oxygenation that can be achieved by a given inspired concentration of oxygen. The optimal concentration of oxygen is one which allows maximum use of the oxygen-carrying capacity of arterial blood. This should result in an oxygen tension of at least 100 to 150 mm Hg, and the hemoglobin content should be such that at this tension the arterial oxygen content should be a minimum of 15 to 20 ml per 100 ml of blood.

COMPLICATIONS OF OXYGEN ADMINISTRATION

ATELECTASIS

The administration of oxygen, particularly of more than one atmosphere of pressure, can cause such undesirable effects as pulmonary atelectasis. When the alveoli of the lungs are filled with oxygen, subsequent alveolar obstruction may result because of complete absorption of the gas with a consequent alveolar collapse. A similar sequence of events occurs when the body cavities are filled with oxygen and this pathway of exchange to the atmosphere becomes obstructed. However, this should not prevent the use of a high concentration of oxygen when indicated.

OXYGEN APNEA

If the response of the respiratory centers to carbon dioxide is depressed and respiration is mainly activated by the carotid and aortic body receptors, the administration of oxygen may cause apnea. In this case controlled artificial respiration is mandatory.

RETROLENTAL FIBROPLASIA

Retrolental fibroplasia is caused by extreme proliferation and secondary shutdown of the capillaries in the retina. It occurs in some premature infants who have been exposed to high concentrations of oxygen at birth. Retinal changes may begin to appear between the third and sixth weeks of life. It should be emphasized that it is the cerebral arterial PO_2, not the inspired PO_2, that is of importance in the etiology of this disease. Thus, a cyanotic infant in the premature group should not be deprived of oxygen for fear of causing retrolental fibroplasia. The limitation of the inspired oxygen concentration to 35 to 40 percent should serve as a guide to the oxygen therapy of the noncyanotic premature. Retrolental fibroplasia has occurred when the oxygen concentration has been limited to 21 percent, which is the concentration of the ambient atmosphere.

OXYGEN POISONING

A high concentration of oxygen administered for about 12 hours or longer can irritate the respiratory tract and produce mild pulmonary congestion, transudation, and exudation, which may progress to atelectasis. This syndrome is not experienced in subjects breathing less than 50 percent oxygen or in those breathing 100 percent oxygen at half atmospheres for 24 hours or longer. Thus, it is assumed that the important factor in the causation of this symptom complex is the oxygen tension, not the concentration of oxygen in the inhaled gas. In the devices used in pediatric inhalation therapy, 50 percent oxygen is rarely exceeded. The central nervous system is affected by pure oxygen inhaled at a pressure greater than 2 atmospheres. This type of oxygen toxicity is being evaluated at present.

METHODS OF ADMINISTRATION

MASKS

To increase the percentage of oxygen in the atmosphere, masks of simple design with expiratory ports may be used (Fig. 2).

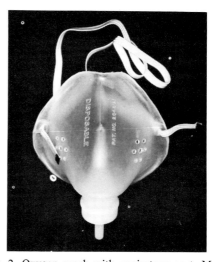

Fig. 2. Oxygen mask with expiratory port. Masks of simple design with expiratory ports may be used to increase the percentage of oxygen in the atmosphere.

Should 100 percent be required, masks of the Rendell-Baker-Soucek type are needed with an Ayre's valveless system or a nonre-

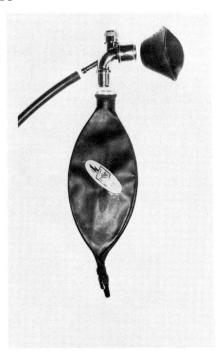

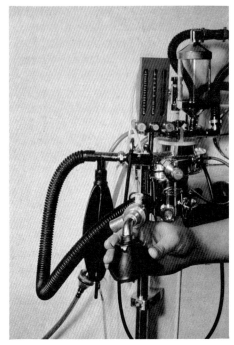

Fig. 3. Rendell-Baker mask, Rendell-Baker kidney piece, bag, and oxygen inlet. Masks of the Rendell-Baker type are needed with an Ayre's valveless system to produce 100 percent oxygen.

Fig. 4. Mask elbow, Sierra nonrebreathing valve, angle hose and T piece bag. A nonrebreathing valve of the Sierra type provides another means of supplying 100 percent oxygen.

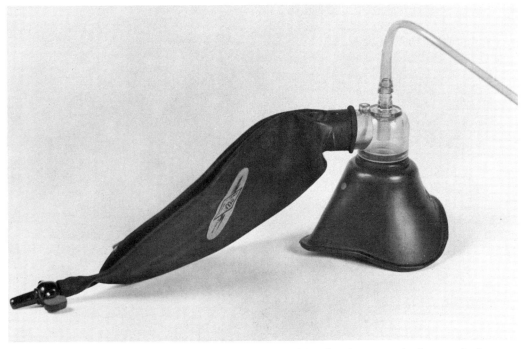

Fig. 5. Rigid Hustead-Browne valve with mask and bag. This valve shows promise in resuscitation.

breathing valve (Figs. 3 and 4). A new system has recently been introduced for use with masks, and preliminary studies indicate that this rigid elbow shows promise in resuscitation (Fig. 5).

Face hoods and nasal catheters have little or no place in pediatric inhalation therapy.

TENTS

The requirements of an efficient oxygen tent are the following: (1) It should be possible to vary the volume of a tent according to the size of the child. (2) It should be possible to raise the side rails of the cribs to the fullest extent. (3) The temperature of the environment of the child should be controllable. (4) The elimination of carbon dioxide should be efficient. (5) Humidification in the tent should be 100 percent, and the particle size of the mist should be 1μ to 8μ, with no particles over 10μ, which will condense and wet the patient. (6) If a mechanical nebulizer is selected for humidifica-

tion, it should be possible to drive it by either oxygen or compressed air. If an ultrasonic nebulizer is used, it should be possible to scavenge the nebulizer cup by either oxygen or compressed air. Both the mechanical nebulizers and the ultrasonic nebulizers should have variably controlled outputs. (7) Everything in contact with the patient should be either disposable or autoclavable.

It is vitally important that inhalation therapy equipment should not be a source of infection. Gas sterilization is the only possible method of adequately sterilizing an oxygen tent that recirculates the tent environmental gases through the basic machinery, but it is impractical for large units. A pediatric air-oxygen tent was devised at The Children's Memorial Hospital based on the adult aquastream oxygen tent, which is a nonrecirculating tent with a one-way, high flow gas system. If the flow is set at 13 per minute, carbon dioxide does not build up in the canopy. The Allan-Walsh Children's Memorial Hospital Mark I and II air-oxy-

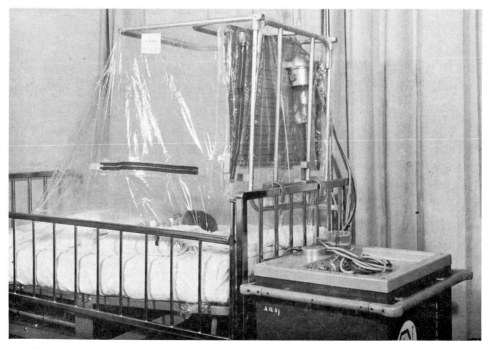

Fig. 6. Allan-Walsh tent fitted to a fully elevated adult-size bed. The tent is at its maximum size. There is an ultrasonic nebulizer on top of the console. Holes have been made in the canopy. The aquastream Allan-Walsh tent can be used for adults because the volume of the tent can be varied according to the size of the patient. The De Vilbiss ultrasonic nebulizer is used to augment the mist therapy.

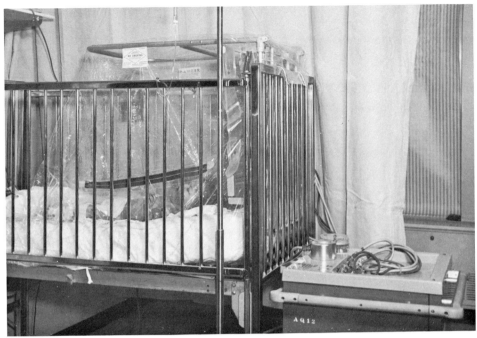

Fig. 7. Allan-Walsh tent fitted to a crib. The canopy is kept as small as possible. With the aquastream Allan-Walsh pediatric air-oxygen tent, it is possible to raise the side rails of the cribs to the fullest extent, as shown. The temperature of the environment can be controlled. The high flow of gas eliminates carbon dioxide. The mechanical nebulizer or ultrasonic nebulizer can be driven by either oxygen or compressed air. The output can be varied.

gen tents provide all the requirements for a suitable pediatric air-oxygen tent. From the illustrations it can be seen that it is possible to vary the volume of a tent according to the size of the patient (Fig. 6). The side rails of the cribs can be raised to the fullest extent (Fig. 7). The heat exchanger ensures that the temperature environment of the child is controlled. When the Mistogen mechanical nebulizer is driven by 13 liters of oxygen through a jet of 0.0025 mm, an output of 2 g per minute is obtained, and the particle size distribution of the mist is from 1μ to 8μ, with no particles over 10μ. Thus, no raining out occurs to wet the patient. The canopies are disposable and are 2-mm thick, which prevents the canopy from being drawn onto the patient's face. Everything else in contact with the patient, the frame, the heat exchanger, the nebulizer, and the leads to the nebulizer and heat exchanger can be autoclaved (Fig. 8). (Any lead to a nebulizer should be sterilized because when the gas flow is shut off there is a backflow of liquids that may

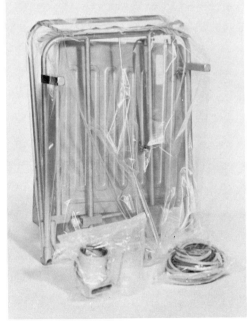

Fig. 8. Heat-back exchanger and Mistogen and tubing leads packaged in plastic. Anything in contact with the patient should be either disposable or autoclavable. The leads to the nebulizer should be sterilized because when the gas flow is shut off there is a backflow of liquid that could contaminate the tubing.

contaminate the tubing.) These oxygen tents have been in use for two years and have proved to be efficient and reliable.

A new method of oxygen tent therapy using the De Vilbiss ultrasonic nebulizer combined with a half-top canopy and with the nebulizer cup's being scavenged with oxygen is presently being investigated (Fig. 9). The dense aerosol itself acts as the heat exchanger. In all oxygen tents the percentage of oxygen in the atmosphere cannot be increased over 40 or 50 percent. Should higher concentration be required, mask therapy is indicated. Oxygen concentration analyzers must be frequently used to check the actual concentration in the tent. Another method of obtaining high oxygen concentration when a tracheostomy has been performed is to scavenge an ultrasonic nebulizer with a 15 liter flow of oxygen and direct it to a tracheostomy collar. This results in a concentration of oxygen of 80 percent.

Oxygen should be humidified, not administered as a dry gas.

The rationale on which the use of humidifiers and nebulizers is based involves the physics of fluids and gases and the physiology and pathology of the respiratory system.

The actual mass of water contained in a certain volume of air is known as the absolute humidity. There is a limit to the amount of moisture that a volume of air can hold at a given temperature, and this is defined as the maximum humidity of the air. Humidity deficit is the difference between maximum humidity and absolute humidity at any given temperature. The amount of moisture air contains varies directly with the temperature; that is, it increases with a rise in temperature and decreases with a fall. Relative humidity is defined as the ratio between the mass of vapor actually present in the atmosphere and the maximum that the atmosphere is capable of holding at a given temperature.

To saturate a dry gas at 30° C, 44 mg of water must be added for each liter of gas. This corresponds to approximately 650 g per 24 hours at a minute volume of ten liters.

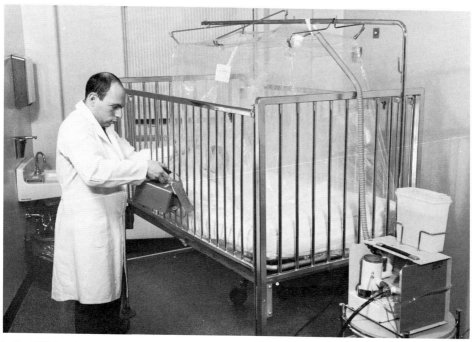

Fig. 9. De Vilbiss ultrasonic nebulizer combined with a half-top canopy and with oxygen scavenging the nebulizer cup. This machine produces such a dense aerosol that it itself acts as the heat exchanger. When the nebulizing cup is scavenged with oxygen a very dense layer of aerosol is produced. This is presently being assessed as a means of increasing the oxygen in the atmosphere along with producing mist therapy.

Because the water content of a saturated gas depends on its temperature, the amount of water must be increased from 18 mg/l to 44 mg/1 on heating the gas from 21° C to 37° C. The heat loss of evaporation must also be considered, since it causes the temperature of the humidifier reservoir to fall below the surrounding temperatures.

Density and buoyancy are important factors affecting suspension of particles. Density is defined as the ratio of the mass of a body to its volume. Therefore, the lower the temperature of a gas at a constant pressure, the greater its density. Archimedes' principle states that all bodies completely or partially immersed in a fluid are buoyed up by a force equal to the weight of the fluid displaced. Therefore, if the weight of a body is less than the weight of the fluid it displaces, the body will float. Gases and fluids are governed by the same laws.

Viscosity, defined as the internal resistance to deformation of a fluid, plays the paramount role in determining the laminar flow rate of a substance through a tube. In turbulent flows the density of the fluid rather than the viscosity plays the important role in determining volume flow rate.

Room air normally has a humidity deficit. When the air is inspired, it is warmed from approximately 21° C to 37° C in the proximal airways. This further increases the humidity deficit, for even if the air were fully saturated at 21° C, heating it to the body temperature would produce a humidity deficit. Normal humidification of inspired air is accomplished by the mucous membrane of the nasopharynx. The mucous membrane of the oropharynx plays an insignificant role in this process. Following a tracheostomy a secondary mechanism develops in the tracheobronchial tree and substitutes for the bypassed nasopharynx. It consists of a gradual change in the ability of the tracheobronchial mucosa to provide humidification. In the adult, 1 liter of water is used in 24 hours to supply this humidifying mechanism; in a child there is a higher requirement per square meter of body surface because of the higher metabolic rate. Diseases producing pyrexia and increased minute volume further increase the demand.

Normal humidification can be bypassed by rerouting the inspired air through an endotracheal tube or a tracheostomy. Infection, allergy, or injury of the nasopharyngeal mucous membrane may have a direct effect on humidification. In the patient with tracheobronchitis the cilia are directly involved and require additional lubrication to retain mobility. Under these circumstances the humidifying mechanism is subjected to an increased demand. The importance of ciliary activity related to the airway size in infants is frequently overlooked. The resistance of the neonatal airway is 30 cm of water per liter per second compared to that of the adult, which is 2 cm of water per liter per second. The size of the neonatal tracheobronchial tree is directly related to the increased resistance.

The consistency of dried mucus is similar in the neonate and the adult. The adult has a relatively large airway and can better tolerate the obstruction caused by dry secretion than can the infant with his smaller system. Humidification is the most effective method of preventing such obstruction. The size of the smaller bronchi in the infant is so critical that swelling of the mucous membrane alone can lead to atelectasis.

An endotracheal tube is constantly in motion, and adequate humidification serves as a lubricant to prevent trauma of the larynx and trachea. This is important in the prolonged use of nasotracheal intubation in attempts to avoid tracheostomy. The advantage of such intubation is still under assessment.

It is important to realize that humidity is gaseous water in a carrier gas, whereas mist therapy is actual particulate water suspended as a mass in the carrier gas. It is rare to have less than 100 percent relative humidity below the carina, even in the tracheostomized patient. Thus, humidification per se can be supplied only to the upper airway. On the other hand, mist therapy can be applied to any part of the airway. A humidifier can supply humidity, whereas a nebulizer supplies both mist therapy and humidity, since evaporation takes place from the surface of each particle of water.

MIST THERAPY

Mist therapy is the inhalation of particulate matter, and where the particles are deposited depends on physical factors. The primary mechanism for the deposition of large particles in the 8μ to 10μ range is inertial impaction. Very small particles under 1μ are deposited by Brownian motion. Particles from 1μ to 8μ are deposited by sedimentation. The site of deposit of a particle largely depends on its size. However, it should not be overlooked that the tracheobronchial tree is in itself a baffling system. Thus, a discussion of the particle size produced by any nebulizer is largely academic, since the mist is promptly baffled by the tracheobronchial tree. Mist therapy is in all probability the most important therapeutic means available

for the treatment of such obstructive lung disease as cystic fibrosis. The mist must be of sufficient density that despite heating to 37° C, 100 percent humidification will be maintained. Surface area is directly proportional to evaporation. One method to ensure 100 percent humidification is to decrease vapor tension (i.e., raise the boiling point of the water) by adding 10 percent propylene glycol. Water will then evaporate normally from the mucous membrane but not from the treated particle. In both children and adults, consideration must be given to the quantity as well as the quality of the mist. The mist produced by efficient mechanical nebulizers has a wide range of particle size, with a predominance of particles of from 1μ to 8μ. These mixed mists are unstable and have a high incidence of undesirable rain-out. On the other hand, mists produced by an ultrasonic nebulizer are extremely stable because the particles are reasonably uniform in size. It is theoretically possible to produce a mist that is sufficiently dense and stable without the addition of 10 percent propylene

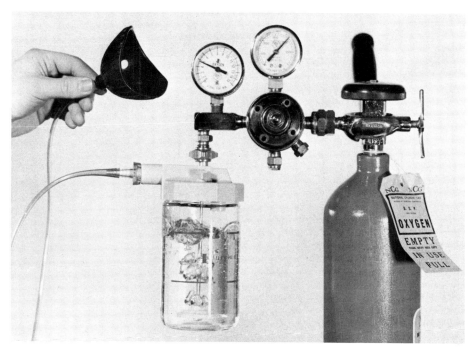

Fig. 10. Emergency oxygen setup with bubble humidifier. Oxygen for mask therapy should be passed through a bubble humidifier.

glycol and which can be deposited in a particular segment of the tracheobronchial tree.

METHODS OF HUMIDIFYING AND PRODUCING MIST THERAPY

HUMIDIFIERS

In all humidifiers the gas to be humidified passes over a large surface area of water. The humidity produced is in gaseous form without particulate matter. This process may be amplified by bubbling the gas through the water or passing it through a grid. Oxygen for mask therapy is passed through a bubble humidifier that will provide 21 percent saturation at body temperature (Fig. 10). One can increase the efficacy of a humidifier by raising the temperature of the water and thus augmenting evaporation from the surface. A heated humidifier can prevent a humidity deficit when an aerosol is introduced into the body by bringing the tem-

perature of the aerosol above body temperature and by allowing for precipitation when its temperature drops to that of the body. The heating element in the Mivab humidifier on the Engström respirator has a constant heat production, whereas the Puritan cascade heated humidifier has a variable and controllable temperature output (Figs. 11 and 12). In a heated humidifier, humidification is supplied independently of gas generation, and the resultant vapor is carried to the patient by the ventilatory gas flow. The output of the humidifier will vary in relation to the ventilatory gas flow, temperature of the water, room temperature, and relative humidity of the ambient air. Therefore, it cannot be a quantitative method of humidification. In a closed system a heated humidifier can supply an adequate quality of humidification to infants and small children, but these are the patients whose humidifica-

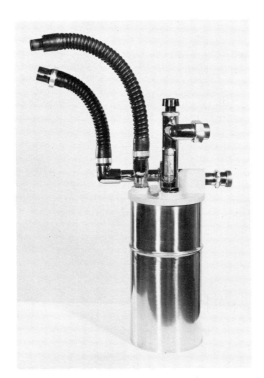

Fig. 11. Mivab heated humidifier on the Engström respirator. It has a constant heat production.

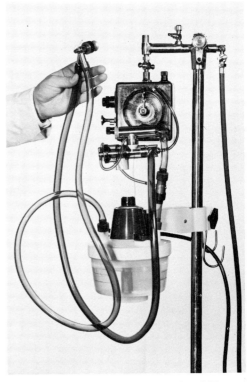

Fig. 12. Puritan cascade heated humidifier on Bird Mark VIII respirator. The humidifier has a variable and controllable temperature output. The temperature should be monitored at the entrance to the patient.

tion requirements are critical and should be supplied by a quantitative method that does not dilute the ventilatory mixture. It may be possible to overhydrate an infant by over-humidifying the atmosphere, especially in a closed circuit. When a heated humidifier is used, it is mandatory to monitor the temperature of the vapor at the patient, not at the humidifier. This temperature should be maintained at or below 105° F at the patient's level.

We put great emphasis on the differentiation between a humidifier and a nebulizer, not only to show the difference between humidification and mist therapy but also to illustrate the difference between a humidifier and a nebulizer in regard to their potential ability to infect patients. In our study of bacteriological kinetics we have not found it possible to transfer bacteria from a humidifier to the patient's direct environment. We believe that this is so because a humidifier only supplies a gas in the carrying gas—no particulate matter is moved. No matter how much the large humidifier, the Air-Shields Isolette C-86 Intensive Care Model with ISC control, is contaminated, we have not been able to trace the contaminants to the immediate environment of the patient. This is in contrast to our experience in studying the bacteriological kinetics of nebulizers.

NEBULIZERS

VENTURI MECHANISMS

The Bernoulli theory states that if a tube is constricted and a gas is allowed to flow through the tube, negative pressure will be created at the point of constriction. Venturi used this theory in designing a mechanism to draw water up into a tube. This type of mechanism, illustrated by the Mistogen nebulizer, requires high gas flows to generate the mist (Fig. 13). Even the best of these nebulizers do not have outputs greater than 2 g of water per minute. When the water is displaced from the reservoir, unfiltered air is introduced into the container. If a compres-

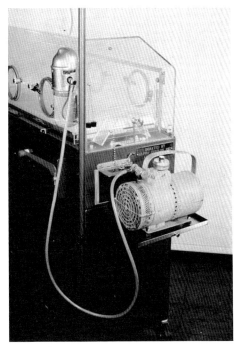

Fig. 13. Mistogen nebulizer being driven by a compressor. The Mistogen mechanical nebulizer with a 1/25,000 jet has a variable and controllable output. High flows of gas are necessary to drive this nebulizer efficiently.

sor is used to drive this nebulizer, another potential source of contaminents is added. There will be a backflow into the leads from the nebulizer when the compressor is switched off. Solutes are concentrated in the reservoir jar, and these may include bacteria that will propagate. Therefore, such nebulizers should be autoclaved and used under sterile conditions. The output of such a mechanical nebulizer depends on the flow, diameter, and length of the jet orifice. The most efficient jet is 0.0025 mm in diameter and has a flow of 13 liters per minute. A compressor that produces such a flow through this small jet is unpleasantly noisy and under certain circumstances may cause damage to the infant's middle ear. The noise level that infants in incubators are subjected to when compressor-driven nebulizers are used is twice the maximum tolerated by the standards of the steel fabricating industry.

The Air-Shields Venturi nebulizer has a lower output than the Mistogen and overcomes the problem of the introduction of unfiltered air by using air from the incubator that has been filtered (Fig. 14). Unfor-

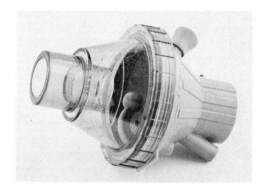

Fig. 15. Mainstream Bird mechanical micronebulizer. This machine operates on a Venturi principle, with the jet stream blowing tiny droplets off the tip of the capillary tube, driving them against a solid object, and causing them to disintegrate into particles.

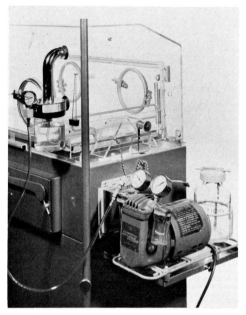

Fig. 14. Air-Shields mechanical nebulizer for use with isolettes. Displaced air is drawn from the incubator itself and this is filtered free of microorganisms.

tunately this nebulizer was designed for use with a pressure gauge, which makes the apparatus unautoclavable. Cold sterilizing of this equipment is inefficient because air locks make it impossible for the sterilizing solution to penetrate into the jet. Acetic acid has been used to sterilize this type of nebulizer, with questionable results.

MAINSTREAM MECHANICAL NEBULIZER

A mainstream mechanical nebulizer consists of a capillary tube partially submerged in the fluid to be nebulized and a jet orifice that passes a gas stream across the tip of the capillary tube, thereby creating a negative pressure at this point (Venturi principle) and thus sucking the fluid up in the capillary

tube (Fig. 15). The jet stream blows tiny droplets off the tip of the capillary tube, driving them against a solid object and causing them to disintegrate into particles of sizes determined by the structural design and by the inlet pressure. The jet stream necessary to drive the nebulizer dilutes the ventilatory mixture that reaches the patient, so the exact amount of each constituent of the aerosol mixture is unknown. Since the greatest advance in ventilation in the past two decades has been the change from qualitative to quantitative techniques, this gain should not be negated by an inadequate humidifying mechanism. Nebulization must be independent of gas flow, and the amount of water nebulized must be measurable. The mainstream mechanical nebulizer has serious deficits, for even the best model cannot produce more than 70 percent humidity.

SIDEARM MECHANICAL NEBULIZER

The sidearm mechanical nebulizer is built on the same principle as the mainstream type, but its efficiency is low, having an output of no more than 16 percent relative humidity (Fig. 16). To overcome this deficit the nebulizer could be pressurized to increase the output considerably, but the other serious deficits mentioned above would still remain.

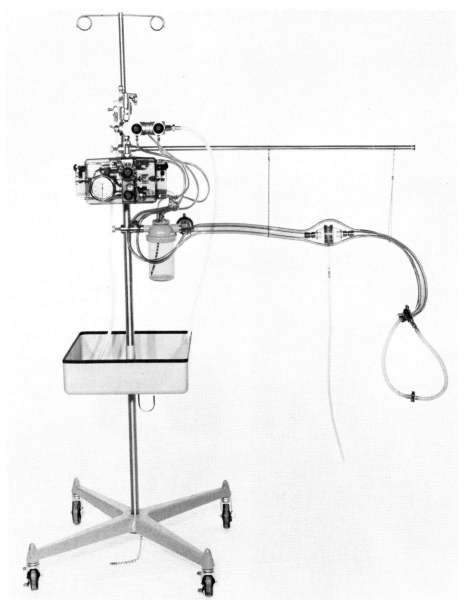

Fig. 16. Pressurized Bird sidearm mechanical nebulizer. To increase the output of aerosol the nebulizer may be pressurized.

OTHER NEBULIZERS

There are other types of mechanical nebulizers working on the principle of the water droplets being shattered, either by a gas flow propelling them against baffles or by centrifugal force pulling them to the sides of a container. All types have serious defects —low outputs, lack of mist density, inability to be sterilized, and, in some, dilution of ventilating mixtures caused by the high gas flow necessary to generate the mist.

ULTRASONIC NEBULIZER

The invention of the ultrasonic nebulizer has made possible an advance in pediatric respiratory therapy. Comparison of ultrasonic nebulization with other methods of aerosol generation illustrates how this was accomplished.

The ultrasonic nebulizer consists of a generator with a 110 v input line. This generator supplies a known amount of electric energy to a piezo-electric crystal which transforms the electric power into ultrasonic energy. The crystal vibrates at or near its inherent frequency—for example, 1.3 mc in the De Vilbiss, 1.4 mc in the Mistogen, and 3 mc in the Mivab. To obtain a large output of mist in the De Vilbiss unit, a focused crystal is employed in addition to a lens system. The way the ultrasonic energy produces mist is unknown and is the subject of much controversy. The aerosol produced by the ultrasonic nebulizer is independent of gas flow. Gas is necessary only to remove the aerosol from the nebulizing chamber. In the De Vilbiss unit all air from the blower system can be filtered free of microorganisms, and the fluid input can be a closed system. The nebulizing cup and the outlets can both be autoclaved (Fig. 17). The Mistogen apparatus can also be autoclaved (Fig. 18). The output of the Mivab ultrasonic nebulizer can be varied from 0 to 0.72 ml per minute (Fig. 19). Herzog and his colleagues devised a nomogram in an attempt to quantitate the fluid requirements of the respiratory tract (Fig. 20). Unfortunately, when the studies were performed an additional Engström heated humidifier was left in the circuit. As

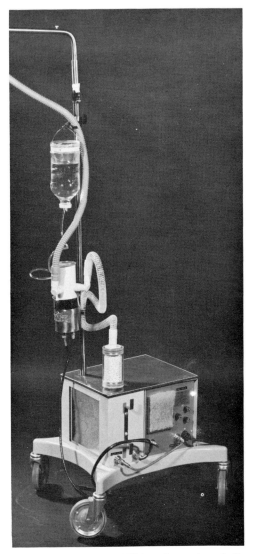

Fig. 17. The new De Vilbiss ultrasonic nebulizer on its own cart. A half-top canopy is being used. All air from the blower system can be filtered free of microorganisms, and fluid input can be a closed system. The nebulizing cup and the outlets can both be autoclaved.

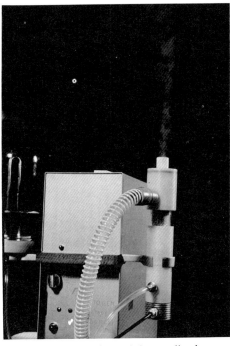

Fig. 18. Mistogen unit used for medicating a patient. Drugs may be nebulized by the ultrasonic nebulizer.

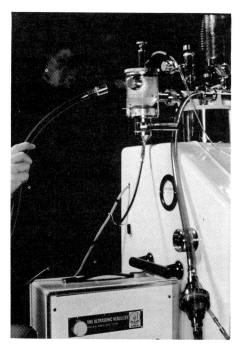

Fig. 19. Mivab ultrasonic nebulizer, developed for use with the Engström respirator, as shown.

has been already pointed out, the output of a heated humidifier is not constant but will vary with the flow and ambient temperature. However, it should be remembered that this

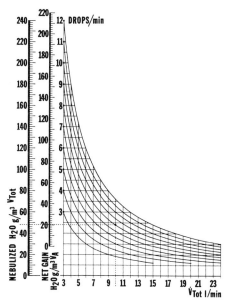

Fig. 20. Hertzog nomogram, designed to aid the quantitation of the fluid requirements for the respiratory tract of the patient.

was one of the first attempts to quantitate ventilation and water requirements. The Mistogen ultrasonic nebulizer has a fixed output of slightly over 2 ml per minute, or 1 ml per minute when a medication chamber is incorporated. Because of this low output, the instrument is relatively unsuitable for tent therapy. The De Vilbiss 880 has a variable output from 0.5 ml per minute to 6 ml per minute. It can be calibrated to deliver accurate amounts of mist at each of four stops.

Because of its ability to produce large volumes of stable mist, the De Vilbiss ultrasonic nebulizer has revolutionized tent therapy for children. Since mechanical nebulizers have limited outputs, it is necessary to keep the volume of the tent small, which creates a physiologically undesirable closed-in feeling. With the ultrasonic nebulizer it is possible to use a half-top canopy that allows ready access to the surrounding atmosphere. This eliminates the need for heat exchangers such as are found in the present humidifier tent combinations exemplified by the croup tent or croupette in an air-conditioned hospital.

To a large extent heat exchange in the half-top canopy occurs from evaporation of some of the large mass of dense mist.

The half-top canopy and ultrasonic nebulizer combination is attractive because of its efficiency and economy. Since 65 percent of the overhead costs of American hospitals is in the form of salaries, any apparatus that can save personnel time and be in itself relatively inexpensive is a contribution to medical care. In addition, the half tents are disposable and therefore minimize the danger of cross contamination through the reuse of equipment. The nebulizing cups and leadouts can be autoclaved. Sterile solutions are introduced through a closed system, and the air or oxygen is filtered free of any organisms.

During a 6-month period the ultrasonic nebulizer has been useful in treating 134 patients with the following conditions:

(1) Upper respiratory infection
(2) Croup
(3) Pneumonia

(4) Bronchial asthma

(5) Bronchiolitis

(6) Laryngotracheobronchitis

(7) Cystic fibrosis

(8) Tracheo-esophageal fistula

(9) Removal of papilloma

(10) Excision of thyroid nodule

(11) Removal of foreign body from bronchus

(12) Congenital heart disease

Some of the other uses for ultrasonic nebulization include humidification for roller-type oxygenators, collection of sputum for cytological and bacteriological study, and diagnostic and therapeutic nebulization of drugs. Contrary to common opinion, we have found that the clinical composition of pharmaceutical agents tested is not changed by the nebulizing process.

HUMIDIFICATION, NEBULIZATION, AND THE INTENSIVE CARE INCUBATOR

The intensive care incubator is an essential instrument for postoperative infant care. It should be fitted with controls so that the skin temperature can dictate the environmental temperature (Fig. 21). The infant is readily accessible because it is placed on a sliding tray built into the incubator (Fig. 22). This incubator is designed to operate normally with 40 percent oxygen or, when the flag is raised, at approximately 80 percent oxygen. It is important that the body of the infant be covered when mist therapy is used, since there is considerable heat exchange from the mist. The humidifier incorporated into the incubator is inadequate to meet the humidity demands of the infant postoperatively. Formerly Mistogen nebulizers driven by compressors were used. Since there is a recirculation of at least 60 l of gas per minute in the C-86 Intensive Care Isolette, this would require an output of approximately 2.5 ml per minute to achieve 100 percent humidification from the nebulizer. On the other hand, the ultrasonic nebulizer of the De Vilbiss type has a variable output which is more than sufficient for this type of incubator. Since the introduction of this nebulizer, the incidence of encrustation of the tracheobronchial tree in the postoperative infant has diminished. Also, the ultrasonic nebulizer has greatly facilitated the weaning of an infant from a ventilator after either an endotracheal or a tracheostomy tube has been used.

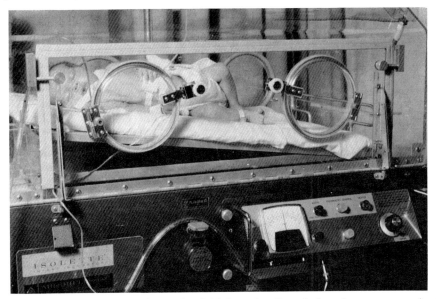

Fig. 21. Infant incubator ISC on patient. The C-86 Intensive Care Isolette has a servomechanism by which the temperature of the infant's skin dictates the environmental temperature.

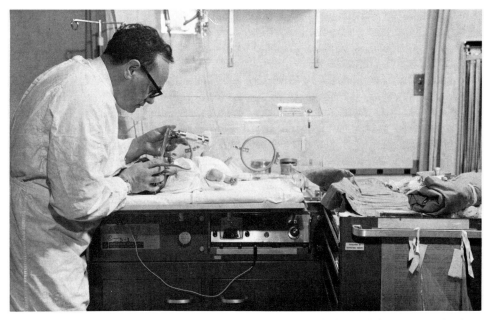

Fig. 22. A C-86 incubator with the infant on a slide-out tray. Intubation is being attempted. The most important feature of an intensive care incubator is the accessibility of the patient.

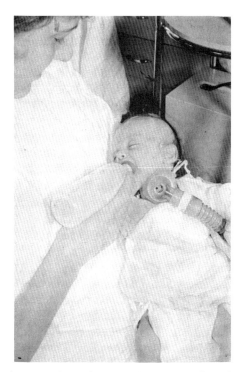

Fig. 23. Infant with a tracheostomy collar ultra-sonic nebulizer. When the infant is removed from the incubator the ultrasonic nebulizer is used in conjunction with the tracheostomy collar.

When the infant is removed from the incubator the ultrasonic nebulizer is used in conjunction with a tracheostomy collar (Fig. 23).

RESPIRATORY INSUFFICIENCY

DIAGNOSIS

The diagnosis of respiratory insufficiency should involve consideration of every facet of gas exchange and gas transport. Oxygen transport depends mainly on the fraction of oxygen in the inspired air, on alveolar ventilation, or diffusion of gases from the alveoli to capillary blood, and on the relation of the distribution of ventilation to the distribution of pulmonary blood flow, hemoglobin content, and volume and distribution of cardiac output. The percentage of oxygen in the inspired air can be measured easily, and this should be done frequently with an oxygen analyzer. This datum, along with hemoglobin content and arterial oxygen tension (PO_2), gives an estimate of the magnitude of the physiological shunt, if any, by comparing the difference in oxygen tension between alveolar and arterial blood. A decreased arterial oxygen content requires a compensatory increase in cardiac output or red cell mass. In children and especially in infants there is frequently peripheral vasoconstriction in the hypoxic state, reflecting the inadequacy of cardiac output and tissue perfusion, which, on the other hand, are the sources of metabolic acidosis. Normal ventilation is the minute volume of ventilation, which in a normal child can be predicted to maintain a normal arterial carbon dioxide tension. In respiratory insufficiency the physiological dead space frequently is increased. Therefore, the predicted figure will be inaccurate, and ventilation will have to be increased above that predicted to maintain a normal arterial carbon dioxide tension. This must be monitored directly. Measurement of tidal and minute volumes can be quite misleading and should be used only as an adjunct to that of arterial carbon dioxide tensions. Measurements of tidal volume can be useful in determining the volume of ventilation necessary to maintain normal arterial carbon dioxide tensions, especially when the patient is being weaned from a ventilator. If respiratory volumes necessary to maintain normal arterial carbon dioxide tensions are known, the precise time to discontinue the ventilator can be predicted.

In the postoperative surgical patient it is not uncommon to have a pathological relationship between ventilation and perfusion (e.g., atelectasis). The alveolar-arterial oxygen tension difference gives a good estimate of pulmonary ventilation perfusion abnormality. The cardiac output and the arterial-venous oxygen content difference must, of course, be within a fairly normal range. The physiological dead space is difficult to measure, especially in the infant. If the volume of ventilation needed to maintain a normal arterial carbon dioxide tension exceeds that which has been predicted, it is most likely caused by an increased physiological dead space, although it may be due to an elevated metabolic rate as well. Again, the work of breathing is difficult to measure in the infant, but every effort should be made to estimate this parameter. It has been the custom to estimate this in relation to the infant's effort and to consider it positively in relation to respiratory insufficiency even when the PO_2 and PCO_2 are within normal limits. Lung compliance, defined as the volume change per unit of pressure change, together with airway resistance, should be carefully evaluated as well.

A diagnostic procedure for respiratory insufficiency in infants and children, although following basically the same pattern as that for adults, has some salient differences. The history is usually obtained secondhand from the parents and other observers. The importance of the history of restlessness cannot be overemphasized. The normal neonatal pattern of ventilation is cyclical. The temperature should always be checked, since this is a common cause of respiratory depression in the infant. Cardiopulmonary auscultation especially can be misleading. It is very difficult to diagnose atelectasis by auscultation in the infant. It is also difficult to estimate the ventilatory exchange. The important vital signs are the cardiac rate, arterial blood pressure, respiratory frequency, and respiratory effort. The hemoglobin content should always be checked, along with the serum electrolytes. Hypokalemia is not an uncommon cause of respiratory depression, and the chloride ion is essential for oxygen transport to the cells. Chest x-ray films help in the diagnosis. An image intensification system would be extremely valuable if it could be located in the intensive care unit. Urinary output and acidity may be indexes of lowered cardiac output or low blood volume. The arterial oxygen and PO_2 tension are measured directly. The efficiency of alveolar ventilation can be deduced from the arterial carbon dioxide tension (PCO_2). The arterial pH, along with the arterial carbon dioxide tension, is essential in determining the acid-base balance. The alveolar-arterial oxygen tension difference demonstrates to some degree the relation of ventilation to perfusion in the lung. In estimating respiratory work the lung compliance, air resistance, and oxygen consumption can be measured. It should be remembered that there is a small respiratory reserve volume in the infant.

TREATMENT

The treatment of hypoxia has been discussed under oxygen therapy. In the treatment of inadequate ventilation, a nasotracheal or endotracheal tube will reduce the physiological dead space to an extent that may be sufficient to compensate for small degrees of hypoventilation. In case this is inadequate, artificial ventilation must be applied. A hand-inflated bag may be used for the treatment of short periods of hypoventilation, but a ventilator should be employed for prolonged artificial ventilation (Fig. 24).

RESPIRATORS

Respirators may be divided into two groups: (1) body respirators, producing ventilation through pressure changes around the whole body (Emerson iron lung and Air-Shields negative pressure isolette) or over certain parts of the body (Cuirass-Moynahan respirator) and (2) devices producing ventilation through pressure changes directly on the airways.

Body respirators have generally fallen into disfavor because it is difficult to lower an elevated PCO_2 with this type of machine. The Air-Shields negative pressure isolette combines environmental control of temperature and humidity associated with ventilation (Fig. 25). Fitting the plastic diaphragm around the neck is difficult and may be traumatic. Assessment of this respirator with special reference to the respiratory distress syndrome of the newborn is presently in progress. Artificial ventilation of the very small premature infant in the 1-kg weight group is difficult because of the management problems of either a nasotracheal or a tracheostomy tube. Thus, the development and assessment of the Air-Shields negative pressure isolette respirator is worthwhile. The tank type and Cuirass type of respirators are infrequently used.

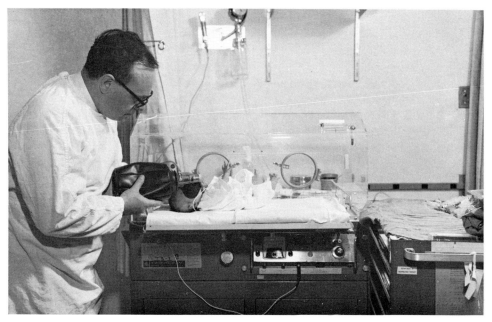

Fig. 24. Self-inflating bag being used to resuscitate a child. It is used for the treatment of short periods of hypoventilation.

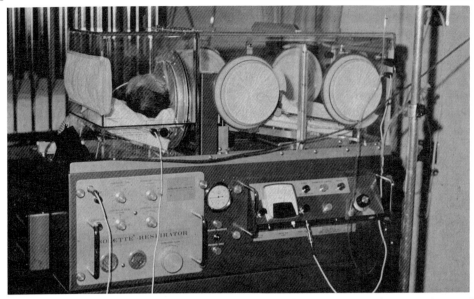

Fig. 25. Infant in the Air-Shields negative pressure isolette, which combines environmental control of temperature and humidity with ventilation.

POSITIVE PRESSURE RESPIRATORS

A simple classification of positive pressure respirators is into pressure-limited ventilators and volume-limited ventilators.

PRESSURE-LIMITED VENTILATORS

Pressure-limited ventilators inflate the child's lungs until a preset pressure is reached. When the inspiratory phase stops the expiration begins; thus, any leak in the system up to a moderate degree will be automatically compensated for. The tidal volume produced by the preset pressure will be a function of the elasticity and airway resistance of the patient's lung and of the inspiratory flow rate. The most common types of pressure-limited ventilators are the Bird and the Bennett. They are both flow generators, the inspiratory flow pattern of gas being determined entirely by the ventilator. They differ in that the Bird has an adjustable inspiratory flow rate. In the infant the pulmonary compliance and airway resistance can change frequently and rapidly, and it is extremely difficult to measure the expired minute and tidal volumes, which would aid in the resetting of the pressure and inspira-

tory flow rate adjustments. This need for manual readjusting is the biggest flaw of pressure-limited ventilators.

THE BIRD MARK VIII VENTILATOR WITH Q-CIRCLE. The Bird Mark VIII ventilator with Q-circle operates on a push-pull system (Fig. 26). The inspiratory tidal volume is pushed into the patient, and the negative pressure on the expiratory lead removes most of the resistance to expiration. The ventilator should not be used with the small-line infant Q-circle but always with the larger tubes of the child Q-circle. This will give the ventilator a better time constant. The machine is connected to the patient by a naso-endotracheal tube or a tracheostomy cannula. We have changed the Bird Y piece to the American standard 15-mm size, which attaches to a standard endotracheal tube connector or a tracheostomy tube adapter. Usually we use the Aberdeen–Great Ormond Street single-lumen plastic tracheostomy cannula in the infants when the Bird connectors are employed (Fig. 27). It is important that a reasonably good fit be obtained either with the nasotracheal tube or with the tracheostomy cannula. Securing the nasotracheal tube to the patient can be difficult. Jackson-Rees

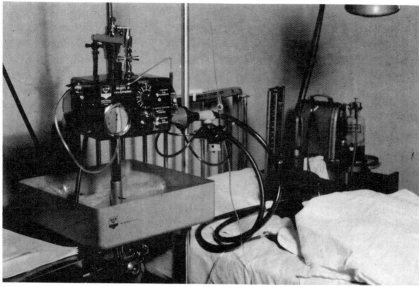

Fig. 26. Bird Mark VIII with Q-Circle, adult Q-Circle. The Bird Mark VIII with Q-Circle is a pressure-limited flow generator respirator with an inspiratory flow rate adjustment.

binds the respirator leads to the head of the patient. We have been unable to find a good method of securing the tubes to the body when a tracheostomy cannula is used. The

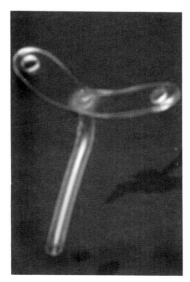

Fig. 27. Aberdeen-Great Ormond Street single lumen plastic tracheostomy cannula, which is used for infants.

patient must be observed continuously to ensure that the connection does not come apart.

The controls of the Bird Mark VIII are empirical and interrelated. For controlled ventilation of an infant our procedure is as follows:

(1) The negative pressure control is set to give −2 cm of water. This is accomplished by turning the negative pressure control very slightly until the Venturi effect of the expiratory valve is heard to be activated.

(2) The sensitivity control on the left is placed approximately at the number −2. This control should echo the setting of the negative pressure control unless the retard cap is used for low compliances, in which case it will have to be moved, approximately to the −10 position.

(3) Taking the high resistance of an infant's airway into account, the pressure control is adjusted to give a positive pressure of approximately 30 cm of water.

(4) The inspiratory flow control is turned to approximately the 40 mark, and the expiratory time control is adjusted to give a 1:2 ratio between inspiration and expiration, including expiratory pause.

The inspiratory and expiratory controls

are adjusted together to give the desired rate. The sensitivity control is readjusted to give the desired amount of sensitivity. The patient should be examined for the efficacy of ventilation.

In our opinion the Bird mainline micronebulizer does not provide adequate humidification. The Puritan-Bennett cascade heated humidifier has been used in conjunction with the Bird Mark VIII with excellent results,

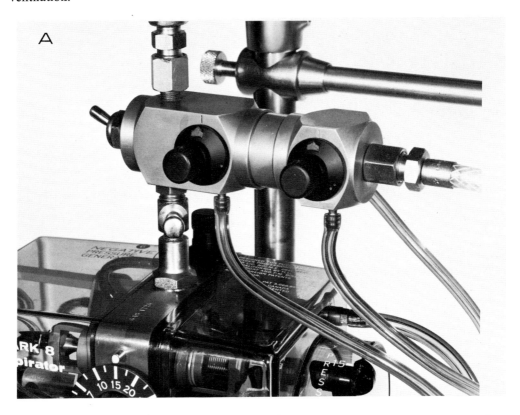

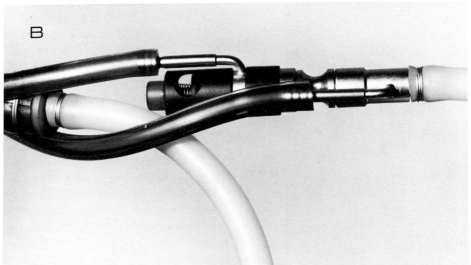

Fig. 28. New Bird large volume pressurized sidearm humidifier with the new double Venturi circuit. A. Flow booster. B. Close-up of double Venturi circuit.

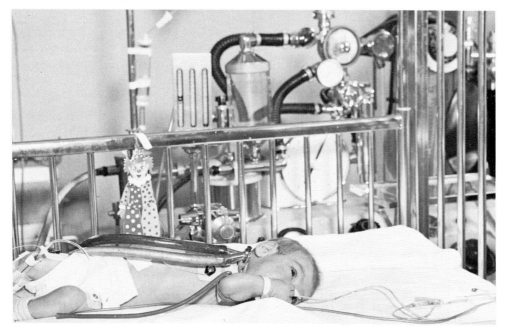

Fig. 29. Engström model 200 being used on an infant. It is our choice of mechanical respirators.

with the temperature at the entrance to the patient being continuously monitored.

The new Bird large volume pressurized sidearm humidifier appears to supply adequate humidification. The new De Vilbiss 900 ultrasonic nebulizer has been designed for use with ventilators. A new double Venturi circuit is presently under evaluation (Fig. 28). The aim in this circuit is to minimize the time delay between the patient and the machine. It is especially suitable for assisting rather than controlling ventilation.

VOLUME-LIMITED VENTILATORS

A volume-limited ventilator will provide a constant minute volume, regardless of changes in pulmonary compliance and airway resistance, if sufficient power is available. The expired minute volume should be measured with a spirometer, especially when there is a small leak in the system. There should be a safety valve incorporated that will bleed the system when a preset pressure has been reached. Our choice of respirators is a volume-limited respirator. The Engstrom

model 200 was selected for the following reasons (Fig. 29):

(1) Its dependability is outstanding, so that artificial ventilation can be carried out for weeks and months with minimal or no service to the machine.

(2) It has the capacity to overcome low compliances and high resistances.

(3) It is easily synchronized with the spontaneous respiration of the patient.

(4) Untoward effects on the patient's circulation are minimal or nonexistent.

(5) Distribution of the pulmonary ventilation is excellent.

(6) It has an outstanding time constant.

(7) There is an automatic variation of flow, pressure, and power with the load (thus the respirator cannot be classified either as a flow generator or as a pressure generator).

(8) The predetermined ventilatory gas volume can be administered within the time available for inspiration with only small pressure fluctuations and low intrapulmonary mean pressure.

(9) The flow curve is interrelated with the pressure curve and has the characteristics that will allow gas to flow through a constric-

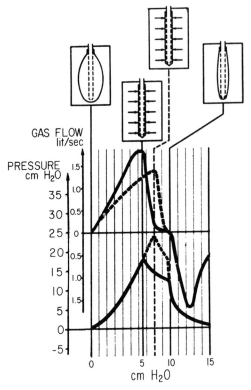

Fig. 30. The flow curve is interrelated with the pressure curve and has the characteristics that will allow gas to flow through a constriction.

tion (Fig. 30). There is also a short static pressure period which allows intrapulmonary pressure equilibration and the final distribution of gas to parts of the lungs with an increased time constant.

(10) The new pediatric dosage valve is accurate, and the wide scale is advantageous when small volumes are demanded (Fig. 31).

(11) It is possible to adapt an anesthesia circuit to the machine that will allow quantitative anesthesia to be administered in conjunction with quantitative ventilation and humidification. Using the respirator as an anesthetic machine ensures that the staff will be familiar with it. When it has to be used ın the intensive care area, the required settings of the machine and the stabilization of the patient in regard to ventilation is readily accomplished.

(12) There is an excellent spirometer in the expiratory channel, so that the actual minute volume can be determined.

(13) Essentially it consists of a nondistensible system. An accurate pressure gauge in the system with the minute volume reading on the spirometer gives a continuous measurement of compliance (Fig. 32). A nurse can monitor the minute volume and changes in compliance and resistance. She can be guided by these parameters and by the breath sounds, which she monitors with a stethoscope, as to when and how frequently to perform endotracheal and bronchial suctioning.

(14) Accurate oxygen flow meters along with an accurate air dosage meter ensure that the inspired oxygen concentration can be varied from 20 percent to 100 percent.

(15) There is a one-way valve that can be opened to the atmosphere, permitting the patient to inspire freely during any phase of the inspiratory cycle, over and beyond the gas available in the free-hanging bag.

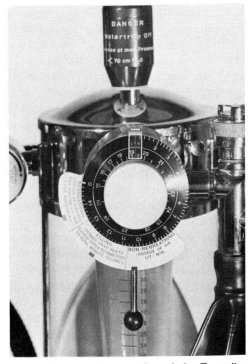

Fig. 31. The new dosage valve of the Engström.

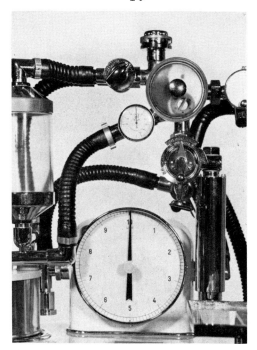

Fig. 32. Pressure gauge and spirometer. The expiratory minute volume is measured on the spirometer and, together with the pressure generator and with the predetermined rate being known, gives a continuous measurement of compliance.

(16) A heated humidifier is incorporated which gives adequate humidification for small children. An ultrasonic nebulizer can also be incorporated either for additional humidification or for mist therapy.

This respirator does not have an automatic cycling device, but it should be remembered that although the minute volume is constant, the tidal volume need not be so. Also, in our technique we hand ventilate and oxygenate before and after suctioning. This not only prevents deoxygenation of the patient when suctioned but also produces a sighing cycle. The inspiratory-expiratory ratio is constant, being 1:2. Under certain circumstances it may be preferable to have a variable ratio. The maximum rate of respiration that can be achieved with this machine is 35 per minute.

USE OF THE ENGSTRÖM 200 RESPIRATOR. In using the Engström 200 respirator, the machine is first checked for leaks and calibration. This is accomplished by block-ing the expiratory flow and placing a known volume into the circuit with the Y piece to the patient occluded. Using Boyle's law it is easy to check the calibration. If the pressure as demonstrated on the gauge remains stable, there can be no leak in the system because the volume applied is constant.

If the height and weight of the patient are known, his surface area can be calculated. A nomogram was evolved to predict the required minute volume of the patient in relation to the machine, taking into consideration the dead space of the machine itself (Fig. 33). The flow meters and dosage valve are adjusted to give the desired concentration of oxygen and the predetermined minute volume. The rate is preobtained from the nomogram. It has been our experience that the nomogram is inaccurate, especially for infants. This is especially true when the machine is used for the administration of anesthesia. Perhaps an additional factor here is our reluctance to administer relaxants and our consequent use of moderate hyperventilation. The only accurate method of ensuring that the correct minute volume is delivered to the patient still remains the determination of arterial PCO_2.

It has been our experience that the Bird large diameter tubing used in the child Q-circle is superior to that provided with the Engström machine (Fig. 34). Care is taken that the total volume contained in the tubes is identical to that contained in the prescribed Engström inspiratory and expiratory tubing for children. In addition, we have incorporated a Bird water trap in both the inspiratory and expiratory leads. A Bird Y connector modified to American standards is used to attach to an endotracheal catheter connector or a tracheostomy tube.

The patient rapidly synchronizes with the machine if adequate oxygenation is provided. No relaxants or sedatives are necessary in the vast majority of cases.

Additional factors influence postoperative respiratory insufficiency. Preexisting pulmonary disease is the most common cause. Many congenital cardiac defects have pul-

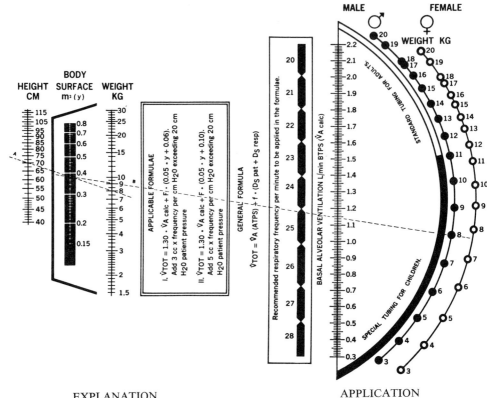

EXPLANATION

$\dot{V}$ Tot = total ventilation liter/min to be adjusted on the respirator. Calculated for a patient without fever.

$\dot{V}_A$ calc = alveolar ventilation calculated with the help of the nomogram liter/min (B T P S).

f = respiration frequency per minute (adjusted on the respirator).

y = body surface in m².

$D_s$pat = dead space of the patient after tracheotomy, in liters, i.e.,

0.05 · y (with the body surface as parameter).

1.30 · $\dot{V}_A$ calc = includes the correction of $\dot{V}_A$ calc to 24° C and a correction for divergents from the standard metabolic conditions.

$D_s$resp = the "functional" dead space of the respirator in liters when using different patient tubes:

I	II
0.06	0.10

respectively.

APPLICATION

1) calculate y from height and weight (example line A)

2) calculate $\dot{V}_A$calc from y, body-weight and sex (example line B)

3) place the values of $\dot{V}_A$ calc and y in the formulas I or II, where I is to be used for special tubing for children, full-drawn semicircular line, and II for standard patient tubes for adults (large size) the open semicircular line.

EXAMPLE

Male patient: height 70 cm weight 8 kg will give a body surface of 0.38 m² · (dotted line A)

Following dotted line B from body-surface to body-weight male patient 8 kg.

$\dot{V}_A$calc = 1.4 liters/min. To get $\dot{V}$To + proceed as follows: The body-surface (y) was found to be 0.38 m².

If according to recommendation the frequency (f) has been set at 25 cycles per minute and the special tubing for children is used (formula I), then $\dot{V}$Tot in liters per minute will be:

1.30 · 1.14 + 25 · (0.05 ·0.38 + 0.06) = 3.46 liters/min.

Fig. 33. Practical ventilation nomogram for the Engström respirator for infants and children. (Courtesy of C. G. Engström, P. Herzog, and O. P. Norlander.)

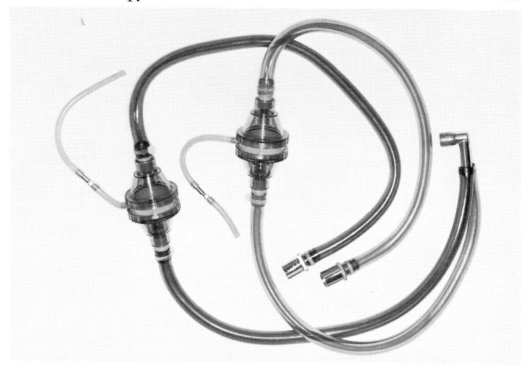

Fig. 34. Bird large tubing with the water trap and the Y piece modified to 15 mm. Bird large diameter tubing is used with a water trap on the inspiratory and expiratory side, and the Bird Y connector is modified to American standards.

monary changes which influence the postoperative management. Patients with obstructive lung disease can be well managed before, during, and after surgery but there will be an increased incidence among them of postoperative respiratory problems. In the infant age group there is a frequent occurrence of respiratory depression because of their limited respiratory reserve, their small airways, and the distinctive diaphragmatic component of the breathing mechanism. Abdominal distension will splint the diaphragm. A wound in the chest or in the upper abdomen can cause splinting of the respiratory movement because of pain. When a pain-relieving drug must be used, it is administered intravenously in approximately one tenth of the intramuscular dose. The patient should be observed until the maximum effect has been obtained. Generally we do not use relaxants during surgery because of our concern over postoperative respiratory insufficiency.

PREVENTION OF RESPIRATORY COMPLICATIONS

In an effort to prevent respiratory complications the temperature should be monitored and controlled both in the operating room and in the intensive care area. In infant management the temperature of the skin should dictate the environmental temperature in a closed-loop system. Anemia is treated along with deficits in blood volume, imbalance of electrolytes, and acid-base ratios. Acidosis interferes with adequate myocardial function and autonomic response. Patient care includes frequent changes in position, active or passive deep breathing, and the encouragement of coughing. Chest movement should not be restricted by bandages or casts, and in the infant the abdominal movement must not be diminished. In the patient with either obstructive or restrictive pulmonary disease, every effort is made preoperatively to achieve maximum pulmonary function. Infants tolerate obstructive lung disease to only a small degree. Adequate tracheobronchial toilet is essential. The airway in infants should be protected from aspiration by giving frequent small feedings and propping the infants up in the optimum position.

Preoperatively, respiratory care is fully explained and demonstrated to the older patients. This helps to eliminate apprehension and ensures the patient's cooperation.

In the patient with obstructive lung disease, retained secretions are mobilized by ultrasonically nebulized water, $\frac{2}{3}$ normal saline, and bronchial dilators. Intermittent positive pressure breathing may be of use in introducing bronchial dilators and playing a part in physical chest therapy. Physical chest therapy is extremely important in the postural drainage of patients. Larger children can be taught breathing exercises. If the patient is old enough to comprehend, he should be instructed in the use of a tracheostomy or nasoendotracheal tube postoperatively. All patients should receive an increased concentration of oxygen in the inspired air following major surgery. Patients should be wide awake before they are moved from the op-

erating room. If there is any doubt about the adequacy of ventilation, the endotracheal tube is left in place while the patient is being moved to the recovery or intensive care area. All cardiac patients are transported with oxygen being administered by a bag and mask.

In pediatric intensive care, chest physical therapy is best administered by the intensive care nurses and inhalation therapists under the supervision of a nurse respiratory therapist. Chest physical therapy should be administered on a 24-hour-a-day schedule, seven days a week. The aim in chest physical therapy is the removal of secretions by postural drainage and by manual assistance to coughing. Manual vibration is extremely helpful in the infant in shaking loose secretions. Manual percussion is also employed, with care being taken not to use too much force. Following this type of therapy, tracheobronchial suction is carried out. Postural drainage is employed to aid in the removal of secretions. In infant management it is necessary to change the position every 30 minutes.

DAVID ALLAN

9

Intensive Care

PHYSICAL LAYOUT

The intensive care area should be arranged to provide the supervising personnel with a clear view of the patients. This can be accomplished by having partitions constructed with clear thick glass above the 3-ft level from the floor. The supervisor can thus detect problems and direct personnel to the critical areas without loss of time. In order to provide privacy for the patients, curtains should be arranged so that the individual patients can be completely enclosed when necessary. The actual space for the patients should be three times that allowed for in normal hospital planning. This generous allotment is needed for the special equipment used in the intensive care area. With a critically ill postoperative patient there must be space around the patient's crib or bed for respirators, suction equipment, monitoring devices, and resuscitation equipment. Every effort should be made to provide space by placing as much of the equipment as possible on shelves off the floor. The floor should be well constructed so that it can tolerate such heavy equipment as portable x-ray units required for emergency roentgenograms. Each patient should have either ceiling or wall equipment for one oxygen outlet, one compressed-air outlet, three suction outlets, and two electrical outlets. In the area where the infants are to be cared for, a filtered air system is preferable to the type usually employed in hospitals.

Every effort should be made from a design and construction standpoint to reduce noise. A great deal of equipment has to be used and there are many people involved, and unless special attention is given to this problem the noise level will reach a point where it is disturbing to the patient and to the nurses caring for the patient. There is some evidence that damage to the patient's hearing has taken place when there has been a long exposure to a constant high level of noise.

Adequate storage space is a second important consideration in planning for an intensive care unit. Fluids, intravenous sets, linen and monitoring units, respirators, and x-ray equipment require a large storage area, and for efficiency they should be adjacent to the patient care area. Unless adequate space is provided for the equipment, it becomes a real problem to move it from a distant area to the intensive care unit. The nursing station should be adequate in size. There is a tendency in building intensive care units to make this part of the space too small. There are many people involved in the care of the patients, and consequently an area where they can be accommodated when writing progress notes or sitting in a group to discuss the patients' problems is essential. These are requirements that are often overlooked but extremely important for the smooth function of an intensive care area.

Adjacent to the intensive care area there should be sleeping rooms. These should be provided for the surgical resident on call, the anesthesiologist on call, and, if possible, for parents who have children who are severely ill. Unless this space for parents is provided, we find that parents are apt to stay awake all night and become irritable from fatigue and be of little value in reassuring their children.

A room should be provided that is equipped for minor operations. This room should have a good operating room light, suspended from either the ceiling or the wall. The room should be stocked to provide for minor operations, such as tracheostomies, insertions of chest catheters, and opening of potentially infected wounds. Such a facility in the intensive care area saves the patient who is in extremely serious condition from being moved from the intensive care area to the operating room and back again. Where these facilities are provided the patient can actually be cared for during the period of great risk in this specially equipped room, so that not only is he isolated from the other patients, but everything is available for the performance of minor procedures without the added danger of being transported.

ISOLATION TECHNIQUE

It is important in caring for the neonate and premature infant to provide isolation technique. Certain areas of the unit must be set aside for this age group, and mask and gown technique must be instituted to reduce cross infection. The technique also decreases the casual traffic through this part of the unit. However, considerable thought must be given to the fact that the child must not be isolated from observation and treatment. Therefore, the design of isolettes must be such that the child can be removed from the isolette and given emergency treatment with speed and convenience. These units must be placed so that they are under constant surveillance by the nursing staff. In addition, small special rooms should be set aside where infected cases can be adequately isolated. This is extremely important, for there are many situations during the postoperative care of children when infection becomes a part of the problem, and instead of the need for intensive care being reduced, it is augmented.

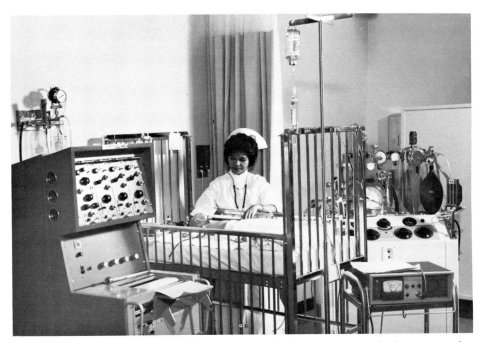

Fig. 1. Patient in intensive care unit. Respirator and monitoring equipment make it necessary that additional floor space be provided for each patient.

SPECIAL EQUIPMENT

The pediatric intensive care unit has requirements that are different from those of an adult unit. A central monitoring system that has merit in adult units has limited value in the care of infants and children. The reason for this is that changes occur extremely rapidly in children and infants, and personnel must be at the patient's bedside rather than at a distance in order to provide the immediate help that is required in emergencies. Monitoring equipment that can be used at the bedside has real merit (Fig. 1). The most important monitoring aid besides the five senses and the stethoscope is a means by which brachycardia can be instantly recognized. Units are now available that have small oscilloscopes (useful for diagnosing arrhythmias) and a sound and sight impulse from the R wave of the QRS complex. An alarm system for either tachycardia or brachycardia is incorporated in the equipment. Such a monitoring system gives early warning of cardiac arrest and permits the attending nurse to call for assistance when changes occur prior to arrest.

Resuscitation apparatus is the most important equipment for the intensive care unit. This equipment is most useful when mounted on a mobile cart. An important part of this equipment is a plywood board that can be placed under the patient so that external cardiac massage will be effective. When massage is attempted without this board, there is insufficient resistance from the mattress to permit efficient external cardiac massage. Laryngoscopes and all types of intubation equipment, plus various medications, are provided on this cart. There is also an emergency tracheotomy setup. It is important that a check list be appended to this cart and that it become the duty of a responsible individual to check this equipment daily so that when an emergency arises all equipment is available and in workable condition.

LABORATORY FACILITIES

With the use of respirators, the need for frequent sampling of venous and arterial blood for gas analysis becomes urgent. In addition to having facilities for the determi-

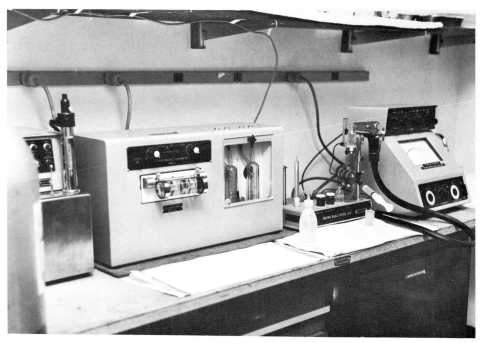

Fig. 2. Blood gas analysis laboratory adjacent to intensive care area. The Astrup technique is shown.

nation of PO_2 and PCO_2 there should be facilities for electrolyte determination. Therefore, in addition to the gas analytical laboratory, there should be equipment for measuring sodium, potassium, and chloride from serum (Fig. 2). The accuracy of gas analysis reading is dependent upon how promptly the determinations are made after the blood is drawn from the patient. By having the laboratory adjacent to the intensive care area, these determinations can be made within minutes after the blood is drawn, so that distortion from prolonged storage is obviated. It is advantageous to have personnel able to make these determinations as needed day and night.

PERSONNEL

The organization of intensive care units is a relatively recent development and was initially intended to provide for the care of postoperative patients. The unit has evolved into an area where care is provided for severely injured and acutely ill children as well as for postoperative patients. The development of this unit concentrated skilled nursing personnel and all types of inhalation-therapy equipment and monitoring devices in one area. The quality of the nursing personnel is the most important ingredient in a good intensive care unit. The nurses must be dedicated, alert observers who are deeply interested in the care of the patient. The efficient operation of an intensive care unit depends to a large extent upon the supervisory nurse. She must be a mature person with experience in administration and in the care of extremely ill children. By concentrating acutely ill patients, severely injured patients, and postoperative patients in one area, the personnel gain skill by constant experience in the care of these patients. The use of respirators to assist in maintaining the patient's pulmonary function is now a common practice. Environmental control apparatus, such as incubators, tents, and humidity devices, as well as intricate monitoring instruments, are now in daily use. This has created a need

for people trained in the operation of these special devices. Usually individuals who have completed nursing school can be given additional training in inhalation therapy, and they can become a great asset to the intensive care unit. There must be many nurses available to care for acutely ill patients, particularly for those requiring respirators and other devices. In special situations a patient may require two or more nurses in constant attendance. It is unwise to reduce personnel during the evening and night shifts, for it is during these periods that crises arise. The level of professional care in the intensive care unit is to a large extent dependent upon the number and quality of house staff available. At times it is necessary to have a resident surgeon in constant attendance for optimum postoperative care in a complicated situation.

PROFESSIONAL SUPERVISION

The professional supervision of the postoperative patient is no longer dependent entirely upon the surgeon. Rather it concerns a group of individuals each of whom brings special skill and knowledge to the problems that occur in the postoperative child. Formerly the anesthesiologist restricted his activities to the administration of anesthesia. Today he has assumed a more active role in the care of the patient. He gives advice regarding the type of anesthesia, the length of operation that is safe, the preoperative preparation of the patient, and the postoperative care. Problems regarding airway patency and pulmonary function are common in the postoperative patient. The anesthesiologist is an expert in maintaining airways and in the use of artificial respiratory apparatus that are increasingly important in the care of the severely ill postoperative patient. The airway emergencies arise with such speed that remedial actions are required within minutes in order to save the patient. It is advantageous to organize the staff in anesthesiology in such a manner that a senior person is on 24-

hour duty in the hospital; thus he is available to administer anesthesia in emergency cases and to be a consultant and play a direct role in the care of the acutely ill patient, particularly those with respiratory problems. The severely injured child presents many of the same problems that confront us in the postoperative patient, and here again the respiratory function and airway patency are often important problems that require the services of a senior anesthesiologist.

The pediatrician is important in the management of the intensive care unit. This is particularly true of pediatric specialists, such as the hematologist, the cardiologist, the endocrinologist, and the expert on infectious diseases. They furnish diagnostic help and aid in the therapy of the gravely ill patient. A pediatrician with general interest in the field of child care and with extensive experience in the actual care of the severely ill child is a great asset. The presence of the anesthesiologist, pediatrician, and pediatric specialist in the intensive care unit does not relieve the surgeon of his responsibility. The postoperative patient is particularly a problem for the surgeon, for he knows exactly how the operative procedure was performed and what complications most likely may arise. Unless he is available and part of the team that cares for the postoperative patient, serious complications may be overlooked until they are so advanced that treatment is ineffective. But when the surgeon is available and is on the lookout for complications that he knows from experience may arise, he can detect these early and institute corrective measures that help minimize their effect. It is obvious from this analysis of the intensive care unit that it is no longer the domain of the surgeon alone. Its management is a cooperative effort, and its operation should be under the direction of a committee on which all of the interested people are represented.

The ultimate responsibility for the patient's care must reside with one individual and his representatives. Unless this arrangement is clearly understood the patient will suffer because there will be no way to place responsibility when essential things remain undone. This person should be the surgeon involved in the operative care of the patient.

EQUIPMENT

The equipment in the intensive care unit is highly important. That relating to the environmental control and respiratory assistance will be described in the chapter on inhalation therapy. In addition, monitoring devices are needed, such as equipment to record electrocardiographs, electroencephalographs, venous pressures, and arterial pressures.

The recording of central venous pressure is a definite aid in the care of the patient in the intensive care unit. The decision whether to give more blood and fluid often hinges on the ability of the heart to tolerate an additional load. Venous pressures of 15 cm of water and above are an indication that cardiac function is not able to cope with the rapid inflow of fluid or blood and that one should curtail such infusions. However, when the venous pressure is 0 to 10 cm of water, the patient can safely be given fluid and blood to support his blood pressure and bolster his urinary output, and the danger of cardiac failure can be minimized by intermittent recording of the central venous pressure. The venous pressure is not an ideal indicator, but it is one that gives considerable information on the status of the circulation and suggests to a certain extent what remedial measures can be safely taken to support the patient.

Equally important is the arterial pressure. There has been a tendency to disregard the use of blood pressure determinations, particularly in small infants. With care and the use of pneumatic cuffs of the proper size reproducible blood pressure determinations can be obtained. It may be difficult to utilize this technique with the extremely ill patient, and direct arterial pressure recordings from an artery by way of a tube to a recording device may be required.

PHYSIOLOGICAL CARE

The maintenance of homeostasis of the body fluids is of the utmost importance. The factors that have been found to be involved in the maintenance of physiological neutrality are numerous. The processes are infinitely complicated, and it is understandable that there are differences of opinions among workers in this field. Authorities vary considerably in their recommendations for therapy in a given situation. The reason for the success of a variety of programs may be attributed to the limiting of application to situations where renal function is normal. Under this condition it is understandable how therapeutic programs varying by as much as 200 percent in volumes of fluids and smaller differences in the composition of solutes are carried out with apparently equally good clinical results. There are complicated problems relating to the establishment of basal requirements of fluids and electrolytes. Most measurements have been made on adults and may contain inaccuracies when applied to neonates, where there are differences in basal metabolism. The kidney's excretory function plays a large role in the maintenance of normal acid-base relations. The excretion of carbonic acid is performed by the lungs, and this has a direct relationship to respiratory alkalosis and acidosis. The intestinal tract has a minor function in the maintenance of the acid-base relationship. To further complicate the problem there has developed a need for taking into account respiratory alkalosis and acidosis in patients. This has brought a whole new set of problems and has still further complicated the understanding of metabolic and respiratory upsets of homeostasis and of the methods of correcting them. The metabolic problems that confront the physician caring for the acutely ill postoperative child are more critical than in adults. The reasons for this are that the water composition and rate of exchange of a child are considerably different from that observed in adults. For instance, an infant weighing 7 kg has an extracellular fluid volume of about 1,400 ml. His intake will be 700 ml, and his outgo will be an equal amount. In comparison an adult of 70 kg has an extracellular fluid compartment of 14,000 ml, and the intake in such an individual is 2,000 ml, with an equal outgo (Fig. 3). This comparison shows that

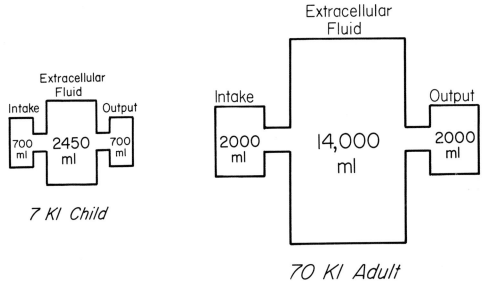

Fig. 3. Diagrammatic representation of fluid metabolism in an infant compared to that in an adult. (Adapted from Gamble. Chemical Anatomy Physiology and Pathology of Extracellular Fluid. Courtesy of Howard University Press.)

the percentage of exchange is 50 percent in a small child compared to 15 percent in an adult. This accounts for the more rapid and severe dehydration that is observed in infants during illness when fluid intake is limited and accompanied by vomiting. Diarrhea adds to the rate of fluid loss, and life-endangering fluid and electrolyte derangements may occur with surprising speed. Another way to appreciate this difference is that in the weight breakdown of the infant there is a 5 percent plasma water which is about the same as in the adult. The solids are considerably different, 25 percent weight of the infant being solids while 40 percent of the adult is solids. The cell water content is about the same, being approximately 40 percent (Fig. 4). The interstitial water is twice as great in the infant as in the adult, being 30 percent in infants and 15 percent in adults. This can be indicated as H_2OI. For many of the computations necessary in correcting fluid and electrolyte disturbances the extracellular water (usually indicated as H_2OE) is essential, and this is taken to be about one third of the water composition of the body, or 20 percent of the total body weight in adults. In infants 35 percent of the total weight is extracellular fluid. These figures are not to be taken as absolute values, for they have been determined by indirect methods and differ depending on what measuring tech-

nique is used. Nevertheless from a practical standpoint they have a definite use.

In the general metabolic process the kidney plays a large role in the homeostasis of electrolyte and fluid balance. The speed of kidney function is not as great as one would expect, and the correction of metabolic aberrations may take 24 hours to accomplish, even with normal kidneys. With defects in the renal function the rate of correction is slower. An important basic fact is that the intracellular electrolytes are potassium, magnesium, and phosphate, whereas the ions of extracellular fluid are sodium and chloride. The cell membranes preferentially maintain some barrier to sodium so that there is a retention of intracellular potassium, and it is only under abnormal situations of depletion or injury that the membrane yields and sodium enters the cell. In the average sick patient, metabolic acidosis and alkalosis is a prime concern, and a considerable number of routine biochemical determinations done in hospital laboratories are designed to yield information regarding these problems. A good amount of information can be gained from the solution of the Henderson-Hasselbalch equation. Gamble has diagrammatically presented this information in Figure 5. In metabolic acidosis at a pH of 7.2 one can note the diminution in the amount of sodium bicarbonate in comparison with that in a

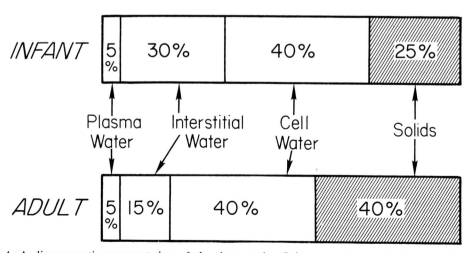

Fig. 4. A diagrammatic representation of the three major fluid compartments in the normal infant and normal adult, taken from Keitel. The major portion of change occurs in the first two years of life.

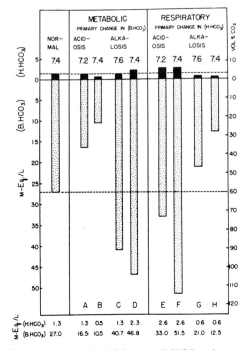

Fig. 5. Plasma (H.HCO₃ and B.HCO₃) in reaction disturbances. (From Gamble. Chemical Anatomy, Physiology and Pathology of Extracellular Fluid. Courtesy of Harvard University Press.)

normal person at a pH of 7.4. This will tend to correct itself, and the carbonic acid and bicarbonate will tend to reach their normal relationship of 1:20. In doing this the carbonic acid will be decreased as well as the bicarbonate, thus safeguarding the pH and returning it to 7.4. In metabolic alkalosis at a pH of 7.6 there is a considerable increase in the bicarbonate level. In the establishment of the normal relationship of carbonic acid and bicarbonate there is an increase in both elements, and the pH is protected and returned to 7.4. In respiratory acidosis at a pH of 7.2 there is an increase in both the bicarbonate and the carbonic acid. In establishing the normal 1:20 ratio of these two substances there is a considerable increase in the bicarbonate, and consequently the pH returns to 7.4. In respiratory alkalosis at a pH of 7.6 there is a decrease in bicarbonate and carbonic acid, and these diminish still further in arriving at the proper ratio of carbonic acid to bicarbonate and in returning the pH to 7.4. It can be seen from this description that by having a determination of

pH and CO_2, one can determine what sort of difficulty the patient is in. However, these measurements are time-consuming, and there are no nomograms that can be consulted to give information concerning the amounts of deficient or excess base. The use of the Astrup electrode (Astrup, 1956) has enabled rapid determinations to be made. It has been found that more reproducible results can be accomplished with the use of arterial blood samples. The Astrup technique is based upon the fact that two pH readings are taken, the first as the blood comes from the patient and the second after equilibration with a constant volume partial pressure of CO_2. With the Anderson nomogram (Anderson and Engel, 1960), one can then arrive at a definite base excess or deficit. This is an extremely quick and accurate method for arriving at the solutions of problems that present in the areas of respiratory acidosis and alkalosis. This is of prime concern to the surgeon who is faced with airway difficulties as well as with cardiovascular problems in his patient during operation and in the immediate postoperative period.

The use of arterial catheters for the measurement of pressure and as a source of arterial blood samples has proved helpful in adults. In infants and small children, in order to insert them into the arteries, the catheters must be of such small size that even keeping them filled with heparin solution when not in use does not prevent clotting and limiting their usefulness to within 24 to 48 hours. The use of arterial-venous shunts, for renal dialysis, has some promise, particularly with the newer types of soft, nontraumatic tubing. A compromise technique has been worked out in which warming of the heel or the lobe of the ear, thus expanding the capillaries, makes possible a skin puncture that will yield blood that is primarily arterial in composition. Although this is not ideal it does give some information in situations where arterial samples are unprocurable. However, when peripheral circulation is impaired as in shock, skin punctures yield samples that do not represent arterial blood.

In order to clarify matters it is well to have

definitions. The use of the terms "alkalosis" and "acidosis" is not realistic inasmuch as it is widely appreciated that one can have an acidosis of respiratory origin coexistent with a metabolic alkalosis. There are all sorts of combinations, and one must therefore have a clear-cut understanding of these terms. Nunn has made the following suggestions: acidosis is a condition that tends to cause acidosis if uncompensated; alkalosis is a condition that tends to cause alkalosis if uncompensated. The following is a list of definitions used in the quantifications of metabolic acid-base relationships by Nunn.

Standard bicarbonate is the bicarbonate concentration in the plasma of fully oxygenated blood that has been equilibrated at PCO_2 equal to 40 mm Hg at 38° C. The normal range is 22 to 26 mEq/l.

Reduced hydrogen ion concentration is the pH of fully oxygenated blood that has been incorporated at a PCO_2 of 40 mm Hg at 38° C. The normal range is 7.36 to 7.44 units.

Alkali reserve of carbon dioxide combining power is the bicarbonate concentration of plasma after separation from the cells that has been incorporated at a PCO_2 equal to 40 mm Hg at 38° C.

Buffer base is the sum of buffer anions in the blood. It includes bicarbonate, protein, and phosphate. Although it can refer to plasma it usually refers to normal blood. The normal range is 44 to 48 mEq/l.

Normal buffer base of blood is the blood's buffer base when the PCO_2 equals 40 mm Hg and the pH is 7.4 to 7.38. It varies with hemoglobin as follows: normal buffer base equals $40 \times 8 + 0.36 \times$ (hemoglobin concentration in grams per 100 ml).

Base excess is the excess of the buffer base over the normal buffer base of blood at its existing hemoglobin concentration.

Base deficit is the deficit of buffer base compared with normal buffer base of the blood at its existing hemoglobin concentration. The normal range is +2.5 to +1.5 mEq/l.

In order to understand respiratory acidosis and alkalosis one must appreciate the fact that determinations must be secured on oxygenated blood—that is, it is only after the lung has performed its function on the blood that samples are valid on which to base determinations that measure the efficiency of pulmonary function. The relationship of pH to carbonic acid and bicarbonate of blood is expressed by the Henderson-Hasselbalch equation. One can readily see that this equation can be solved, provided two values are available. The direct measurement of PCO_2 is difficult, and, therefore, measurements of pH have been relied upon because of the ease and accuracy of determination. The arterial blood samples must be drawn without any bubbles in the sample, for this may produce changes by equilibration with the CO_2 in the air and lead to erroneous results. The sample must be analyzed promptly within 10 to 15 minutes after the blood is drawn. First the pH of the sample is determined, and then CO_2 of 45 mm Hg tension is passed through the sample and a second pH is measured. Equilibration is then accomplished with 35 mm Hg tension, and the third reading is made. Thus, two of the values of the Henderson-Hasselbalch equation are known, and its solution is now possible. To solve the equation mathematically is time-consuming, and, therefore, nomograms have been made that permit rapid solution. The Anderson nomogram (Fig. 6) is used by many clinics and gives a considerable amount of information, including the bicarbonate excess or deficit. Although this information is used in emergencies, the surgeon must not rely on it completely; rather, electrolyte determinations should be made so that these values, if abnormal, can be corrected as well as the bicarbonate. The PCO_2 value arrived at is of prime value in appraising respiratory function and, when respiratory assistance is used, in checking on the efficiency of the apparatus.

CORRECTION OF DEHYDRATION

A common problem that confronts the clinician and surgeon is the dehydrated patient. To determine the degree of hydration

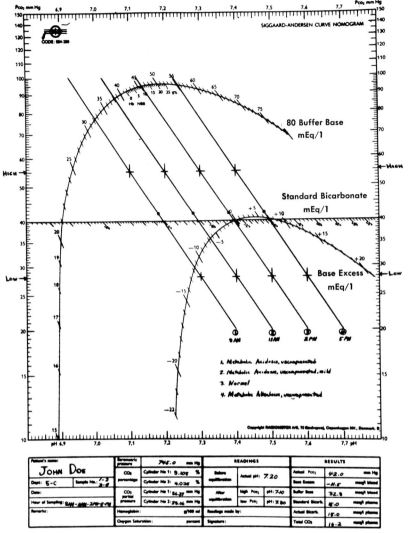

Fig. 6. Anderson nomogram.

has and will continue to be a problem that cannot be solved by direct measurement; rather it must depend to a large extent on clinical judgment. In the past we have relied upon skin turgidity, the amount of urine output, the concentration of the urine, and the condition of the mucous membrane of the mouth. All of these are aids that serve the experienced clinician. However, they lack the precision that is desirable in the small baby where there is less tolerance of error. By measuring the child's length and his head circumference and plotting these on a nomogram the average weight can be determined.

Subtracting the babies' actual weight gives the loss from dehydration providing the child's weight was within normal limits before the illness. Parents often know the pre-illness weight of small children and infants, and this gives a direct reliable figure that can be used in computing the percentage of dehydration. Having determined the percentage of dehydration one can then calculate replacement on the basis of restoration to a normal weight. For instance, a 3 kg baby has by estimation or by computation a 20 percent dehydration; 20 percent of 3,000 g is 600 g, or 600 ml of fluid required for complete hydration. It is important that additional fluids be added for maintenance requirements during the period of infusion.

Although these methods have merit in children dehydrated from low fluid intake, vomiting, and diarrhea, they are faulty in dealing with the patient with an intestinal obstruction, where the so-called third compartment, the intestinal tract, has trapped large amounts of fluid that are not available for metabolic use despite their presence in the body. Because of the intestinal dilation and some increase in intraluminal pressure this fluid remains isolated from the general circulation. With peritoneal infection large amounts of fluids are poured into the peritoneal cavity and are lost to the metabolic processes. In such situations, total body weights are misleading, and the clinician and surgeon must depend upon a general appraisal of the child to arrive at an estimate of the percentage of dehydration.

The derangement of electrolytes need not be estimated, although some prediction can be made from the history. If there has been excessive vomiting, the possibility alkalosis may develop is real. However, such estimates are not too essential, for today in a modern hospital the various electrolytes in the blood can be determined rapidly and accurately. With these values available plus the percentage of dehydration, either on the basis of direct measurement or estimation, the restoration to a normal hydration and electrolyte composition can be achieved. The volume of fluids to be given can be computed directly on the percentage of body weight loss. The electrolyte replacement should be computed on the basis of the electrolyte measurements. Since the chloride ion is largely in the extracellular fluid it would appear that the computation of its deficiency should be based on about 35 percent of the body weight in infants. Sodium has a potent effect on water metabolism. As a deficit of sodium develops there is a shift of water from the extracellular fluid into the cell as a compensatory mechanism. As sodium is added to the extracellular fluid, fluids leaves

the cell to enter the extracellular compartment. Consequently, sodium replacement must be computed on more than the extracellular fluid. It is customary to use 60 percent of body weight for this calculation. It is prudent to plan only a 50 percent correction in 24 hours, a practice that has proven wise from clinical experience. One must remember to add maintenance volumes to the computed deficits.

In the case of acidosis or alkalosis both intracellular and extracellular fluids are involved, and replacement should be computed on a more generous percentage basis of 70 percent of body weight. For instance, the difference between the normal values and the determined values can be computed. The percentage of body weight can then be used to determine the total volume where these deficits are present. On the basis of this, the total deficit can be determined. For example, a patient weighing 6.0 kg has a chloride of 80 mEq (100 is normal), and there is a deficit of 20 mEq per 1,000 ml. The infant's weight is 6,000 g, 35 percent of which, or 210 ml, is extracellular fluid. Twenty times 2.1 is 42 mEq. Fifty percent correction would be $\frac{1}{2}$ of 42, or 21 mEq, which is to be given in addition to the basic requirement of 27 mEq per square meter per 24 hours.

Some institutions use standard prepared solutions for correction and designate these by symbols. This works well within the institution, but the physician cannot function well in other hospitals where other systems are used. It would appear more wise to use standard solutions and mix these or add electrolytes to fit each patient's needs.

The computation of a potassium deficit is difficult because here we are dealing primarily with an intracellular substance, with a small component in the extracellular fluid, which is the level measured. However, when there is evidence of urinary output and the serum potassium is 3.5 or lower, 2 mEq/l of potassium can be given per kg of weight for safe restoration. Precautions should be taken when potassium is given to limit the concentration in fluids to 25 mEq/l. When there are indications of decreased renal function and when dealing with prematures there is danger in the administration of potassium unless the situation is carefully analyzed.

There are electrocardiac changes in potassium concentration disturbances. The tracings may indicate hyperkalemia, but they cannot be relied upon for they may be lacking. The changes are prolongation of the P-R interval, widening and disappearance of the P wave, peaked and narrow T waves, and cardiac irregularities.

The clinical findings of hypokalemia are diffuse and include weakness, mental clouding, and ileus. There may also be apathy or increased irritability and cardiac arrhythmia.

For the correction of metabolic acidosis, soda bicarbonate or sodium lactate can be used. Patients with liver disease, salicylate toxicity, glycogen storage disease, or shock may fail to metabolize lactate normally, and for this reason sodium bicarbonate is the more effective agent. Caution should be used and correction limited to 50 percent of the computed deficit, for the patient may develop postacidotic tetany and alkalosis, which may be related to the rise in pH and the decrease in ionized calcium.

The treatment of metabolic alkalosis is a more complicated problem. There is no ideal substance to give to correct alkalosis. Large quantities of chloride must be provided when there has been an excessive loss of hydrogen chloride in metabolic alkalosis. Since such patients also lose sodium and potassium, the administration of sodium chloride and potassium chloride is permissible, for the patients are able to excrete a moderate excess of sodium and potassium, and the hypochloremia is corrected. Provided there is no disturbance of ammonium metabolism, ammonium chloride may be used as another source of chloride.

When potassium depletion is associated with the alkalosis, there is an abnormal gradient of potassium between cell and plasma. Therefore, potassium chloride is used for correction, and when the potassium defect is corrected the loss of hydrogen stops and the

alkalosis is corrected. Oftentimes with alkalosis there may be an associated tetany with low ionized calcium. The correction of this depends upon a number of factors in addition to the low calcium. One must know the serum protein level because calcium is in combination with the proteins, and when total proteins are reduced more ionized calcium is available. It should also be remembered that the ionization of calcium depends on pH, so that with acidosis there is a greater number of calcium ions. Alkalosis, however, depresses the ionization of calcium and hastens the appearance of clinical tetany. In such situations it is advisable to consider the use of calcium chloride provided it is given judiciously. Here, the administration of calcium chloride not only elevates the calcium content of the blood but supplies chloride, which will help correct the alkalosis and thus indirectly increase calcium ionization. Calcium chloride is more dangerous than lactate because of its tendency to produce cardiac irregularities unless used with care. Where there is not an acute problem, and where the need is less urgent for calcium, calcium gluconate is safer to use. Attention should also be called to the fact that with alkalosis it may be helpful to have the patient breathe an increased concentration of carbon dioxide, which again will help correct the alkalosis.

POSTOPERATIVE PARENTERAL FLUID AND ELECTROLYTE NEEDS

It is assumed that the patient has been brought to a normal equilibrium preoperatively. Consequently, postoperatively, the planning should be for maintenance rather than for replacement. There has been a tendency in the past to plan fluid therapy postoperatively on the basis of electrolyte deficits determined by actual analysis of venous blood samples and estimated fluid losses. A better plan is to provide basic maintenance requirements and to project therapy on this basis. This does not mean that electrolyte determinations should be dispensed with. Rather, they should be used liberally to check the therapy. The first step to be taken in planning maintenance fluid requirements is to formulate a basis upon which to compute fluid needs. This can be done in one of several ways: on the basis of weight, on the basis of metabolism, and on the basis of surface area. No method is perfect; all have defects. However, after considering all the methods we have selected surface area as most advantageous. It is perfectly true in small infants that fluid requirements can be computed directly upon weight. However, as the child grows in weight one cannot use the weight directly as a gauge of fluid requirement, for it would result in giving older children excessive amounts of fluid. When weight is used, one has to reduce the amount of fluid per kilogram as the child becomes progressively heavier. Such systems are satisfactory despite the fact that the values are arbitrary. The system suggested by Holliday (1957) based on caloric expenditure is excellent and can be computed provided the basic values are remembered. The system is based on 100 ml of water per 100 cal of estimated caloric expenditure. The following is the estimated caloric expenditure based on the patient's weight:

$$0–10 \, kg = 100 \, cal/kg,$$
$$10–20 \, kg = 1,000 \, cal + 50$$
$$cal/kg \text{ for each kg over 10,}$$
$$20 \, kg \text{ and over} = 1,500 \, cal + 20$$
$$cal/kg \text{ for each kg over 10.}$$

In the use of this method the following values for electrolytes are suggested for maintenance:

$$Na—3 \, mEq/100 \, cal,$$
$$Cl—2 \, mEq/100 \, cal,$$
$$K—2 \, mEq/100 \, cal.$$

The surface area method of computation is equally good, and we have found it satisfactory after many years of use (Fig. 7).

Next, one must decide what the fluid requirement for maintenance per 24 hours per square meter is. This would ideally be arrived at by computing the insensible water loss and the normal amount of urine volume per 24 hours. Lowe has used 500 ml per square meter per 24 hours as the average insensible water loss.

Computation of urine output is more complicated and has been arrived at by calculating that under basic conditions the total solutes to be excreted is approximately 230 mOsm per square meter of body surface per 24 hours. To remove this quantity of solute would require 580 to 780 ml of water per square meter per 24 hours according to Lowe, and he has recommended 1,500 ml per square meter per 24 hours. We have used a lower figure, 1,200 ml per square meter per 24 hours.

The great value of frequent weighing of the patient should not be forgotten, particularly in infants where the technique is simple and the need for information is great. In the average postoperative patient, daily weights are sufficient. However, in the severely ill neonate with short intestines, where the loss from frequent stools may be large or where an ileostomy is present, weights at 8- to 12-hour intervals will be helpful in gauging the volumes and rates of parenteral fluid infusions.

The requirements of electrolytes on the basis of amount per square meter per 24 hours are: sodium 40 mEq, chloride 27 mEq, and potassium 21 mEq per square meter per 24 hours. With these figures available, it is possible to write orders on the basis of basic needs for these maintenance requirements. As an additional caution, it should be mentioned that when the patient is being maintained in a humidified atmosphere, the amount of fluid required should be somewhat less. This is particularly true if ultrasonic nebulization is used where the droplet size is extremely small and therefore penetrates deeply into the pulmonary tree. Nomograms regarding the amount of absorption through the pulmonary system are not available. Here one must carefully weigh the patient to

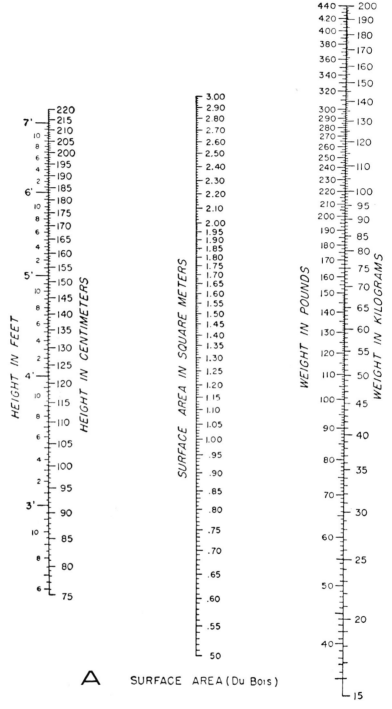

A   SURFACE AREA (Du Bois)

Fig. 7. Charts of body surface area in relation to weight and height. The body surface area is an accurate basis for determining volume of postoperative fluids; 1,200 ml is required for each square meter of surface area per day. A. Chart for estimating surface area of infants.

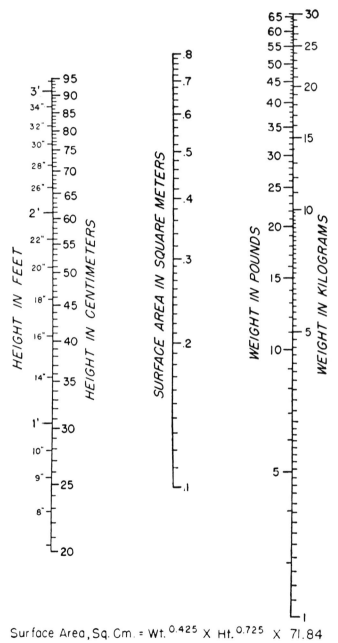

B   Surface Area, Sq. Cm. = Wt.$^{0.425}$ X Ht.$^{0.725}$ X 71.84

Fig. 7 (cont.). B. Chart for estimating surface area of children. (From Crawford, et al. Pediatrics, 5:783, 1950.)

be sure that overhydration does not take place. Added to these basic maintenance volumes and amounts of electrolytes are such losses as fluids drained by nasogastric tubes and from chest catheters or wounds (Table 1, from these basic solutions, dilu-

TABLE 1.   STOCK SOLUTIONS AND CONCENTRATES

SOLUTIONS

250–500 ml volumes

Dextrose 5 percent water
Dextrose 5 percent—0.2 percent sodium chloride
Normal saline
Lactated Ringer's

CONCENTRATES

3 ml–30 ml per volumes mEq

Ammonium chloride
Potassium acetate
Sodium lactate
Dextrose 50 percent
Sodium chloride
Potassium phosphate
Potassium chloride

Sodium bicarbonate—50 ml contains 44.6 mEq

tions and additions can be made to provide for the intravenous setup).

For the first time infants have been reported to have gained weight and develop normally over periods of weeks with feedings limited to the intravenous route. Wilmore (1968) achieved this with a solution of 25 percent glucose and 5 percent fibrin hydrolysate supplemented with minerals and vitamins. This hypertonic solution was apparently less destructive to veins, provided the solution has a pH of 7.4. The acidity of the solution was changed to neutral with the addition of sodium chloride. The solution was injected through a catheter inserted in a neck vein and advanced into the vena cava.

OBTAINING BLOOD FOR CHEMICAL ANALYSIS

After the child has been accustomed to the hospital, his physical preparation for operation is begun. The seriously ill child should have blood drawn and sent to the laboratory for emergency analysis as soon after admission as possible, in order that his electrolyte balance may be appraised. Basic blood determinations include carbon dioxide, sodium, potassium, chloride, and blood urea nitrogen. It is possible to secure 2 to 10 ml of blood from small infants by a femoral or jugular venipuncture, but to repeat this daily on small, sick babies may be harmful. It can be avoided by using microtechniques in the laboratory, so that sufficient blood is obtained from the heel prick to permit blood urea nitrogen, chloride, potassium, sodium, and carbon dioxide determinations.

When several millimeters of blood are required from an infant, jugular or femoral venipuncture must be performed. The insertion of a needle into the superficial or deep jugular vein is difficult, and complications may occur. As in any venipuncture, vessels may be lacerated and bleeding may follow, although the bleeding is usually not of a dangerous amount. The lung apex may be damaged and pneumothorax produced. Femoral venipuncture is easier, but complications may be more serious. If the femoral artery is torn, there may be extensive concealed hemorrhage. This may also occur after the laceration of the femoral vein. Arterial injury may result in spasm sufficient to produce transient ischemia of the leg. Gangrene of a part of the limb has occurred, and infants known to be bleeders have died from hemorrhage following femoral venipuncture. Formations of arteriovenous communications have been reported after femoral vein puncture. This apparently has occurred when the vein has been entered 3 or 4 cm below the inguinal ligament, where one vessel lies behind the other. However, there are occasions when it is a necessary procedure. The infant must be held securely. The femoral artery is located by palpation as it emerges below the inguinal ligament and is carefully avoided. The needle is inserted medial to the artery, and negative pressure is applied by the syringe as the needle is being withdrawn. Repeated insertions of the needle should be avoided.

Sufficient blood samples for crossmatching can be secured from a heel prick. A few drops of blood can be placed in 2 or 3 ml of saline for cell suspension. A larger amount can be collected in a micro Hinton tube, centrifuged in the tube, and made available for completion of the crossmatch.

PARENTERAL FLUID HYDRATION

Investigations have indicated that hypodermoclysis as a method of hydration should be avoided whenever possible. Two and one half to 5 percent glucose solution in a clysis may actually dehydrate the patient, aggravate an existing electrolyte imbalance, and even contribute to shock. This is because the hypotonic fluid (in regard to electrolytes) causes a passage of electrolytes from the vascular fluid to the tissue spaces where the clysis has been administered, further aggravating the state of hydration and causing harmful electrolyte shifts. Absorption of fluid from the subcutaneous tissue is slow, and general utilization of the fluid will be delayed and valuable time lost in hydration of the patient. The use of drugs such as hyaluronidase to hasten the diffusion of fluid in the subcutaneous tissue may actually intensify the ill effects of the clysis. Another important reason for avoiding clysis is the prolonged discomfort it entails.

The intravenous administration of parenteral fluids in infants and children is not too difficult, and it avoids the disadvantages and dangers of clysis. The most accessible vein for intravenous therapy to newborn infants and babies up to 9 or 12 months old is in the scalp (Fig. 8). To facilitate inser-

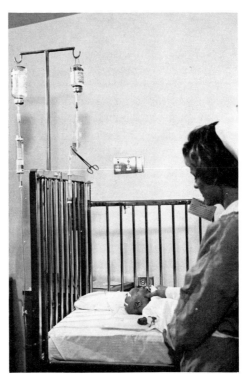

Fig. 8. Scalp intravenous setup.

tion of the needle, the baby is securely wrapped in a blanket and placed on a table so that its head rests on the edge. The baby is given a sugar nipple, and the hair is shaved from the frontal area of the baby's head. The nurse holds the infant on the table under her arm so that she can use both hands to control the infant's head. The skin is prepared by scrubbing with aqueous Zephiran Chloride (1:1,000). A 24 beveled needle from which the bulb has been removed is inserted into a polyethylene tubing. This equipment is now commercially available in sterile disposable units. Such a needle can be taped in place more easily than a needle with a bulb and adapter. The needle is then inserted into a vein in the frontal area and threaded into the lumen for a short distance. Immobilization is more effective when a vein in the frontal region is used rather than one in the temporal region. The polyethylene tubing can then be attached to the intravenous set. By having a three-way stopcock in the set, fluid and medications can be rapidly administered to the infant with a syringe.

Intravenous administration is safe with relatively well babies. But in extremely sick patients, particularly those with pulmonary disease, the rapid infusion of intravenous fluid may produce life-endangering pulmonary edema. Such a catastrophe can be avoided by administering the fluid or blood by gravity, using the needle in the scalp vein for a constant intravenous drip.

To prevent rapid infusion of harmful volumes of fluid, various commercial devices, such as compartmental plastic containers, are available that can be cross-clamped and thus limit the infusion to small increments (Fig. 9).

When dehydration is corrected preoperatively, the patient is well hydrated at the end of the operation. To prevent the administration of excessive amounts of fluid, specific amounts should be ordered in addition to a specific rate of flow. Otherwise, if the rate of flow inadvertently increases the baby may receive a disastrous quantity.

Children one year of age and over have veins in the extremities adequate for intravenous infusion. In older children, the antecubital veins can be used. But these veins should be avoided in younger children who are less cooperative and in whom the inevitable motion at the elbow frequently dislodges the needle. The arm below the elbow,

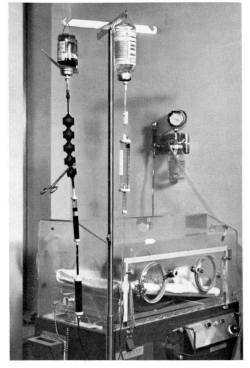

Fig. 9. Special infusion set that provides safeguards against the infusion of large quantities of fluid or blood. The fluid administration set has a microdrip so that the rate of infusion can be controlled. The blood transfusion set has a series of plastic containers, each segment containing 10 ml. A clamp is placed across a segment to limit the infusion.

the hand, and the wrist are areas where the veins are more superficial and immobilization is more successful.

While intravenous needles in the scalp or

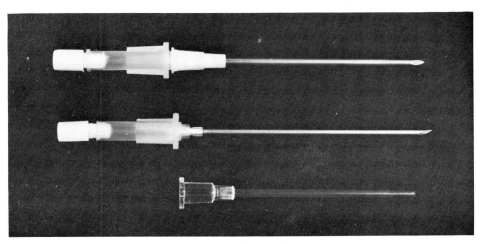

Fig. 10. Plastic cannulas.

arm veins are satisfactory in both infants and children before and after operation, in the course of surgery on infants it is imperative to have a dependable intravenous route open for the injection of fluids, blood, and medication. Various plastic cannulas are available for older children with larger veins (Fig. 10). These are superior to needles, for they are less likely to be dislodged or to injure the vein wall. In smaller children and infants an open system into the patient's vascular system can be guaranteed only by exposing a vein surgically and tying a metal cannula or plastic cannula into the vein. The catheter or cannula should be removed if possible within 48 hours to prevent the complication of phlebitis.

GASTRIC AND INTESTINAL SUCTION

Routine preoperative gastric intubation and the administration of an enema for all cases having a laparotomy is no longer advised. These procedures are often unnecessary and upsetting to the child. But there are numerous indications for the insertion of a Levin or Miller-Abbott tube both before and after operation. Patients who are vomiting and whose symptoms indicate possible abdominal surgical disease should have a Levin tube inserted. Intubation is especially valuable in small, severely ill infants. Because such infants are so weak, there is danger of aspiration of vomitus, and the resulting pulmonary complication may be fatal. There may be a need for a gastrostomy for decompression in severely ill patients who have undergone abdominal surgery. By this means effective gastric decompression is provided without the disturbance of airway that is almost inevitable when a nasogastric tube is used. Against these advantages must be balanced the complications of gastrostomy. Since these complications are real possibilities it is unwise to use gastrostomy routinely when abdominal surgery is performed, for in most situations nasogastric suction is adequate and without complication. However, in

selected cases gastrostomy has a definite place. If on physical examination there is great distension, or a roentgenogram of the abdomen outlines distension of the small intestine, a Miller-Abbott tube should be used rather than a gastric tube. Before a Miller-Abbott tube is inserted it must be examined carefully for leaks, particularly at the point where the balloon is attached to the tube. The length of the tube to be inserted initially is roughly determined by measuring the distance from the patient's nose to his stomach. The tube is lubricated and inserted through a nostril. Older children should drink water while the tube is being inserted. When it is in place, 1 ml of mercury should be injected into the balloon and the patient fluoroscoped so that the tip may be positioned properly and an attempt made to pass it into the duodenum. When this is not possible, the tip can be properly positioned to facilitate the tube's spontaneous entrance into the duodenum. It is advantageous to have the radiologist arrange the tube so that it will lie along the greater curvature with the tip at the pylorus. The patient is then returned to the ward with the tube taped to the nostril, and he is propped up on his right side.

Giving small amounts of fluid and keeping the patient on his right side may hasten the passage of the tube into the duodenum. Twelve to 24 hours after the tube has been inserted, an abdominal roentgenogram should be taken or fluoroscopy performed. Frequently, these examinations will show that the tube has entered the second or third portion of the duodenum, and orders should be written to advance the tube an inch every hour. If the tube is curled in the stomach, it must be repositioned. The patient must either be fluoroscoped or have a plain abdominal roentgenogram made daily to guard against loops of tubing accumulating in the stomach and even prolapsing through the pylorus. One extra loop of tubing in the stomach is sufficient to prevent progression of the tip of the tube. When the tube advances slowly into the small intestine, it is advisable to inflate the balloon with 5 to 10 ml of air to accelerate its progress. If a leak occurs in the bag and mercury is released into the intestinal tract, the mercury will pass through with the fecal contents and produce no ill effects on the patient. If the tip of the tube remains at a fixed point in the intestine for 24 hours, a small amount of 30 percent Urokon sodium solution (sodium 3-acetylamino-2,4,6-triiodobenzoate) is injected through the tube and roentgenograms are taken to outline any point of mechanical obstruction. This is particularly useful when it has been impossible to distinguish clinically between reflex ileus and partial intestinal obstruction.

No rubber tubing of satisfactory length and diameter has been available for intestinal intubation of infants. The child's size Miller-Abbott tube is too large to insert through a small baby's nostril, and the 8F urethral catheter is not long enough. Recently, we have devised a tube of polyvinyl plastic that has a slightly smaller outside diameter than an 8F catheter and a thin wall that makes the lumen equal to that of a small Miller-Abbott tube. A finger cot is attached to the tube with multiple turns of 6-0 silk; 0.5 ml of mercury is placed in the balloon before the second side is attached to the tube. Four or five openings are made in the tubing behind the balloon so that the intestine will be decompressed in back of the balloon as well as at the tip. The tube can be inserted through an infant's nostril and is readily swallowed. It is not radiopaque, but it can be made so by injecting Lipiodol into it. A 15 blunt intravenous needle will fit into the tubing and serve as a convenient link to the suction apparatus (Fig. 11).

Innumerable mishaps can deprive the patient of the advantages of intestinal intubation, and only constant vigilance on the part of the doctor will assure that the tube is functioning properly. It should be irrigated every two hours with 10 ml of saline to prevent plugging. Ten millimeters of water are repeatedly injected through the tube and withdrawn until the injected fluid returns

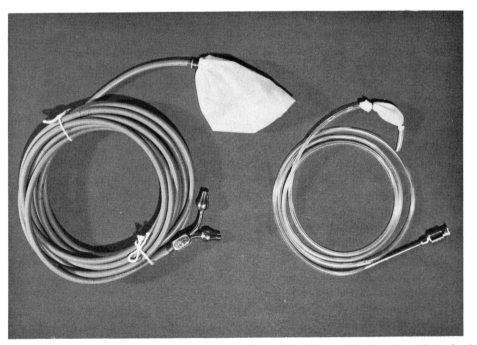

Fig. 11. Right, a polyvinyl intestinal tube. Note that it is considerably smaller than the child's size Miller-Abbott tube at the left.

freely and with little discoloration. If the fluid cannot be withdrawn, the tube is probably kinked. Under these circumstances the situation can be treated by withdrawing the tube several inches and repeating the irrigation. If this does not permit the withdrawal of injected fluid, fluoroscopy should be performed to correct any kinking or prolapse without pulling the tip back into the stomach. Irrigations should not be relegated entirely to the nursing service. Once or twice a day the attending doctor should test the tube function by irrigation. The tube should not be removed until the patient has passed flatus and fecal material and until a 24-hour period of clamping the suction lumen has produced no pain or distension.

Some years ago it was proposed that intestinal distension could be controlled partially by maintaining the patient in a 90 percent oxygen concentration. It demonstrated experimentally that this concept was valid. When the nitrogen in the air of the room is displaced with oxygen, the concentration of nitrogen in the alveolar spaces is reduced far below the normal 80 percent. In this indirect way, the intestinal gas is speeded from the bowel to the lung by way of the bloodstream. A further advantage is that the gas swallowed by the patient is 90 percent oxygen, which has a far more rapid rate of diffusion than nitrogen. The proper tent must be used so that a 90 percent concentration of oxygen is maintained over long periods of time. To increase the effectiveness of this treatment, the nursing care must be so organized that the tent will be disturbed only at four- to six-hour intervals. If the tent is opened frequently, it is impossible to maintain a sufficient concentration of oxygen to be effective in the treatment of intestinal distension.

Oxygen is of great help to patients with respiratory diseases, congenital defects of the heart, and obstructive lesions of the respiratory tract. However, oxygen is frequently given to the patient without any clear indication, and a great deal of effort and money are wasted in this manner.

PHYSICAL POSTOPERATIVE CARE

As soon as the operation is completed and the patient can be moved, he should be taken to an intensive care unit. A careful chart of the patient is kept with recordings of pulse, respiration, and blood pressure every 15 minutes until the patient is conscious. The constant care of severely ill infants is begun in the operating room and continued in intensive care. These infants are so weak that they cannot clear their air passages; consequently, mucus can collect and produce laryngeal spasm. Unless a nurse is in attendance at all times to suction the patient's oropharynx and to clear the air passages, death may occur. Undoubtedly the results of the complicated surgery required for such conditions as atresia of the esophagus and tracheoesophageal fistula, as well as extensive resections and anastomoses in the abdominal cavity, can be improved by having a nurse in constant attendance until a good recovery has been made.

Immediately after the operation, the patient is placed on his side as a matter of routine. Some patients may require a special position because of a particular disease or operation. In generalized peritonitis, it is well to maintain the patient in the low Fowler's position immediately after operation. Most patients who have had chest operations can be placed on either side, but if this is not tolerated the low Fowler's position will usually be comfortable.

Patients who have undergone operations in the abdomen or in the extremities and who have pain postoperatively should be given morphine or Demerol. Those who have had chest operations and who suffer postoperative pain should be given codeine because this drug produces less depression of the respiratory system than does morphine. In the rare instances when small infants and young children are irritable postoperatively, small doses of phenobarbital are usually helpful. Generally, little if any postoperative sedation is necessary.

All patients who have had abdominal operations should have a Levin tube with a Wangensteen suction apparatus in place until normal peristalsis returns. The time for removal of these tubes is determined by the amount of gastric drainage that the tube produces. Usually, as peristalsis becomes active the amount of drainage decreases abruptly. Occasionally a patient will have good peristalsis and no abdominal distension, but the Levin tube will draw back larger quantities of bile-stained secretions. If the tube position is checked, it will often be found that the tip has slipped into the duodenum. Withdrawing the tube 2 or 3 inches will stop the drainage of bile-stained fluid. Postoperatively there are several advantages to the routine use of a Levin tube in abdominal cases. In the first place, it removes anesthetic-saturated fluids from the stomach and thus contributes to a more comfortable postoperative course and hastens the return of gastrointestinal function. Furthermore it relieves the patient of the discomfort of vomiting and retching postoperatively. A Miller-Abbott tube should be used when there is marked abdominal distension or when intestinal obstruction is anticipated in the postoperative course.

TREATMENT OF OLIGURIA OR ANURIA

Patients who developed renal failure as a result of mismatched blood transfusions, drugs, or following manipulation of the urinary tract were formerly treated with rapid infusions of hypotonic solutions in an effort to increase urine flow. Since such therapy rarely produced the desired result, the additional fluid was retained and produced edema, hyponatremia, and water intoxication. The rational method of treatment requires the following: information concerning current and recent drug, anesthetic, and fluid intake; a clinical estimate of the current state of dehydration; and an estimate of the patient's insensible water losses from the skin and respiratory tract.

It is important to be certain that oliguria is not the result of underhydration. Oliguria associated with poor skin turgor, sunken eyes, and an anterior fontanel should be treated with an isotonic salt solution infused at a rate of 20 ml/kg/hr until the skin turgor is normal. If urine output does not improve when the patient has been hydrated, further treatment should follow the principles given below for care of renal failure. Oliguria may result from inappropriate antidiuretic hormone release, which may be induced by such drugs as morphine, barbiturates, and certain inhalation anesthetics. The scanty urine produced has a very high specific gravity and osmolarity, while the patient's plasma exhibits hyponatremia and hypo-osmolarity if water intake is not restricted. The best treatment for this condition is prevention by restricting the water intake in clinical situations where such a response can be expected to occur. Should hypo-osmolarity, hyponatremia, or edema develop, severe restriction of water intake will lead to gradual improvement. If the patient has symptoms of water intoxication, a prompt diuresis can usually be obtained by oral administration of a small dose of dilute ethyl alcohol. If the patient is receiving artificial ventilation, inhalation of a gas mixture containing 5 to 8 percent carbon dioxide for a few minutes may also initiate a diuresis. Both alcohol and CO_2 inhalation act as inhibitors of antidiuretic hormone release.

Recently, infusions of a hypertonic solution of an inert carbohydrate substance, mannitol, have been used to promote an osmotic diuresis and relieve oliguria. This therapy has been effective in relieving oliguria associated with postoperative water retention and in the early oliguric phase of acute renal failure caused by transfusion reactions, nephrotoxic drugs, or other toxins. This therapy might be particularly effective in relieving oliguria secondary to crystalluria, which may accompany the administration of such a drug as sulfonamide. The usual dose is 1 g per kg of body weight given intravenously as a 15 to 20 percent aqueous solution. It should be remembered that the resulting diuresis will increase sodium as well as body water losses, and additional amounts of salt and water must be provided to meet these increased losses. If a diuresis does not occur following infusion of hypertonic mannitol, nothing is to be gained by repeating the infusion, and the patient should be treated as outlined in the following paragraphs.

If oliguria secondary to dehydration or inappropriate antidiuretic hormone release can be excluded, and if renal failure seems to account for a diminished urine output, water intake should be restricted to amounts sufficient to replace current net water losses. With complete anuria, such losses would represent the insensible loss less the water produced by metabolism. The net water requirement can be estimated to be about 300 ml of the estimated caloric expenditure per day. This estimate should be checked by frequent weighing of the patient, often more than once daily. If water intake is not excessive, the patient should lose weight slowly, since catabolism of body tissues will occur as a result of a low caloric intake. Catabolism of body protein can be minimized by the provision of maximum calories in the form of fat or carbohydrate. Intravenous fluids can be given as 10 to 15 percent solutions of dextrose or dextrose and invert sugar. The calories that can be provided are limited by the amount of water that can be given and by the size of the vein receiving the infusion. A small vein will rapidly develop phlebitis and thrombosis if the tonicity of the infusote is above that provided by a water solution containing 8 percent dextrose. Older children may be able to tolerate hard candy and butterballs given orally.

Blood chemistries taken daily will be useful in the early detection of hyponatremia, severe acidosis, and hyperkalemia; and serial determinations of pH, CO_2 content, sodium, and potassium are necessary. Serial electrocardiograms will often give the earliest indication of potassium toxicity. Should water intoxication and hyponatremia, edema, hy-perkalemia, or severe acidosis develop, either hemodialysis or peritoneal dialysis should begin promptly. The appearance of pulmonary edema demands prompt measures to reduce the plasma volume, including peripheral tourniquets, phlebotomy, and dialysis against a hypertonic dialysing fluid to remove water.

If the kidney recovers from the anuric or oliguric phase of acute renal failure, some improvement of urine output can be expected within 8 to 14 days. Care should be taken to provide additional fluid as needed to prevent dehydration during the diuretic phase that may occur following the oliguric phase.

Great care should be taken to avoid the use or to modify the dosage of any drugs normally excreted by the kidney that must be used in treating the oliguric or anuric patient. The best rule to remember is to avoid the use of any drug for which there is not a clear-cut indication.

VASCULAR AND PULMONARY COMPLICATIONS

Fortunately, vascular and pulmonary complications, which are so dangerous and so common in adults, are unusual in children. Occasionally, after long operations, atelectasis may occur in the first 52 postoperative hours, and when it develops the child will have a sudden onset of rapid respirations, slight cyanosis, and tachycardia. Palpation of the neck may reveal some tracheal deviation. In the area of the atelectasis there will be a dullness to percussion and a depression of breath sounds. It is difficult to obtain sufficient cooperation from children for effective coughing to correct this condition. Almost invariably the insertion of a catheter through the nose into the pharynx produces sufficient coughing to effectively dislodge the plug of mucus that has produced the atelectasis. Suction on the catheter promptly removes any material that may be coughed up. Should this method fail, it may be necessary to insert the catheter into the trachea with the aid of a laryngoscope. This can be accomplished in babies but is more difficult in older children. With severe atelectasis, which cannot be effectively treated by these measures, it is necessary to proceed with bronchoscopy and with direct suction applied to the affected lobe, even if a general anesthetic is necessary to carry out this maneuver.

It is rare to have postoperative pneumonia in children. Usually the atelectasis clears with effective treatment, and there are no further sequelae. Cardiac complications are seldom encountered except for paroxysmal tachycardia on rare occasions. This can be treated effectively by digitalizing the baby. Occasionally a child with a congenital heart anomaly may have some degree of failure postoperatively. This is evidenced by enlargement of the liver and by pulmonary rales. When this complication arises in the postoperative child, digitalization is usually effective in controlling the situation.

Such complications as phlebothrombosis and pulmonary embolism are practically unheard of in children and need not concern the surgeon during the postoperative period except after splenectomies, when patients may develop thromboses, particularly in the mesenteric vessels. A guiding principle in the postoperative care of children is to anticipate complications and to treat them effectively in the incipient stage so that a full-fledged complication never becomes established.

ANTIBIOTIC THERAPY

There are several general decisions that must be made in the antibiotic therapy of a patient: whether or not to use antibiotics, what antibiotic should be selected, what dosage should be used, and what should be the duration of therapy. This section outlines the principles involved in answering these questions and lists recommended choices and doses of antibiotics that are generally accepted in present practice.

WHEN SHOULD ANTIBIOTICS BE USED?

Sometimes it is difficult to decide whether an antibiotic should be used. In such situations the age of the patient is often the decisive factor. A minor infection or a possible early infection often should be treated with antibiotics when the patient is a newborn or a young infant, whereas an older child would simply be observed.

Skin or soft tissue infections frequently require careful clinical judgment about the need for antibiotics. Operative drainage of pus is ordinarily sufficient, but a delay in improvement or the presence of cellulitis may justify the use of an antibiotic. For minor skin infections, a drug should be used that is not ordinarily reserved for serious infections. The widespread use of penicillinase-resistant penicillins could hasten the selection of genetic mutants of staphylococci that produce beta-lactamases (penicillinase) capable of inactivating these newer penicillins. Therefore, erythromycin or a similar antibiotic is preferable for minor infections caused by penicillin-resistant staphylococci.

The use of prophylactic antibiotics directed at preventing infections caused by specific organisms, such as the streptococcus and meningococcus, is well established. However, attempts to prevent bacterial infection in general, such as in the comatose patient, not only are likely to fail, but often select antibiotic-resistant organisms for superinfections and do more harm than good. However, the long-term prophylactic use of urinary antiseptics, such as nitrofurantoin, appears to be both safe and effective. Few controlled studies have been done to evaluate the routine use of antibiotics following cardiac surgery, although this practice is now frequent.

The major risk of prophylactic antibiotics is that they predispose the patient to superinfection. The replacement of normal bowel flora with resistant organisms often occurs after the oral administration of broad-spectrum antibiotics and may be related to the

TABLE 2.   CHOICE OF ANTIBIOTICS BASED ON CLINICAL DIAGNOSIS,
UNTIL CULTURE AND SENSITIVITY RESULTS ARE KNOWN

CLINICAL DIAGNOSIS	ANTIBIOTIC	EXPECTED ORGANISM
Skin and Bones		
Furuncle, abscess	Erythromycin	Staphylococcus
Wound infection	Penicillin	Streptococcus
serious	add kanamycin	Staphylococcus, coliforms
Cellulitis	Parenteral penicillin	Streptococcus
unresponsive to penicillin	treat as an osteomyelitis	
Septic arthritis or osteomyelitis	Methicillin*	Penicillin-resistant staphylococcus
if no improvement	add chloramphenicol	Coliform
Eye, Ear, Nose, and Throat		
Exudative pharyngitis	Penicillin	Streptococcus
Orbital cellulitis	Penicillin	Streptococcus
Otitis media	Penicillin	Streptococcus or pneumococcus
in a preschool-age child	Ampicillin	Haemophilus
Mastoiditis or sinusitis,	Methicillin*	Staphylococcus
serious	add chloramphenicol	Coliform, hemophilus
Severe croup	Ampicillin	Hemophilus
Chest and Abdomen		
Typical pneumonia	Penicillin	Pneumococcus
Severe pneumonia or empyema	Methicillin*	Penicillin-resistant staphylococcus
Postoperative pneumonia	add kanamycin	Coliform
Peritonitis or abdominal abscess	Penicillin and kanamycin	Streptococcus, anaerobes, coliforms, staphylococcus
Urinary		
Acute urinary infections	Sulfisoxazole	Coliform
Recurrent or chronic urinary infection	Nitrofurantoin	Coliform
Urinary infection occurring during above therapy	Ampicillin	Enterococcus
Central Nervous System		
Purulent meningitis, complicating head injury	Penicillin and chloramphenicol	Anaerobes, coliforms, or hemophilus
Brain abscess	Penicillin and chloramphenicol	Anaerobes, pyogenic cocci or coliforms
General		
Septicemia	Methicillin* and kanamycin and polymyxin B	Staphylococcus Coliform Pseudomonas (especially with burns)

* Or an equivalent penicillinase-resistant penicillin listed in Table 4.

severe fulminating infections that are sometimes observed after operations on patients
who have received antibiotics for 7 to 10
days before surgery.

Before the surgeon orders any antibiotic,
he should first determine if all useful cultures
have been obtained. Once antibiotic therapy
has been begun, negative cultures are of no
value. Pus and exudates should always be
cultured. When pus or exudate is not present, other cultures may be of value; for
example, in pneumonia or cellulitis, cultures
of the throat and blood should be done before starting antibiotics.

WHAT ANTIBIOTIC SHOULD BE CHOSEN?

Preliminary simple bacteriological techniques practiced by the surgeon can be extremely useful guides to the selection of antibiotics. Pus or exudate should always be
gram stained, a brief procedure that does

not require timing of the stains. Immediate
plating of the pus usually will save a day in
identifying the organism and in obtaining
sensitivity results. Facilities for the surgeon
or an assistant to inoculate and incubate a
simple blood agar plate should be available
in every hospital when a technician is not
available. When an incubator and blood agar
plates are not available, a swab of pus or
exudate may be stored in a tube of broth in
a refrigerator.

If no material is available for gram stain,
the initial choice of an antibiotic is based on
the clinical diagnosis, which implies a probable infecting organism. Table 2 lists recommended choices of antibiotics for most clinical situations, classified by the anatomic
areas involved. No table can cover every
situation, and the surgeon must occasionally
make exceptions to these choices. When
antibiotics have been begun because of a
clinical diagnosis, they should not be discontinued merely because of negative cul-

TABLE 3.   CHOICE OF ANTIBIOTICS BASED ON LABORATORY REPORTS

ORGANISM	BEST DRUG IF SENSITIVE		
	SERIOUS INFECTION	ALTERNATE DRUG	MINOR INFECTION
Pneumococcus, gonococcus, group A streptococcus, clostridia (gangrene or tetanus), penicillin-sensitive staphylococcus	Penicillin	Erythromycin	Penicillin
Penicillin-resistant staphylococcus	Methicillin*	Oxacillin*	Erythromycin
Escherichia coli, proteus, klebsiella-aerobacter, achromobacter, mima, herellea, alcaligenes	Ampicillin, cephalothin, or kanamycin	Chloramphenicol	Sulfisoxazole (urinary)
Enterococcus, alpha streptococcus, or gamma streptococcus	Ampicillin	Streptomycin with penicillin	Nitrofurantoin (urinary)
Pseudomonas	Polymyxin B or colistin	Gentamicin	Tetracycline
Enteropathic Escherichia coli	Neomycin (oral)	Colistin (oral)	Neomycin (oral)
Salmonella	Chloramphenicol	Ampicillin	Ampicillin
Haemophilus influenzae	Ampicillin or chloramphenicol	Tetracycline	Sulfisoxazole
Shigella	Ampicillin	Tetracycline	—
Meningococcus	Penicillin	Ampicillin	—
Tularemia, brucellosis	Streptomycin	Tetracycline	—

* Or equivalent penicillinase-resistant penicillin listed in Table 4.

tures, unless the clinical diagnosis is also changed.

Clinical evaluation of the severity of the illness is necessary. The most potent drug should be used in a serious illness in spite of some risk toxicity, but the antibiotic of least toxicity or no antibiotic at all should be used for a minor illness.

After the bacteriology laboratory results have been reported, many drugs may appear to be effective on the basis of in vitro susceptibility tests. The antibiotic recommendations in Table 3 are based both on the usual susceptibility test results and on clinical experience with the particular organism. Alternate drugs are listed, and occasionally a less toxic drug is advised for minor infections. Susceptibility testing is unnecessary for group A streptococcus and pneumococcus, which are always susceptible to penicillin and erythromycin.

Occasionally, the simultaneous use of more than one antibiotic is advisable. When no single antibiotic is effective against all of the usual bacteria that may cause a serious clinical syndrome, then a combination of two (or, rarely, three) antibiotics may be advisable until laboratory reports are available. Synergism or antagonism between two antibiotics has rarely been documented in controlled clinical studies. The necessity to select therapy effective against more than one possible organism, before the infecting organism is known, is a much more important reason for the use of two antibiotics than considerations of synergism or antagonism. The use of fixed combinations of drugs in proprietary preparations limits dosage flexibility and is not advisable.

New antibiotics should not be used routinely until proved to be superior to older antibiotics. The physician should wait for extensive unbiased observations of their effectiveness and toxicity that have been published in authoritative journals before changing from standard therapy to the latest antibiotic on the market.

It is helpful to be able to put a new drug in a category with an older antibiotic with which the physician is familiar in order to know what antibacterial spectrum and toxicity to expect. For this purpose, Table 4

TABLE 4.   CLASSIFICATION OF ANTIMICROBIAL DRUGS BASED ON STRUCTURE AND SPECTRUM, WITH SELECTED EXAMPLES

Penicillin Group
aqueous penicillin, procaine penicillin penicillin G, penicillin V, phenethicillin

Penicillinase-resistant Penicillin Group
methicillin, oxacillin, cloxacillin, nafcillin

Macrolide Group
erythromycin, oleandomycin, novobiocin, lincomycin

Sulfonamide Group
sulfisoxazole, trisulfapyrimidines

Tetracycline Group
tetracycline, oxytetracycline, chlortetracycline, demethylchlortetracycline

Dioxystreptamine Group
kanamycin, streptomycin, gentamicin

Polymyxin Group
polymyxin B, colistin

Urinary Antiseptic Group
nitrofurantoin, nalidixic acid, methenamine mandelate

Chloramphenicol

Ampicillin

Cephalothin

classifies currently used antibiotics into groups and lists selected examples in each group.

Gentamicin has a spectrum similar to kanamycin and neomycin. It is not a polymyxin, but like polymyxin B and colistin it is usually effective against pseudomonas.

Only a small proportion of gram-negative enteric organisms are susceptible to cephalothin or ampicillin. However, either of these antibiotics is the best choice when effective in vitro because of low toxicity, especially when renal function is impaired, since high serum concentrations of these antibiotics are not toxic. Cephalothin is as effective and nontoxic as the penicillinase-resistant penicillins and has a chemical structure that is closely related to penicillin. Cephalothin is very useful for a sensitive Klebsiella-Aerobacter. Ampicillin is useful for Salmonella carriers, enterococcus infections, and Hemophilus infections.

Generic names are used for simplicity in these tables. Since each drug may be marketed under several trade names, the physician will usually find it easier to learn and remember generic names. If generic names are used in prescriptions, the patient's drug cost may be decreased.

WHAT DOSES SHOULD BE USED?

Pediatric doses and doses for newborns and premature infants are shown in Table 5. In serious illnesses, the most potent drug

TABLE 5.   PEDIATRIC DOSES OF SELECTED ANTIMICROBIAL AGENTS

DRUG	ROUTE OF ADMINISTRATION	PEDIATRIC (MG/KG/DAY)	NEWBORN
Ampicillin	Oral	50–100	ID‡
Ampicillin	IM* or IV†	50–200	
Cephalothin	IM or IV	40–80	ID
Chloramphenicol	Oral or IM	50–100	25–50
Chloramphenicol	IV	100	25
Cloxacillin	Oral	50	ID
Colistin	IM	1.5–5	1–2
Colistin	Oral§	10	5
Erythromycin	Oral	40	20–40
Gentamicin	IM	1	ID
Isoniazid	Oral	10–30	10–30
Kanamycin	IM	15–25	5–15
Lincomycin	Oral	30–60	ID
Methenamine mandelate	Oral	50	ID
Methicillin	IM or IV	100	100
Nafcillin	Oral, IM, or IV	50–100	ID
Nalidixic acid	Oral	50	NR‖
Neomycin	Oral§	50–100	50
Nitrofurantoin	Oral	4–8	NR
Oxacillin	Oral or IM	50–100	50–100
Penicillin	Oral or IM	10–25 (20,000–50,000 units)	10–25 (20,000–50,000 units)
Penicillin	IV	20–500 (40,000–1,000,000 units)	20–50 (40,000–1,000,000 units)
Polymyxin	IM	2.5	1–2
Streptomycin	IM	20–40	10–30
Sulfisoxazole	Oral	100–150	50—NR
Sulfisoxazole	IV	150–200	NR
Tetracycline	Oral	20–40	10–20
Tetracycline	IV	10–15	5

* IM = intramuscular.
† IV = intravenous.
‡ ID = insufficient data.
§ Not absorbed when given by mouth.
‖ NR = not recommended.

should be given at maximum dosage by the most reliable route (usually intravenous infusion) for the best evaluation of clinical response. Oral absorption of antibiotics may show extreme variations, so that parenteral administration is advisable in serious illnesses. When renal impairment is present, lower doses are advisable, particularly for kanamycin, polymyxin, or chloramphenicol, which have toxicities directly related to an excessively high serum concentration.

Most antibiotics should be given every 6 hours at the onset of an illness, but after improvement they may be given 3 times a day for convenience. For newborn infants, intramuscular antibiotics may be given every 8 or every 12 hours. The lower dose listed for newborns can be used for prematures in the first week of life.

HOW LONG SHOULD A DRUG BE CONTINUED?

No simple formula can be given for the duration of antibiotic therapy. The drug should be given for long enough to provide a margin of safety after a satisfactory therapeutic response, which usually requires a total period of at least 5 days. If a satisfactory therapeutic response does not occur within 48 hours, or if the patient becomes worse clinically at any time after 24 hours of therapy, continued use of the drug should be reevaluated.

TABLE 6.   COMMON DRUG TOXICITIES

DRUG	MOST COMMON SEVERE EFFECT	OTHER EFFECTS	SPECIAL NEWBORN TOXICITIES
Penicillin	Exfoliative dermatitis Anaphylactoid shock	Serum sickness Angioneurotic edema Rash; fever	Hyperkalemia
Oxacillin, methicillin	Superinfection		
Ampicillin		Diarrhea	
Erythromycin		Allergic hepatitis	
Chloramphenicol	Aplastic anemia	Bone marrow depression	Gray syndrome (shock and death)
Sulfas	Exudative dermatitis	Pancytopenia Hematuria	Kernicterus
Streptomycin	Vestibular damage	Deafness	Central nervous system depression Deafness
Polymyxins		Nephrotoxicity Paresthesias	
Kanamycin	Deafness	Curare effect (IP)* Nephrotoxicity	
Neomycin		Curare effect (IP)*	
Tetracycline	Superinfection Liver toxicity	Diarrhea Phototoxicity Renal dysfunction Tooth staining Bulging fontanel	Tooth staining
Gentamicin	Vestibular damage	Nephrotoxicity	
Nitrofurantoin		Vomiting Hemolytic anemia Paresthesias	

* IP = intraperitoneal.

Criteria for the clinical evaluation of the response can usually be determined at the time the drug is begun. The most useful guides to clinical response are body temperature, respiratory rate, general appearance, and the local signs of the particular infection, such as the extent of cellulitis, tenderness, and edema. The physician should not hesitate to add another antibiotic or to change antibiotics when the expected improvement does not occur, but these changes should not be made without a careful reevaluation of the working diagnosis. Reevaluation should include such considerations as loculated pus, superinfection with a resistant organism, an unrecognized complication, another diagnosis, or more extensive involvement by the infection than was originally recognized, such as osteomyelitis underlying a cellulitis. Pulmonary superinfection is particularly common in infants with pulmonary congestion secondary to congenital heart disease and in patients with tracheotomies. Such patients should have cultures of the throat or tracheal secretions done routinely twice a week during antibiotic therapy so that sensitivities will be available immediately if clinical evidence of superinfection emerges.

An antibiotic should usually be discontinued at the first clinical or laboratory sign of a known associated toxic effect. The toxic effects most frequently associated with commonly used antibiotics are shown in Table 6. Hypersensitivity to penicillin is uncommon in infants and children. The occurrence of a rash during penicillin therapy for cellulitis or a wound infection may represent scarlatina from erythrogenic toxin of the infecting streptococcus and may occur after several days of penicillin therapy.

Kanamycin is ototoxic and should not be used longer than a week.

Neomycin, and occasionally polymyxin B, colistin, streptomycin, and kanamycin, when instilled into body cavities, have been associated with paralysis from a neuromuscular blockade, especially after ether anesthesia. This paralysis may also occur rarely after parenteral administration and may produce apnea. The neuromuscular blockade associated with streptomycin and neomycin can be reversed by neostigmine. For further details of the pharmacology and clinical toxicity of antimicrobial agents, the reader is referred to several excellent reviews.

SURGERY IN BLEEDERS

Surgeons have always been interested in diseases that are associated with postoperative bleeding. These conditions are uncommon, hemophilia occurring 2 to 3 times per 100,000 population. Failure to detect bleeding tendencies in the preoperative evaluation of the patient means a prolonged miserable hospital stay and on occasion the patient's death. The bleeding defects can be placed into three categories: platelet defects, vascular fragility, and plasma coagulation defects. In this discussion, we are considering only generalized defects and not the localized lesions that may cause bleeding, such as telangiectasis or hemangioma.

PLATELET DEFICIENCY

Seventy-five percent of patients with idiopathic thrombocytic purpura are under 12 years of age. The etiology is considered to be an immunological abnormality analogous to autoimmune acquired hemolytic anemia. A high percentage have a good prognosis and will have a permanent remission in 6 to 12 months. These patients make themselves known by showing extensive subcutaneous hemorrhages from slight trauma and petechial hemorrhages. These subdermal hemorrhages are not palpable. The diagnosis is readily established by a platelet count. Counts below 60,000 may be associated with bleeding. After onset, steroids are of some help in inducing a rise in platelets, and in severe cases this may be a helpful adjunct in the treatment of the patient. If there is not a spontaneous remission in 8 to 12 months, splenectomy is indicated. It may be wise to continue low dosage of steroids prior to and during the operation. Prompt discontinuation of these postoperatively is important if possible. There are a number of secondary causes that produce thrombocytopenia, such as lupus erythematosis, leukemia, and congestive splenomegalia with esophageal varices. These conditions are usually quite obvious and do not present a problem to the surgeon. Thrombocytopenic purpura is usually so evident clinically that the surgeon is warned of the condition before he subjects the patient to operation.

VASCULAR DISEASE

Anaphylactoid purpura, or Henoch-Schönlein syndrome, is actually a disease of the small vessels, which do not retract properly in response to trauma, leading to continued bleeding. The onset of this disease is variable; abdominal pain may precede the appearance of petechial hemorrhages. Usually the skin lesions are obvious, giving the surgeon effective warning. This is actually an inflammatory disease, and the subcutaneous hemorrhages are consequently palpable. The worrisome thing in taking care of these patients is that with abdominal pain, particularly with the onset of the attack, there may be intussusception, which can be a problem to deal with. Steroids may be helpful, particularly when there is abdominal pain. An effort should be made to reduce the intussusception without operation. However, when the situation has progressed to a point where reduction of an intussusception is not accomplished by barium enema, operation must be undertaken, and resections can be successfully performed.

Ehlers-Danlos syndrome is an extremely rare disease that should be mentioned. It is the so-called India rubber man disease. In these patients there is not a great problem with hemorrhage; rather, the problem is failure of wound healing. It is primarily a disease of the connective tissue. These patients can have the skin over various bony prominences stretched considerably because of the defect in the connective tissue. It is an au-tosomal dominant genetically determined disease.

PLASMA FACTOR DEFICIENCY

The patients with plasma factor deficiencies constitute the most important group of patients that a surgeon must be aware of in order to prevent serious postoperative bleeding. Von Willebrand's syndrome is an unusual disease that is very much like hemophilia. It is a pseudohemophilia and occurs in girls as well as in boys. Originally thought to be caused by a vascular defect, it is now known to be the result of a deficiency of a plasma factor essential for normal platelet adhesiveness and a deficiency of factor VIII. It affects both sexes, is inherited as an autosomal dominant trait, and is found in the family history of over 80 percent of patients. These patients have a history of bleeding readily. Coagulation studies are normal, but there is an increase in bleeding time. When surgery is needed in such patients, it is well to prepare them with fresh plasma and to give very small doses of prednisone. It is not absolutely imperative to have fresh plasma, since stored plasma will have a sufficiently active factor in most instances to return the bleeding to normal.

HEMOPHILIA

Hemophilia is a clinical syndrome now recognized etiologically as a group of entities each arising from a distinct inborn error of metabolism, manifested as defects in the production of specific proteins essential in the clotting process. There are three forms of this disease. The classical hemophilia, AHF, the Christmas disease, PTC, and hemophilin C. The splitting of hemophilia into two groups has been done on the basis of the fact that a patient with Christmas disease will have the factor necessary to correct the bleeding in a typical patient with classical hemophilia. These are sex-linked recessive traits. Consequently, the defect is carried in females but occurs in males. The Christmas and classical groups comprise 90 percent of the hemophilia, with the Christmas type accounting for 10 to 15 percent of this number. Hemophilia C (PTA deficiency) is less severe than the commoner types and is transmitted as an autosomal dominant and affects both sexes.

In detecting hemophilia, the history and examination of the patient are far more important than any screening test. It has been demonstrated in studies that in some instances laboratory tests failed to detect the disease where careful history and physical examination established the diagnosis. For unknown reasons newborns with hemophilia may not exhibit a bleeding tendency. This explains why such a newborn may have a circumcision shortly after birth with no significant bleeding. Because of the genetics of this disease, the family history is extremely important. One must be aware of the fact that there can be a negative family history where the mother proves to be an only child. Therefore, it is important to inquire about the disease in more than one generation. In examination of the patient, any evidence of joint diseases that cannot be accounted for should suggest the possibility of the patient being a hemophiliac. Bleeding into the joints with disability and limitation of motion is a common complication.

The treatment of this disease is to supply the factors that the patient lacks. These have a short half-life and consequently must be given to the patient quickly after they have been withdrawn from the donor, or fresh frozen plasma must be quickly unfrozen. Plasma concentrate can be used. The corrective substance most readily available in most hospitals is fresh frozen plasma. This is effective providing sufficient volumes of fresh or frozen plasma are given. Large quantities have to be given, and this may pose a problem in the pediatric patient. Concentrated AHF, but not PTC or PTA, is available. One form has been prepared by repeated freezing and has a concentration five to ten times that of fresh plasma. There is a glyceine precipitate material available that is expensive. In the actual treatment of the patient, 10 ml of plasma per kilogram of weight should be given as an initial injection. Following that, a program should be set up with about 5 ml of fresh frozen plasma per kg given every 4 to 6 hours. The problem is that the volumes required may exceed the amount of fluid that the patient can tolerate. It is important to continue the above outlined therapy until complete healing has taken place. Unless this is done, secondary bleeding will take place, and then the situation will have to be treated as a fresh case of bleeding and therapy continued over sufficiently long periods of time for rehealing to be complete. Surface incisions completely heal in 5 or 6 days, and it is possible in such situations to discontinue the treatment 2 to 3 days later. However, the lesions of the tongue and mucous membrane of the mouth must be treated for longer periods of time, since complete healing in the presence of saliva may be delayed.

One can gain some idea of the effectiveness of the treatment by measuring clotting time. For such determinations fresh venous blood is required. If blood is secured with a skin puncture, there is admixture of the thromboplastic material in the tissue, which will correct the defect in the blood. This makes it difficult to secure blood in small infants to establish the diagnosis. One must go by history in such situations and wait until the child is large enough to be a subject for withdrawal of venous blood from peripheral vessels rather than from the vessels of the neck or the groin. Fatal retroperitoneal hemorrhage has been reported from femoral vein puncture. In treating these patients it is always better to insert needles into peripheral veins than to perform cutdowns. When cutdowns are made, this adds an incision that may bleed and produce a problem; furthermore, veins are destroyed. The patient's life may depend on someone's being able to promptly insert a needle into a vein. Consequently, needless destruction of peripheral veins is to be avoided. There are two periods of danger after surgery in hemophilia. Hemophiliacs do not bleed excessively during operation but often begin to do so about 24 hours after operation. This may be because of the tissue thromboplastic material that is released from the operative site. At the end of 24 hours, these local effects have disappeared, and the first postsurgery danger period confronts the patient with hemophilia. There seems to be another period when there is danger from bleeding, and this is about one week after trauma or surgery. On rare occasions, antibodies to the specific antihemophilic factor may develop. This is seen in adults on rare occasions and is even more unusual in children. When it does occur, it is a grave problem, since no matter how much of the active substance is given the patient's antibodies neutralize it and he continues to bleed. In these situations, death is the usual outcome.

Some parents assume that the hemophilic child will be better protected if he is obese, their reasoning being that this cushions the patient against trauma. Actually, it is poor practice to allow a patient with this disease to become obese, simply because it is difficult or impossible in such children to insert needles into veins, which may be lifesaving during episodes of bleeding.

A number of preparations have been used as long-term medications in hemophilia, the first being a peanut flour extract with 90 percent ethyl alcohol. So far the results are promising but not conclusive. Although treatment of hemophiliacs to control bleeding is improved over the methods used a few years ago, surgery should not be undertaken in a hemophiliac except in an extreme emergency or in a life-threatening situation.

There has been much discussion about fibrinolysins being present in patients who have severe bleeding, particularly during prolonged operations. This is a poorly documented entity, and it is now thought that a hypercoagulation syndrome may play a part in these patients. The measurement of low levels of fibrinogen in the blood may actually be the result of hypercoagulation, and it is now thought that perhaps some of these patients should be treated with heparin. It is a rare condition, and most surgeons are very unlikely to encounter it.

ORVAR SWENSON
THOMAS J. EGAN
HUGH L. MOFFET

REFERENCES

ABBOTT, W. E., et al. The danger of administering parenteral fluids by hypodermoclysis. Surgery, 32: 2, 1952.

ABILDGAARD, C. F., et al. Screening tests for disorders of thromboplastin formation. Pediat. Clin. N. Amer., 9: 819, 1962.

ANDERSON, O. S., and ENGEL, K. A new acid-base nomogram. Scand. J. Clin. Lab. Invest., 12: 177, 1960.

ASTRUP, P. A simple electrometric technique for determination of carbon dioxide tension in blood and plasma. Scand. J. Clin. Lab. Invest., 8: 33, 1956.

ATUK, N. O., MOSCA, A., and KUNIN, C. The use of potentially nephrotoxic antibiotics in the treatment of gram-negative infections in uremic patients. Ann. Intern. Med., 60: 28, 1964.

BERGSTROM, W. H. Fluid and electrolyte problems. Pediat. Clin. N. Amer., 11: 795, 1964.

BIGGS, R. Proc. Roy. Soc. Med., 57: 1171, 1964.

BOUDREAUX, H. B., and FRAMPTON, V. L. Nature, 185: 469, 1960.

BRUCK, E., ACETO, T., Jr., and LOWE, C. U. Intravenous fluid therapy for infants and children. Physiologic principles and a practical regimen with examples of application. Pediatrics, 25: 3, Part I, 1960.

CARROL, W. W. Parenteral fluids in gastrointestinal surgery. Surg. Clin. N. Amer., 34: 1, 1954.

DOWLING, H. F. Present status of therapy with combinations of antibiotics. Amer. J. Med., 39: 796, 1965.

EVANS, F. T., and GRAY, T. C. Modern Trends in Anesthesia, II. Hydrogen Ion Regulation and Biochemistry, London, Butterworth & Co. (Publishers), Ltd., 1962.

FOSTER, F. P. Antibiotic management of severe infections. Postgrad. Med., 33: 32, 1963.

FRIIS, H. B. Changes in body water compartments during growth. Acta Paediat., 46: 110 (Suppl.), 1957.

GAMBLE, J. L. Chemical Anatomy Physiology and Pathology of Extracellular Fluid. Cambridge, Mass., Harvard University Press, 1964.

HARTMANN, J. R., et al. GP, 32: 144, 1965.

HOLLIDAY, M. A., and SEGAR, W. E. The maintenance need for water in parenteral fluid therapy. Pediatrics, 19: 823, 1957.

KAGAN, B. J., ed. Symposium on antimicrobial therapy. Ped. Clin. N. Amer. 8: 967, 1961.

KEITEL, H. G. The Pathophysiology and Treatment of Body Fluid Disturbances. New York, Appleton-Century-Crofts, 1962.

LOWE, C. U. Pre-operative and Post-operative Care of Infants and Children. Boston, Little, Brown and Company, 1960.

———— ROURKE, M., MacLACHLAN, E., and BUTLER, A. M. Use of parenteral potassium therapy in surgical patients. Its role in preventing chloride loss. Pediatrics 6: 2, 1950.

MacFARLANE, R. G. Proc. Roy. Soc. Med., 58: 251, Apr. 1965.

MARSHALL, M., and JOHNSON, S. H. Use of nitrofurantoin in chronic and recurrent urinary tract infection in children. J.A.M.A., 169: 919, 1959.

MARTIN, W. J. Newer antimicrobial agents having current or potential clinical application. Med. Clin. N. Amer., 48: 255, 1964.

NUNN, J. F. Nomenclature and presentation of hydrogen ion regulation data. In Evans, F. T., and Gray, T. C., eds. Modern Trends in Anesthesia. London, Butterworth & Co. (Publishers) Ltd., 1962.

PAINE, T. F. Gram staining without the clock. New Eng. J. Med., 268: 941, 1963.

PAPPAS, Λ. M., et al. J.A.M.A., 187: 772, 1964.

PERKINS, R. L. Apnea with intramuscular colistin therapy. J.A.M.A., 190: 421, 1964.

PETERS, J. P. Water balance in health and in disease. In DUNDAN, G. G., ed. Diseases of Metabolism, 3rd ed. Philadelphia, W. B. Saunders Company, 1952.

———— and VAN SLYKE, D. D. Hemoglobin and Oxygen. Carbonic Acid and Acid-Base Balance. Baltimore, The Williams and Wilkins Company, 1931.

PETERSDORF, R. G., et al. Symposium on the chemoprophylaxis of infection. J. Pediat., 58: 149, 1961.

POLLOCK, M. R. Enzymes Destroying Penicillin and Cephalosporin. Antimicrobial Agents and Chemotherapy—1964. SYLVESTER, J. C., ed. Ann Arbor, Michigan, American Society for Microbiology, 1965, pp. 292–301.

REED, W. A. Antibiotics and cardiac surgery. J. Thorac. and Cardiov. Surg. 50: 888, 1965.

RICKHAM, P. P. The Metabolic Response to Neonatal Surgery. Cambridge, Mass., Harvard University Press, 1957.

ROBERTS, H. R., PENICK, G. D., and BRINKHOUS, K. M. J.A.M.A., 190: 546, 1964.

SCHWARTZ, W. B., LEVINE, H. D., and RELMAN, A. S. The electrocardiogram in potassium depletion. Amer. J. Med., 16: 3, 1954.

SMITH, N. J., and VAUGHAN, V. C., III. In NELSON, W. E., ed. Textbook of Pediatrics, 8th ed. Philadelphia, W. B. Saunders and Company, 1964, p. 1062.

SWANSON, W. W., and IOB, L. V. Loss of minerals through the skin of infants. Amer. J. Dis. Child., 45: 1036, 1933.

SWEENEY, W. M., DORNBUSH, A. C., and HARDY, S. M. Antibiotic activity in urine and feces after oral and intravenous administration of demethylchlortetracycline. New Eng. J. Med., 263: 620, 1960.

VON WILLEBRAND, E., and JURGENS, R. Von Willebrand's Disease. Brit. Med. J., 2: 963, 1964.

WEINSTEIN, L. Superinfection: A complication of antimicrobial therapy and prophylaxis. Amer. J. Surg., 107: 704, 1964.

———— Chemotherapy of microbial disease. In GOODMAN, L. S. and GILMAN, A., eds. Pharmacological Basis of Therapeutics. New York, The Macmillan Company, 1965, pp. 1144–1342.

WILMORE, D. W., and DUDRICK, S. J. Growth and development of an infant receiving all nutrients exclusively by vein. J.A.M.A., 203: 860, 1968.

10

Types of Incisions

OPERATING ROOM EQUIPMENT

Of interest to the pediatric surgeon is a special child-sized operating table several inches narrower than the adult-sized table. The smaller operating table places the surgeon closer to the patient, so that he can see better. More important, not having to bend over a wide table contributes to his comfort. The narrow table offers the same advantages to the assistant and makes him a more efficient helper. These narrow tables, although only $13\frac{1}{2}$ inches in width and therefore ideal for infant surgery, can accommodate children up to 12 or 14 years of age (Fig. 1).

The operating room must be supplied with instruments of suitable size for infants. The retractors may be small; hemostats should have fine, delicate points so that a minimum of tissue is crushed while securing hemostasis. The needle holders must be small enough to handle the fine, short needles, which are essential to sewing and working in small wounds. Tissue forceps must be of the plastic type with fine points (Fig. 2). The best dissecting scissors are the Metzenbaum, which have relatively blunt points and are slightly curved. The Metzenbaum scissors can now be obtained in a variety of lengths (Fig. 3).

A fine grade of silk is the suture material of choice. Cotton is satisfactory as far as strength and tissue tolerance is concerned; however, cotton is harder to handle and for this reason silk is preferred. Only rarely is silk stronger than 4-0 needed in operations on infants and children. On infants, particularly premature infants, 5-0 and 6-0 silk is all that is needed. Six-0 and 7-0 is now procurable, and, with small, curved, atraumatic needles, this is an ideal suture material for various types of anastomoses. Six-0 silk is excellent for subcuticular closure of the wounds. It is now possible to obtain catgut, plain or chromic, as fine as 5-0. For wounds that are infected, or in operations where the likelihood of infection is great, fine chromic catgut should be used rather than silk.

SKIN PREPARATION

The most satisfactory preparation for the operator's hands is a six-minute scrub with Phisohex.* When the operator or any member of the operating team changes from one case to another, a three-minute scrub is sufficient.

An infant's skin is sensitive, and the use of harsh chemicals to disinfect it in preparation for operation should be avoided. An adequate preparation can be secured without danger of injury to the skin by the following routine. At operation, three scrubs of Phisohex are applied with gauze sponges held by long sponge forceps. This is primarily a mechanical cleaning, and the skin should be actively scrubbed for three minutes with each sponge. Following the three scrubs with Phi-

* Entsufon, lanolin, petrolatum, and hexachlorophene 3 percent.

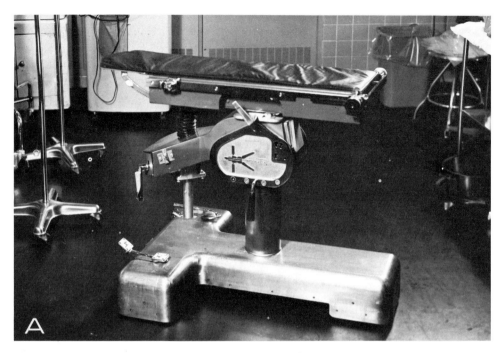

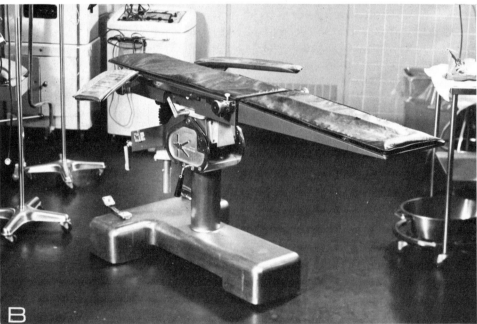

Fig. 1A. Infants' operating-room table. Its great advantage is that the width is 13½ inches, which permits the operator and assistants to be closer to the patients. Consequently, they do not need to bend over to perform operations, which they must do when using adult tables, which are 22 inches wide. B. Same table with extension in place, making table suitable for older children.

sohex, the area is scrubbed with three sponges soaked in 1:1,000 aqueous Zephiran for a total of three minutes. The immediate area of the incision is dried with a sponge.

After the incision has been made, the skin that is exposed between the incision and the walling-off towels should be covered by gauze sponges. In operations that last more than

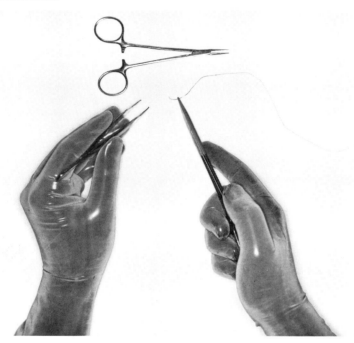

Fig. 2. Small instruments suitable for pediatric surgery.

one hour it is well to sew the gauze pads to the subcutaneous tissue along the edge of the skin incision with a continuous silk suture. This prevents contact with the skin, which is the least aseptic portion of the operative field.

Soft, pliable, yet tough plastic material has

recently become available, with one side covered with an adhesive material so that it adheres to the skin. This type of material for covering an area, particularly when it is close to a drainage area, as in an ileostomy or colostomy, has definite advantages.

The theoretical advantage of this type of

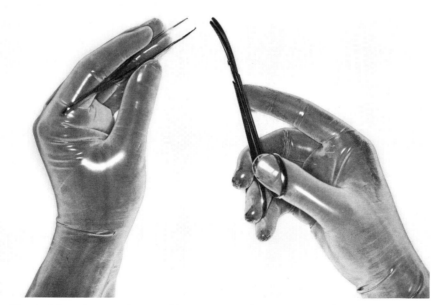

Fig. 3. Metzenbaum scissors, which are useful in infants' and children's surgery.

draping is that the skin surface, which is potentially the most contaminated part of the operative field, is eliminated from the operative area.

SURGICAL INCISIONS

In pediatric surgery there are many occasions for the removal of skin and subcutaneous lesions from various parts of the body. In such situations, a prime consideration is the cosmetic result. Whenever practical, the incision should be placed parallel to the normal lines of the skin in order to secure an optimum cosmetic result (Fig. 4). Many years ago Langer described the normal skin folds or creases in all parts of the body and indicated that superior cosmetic results are obtained when incisions are made parallel to these lines. Keloid formation is less common and less severe in such incisions.

There are a number of requirements that must be provided for in a surgical incision. First the pathology must be conveniently exposed, and the various maneuvers required during the operation should be provided for. A fundamental requirement is adequate exposure without excessive retraction, for vigorous pulling on tissue may produce tissue damage and retard primary healing. To a certain extent, the size of an incision for a given operation depends on the number and

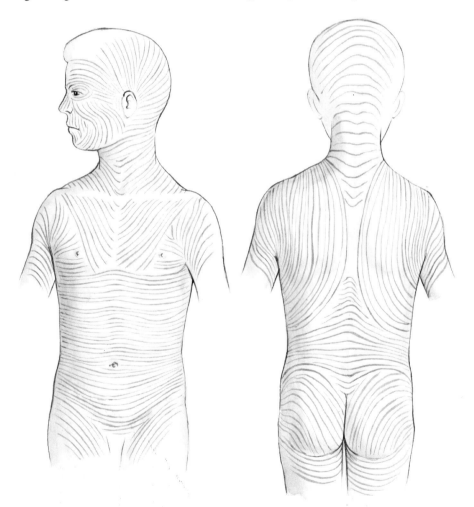

Fig. 4. Normal skin folds or lines. Superior cosmetic results can be achieved by placing elective incisions parallel to these lines.

experience of surgical assistants available to provide exposure. A second requirement concerns the strength of a healed incision and the lack of disturbance of normal function. The comfort of the patient's incision should be given consideration. Of some importance is the cosmetic appearance of the healed incision, particularly in children, who look forward to 60 or 70 years of life.

Adequate incisions are necessary; however, this does not license the surgeon to make excessively long incisions, which may happen particularly when a surgeon primarily concerned with adults performs an operation on an infant. The pathology to be exposed corresponds in size to the patient. For instance, an infant's hernia can conveniently be repaired with a 3 cm, precisely placed, transverse incision rather than with an adult size, diagonal incision. An essential requirement for an adequate yet reasonable in size incision is that it be in the best possible position. It should be remembered that incisions grow with the child, and a long scar on the infant or small child becomes enormous when adulthood is attained.

Another, less important consideration is that incisions made parallel to normal skin folds heal more kindly and give a superior cosmetic result than when these folds are cut across. It is believed that keloid formation is less in incisions made in conformity to the normal skin folds or creases.

The speed with which an incision may be made, consistent with gentleness and regard for tissue, and the time consumed in closing the incision become factors to which consideration must be given. When dealing with feeble patients it is wise to reduce operating time as much as is consistent with the performance of an adequate operation.

ABDOMINAL INCISIONS

ANATOMY

The abdominal wall musculature is composed of the rectus and the oblique muscles, which are the external and internal oblique and the transversalis. The rectus muscles arise from the xiphoid cartilage and from the anterior surfaces of the fifth, sixth, and seventh ribs, and they attach to the os pubis and to the ligaments covering the symphysis pubis. The muscles are encased in a fascial sheath that is defective posteriorly below the semicircular line of Douglas. Actually the sheath is the fascial attachment of the flat or oblique muscles and should be visualized as transverse rather than vertical fibers.

The external oblique takes its origin from the anterolateral surfaces of the lower eight ribs. The most lateral portion consists of fibers that pass vertically downward to the anterior half of the iliac crest. The structure becomes aponeurotic anteriorly and below the umbilicus and joins with the internal oblique and transversalis to form the rectus sheath. The internal oblique arises from the lateral half of the inguinal ligament and from the anterior two thirds of the iliac crest and the lumbar dorsal fascia. The lateral portion or posterior portions insert into the lower three ribs. The more medial portion, which extends obliquely upwards and medially, becomes aponeurotic and helps form the rectus sheath. There are also attachments to the seventh, eighth, and ninth costal cartilages. The transversalis, the deepest muscle, is transverse in its direction and has a wide attachment. The transversalis fascia is deep to the transversalis muscle and is much denser low in the abdomen, particularly in the inguinal region where it is an important structure forming the conjoined tendon.

The blood supply is from the superior and inferior epigastric arteries, which lie posterior to the rectus muscle. Additional sources are the deep circumflex iliacs, the intercostals, and the lumbar arteries. These are rich anastomotic systems that make it rather difficult to make surgical incisions that would endanger the viability of a portion of the abdominal wall.

NERVE SUPPLY

The nerve supply to the abdominal musculature is such that attention to its components is important in making abdominal incisions. Innervation is from the lower six intercostals and first lumbar nerves. There is considerable intercommunication between the components of each nerve and the trunk above and below. The trunks from 6 through 9 pass deep to the costal arch and enter the abdominal wall between the transverse and internal oblique muscles. The same layer is the position of trunks 10 through 12, which pass between the ribs. The anterior branch of the iliohypogastric nerve enters the internal oblique and little medial to the anterior superior spine and runs forward and downward. Because of the rich anastomosis be-

tween the intercostal trunks it is possible to cut one and perhaps two with no ill effects. It is wise to be careful, for there may be variations in the system and some individuals may show ill effects from having two trunks cut.

Of practical importance is the innervation of the rectus. The intercostal nerves enter the rectus along the lateral border and segmentally innervate this and the long muscle. There is not a rich anastomotic system at this level, and therefore cutting nerves at the lateral border of the rectus will denervate corresponding segments of the rectus.

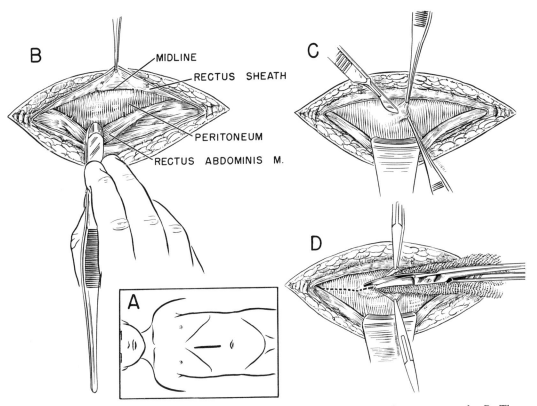

Fig. 5. Laparotomy opening. A. The incision is placed over the midpoint of the rectus muscle. B. The rectus muscle has been separated from its sheath so that it can be retracted laterally. C. The peritoneum is opened with the posterior rectus sheath. This layer is grasped with fine-tooth forceps and tilted upward. The opening is made with a scalpel 1 cm away from the forceps. If any intestine has been caught with the forceps, it will be free to escape from the scalpel blade when the opening is made. The natural inclination of the surgeon is to open the peritoneum between the two forceps, but if intestine is held by the forceps, it cannot escape, and the gut will be opened. D. Fine pointed clamps are attached to the peritoneum for traction. A corner of a gauze sponge is inserted into the peritoneal cavity and pushed ahead of the scissors used to open the peritoneum. This guards against injury to the intestine.

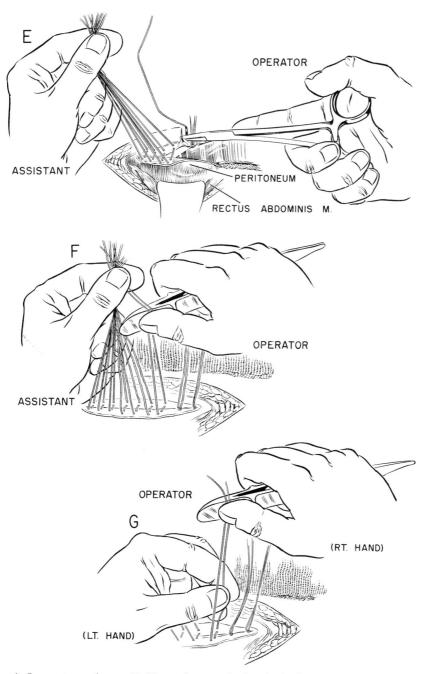

Fig. 5 (cont.). Laparotomy closure. E. The peritoneum is closed with interrupted 4-0 or 5-0 silk sutures. These are placed so that the cut edges of peritoneum are turned out into the wound. All sutures are placed, and then traction on all of them gradually brings the abdominal edges together. The distribution of tension on all the sutures prevents tears in the peritoneum. F. The assistant holds all the sutures between the index finger and thumb of one hand. The operator takes a suture to be tied by grasping it between the end of a tissue forcep and the thumb of his right hand and pulling it free from his assistant's hand. Note the special forceps with the ends tapered to facilitate separating the suture to be tied. G. The operator takes the side of the suture farthest away, with his left hand.

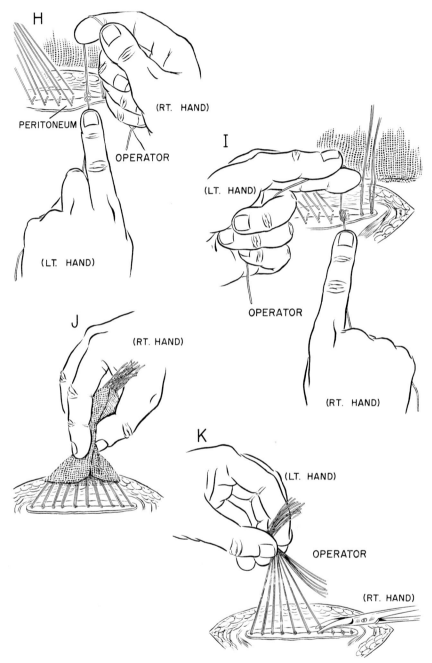

Fig. 5 (cont.). Laparotomy closure. H. The first half of the square knot is tied by extending the right hand across the incision. I. A square knot is tied and the left hand is extended across the incision. J. As each suture is tied, it is laid across a sponge. When all sutures have been tied, the sponge is picked up and all sutures are gathered together. K. The sutures are cut with ⅛ inch ends.

INCISIONS

Rectus muscle splitting is not an ideal incision, for the medial segment of rectus

becomes denervated and may exhibit weakness by bulging. Furthermore evisceration is not uncommon when this incision is used.

Vertical incisions that retract the rectus

ing incisions. Numerous factors play a part in dehiscence, consequently it is difficult to determine which is more prone to this complication. With careful technique and the use of interrupted silk sutures the incidence of dehiscence should be about equal. It is possible to perform a number of abdominal operations in addition to an appendectomy through an enlarged McBurney incision. Reduction of intussusception and excision of a Meckel's diverticulum can be performed with ease through such an incision. The skin incision should be transverse, halfway between the iliac crest and the costal margin, and it should extend from the midaxillary line laterally to the midpoint of the right rectus muscle medially. The external oblique muscle and the internal oblique muscle are opened widely along the course of their fibers. It is important to extend the incision by dividing the fascia of the rectus muscle for 1.5 cm and to push the rectus muscle fibers medially rather than to divide any of them. The peritoneum is then opened in the course of the fibers of the transversalis. With an incision, adequate exposure is gained to reduce an intussusception or to resect an intussusception should it be irreducible.

The McBurney incision is not adequate for a general abdominal examination, such as is required when a patient is being explored for bleeding from the gastrointestinal tract. The advantage of this gridiron incision is that evisceration will not occur postoperatively, and, therefore, provided the patient progresses satisfactorily, discharge from the hospital can safely be permitted on the third or fourth postoperative day. Patients who have had rectus muscle-retracting incisions should be hospitalized for at least seven days to prevent the possibility of evisceration after discharge.

THORACOABOMINAL INCISIONS

These incisions have proved of some value in removing large renal tumors and in performing splenorenal and portocaval shunts. However, recently some delayed changes in the diaphragm have occurred in some patients and lessened enthusiasm for this incision. The patient is placed supine on the table, and a rolled blanket is used to elevate the side of the patient where the incision is to be placed. The abdominal portion of the incision begins 3 to 4 cm above the level of the umbilicus several centimeters lateral to the midline, and it is curved upward on the chest between the tenth and eleventh ribs and continued to the midaxillary line. One half to three quarters of one rectus muscle is divided. The external and internal oblique as well as the transversalis are divided between the rectus muscle and the costal margin. It is necessary partially to divide the diaphragm to permit the wound to separate to an adequate exposure. Often rather large vessels are cut while incising the diaphragm, and these bleed sufficiently to require ligation.

A self-retaining retractor is used to separate the ribs after the intercostal incision has been made and the chest opened. The closure of such an incision begins with two rows of silk sutures being placed in the diaphragm, one approximating the pleural side and the other the peritoneal side. The tenth and eleventh ribs are then brought together by placing two 4-0 catgut pericostal sutures; a catheter is left in place in the chest, and the rib sutures are tied. A running catgut suture is used to approximate the intercostal muscles and to make the chest incisions airtight. The anesthesiologist uses positive pressure to expand the patient's lungs. As this pressure is applied during the patient's expiration, the intercostal catheter is opened and air from the pleural space is permitted to escape from the catheter, the tip of which is under water. During inspiration, the catheter is clamped to prevent fluid or air being sucked back into the chest. This routine is repeated until there are no further bubbles or air expelled during forced expiration. The tube can then be withdrawn, and in most instances there is full expansion of the lung. As there have been no operative procedures within the pleural cavity, it is unnecessary to leave a catheter in place for drainage postoperatively. The abdominal portion of the wound is closed with interrupted black silk 4-0 sutures to the peritoneum, internal and external oblique muscle, and rectus sheath. The subcutaneous tissue is brought together with 5-0 black silk sutures. The skin edges are approximated carefully with a continuous 5-0 plain catgut subcuticular suture, and a collodion dressing is applied. This type of skin closure has a particular advantage in those patients who have had large malignant tumors removed and who require postoperation radiation. The radiologist is not bothered by a large dressing; the fields of radiation can be outlined accurately, and there is no adhesive tape, which may contribute to a burn of the skin during therapy. We have experienced no wound difficulty with this type of closure in patients who received radiation immediately following operation and who had it continued for a period of two or three weeks.

CHEST INCISIONS

The types of incisions to be used in the chest in pediatric surgery differ from those most useful in adult patients. The rib cage in infants and children is pliable, and for that reason one can gain a good exposure with an incision that is not practical in the more rigid adult chest. Lobectomy, pneumonectomy, ligation of the patent ductus, shunts for tetralogy of Fallot, and excision of duplication of the superior third of the esophagus can best be approached through an anterolateral incision. The patient is supine on the operating table with a folded bath towel under the left shoulder. The left arm is suspended over the table on the anesthesiologist's screen. The anterolateral incision, which has been popularized by Gross for patent ductus, is an excellent one. It affords good exposure during operation, produces a minimum of discomfort to the patient in the early postoperative period, and has a good cosmetic result. The incision begins at the midline of the second interspace and curves below the nipple, particularly in fe-

male patients, so that the incision will be under the breast. It then curves upward and terminates at the anterior axillary line.

The pectoralis major and the pectoralis minor are divided between the third and fourth ribs. For lobectomy, pneumonectomy, patent ductus, and shunt operations, the incision is made between the third and fourth ribs. The intercostal incision is extended back between the ribs to the posterior axillary line to permit the ribs to be separated widely. The third and fourth costochondral junctions are then divided with V-shaped incisions, and this usually provides adequate exposure for the procedures listed above. Should the exposure be inadequate, the second or fifth costochondral junction, or both, may also be divided.

The closure of this anterolateral incision is simple. A 3-0 braided silk suture is placed through the ends of the cartilaginous portions of the cut rib. Interrupted 3-0 chromic catgut sutures are placed around the third and fourth ribs at three points. These are tied, bringing the third and fourth ribs together. The silk sutures through the cartilaginous portion of the ribs are tied and a continuous chromic catgut suture used to reapproximate the intercostal muscle. The pectoralis minor and pectoralis major are then reapproximated with interrupted 4-0 black silk sutures as is the subcutaneous tissue. A continuous 5-0 plain catgut suture is placed as a subcuticular suture to complete closure of the incision, and collodion is painted over the incision. When postoperative chest drainage is indicated, the catheter should be inserted through a stab wound and not in the operating incision.

GENITOURINARY INCISIONS

Exposure of the kidney is not difficult. The patient is placed on his side and positioned so that the kidney bar and the break in the table are in the flank. By the use of these devices, lateral flexion can be produced and the space between the iliac crest and the costal margin approximately increased on the side where the operation is to be performed. A transverse incision is used, extending from the erector spinae muscles posteriorly to the anterior surface of the abdomen. The external and internal oblique muscles are divided with the scalpel, and bleeders are grasped with fine hemostats. A large intercostal nerve usually is found between the internal oblique and the transversalis, and care must be exercised in the posterior aspect of the incision to prevent damage to this important nerve. Division of this large nerve trunk may result in weakness of the abdominal muscles on the side of the incision.

When the transversalis is broken through posteriorly, there is direct access to the renal fossa. To secure adequate exposure, the peritoneum is separated from the transversalis fascia with blunt dissection, and then the fascia is divided without opening the peritoneum. The perirenal fascia must be opened, and the kidney is then exposed. If the peritoneum is opened inadvertently, it should be closed with a continuous chromic catgut suture.

In most instances it is prudent to have a drain in place when the incision is closed. Either interrupted silk or continuous chromic catgut sutures can be used to reapproximate the various layers of the incision, depending on whether or not infection is encountered.

Often the kidney is exposed to perform nephrostomy. In order to place the tube through the kidney substance where it is thinnest and where less damage will result, it is advisable to make a small opening in the renal pelvis. A curved probe is inserted through the opening, and by probing against a finger on the outside of the kidney the most suitable place for the nephrostomy can be selected. The probe can be forced through the renal substance and the opening enlarged by inserting the hemostat beside the probe and spreading the renal tissue. The nephrostomy tube is then tied to the end of the probe with a suture and pulled into place as the probe is withdrawn. The suture is cut through the small opening in the pelvis, releasing the probe. This maneuver assures

that the end of the tube is in a good position in the pelvis, and it also prevents unnecessary destruction of renal substance.

The pelvic opening is closed with chromic catgut sutures, care being exercised that the suture does not penetrate the pelvic mucosa. A chromic suture is also used as a purse-string in the renal capsule around the catheter to help maintain it in its optimum position. As an aid in preventing nephrostomy tubes from inadvertently coming out, a heavy silk suture is placed through the skin securely tied to the tube.

Suprapubic cystotomy frequently must be performed. A catheter should be placed in the bladder and a sufficient quantity of fluid injected to make the bladder palpable suprapubically. A vertical or transverse skin incision is made and the fascia between the recti divided. The loose areolar tissue covering the bladder should be pushed toward the dome of the bladder. In doing so the peritoneal fold is pushed away, and the likelihood of its being opened is lessened.

The bladder is opened vertically, and Allis clamps are placed in the edges to support them and to check bleeding. In order to expose the trigone, moistened sponges are placed in the fundus. Narrow ribbon retractors are used to give exposure, one on each side and one against the sponges in the fundus. This draws the trigone into view and permits catheterization of the ureters or other procedures to be performed on the trigone or bladder outlet.

Whether a suprapubic catheter is left in place or the bladder closed tightly depends on what procedures have been performed in the bladder. If bleeding is likely to occur, it is advisable to use a suprapubic catheter; otherwise a tight closure can be performed. If clots form in the bladder, a suprapubic tube is useful as an additional vent and as a means to help dislodge clots. The bladder wall closure is accomplished with a 4-0 plain catgut suture to the mucosa and muscular wall. This material inside the bladder will not be the cause of encrustations.

A row of interrupted silk sutures is then

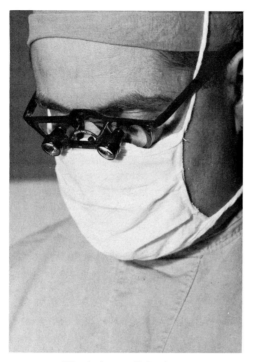

Fig. 6. A magnifying loupe.

placed in the musculature of the bladder. These must not penetrate the mucosa. When a catheter is to be left in the bladder, it should be placed close to the symphysis. A pursestring suture of silk is used around the catheter to prevent urine escaping into the wound. As the abdominal incision is closed, the catheter should be brought out diagonally so that a longer tract is formed in the abdominal wall. When the catheter is removed from such a wound, there is less likelihood of urine leaking for more than a few hours. When the bladder is closed without a bladder tube, a drain should be left in the space between the bladder and the symphysis.

NECK INCISIONS

A transverse incision, particularly when placed in a fold of the neck skin, results in a far better cosmetic result than any other. A diagonal incision, especially when placed along the anterior border of the sternocleidomastoid muscle, provides no better exposure than a transverse incision, and the cosmetic result is regrettable. Consequently, the diagonal neck incision has no place in pediatric surgery.

USE OF MAGNIFYING DEVICES

When fine, highly detailed dissection and reconstructions are performed, magnifying aids are required. The various loupes used by eye surgeons are excellent, since they provide almost two-times magnification with a focal length of about 12 inches (Fig. 6). This enables the surgeon to stand in comfort and permits instruments to be used in the field without undue hazard of contamination.

WOUND HEALING

There are a number of factors that contribute to ideal wound healing. Among those for which the surgeon is responsible are the following:
(1) Asepsis
    (a) Careful preparation of skin
    (b) Change of gown, gloves, and instruments when there is a definite break in technique
(2) Minimal trauma
    (a) Sharp dissection; minimal use of blunt dissection
    (b) Elimination of devitalized tissue by the use of fine instruments
    (c) Gentleness in handling tissue, particularly in infants
(3) Hemostasis
    (a) Individual ligation of bleeding vessels
    (b) Use of fine silk such as 5-0 and 6-0.

ORVAR SWENSON

11

Trauma

Accidental injury is the chief cause of death in children from 1 to 14 years of age. The next most common cause is malignant disease, which accounts for about one third as many deaths as occur from accidents; and infections are now responsible for fewer than one fifth of the total childhood mortality rate. Since the great majority of accident victims can be restored to normal life with proper treatment, it is important to emphasize principles of management that have been found necessary to their optimal care.

The commonest cause of death from trauma during childhood is injury sustained during a motor vehicle accident, followed by drowning and by burns caused by fires and explosions. In the United States in 1960, 93,330 people died of trauma. Of this number 15,708 were under 14 years of age. Zollinger and his colleagues (1962) have reported the etiology of trauma in children admitted to hospitals following accidents as follows: falls, 46 percent; injuries from sharp objects, 15 percent; automobile and bicycle accidents, 9 percent; sports accidents, 6 percent; animal and insect bites, 5 percent; and unclassified, 18 percent (Fig. 1).

The major sites of injury sustained by these children were the head in 41 percent, the neck and cervical area, 0.2 percent; the thorax, 8 percent; the upper extremities, 28 percent; the abdomen, 5 percent; the

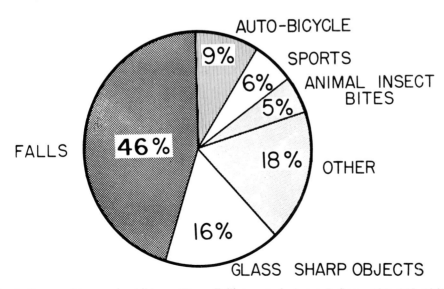

Fig. 1. Causes of trauma in children. (From Zollinger et al. Amer. J. Surg., 105: 855, 1962.)

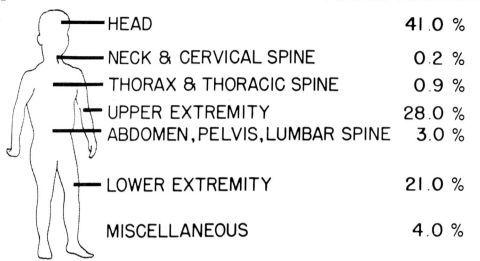

HEAD	41.0 %
NECK & CERVICAL SPINE	0.2 %
THORAX & THORACIC SPINE	0.9 %
UPPER EXTREMITY	28.0 %
ABDOMEN, PELVIS, LUMBAR SPINE	3.0 %
LOWER EXTREMITY	21.0 %
MISCELLANEOUS	4.0 %

Fig. 2. Major sites of trauma in children. (From Zollinger et al. Amer. J. Surg., 105: 855, 1962.)

lower extremities, 21 percent; and miscellaneous, 4 percent (Fig. 2). There is a distinct seasonal incidence of trauma, with the peak coming in the late spring and early summer. As might be expected, injuries are twice as common among boys as among girls. The average age varies considerably according to the etiology. Up to the age of 18 months, burning, neglect, drowning, and poisoning are the most common causes of accidental death. As the child becomes more active he is more likely to be hit by a motor vehicle and to be injured by falls and bicycle accidents. Over one half of childhood accident fatalities occur before the victim has reached the age of five years, a reflection of the relative severity of injury in the young child, the difficulties encountered in the diagnosis, and perhaps also the adequacy of the management both before and after the child's admission to the hospital.

There are three categories of patients to

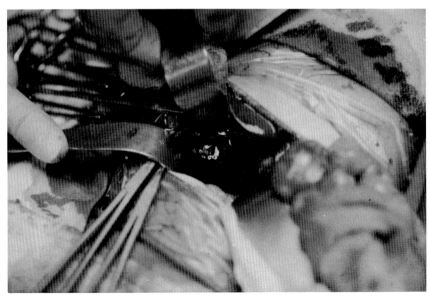

Fig. 3. A hematoma of the liver in a newborn baby. 200 ml of bloody fluid was present in the peritoneal cavity at operation. Recovery was uneventful. (Courtesy of Dr. John Raffensberger.)

be considered under the general heading of trauma in children. During delivery the baby is subjected to considerable stress. Although minor degrees of trauma are common in newborn babies, it is surprising that more abdominal and chest injuries do not occur at this time. Nevertheless, the problem is one which is attracting increasing interest. Another problem is that of the "battered child" who has been subjected to repeated parental abuse. The third category is that of accidental injuries in older children, which may be multiple and which require considerable skill in their diagnosis and management for a successful outcome to be achieved.

BIRTH INJURIES

Although serious injuries during birth are uncommon, it is now recognized that laceration of liver or spleen may occur in neonates whose deliveries have been normal or who have required breech extraction. Neonates sustaining these injuries may appear perfectly normal at birth, and it is not until several hours or even a day or two later that they become pale, have poor pulses, low blood pressure, and distended abdomens. Unless prompt surgical intervention is undertaken, the chance of survival of these neonates is remote (Fig. 3).

Chest injury in the newborn period is limited essentially to the development of a pneumothorax with or without mediastinal emphysema. If the pneumothorax is slight and it does not progress, no treatment is required. When larger accumulations of air are found or the amount is seen to increase, the insertion of a small intercostal catheter into the second intercostal space with a simple underwater seal is usually all that is required.

Head injuries, fractures of various bones, and peripheral nerve damage, such as Erb's palsy, are other injuries that are not infrequent in the newborn. These are discussed in other parts of the book.

THE BATTERED-CHILD SYNDROME

Any hospital dealing with accident cases will have to admit children who have been mistreated by their parents, guardians, or

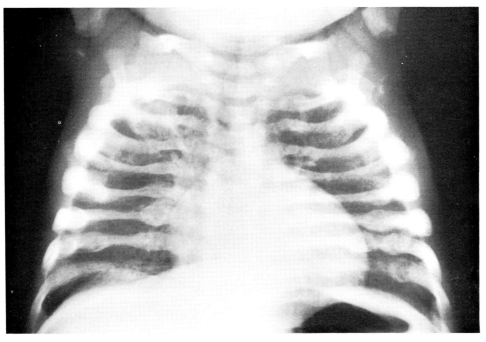

Fig. 4. Multiple healing rib fractures in a small baby, a finding typical of child abuse.

caretakers. The etiology of the trauma is often overlooked on the first admission, and the child is returned to his environment where further maltreatment occurs that may eventually lead to the child's death. Although this type of trauma has been known for centuries, it is only in the past few decades that the syndrome has been identified with reasonable certainty. Coffey, Silverman, and others have published descriptions of the roentgen changes observed in the long bones of children who have undergone this form of trauma. It consists of a distinctive subperiosteal new bone formation and multiple fractures in various shafts of the long bones. Healing rib fractures are also frequently seen (Fig. 4). These patients have usually sustained repeated injuries, and consequently proof of previous mistreatment is often present in bone survey films when the child is admitted with a fresh injury. The changes in the long bones, ribs, and vertebrae are so characteristic that they are pathognomonic of inflicted injury when combined with soft tissue or head injuries (Fig. 5).

The age group involved in parental mistreatment is under three years. Beyond that age the child is vocal, and his ability to tell what has happened causes this type of trauma to diminish. The seriousness of the injuries can be appreciated from the study by

Kempe and his colleagues (1962) that reviewed 302 cases of battered children. Eighty-five of the children sustained permanent injuries, and 33 deaths occurred in the entire group.

It is important for attending physicians and surgeons to appreciate that child mistreatment is not limited to any economic or social group. That the parents are well-to-do and highly educated does not eliminate the possibility that they have abused their child. Usually a vague story of a fall is given by the parents to account for the injury, or a sibling is blamed for having caused it, but the history is inadequate to account for the severe and multiple injuries which the child has sustained. It is extremely rare to have the parents admit to inflicting trauma to their child. Usually they will agree on a story, but sympathetic questioning will at times lead to remarks by either the mother or the father that the other parent is unduly strict with the child or that one or the other of them cannot control his temper. This history, together with the findings on roentgen examination of the extremities, will often establish the diagnosis of parental trauma.

In the past, abused children were treated, and nothing was done to prevent further attacks. Doctors were reluctant to report such cases to the police for fear of subsequent

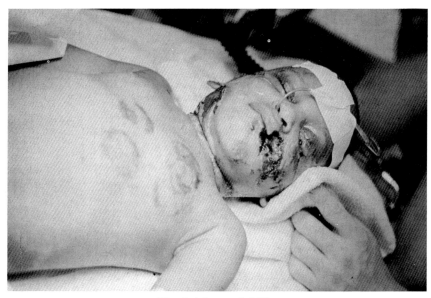

Fig. 5. A battered child.

suits against them by the parents on the grounds of libel. In many states, however, there are now specific laws preventing suits against the doctor for reporting suspected cases of the battered-child syndrome. These states have set up organizations for the investigation of reported cases. Because repeated trauma is the rule it is important to investigate the family and to determine if it is advisable to place the parents under psychiatric therapy or in extreme cases to remove the child from his hostile family, in order, perhaps, to save his life or to prevent permanent physical damage.

ACCIDENTAL INJURIES

Children involved in accidents are in an older age group than the battered children and are beyond the direct supervision of the parents. The average age of these patients is about 8 years. Severe injury is most often caused by their having been struck in the street by an automobile, and the injuries are usually multiple. In such cases the need for hospitalization is apparent. Other minor degrees of trauma, however, may also lead to serious injury. Lacerations of the liver and spleen or perforations of the bowel, for example, not infrequently follow apparently insignificant blunt abdominal trauma.

In the patient who has sustained severe injury, particularly where the injury involves the respiratory or vascular systems, prompt treatment is the greatest factor in the patient's survival. Consequently, it is well for the accident room to have its personnel trained to approach these problems in a systematic manner, in order to ensure that the most important assistance will be promptly and efficiently performed.

AIRWAY

As soon as the patient is observed in the accident room, a rapid general appraisal is essential, with emphasis on the respiratory system. If there are labored respirations or cyanosis, immediate attention to the airway should be given. When careful suctioning of the oropharynx does not relieve respiratory distress, tracheal intubation should be the immediate objective. In most instances the insertion of an endotracheal tube is a faster and a surer way to give prompt relief to airway obstruction than the performance of a tracheostomy. When the trauma is severe, the patient is apt to be sufficiently relaxed for endotracheal intubation not to be difficult. In situations where intubation cannot be accomplished—for example, when a fracture of the larynx has occurred and its lumen is obstructed by hematoma formation—tracheostomy is the next possibility. Performing a tracheostomy on a thrashing, uncontrollable patient, however, is an extremely dangerous operation. Damage to the esophagus or the great vessels of the neck has occurred under such circumstances. The insertion of a large bore (14- or 15-gauge) needle into the trachea may be lifesaving in situations where intubation cannot immediately be accomplished. The most convenient place to insert such a needle is just above the cricoid cartilage, through the cricothyroid membrane. It is important to be sure that the needle does not go through the posterior tracheal wall into the esophagus rather than remaining in the laryngotracheal airway. If an endotracheal tube relieves the obstruction and adequate aeration is established, tracheostomy can be delayed, but when a needle has been inserted it is well to proceed at once to tracheostomy. If the injury has produced a flail chest or the patient is extremely lethargic, with inadequate ventilation, assisted respiration is required to supply the patient with adequate oxygen and removal of carbon dioxide. This is accomplished by the attachment of a mechanical respirator to the endotracheal tube.

ASSESSMENT OF SHOCK

Once the airway has been established, the patient should be carefully undressed. It is well to move the child as little as possible, and therefore it is important to cut garments off rather than to disturb the patient unduly by removing them intact. Many centers place injured patients on a radiolucent plastic carrier so that they are disturbed very little during the subsequent manipulations. The physician should be in attendance while the patient is being undressed, for this provides an opportunity for a cursory examination of the patient. If there is evidence of shock as determined by low blood pressure readings and assessment of the pulse, immediate measures should be taken to counteract the hypotension. A cutdown should be inserted. Ideally this is a tube placed through an arm vein into the thoracic inflow so that the tube can be used to secure venous pressure recordings, as well as to serve as a route for the infusion of fluid and blood. When the intravenous cutdown is inserted, a blood sample should immediately be drawn and sent for typing and the crossmatching of a generous amount of blood. The blood loss may well have been severe or there may be continued bleeding, and in such situations it may be necessary to place two cutdowns in the patient. The extremities used should be those away from the area of damage. When there is a possibility of severe intra-abdominal bleeding, for example, the cutdown should be in the upper extremities to avoid infusing blood which must traverse the area of vascular injury, where it may escape from the circulation and fail to replenish the blood volume. In a patient in shock, normal saline or Ringer's lactate infusions should be started immediately, followed as quickly as possible by plasma or some blood substitute to expand the blood volume. In most institutions blood can be crossmatched and ready for infusion into the patient in less than half an hour. During this critical waiting period it may be lifesaving to give plasma to the patient or to use universal type O blood rather than to chance disaster from the inevitable delay in crossmatching.

EXAMINATION OF THE PATIENT

With the airway established, blood drawn for crossmatching and typing, and infusions being administered to restore the circulation, the physician is now able to conduct a careful and detailed examination of the patient. A great deal of information can initially be gained by talking to ambulance drivers or to people who observed the accident, in order to ascertain the force of contact and the part of the body directly traumatized. It is important early in the observation of the patient to see if he is alert and to obtain his recollections of the accident. If an intracranial injury is likely, a quick neurological examination is essential. At this point, it is important to realize that the care of the severely injured child is a multidisciplinary endeavor and that specialists should be notified for immediate consultation, particularly the neurosurgeon.

After the examination has been completed the patient should be placed under constant observation, with recordings made of the pulse, respirations, and blood pressure as frequently as every 10 to 15 minutes. Blood must be given vigorously to restore and to maintain the blood pressure. When this has been accomplished the infusion can be slowed. A subsequent fall of pressure is evidence of continued bleeding. Returning the blood pressure to normal may be impossible in patients with lacerations of large vessels, and unless this is recognized and appropriate operative intervention is undertaken, no amount of transfusion will save these patients' lives. Transfer to the operating room even during resuscitation may therefore be necessary when the patient's condition is deteriorating.

Detailed examination of the patient will give a baseline for future reexaminations and will also call attention to fractures, which should be splinted as carefully as possible while awaiting x-ray examination. The patient should not be urged to void. There may be a laceration of the bladder that under pressure will lead to extravasation of increased amounts of urine into the peritoneal cavity or retroperitoneal spaces. It is wiser to insert a catheter and to drain the bladder. The presence of blood indicates a laceration of the bladder or kidney. The catheter also permits the urinary output to be measured, which helps one to gauge the adequacy of therapy. Once a catheter is in place, a cystogram to detect bladder lacerations can be accomplished. In gauging the amount of blood and fluid needed, the urine output, central venous pressure monitoring, and measurements of the blood pressure are usually sufficient. We prefer to sustain the central venous pressure between 10 and 15 cm of water. The amount of blood and fluids required to maintain this normal venous pressure may be surprisingly large, often on the order of once or twice the calculated blood volume of the child being treated.

BLUNT ABDOMINAL TRAUMA

Patients with abdominal trauma may have misleading physical signs when first observed in the accident room. Consequently, unless there is evidence of severe internal bleeding, the decision to perform an abdominal exploration should be delayed until the patient has been installed in his hospital bed and re-examined. Often the rigid abdomen observed in the emergency room disappears completely during the first few hours after the patient's admission to the hospital. Continued monitoring of the vital signs is important to detect internal bleeding. The failure of reasonable amounts of blood to sustain the blood pressure is an indication of continued bleeding, and if this is accompanied by abdominal distension or tenderness, the likelihood of serious intra-abdominal injury is considerable. Patients losing blood will complain of excessive thirst, and this should be called to the attention of the surgeon. In addition to examination of the patient's abdomen, supine and upright roentgenograms to detect free air in the peritoneal cavity are extremely helpful. The place of peritoneal tap in the management of these patients has been disputed. It is true that an abdominal tap which yields a copious amount of blood is helpful in planning a mode of treatment. On the other hand, a negative tap must not be relied upon and certainly should not be given major consideration in deferring surgical intervention. One disadvantage of the examination is that the needletracks become painful, and it is often difficult to follow the signs of increasing intra-abdominal tenderness. Recently peritoneal lavage with 500 to 1,000 ml of saline has been used to assess abdominal injuries. If there is gross blood, a rupture of the liver or spleen is likely. A considerable number of white blood cells in the returned fluid usually indicates perforated intestine. The fluid may also be studied for the presence of bile, a sign of a ruptured liver, or for an increased amylase content, which may indicate the presence of traumatic pancreatitis.

In the patient with blunt trauma, careful repeated examination is probably the best insurance against overlooking a serious complication. It is important to examine the serum amylase for a possible rise initiated by pancreatic trauma. In evaluating abdominal films outlining free air under the diaphragm, the amount of free air may be important in placing the site of trauma. It is well known that traumatic perforation of the duodenum yields only a small amount of air under the diaphragm. This may be related to the fact that the tear may be retroperitoneal or into the lesser omental cavity, and consequently the volume of free air in the peritoneal cavity may be slight. When the amount of gas in the intestinal tract is not excessive, such retroperitoneal air may be seen in the upper midabdomen as small irregular collections of gas on each side of the vertebral column. Often the patient with blood in the peritoneal cavity will complain of pain in the shoulders and may have localized tenderness over an area of injury. Some help when a liver tear is suspected can be obtained from a liver scan, especially in the patient who is in good condition despite an abdominal injury. When more active bleeding is suspected an aortogram is held to be superior.

RUPTURE OF THE SPLEEN

It is well known that splenic injury can be sustained from relatively minor abdominal trauma. This may be related to the fact that the patient with a ruptured spleen may have a spleen that is relatively free in the abdominal cavity. Persistent abdominal pain, left shoulder pain, excessive thirst, and a falling blood pressure and hematocrit are indications for operative exploration. Abdominal films sometimes reveal that the stomach is displaced medially by the clotted blood around the spleen. In performing the exploratory operation we prefer to make a gen-

erous vertical incision splitting the rectus muscle on the left side when a ruptured spleen is suspected. This gives an opportunity to examine all of the abdominal contents carefully, a procedure which is more difficult when a lateral or transverse incision is used. If the spleen is ruptured, its removal is indicated despite the fact that bleeding has stopped, because of the likelihood of delayed hemorrhage. Such delayed rupture of the spleen may take place days or even weeks

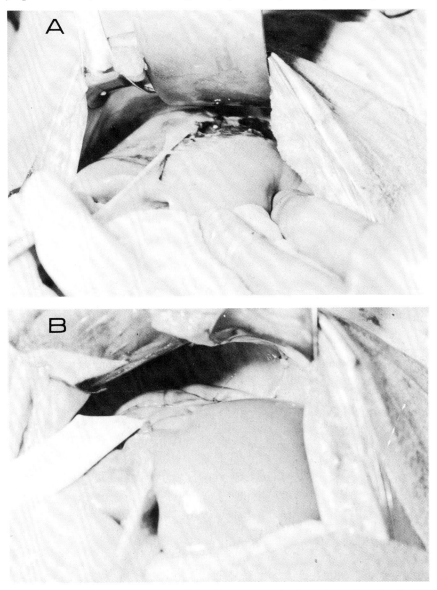

Fig. 6. A. Laceration of the liver. 1,500 ml of blood was present in the peritoneal cavity. B. After evacuation and suture closure. Note the large drain in the defect. The subphrenic space is also drained.

after injury and makes its presence known by the development of anemia and the presence of a mass in the left upper quadrant.

At the time of splenectomy the diaphragm on the left side should be palpated to be sure that a rupture has not occurred. This is particularly important when there has been severe trauma. It is well to examine the liver to be sure that there are not multiple intra-abdominal injuries. The presence of any bile-stained fluid in the peritoneal cavity indicates the need for a thorough examination of the liver and extrahepatic bile structures before the abdomen is closed.

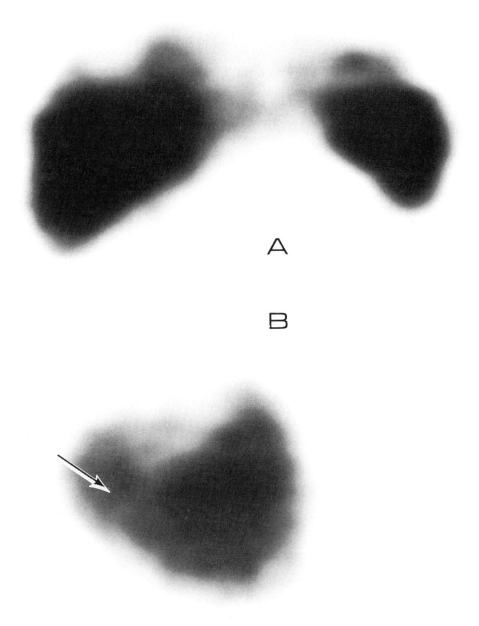

Fig. 7. A. Liver scan. Defect posterior and superior in right lobe is clearly visible. The shadow on the right is the spleen. B. Lateral view showing a large defect. Note the small fracture line running to the inferior surface of liver.

LIVER INJURIES

When there has been a history of trauma predominantly to the right upper quadrant or right lower chest and the patient manifests tenderness in the right upper quadrant, the possibility of liver injury must be taken into consideration. Persistence of the signs of liver injury, despite the fact that there is no fall in blood pressure, is an indication for exploration. When exploration reveals the injury to be a liver laceration, it is important to remove the clot and to suture the tear carefully with deep chromic catgut sutures (Fig. 6). In the past it was common to pack large injuries of the liver with gauze. Experience has established that subphrenic infection frequently occurs and that when such packs are removed there is great likelihood of severe secondary bleeding. This practice has therefore been discontinued. It is far better to use absorbable hemostatic material where such a procedure is necessary. The best program is to control the bleeding with suturing. It may be necessary to remove part of a lobe or, in cases of extensive injury to one lobe, to perform lobectomy. In all patients treated for liver injuries, drains should be left in place in the area of repair and in the subphrenic space because of the great likelihood of a bile leak. Such bile drainage may not be evident at the time of operation but may take place some time after the closure has been completed. It is advocated by some surgeons that a cholangiogram be performed at the time of operation, since occasional ruptures of the common or hepatic ducts have been reported. This catastrophe is extremely rare in children, and unless there is a local indication for a cholangiogram, such as the presence of a great deal of bile in the peritoneal cavity without the evidence of a parenchymal tear, the examination can be safely omitted. One of the complications of trauma to the liver is bleeding into the biliary ducts, a complication referred to as hemobilia. This serious complication can be avoided by the careful debridement and suturing of liver lacerations. Liver scans are useful in demonstrating liver tears. These can now be accomplished with minimal radiation exposure and with great speed, and they provide exact information about the size and site of the laceration (Fig. 7).

INJURIES TO THE PANCREAS

In patients with injuries to the pancreas there will usually be an elevated serum amylase, but frequently it is impossible to make a preoperative diagnosis of pancreatic injury. It is important to examine the pancreas care-

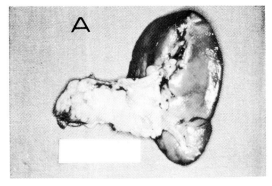

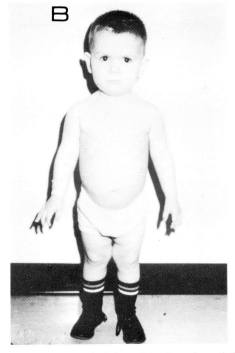

Fig. 8. A. Pancreatic injury. Distal portion of the body was removed together with the spleen. B. Patient after recovery.

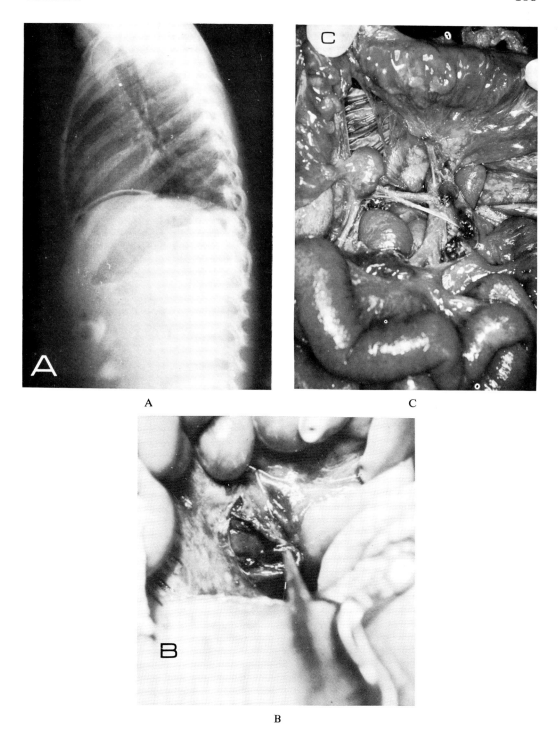

Fig. 9. Intestinal injuries. A. Lateral upright roentgenogram revealing a small amount of free intra-peritoneal air. This is seen in duodenal and intestinal margin tears. B. Large anterior tear of the third portion of the duodenum. C. Photograph taken at post-mortem, revealing an extensive mesenteric tear that had caused overwhelming hemorrhage. (Courtesy of Dr. John Raffensberger and Dr. Jordan Weitzman.)

fully when there is a great deal of fluid in the peritoneal cavity without an obvious source of leakage. We have seen a toddler with a complete transection of the body of the pancreas who developed signs and symptoms which closely approximated those of appendiceal perforation and peritonitis (Fig. 8). Considerable intra-abdominal fluid was present in that case.

The management of injuries of the pancreas is not unusually difficult when there is a transection beyond the head. Resection and removal of the distal portion with careful ligation of the duct and closure of the stump is essential. It is not always necessary in children to remove the spleen in such situations, and there is some advantage in not doing so, in order to guard against overwhelming infections. When the tear involves the head of the pancreas it may be necessary to use a Roux-en-Y procedure and to insert both fractured ends into the intestine for

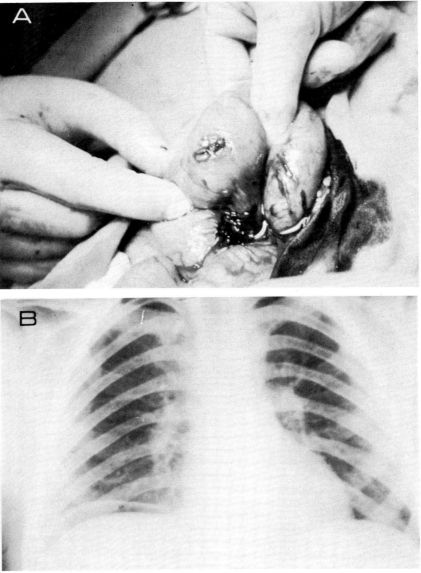

Fig. 10. A. A small traumatic laceration of the free margin of the jejunum. B. Air is clearly visible beneath the right diaphragm.

drainage. It is interesting that extensive resection of the pancreas does not generally affect the patient's glucose metabolism.

INTESTINAL INJURIES

Traumatic perforation of a portion of the gastrointestinal tract is not unusual. The most frequent sites are the third portion of the duodenum and the free margin of the jejunum. The tear in the third portion of the duodenum probably occurs so frequently because the duodenum crosses the vertebral bodies and thus is susceptible to trauma (Fig. 9). In these cases there is usually only a small amount of air in the peritoneal cavity, since the injury is retroperitoneal or communicates with the lesser omental cavity. If the perforation is small it is possible to freshen the edges until free bleeding occurs and to reapproximate them. In order to control bleeding we use a double suture layer, one of 5-0 chromic to approximate the mucosa and to turn in the bowel wall and a second layer of interrupted 6-0 silk sutures to reinforce the closure. When a large laceration is present it is usually best to free up the duodenum from surrounding structures and to resect the portion containing the tear. If good bleeding occurs from the bowel ends, it is safe to do a two-layer closure. Drainage of the area is not necessary or wise. It is important to remove gross contamination by means of irrigation of the peritoneal cavity. If the lacerations are extensive and in the distal part of the small intestine, they should be resected and an anastomosis performed. When they are small (Fig. 10) a simple closure can be accomplished safely after the edges are freshened. In the case of large bowel injury an ileostomy or colostomy above the repair of a primary colon laceration is safer than simple repair alone.

DUODENAL HEMATOMA

Duodenal hematoma is an isolated lesion that occurs surprisingly frequently and can be caused by localized and not too severe trauma. The patient has a history of trauma and then is perfectly well, starting to vomit only a day or so after the injury. This vomiting is caused by the accumulation of a large blood clot under the duodenal serosa of sufficient size to effectively occlude the lumen. One may outline this type of obstruction radiographically and establish a preoperative diagnosis by giving the patient barium by mouth (Fig. 11). In some instances the

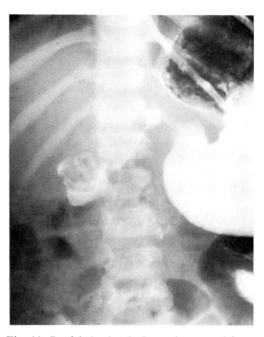

Fig. 11. Partial duodenal obstruction caused by a traumatic hematoma.

patient is seen several days after the injury occurred, and occasionally the hematoma is sufficiently resorbed for operation to be unnecessary. In most instances, however, the obstruction is persistent, and consequently early drainage of the hematoma is indicated (Fig. 12). Simple evacuation of the clot is sufficient to relieve the obstruction and restore the child to good health (Fig. 13). It is not necessary to make any attempt to suture the serosal peritoneum, which has had to be divided to evacuate the hematoma. Such patients do well. They should be able

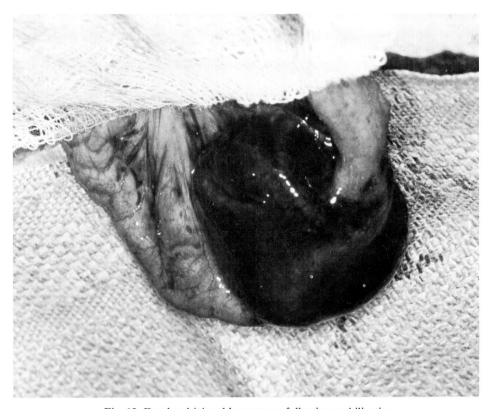

Fig. 12. Duodenal-jejunal hematoma, following mobilization.

to take food on the second or third day after the operation, and they usually make a rapid recovery.

PENETRATING ABDOMINAL WOUNDS

It is important to get as much of the history of the injury as possible in evaluating patients with penetrating abdominal wounds. Often this information is not available, and one must make a decision for or against operation on the basis of the physical findings alone. An auxiliary technique which may help avoid an exploration is to perform a sinogram of the puncture wound with contrast material by means of roentgenograms. If this proves that the sinus does not enter the peritoneal cavity, and the patient is free of symptoms, abdominal exploration will not be needed. In most instances, however, it is safer to perform an abdominal exploration than not to do so. There are relatively minor ill effects from a negative exploration. On the other hand, serious injury to an abdominal viscus, such as a perforation of the intestine or laceration of a vessel or organ, may be overlooked unless the surgeon makes a practice of exploring most patients with penetrating wounds in the region of the abdomen.

CHEST INJURIES

Patients with chest injuries can be divided into two groups, those with blunt trauma and those with penetrating wounds.

PENETRATING WOUNDS

The patient with a penetrating wound may be treated on the basis of the immediate physical findings. A sucking chest wound requires urgent treatment to avoid the danger of a tension pneumothorax. If the patient's condition is satisfactory, roentgenograms should be made. With evidence of an air-fluid level in the chest, an intercostal

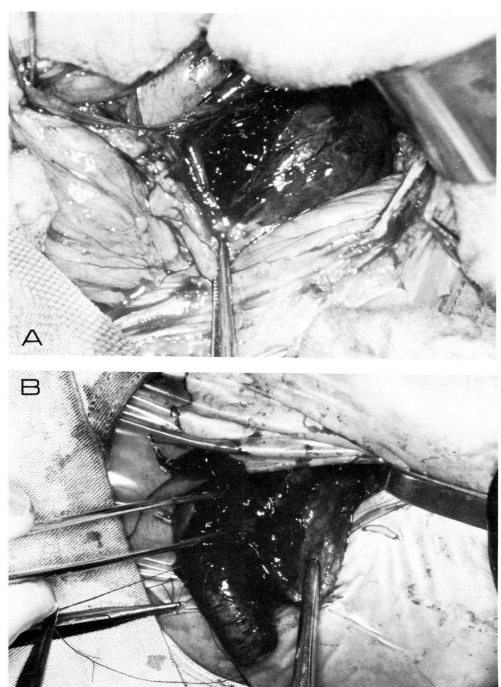

Fig. 13. A. Large hematoma of the third portion of the duodenum. B. The hematoma has been evacuated.

catheter should be inserted and connected to a water seal. This simple maneuver provides drainage of the fluid and air and is a means of measuring continued blood loss. Explo- ration of the chest is usually unnecessary. It is important to recall that negative thoracic explorations are associated with considerable increases in mortality and morbidity, in comparison to negative abdominal explorations. There are probably too many negative chest explorations performed, and intercostal drainage is effective in most instances when there is a fluid-air level on chest roentgenograms. However, when the volume of escaped air is large and cannot be controlled by this method, or when there is continued bleeding, direct exploration is indicated. The presence of foreign material, such as a bony fragment or other debris, within the mediastinum also calls for exploration and debridement.

SUCKING WOUNDS

Sucking wounds of the chest are serious complications of thoracic injuries and must be dealt with promptly in order to restore effective respiration. An emergency measure consists of placing vaseline gauze over the sucking wound. This is covered with a thick gauze dressing. The dressing permits fluid and air to escape but is an effective valve against the reentry of air. Some surgeons recommend using skin clips to approximate the skin and thus converting the chest opening into a closed wound. If a tension pneumothorax is present, as indicated by increasing dyspnea, cyanosis, and deviation of the trachea and heart to the opposite side, the insertion of a needle or intercostal tube may be lifesaving. The patient should be taken to the operating room and a formal closure made as soon as it is practical to do so. Intercostal drainage by a catheter connected to a water seal or to suction is necessary for two or three days after this procedure.

CLOSED TRAUMA

It is important to appreciate that a fracture of the larynx or the trachea may occur with closed chest trauma and that this may be associated with the excessive accumulation of subcutaneous and mediastinal air. Any penetrating wound of the chest, particularly in association with fractured ribs, may produce extensive accumulations of sub-

cutaneous air. If it is possible, an x-ray of the chest should be made to determine the side of the pneumothorax. Insertion of an intercostal tube to decompress the pneumothorax controls the subcutaneous emphysema. When x-rays are not readily available, the insertion of a needle into the suspected side will give evidence of a tension pneumothorax. In a patient who has sustained a crushing injury that has produced a flail chest, or in one in whom a large part of the chest moves paradoxically with respiratory effort, it has been the practice in the past to arrange some type of external fixation—for example, through suspension by sternal or rib traction. Usually these contrivances are not entirely successful in stabilizing the chest. Placing the patient on a respirator is a more effective method. Since it is necessary to keep the patient on a respirator for a number of days until stabilization of the chest occurs, a tracheostomy is essential. It is important to use the respirator in such a way that the pressure never goes into the negative range, so that collapse of the chest will not take place intermittently. Patients with flail chests have been maintained on this type of assisted respiration for over a month with eventual recovery.

Blunt trauma to the chest may produce unexpected lesions of the lung. One may see accumulation of fluid in the chest cavity or a localized collection of fluid with an air-fluid level. Occasionally, intrapulmonary hemorrhage occurs (Fig. 14). Most of these situations, if not progressive, will take care of themselves. In patients with such conditions it may sometimes be necessary later on to do some type of resection or drainage procedure for complete cure. The need for decortication of the lung, however, has decreased considerably because of the use of early intercostal drainage to remove blood from the chest.

FRACTURES

Except for compound fracture, injuries about the elbow, and other lesions which

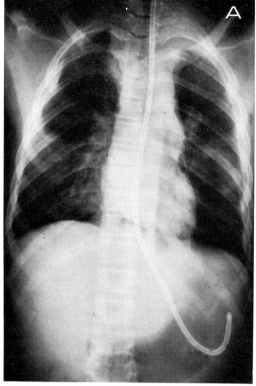

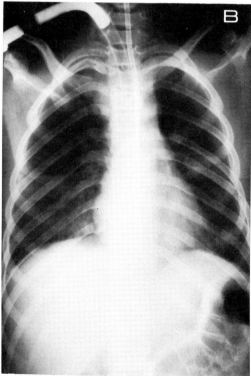

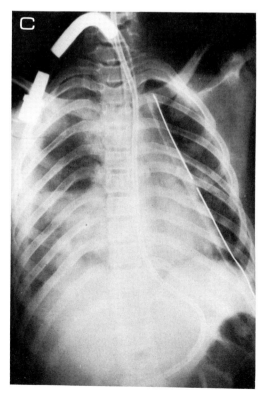

Fig. 14. Injuries caused by blunt trauma to the chest. A. Widened mediastinum from blunt trauma. There is moderate infiltration of the right chest. B. Massive intrapleural and intrapulmonary collection of blood on third day. C. Clearing of chest at the end of the tenth hospital day.

contribute to nerve injury, fractures are not emergencies. External splinting is sufficient until the patient is in a condition that allows reduction and fixation of the fractures.

HEAD INJURIES

Head injuries are dealt with in another section of the book.

INJURIES TO THE URINARY SYSTEM

When a child has sustained injury to the lower abdomen, and specifically when there is a pelvic fracture, it is important to insert a catheter into the bladder. Inability to catheterize the bladder indicates that a tear of the urethra may have been sustained. This possibility can be investigated by means of a retrograde urethrogram, or the test can be omitted and a suprapubic cystotomy performed. When the catheter enters the bladder and clear urine is obtained no further investigation is required. Blood-stained urine

is an indication for a cystogram to verify whether or not the bladder is intact. When the trauma is to the flank area and there is hematuria, an intravenous pyelogram is informative. This examination is not reliable

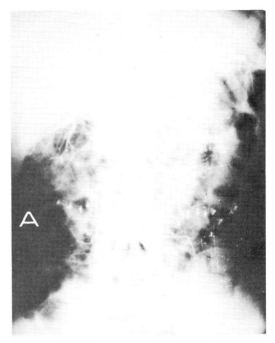

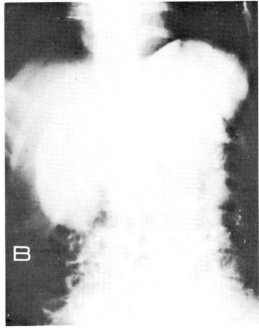

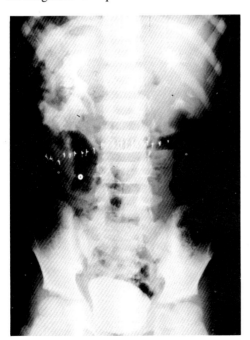

Fig. 15. Extravasation of contrast material from left kidney after trauma. Splenectomy had previously been performed. (Courtesy of Dr. John G. Raffensberger.)

Fig. 16. A. Aortogram outlining all visceral vessels. B. Nephrogram after aortogram. The lower pole of the left kidney is missing.

when the patient is in shock, for under these circumstances kidneys will not be visualized because of inadequate renal perfusion.

Some extravasation of contrast material (Fig. 15) is not necessarily an indication for renal exploration, for experience has proven that remarkable healing with excellent preservation of function is possible under such circumstances. Continued bleeding of sufficient magnitude to contribute to shock is an indication for exploration. A vascular tear is likely to be found in such situations. In a patient with a known kidney injury the development of fever and a renal mass during his convalescence is an indication for exploration. Drainage of an infected hematoma may be all that is required. A severely damaged kidney with minimal renal function may require removal.

Penetrating injuries lacerating a part of the urinary system are rare. We have observed a patient who sustained a gunshot wound of the abdomen which injured a ureter and resulted in a ureterocutaneous fistula. At exploration the two ends of the ureter were mobilized and an end-to-end anastomosis accomplished with a good result.

An aortogram may be of help in outlining renal injury. In many centers dealing with large numbers of trauma cases this procedure is widely used for the early diagnosis of both intra-abdominal and retroperitoneal injuries (Fig. 16).

ORVAR SWENSON
WILLIAM L. DONNELLAN

REFERENCES

AVERY, E. E., MÖRCH, E. T., and BENSON, D. W. Critically crushed chests: A new method. J. Thorac. Surg., 32: 291, 1956.

CAFFEY, J. Multiple fractures in long bones of infants suffering from chronic subdural hematoma. Amer. J. Roentgen., 56: 163, 1946.

CROSTHWAIT, R. W., ALLEN, J. E., MURGA, F., BEALL, A. C., Jr., and DEBAKEY, M. E. Surgical management of 640 consecutive liver injuries in civilian practice. Surg. Gynec. Obstet., 114: 650, 1962.

GILLESBY, W. J. The rib as a secondary missile. U.S. Armed Forces Medical Journal, 3: 1839, 1952.

KEMPE, C. H., SILVERMAN, F. N., STEELE, B. F., DROEGENMUELLER, W., and SILVER, H. K. The battered-child syndrome. J.A.M.A., 181: 17, 1962.

KULOWSKI, J. Motorist injuries to children. J. Pediat., 47: 696, 1955.

MacLEAN, L. D. Traumatic rupture of the diaphragm. Postgrad. Med., 29: 383, 1961.

MADDING, G. F., LAWRENCE, K. B., and KENNEDY, P. A. War wounds of the liver. Texas J. Med., 42: 267, 1946.

MANHEIMER, D. I., DEWEY, J., MELLINGER, G. D., and CORSA, L., Jr. 50,000 child-years of accidental injuries. Public Health Rep., 81: 519, 1966.

MOSELEY, H. F. Accident Surgery. New York, Appleton-Century-Crofts, Vol. 3, 1965.

RICE, R. G., STARBUCK, G. W., and REED, R. B. Accidental injuries to children. New Eng. J. Med., 255: 1212, 1956.

ROAF, R. Trauma in childhood. Brit. Med. J., 1: 1541, 1965.

SILVERMAN, F. Roentgen manifestations of unrecognized skeletal trauma in infants. Amer. J. Roentgen., 69: 413, 1953.

ZOLLINGER, R. W., CREEDON, P. J., and SANGUILY, J. Trauma in children in a general hospital. Amer. J. Surg., 104: 855, 1962.

12

Congenital Anomalies of the Eye

Congenital malformations of the eyes and eyelids are not common, but when they do occur they vary from a complete absence of one or both eyes (anophthalmos) to such a minor deformity as the presence of a congenital pupillary membrane.

OCULAR MALFORMATIONS

The complete absence of one or both eyes may be associated with a structurally complete orbit in an otherwise completely normal child. Cyclopia, which is essentially a fusion of the two eyes resulting in a single eye located in the center of the forehead, is usually incompatible with life because of the associated malformation of the anterior portion of the brain.

One or both eyes may be congenitally small (microphthalmia). Such eyes are usually normal, except that functionally they are frequently quite farsighted (hyperopic). In addition, some of the microphthalmic eyes may contain malformations, such as retinal cysts, congenital cataracts, and a congenital retinal detachment.

Some eyes may be larger than normal (megalophthalmia). Such enlargement may be limited to a large cornea (megalocornea), or the entire eye may be enlarged. These eyes are usually highly nearsighted (myopic), and the child requires corrective lenses for func-

tional vision. Surgery on such eyeballs to reduce the degree and complications of myopia is not generally recommended. An enlarged eyeball should not be confused with an eye that has been pushed forward (exophthalmos) by an orbital tumor. Similarly, a congenitally enlarged eyeball must be differentiated from one enlarged as a result of a primary (congenital) glaucoma or a glaucoma secondary to a retinoblastoma. Occasionally a congenitally cone-shaped cornea (congenital keratoconus) will simulate a congenitally enlarged eyeball.

Common structural eye malformations are the keyhole defects (colobomas) of the iris, lens, retina, and optic nerve (Fig. 1). Such eyes are usually amblyopic. These malformations are otherwise of no significance except for the minor cosmetic defect produced. No surgical repair is possible or indicated for the coloboma.

Congenital clouding or opacification of the cornea may be the result of an intrauterine infection or may follow a forceps injury to the cornea, particularly involving the left eye. It may also be the result of an accidental instillation of a strong solution of silver nitrate or may be the first indication of a congenital glaucoma. Treatment of these opacities varies with the etiology.

A dermoid of the cornea appears as a raised, white plaque in the inferior temporal quadrant of the cornea and may contain fat

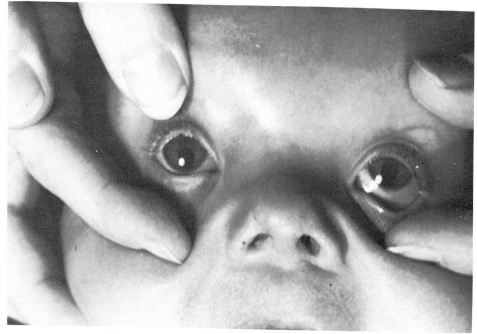

Fig. 1. Bilateral inferior congenital colobomas of the iris.

or hair. Some large dermoids completely obscure the cornea. This treatment of choice is covering the lesion with an artificial plastic eye thus overcoming the cosmetic defect. The small dermoids require no treatment. When they become vascularized and enlarged, excision is advisable.

A bluish discoloration of the sclera is not uncommon as a transient phenomenon in the eyes of newborns. Such blue scleras must not be confused with the same phenomenon in older infants with cardiac malformations or osteogenesis imperfecta.

Abnormalities of the pupil are not uncommon. In 25 percent of the population there is a physiological anisocoria (that is, one pupil is larger than the other). This inequality is of no clinical significance. Another common abnormality is a congenital pupillary membrane. In these cases a strand of persistent iris tissue extends from the iris across the pupil, attaching itself to the anterior surface of the lens. As these pupillary membranes infrequently interfere with vision, surgical removal is contraindicated.

Developmental retinal cysts may occur in the retinal periphery. Surgery is not indicated unless the cyst is enlarging or is producing a detachment of the retina.

ADNEXAL ABNORMALITIES

The most common developmental abnormalities of the eyelids are epicanthal folds, ptosis, and colobomas (Fig. 2). The persistent epicanthal fold is of little clinical significance, except that many children with these folds and with straight, nondeviating eyes are mistakenly referred for therapy for "crossed eyes." Careful examination of such patients reveals that one eye becomes lost under the lid fold on lateral gaze, thus giving the illusion of being crossed.

Congenital ptosis may be unilateral or bilateral (Figs. 3, 4, and 5) and of such a mild degree that no surgical correction is needed. The ptosis may, however, be severe and require surgery to correct the cosmetic defect. Surgery is preferably undertaken when the patient is about five years old. It

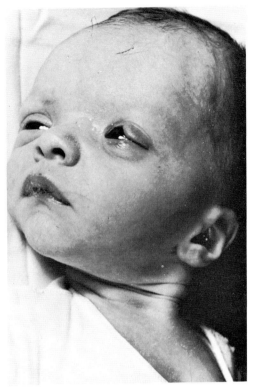

Fig. 2. Congenital coloboma of the left upper lid.

consists essentially of resection of the levator palpebral superioris muscle. Colobomas of the eyelids require early repair to protect the cornea from ulceration.

Failure of the nasolacrimal duct to open is a common abnormality and is caused by epithelial debris or a membrane in the inferior portion of the nasolacrimal canal. The administration of antibiotic drops and massage of the lacrimal sac will open most ducts. If the passage has not opened by the time the child is six months old, probing of the nasolacrimal duct should be performed, preferably under general anesthesia.

Congenital paralysis of the ocular muscles is not uncommon and may involve a single muscle in one or both eyes or may involve all the muscles in one or both eyes (ophthalmoplegia externa). The muscle most commonly involved is the external rectus muscle. This is usually a result of an aplasia of the sixth-nerve nucleus. A convergent strabismus often develops for which surgical correction may be indicated at about the age of four years.

CONGENITAL GLAUCOMA

Congenital glaucoma (hydrophthalmos, buphthalmos) may be defined as an elevated intraocular pressure occurring in infants or children under the arbitrarily set age of 18 years. The normal intraocular pressure when measured under general anesthesia usually measures from 15 to 25 mm Hg with Schiøtz's tonometer. The etiology of congenital glaucoma is unknown. Several developmental abnormalities in the eye, such as the absence of Schlemm's canal, the presence of embryological tissue in the angle of the anterior chamber, and abnormal insertion of the musculature of the ciliary body, may predispose to the development of congenital glaucoma.

Other developmental abnormalities which may be associated with a rise in the intraocular pressure include aniridia (absence of the iris) and spherophakia (globular lens associated with a small cornea).

In addition some of the phakomatoses may be associated with an elevated intraocular pressure including von Recklinghausen's disease, Lindau–von Hippel disease and the Sturge-Weber syndrome.

In all of these conditions the aqueous humor is formed at a normal or increased rate, and its passage from the eye is impeded by the abnormality in the chamber angle of the eye. As a result of this impediment to the outflow of aqueous humor there is an increase in the intraocular fluid volume and a subsequent elevation of the intraocular pressure.

The cardinal symptom of congenital glaucoma is photophobia. Infants and children with this condition are extremely sensitive to light and react to it by keeping their heads down and their eyes tightly closed.

The signs of congenital glaucoma are multiple and varied. The onset may be apparent immediately after birth or may develop years later. As a rule, both eyes are affected, although they need not be simultaneously in-

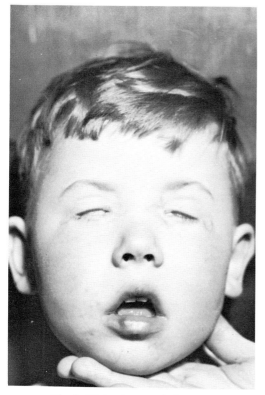

Fig. 3. Bilateral congenital ptosis.

Fig. 4. Ptosis of the right upper lid caused by a plexiform neuroma.

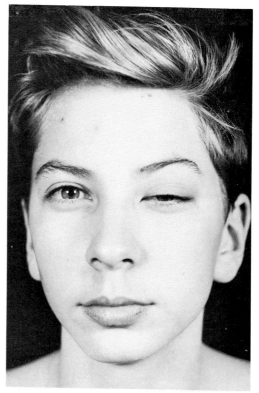

Fig. 5. Ptosis of the left eye resulting from fluid in the region of the superior orbital fissure, secondary to acute ethmoiditis.

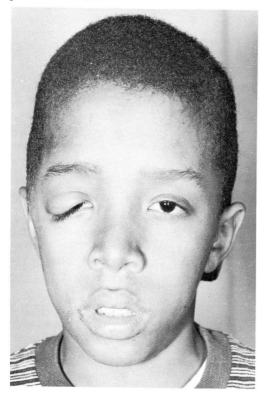

volved. The eyes tend to be prominent, and the corneas are usually enlarged. A horizontal corneal diameter exceeding 12 mm is usually considered pathological. The corneas demonstrate some haziness (Fig. 6), and lying in the posterior layers of the cornea are horizontal lines known as tears in Descemet's membrane. The anterior chamber is deep, and the pupil size will vary depending upon the degree of elevation of the intraocular pressure. The pupil, however, need not be dilated and fixed to light. The lens is clear, and the optic nerve head in the early stages is usually not cupped. Later in the disease the optic nerve does undergo this change.

The diagnosis is suspected from the signs and symptoms and is confirmed by finding an elevated intraocular pressure, measured with the child under general anesthesia. Roentgenograms of the skull, orbits, and foramen are normal. Medical treatment with a miotic, such as pilocarpine, or with the

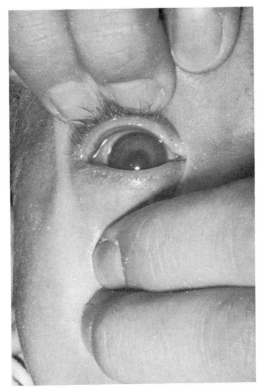

Fig. 6. Enlarged and hazy cornea in congenital glaucoma.

carbonic anhydrase inhibitors is usually ineffective. A goniotomy of the chamber angle, permitting the aqueous humor to have access to Schlemm's canal, seems to be the best treatment. Prognosis must be guarded, although it is generally possible to salvage at least one eye.

Differential diagnosis must be made from other conditions which give rise to an enlarged eye, cloudy cornea, or exophthalmos. Secondary glaucoma must also be excluded. Those conditions which give rise to large eyes include myopia, keratoconus (conical cornea), and megalocornia (congenitally large corneas). Conditions that may give rise to corneal haze include Hurler's disease, cystinosis, silver nitrate burns of the cornea, and damage to the cornea resulting from a forceps injury. Those conditions which may give rise to a secondary glaucoma include intraocular infections, retrolental fibroplasia, and glaucoma secondary to a retinoblastoma.

In congenital glaucoma the anterior chamber is always deep, but the author has never seen a case of secondary glaucoma which was due to a retinoblastoma in an infant or a child in whom the anterior chamber was not shallowed.

CONGENITAL CATARACTS

Congenital cataract is an opacity of the lens which is usually present to some degree at birth. Fortunately many types of congenital cataracts do not interfere with vision and are nonprogressive. These include the opacities which affect the sutures of the lens (sutural cataracts), and punctate, zonular, floriform, and coronary cataracts. Those types of congenital cataracts which interfere with vision are of clinical significance. They include (1) the anterior or posterior polar cataracts, (2) the nuclear cataracts, and (3) the diffuse opacities. The anterior variety usually occurs on the anterior pole (surface) of the lens, and the posterior variety occurs on the posterior surface of the lens; the nuclear cataracts occur in the center of the lens; and a diffuse cataract presents a completely opaque lens.

The etiology is unknown except for those congenital cataracts associated with maternal rubella occurring during the first trimester of pregnancy. Congenital cataracts may be unilateral or bilateral. Unilateral cataracts have few symptoms, but the mother may complain that her baby has a "spot" in one eye. Either a congenital cataract or a retinoblastoma should be suspected in such cases. Diagnosis of a congenital cataract is not difficult. These eyes are usually smaller than normal, and a light directed obliquely at the eye reveals the lens opacity.

The treatment of congenital cataracts varies, depending upon whether the condition is unilateral or bilateral. In either case, if the cataracts do not interfere with vision, no therapy is needed.

In unilateral cases, if the cataract is not removed, the patient goes through life with a white spot in the pupil, and the eye becomes divergent. The optimum time for surgical removal is between two and five years of age. Discission (needling) of the lens, followed in some cases by a linear extraction (washing out of the anterior chamber), is the treatment commonly used. Often needling of the lens must be repeated to obtain a maximum effect.

In treating children with bilateral cataracts, the eye with the more advanced opacity is operated on at the age of six months in order to permit the fovea to develop. Again the operation of choice is a needling of the lens, with or without a linear extraction. After one eye has been successfully treated, the other eye can be either operated on immediately or can be treated as a unilateral cataract.

The prognosis for congenital cataracts is generally guarded because complications, including infections, hemorrhage, secondary cataracts, glaucoma, and retinal detachments, are frequent, and developmental abnormalities are present in as high as 50 percent of the cases. After successful surgery the patient may be fitted with cataract lenses and in later years with contact lenses.

Many children who have had surgery for congenital cataracts are able to carry on quite well in regular school classes. Those who cannot, can be helped in "sight saving" classes. Although some mentally retarded children have congenital cataracts, there is no truth to the general statement that congenital cataracts are associated with mental retardation. Often the development of children with congenital cataracts is slower than normal because of poor vision, but many of these children are above average in alertness, responses to mental stimulation, and intelligence.

RETROLENTAL FIBROPLASIA

Retrolental fibroplasia is a condition seen usually but not exclusively in premature infants and is the result of postnatal oxygen sensitivity. Pathologically this condition may be divided into the acute and chronic stages. The acute stage may be divided into four phases: phase I, in which the retina merely exhibits dilated retinal veins; phase II, in which edema of the retina and retinal hemorrhages usually are present in the superior temporal quadrant; phase III, in which a localized detachment of the retina occurs; and phase IV, in which a complete detachment of the retina also occurs. The acute stage commences about the second week after birth. In the chronic stage there is a complete detachment of the retina, cataract formation, uveitis, glaucoma, and atrophy of the eyeball. The condition is usually bilateral and frequently is more advanced in one eye than in the other. The condition can arrest itself at any time in the acute stage or may progress into the chronic stage, in which case the retinal changes are irreversible. There is no treatment for this condition once it has developed. Treatment, therefore, lies in prevention. Oxygen should not be administered to premature infants unless it is lifesaving. The only valid indication for oxygen is cyanosis and respiratory distress. If oxygen is required it should be administered in a concentration compatible with the relief of symptoms, but should not exceed 40 percent. The oxygen concentration should be measured and recorded every two hours, either by the inhalation therapist or by the nurse in charge of the incubator. The oxygen should be discontinued as soon as practicable. Surgical correction of the retinal detachments associated with retrolental fibroplasia is now being attempted, but the results at present leave much to be desired.

INTRAOCULAR AND ORBITAL TUMORS

The most common neoplasm in the eye of infants and children is a retinoblastoma. This is a malignant tumor arising from the inner layers of the retina. The neoplastic cells tend to duplicate the cells of the retina and to arrange themselves in circular fashion around a blood vessel, forming rosettes. Mitoses are common. The etiology of this tumor is unknown. It seldom occurs after the age of seven or eight years. In the early stages it gives rise to no signs or symptoms, but the child's mother may complain that she sees a white spot in the child's eye. In approximately 25 percent of the cases the tumor is bilateral.

Examination of the eye often reveals a yellowish pupillary reflex or a diffusely thickened retina resembling an orange peel. A polypoid mass may sometimes be seen in the vitreous, or a detachment of the retina may be present. This diagnosis is usually confirmed upon examinaton of the fundus, with the child under general anesthesia. Diagnosis is further confirmed by the finding of an intraorbital calcification, which may be seen in as many as 75 percent of the cases. If the tumor has invaded the optic nerve, there may be an enlargement of the optic foramen. When the diagnosis is confirmed, it is well to have at least one other ophthalmologist concur in the diagnosis before surgical treatment is undertaken. There is only one treatment for unilateral retinoblastoma: immediate enucleation of the involved globe. The most satisfactory treatment of bilateral retinoblastoma is a bilateral removal of the globes. However, since both the physician and the parents are reluctant to agree to a bilateral enucleation it is advisable to remove the eye having the more advanced tumor and to treat the remaining eye with x-ray therapy plus systemic triethylene melamine phosphate. The prognosis varies with the stage of advancement of the disease. If the disease is unilateral and the tumor has not extended into the optic nerve, enucleation will cure the patient. Patients who survive may in turn have offspring who may develop retinoblastoma. Cures as high as 25 percent are reported following the use of x-ray and triethylene melamine phosphate. Loss of vision and damage to the ocular structures occur with the growth of the tumor and following x-ray treatments.

Retinoblastoma must be differentiated from those inflammatory and hemorrhagic conditions which produce a similar fundus picture. It must also be differentiated from those conditions producing orbital calcifications, such as far advanced retrolental fibroplasia and vascular malformation. Enlargement of the optic foramen by a glioma of the optic nerve or a glioma of the optic chiasm should not be confused with the enlargement resulting from extension of the retinoblastoma into the cranium. Retinoblastoma metastasizes by direct extension backward along the optic nerve and by erosion into the retinal vessels, producing systemic metastases particularly in the lungs and long bones.

ORBITAL TUMORS

The most common benign orbital tumor in children is a hemangioma, whereas the most common malignant tumor is a sarcoma. The hemangioma (Figs. 7, 8, and 9) remains quiescent and gives rise to no ocular signs or symptoms. As the tumor enlarges or becomes thrombosed it gives rise to a moderate degree of protopsis. The eye is usually pushed straight forward, and motion is somewhat restricted in all directions. There may be some swelling and edema of the lids as well as distension of the veins of the face and conjunctiva. The remainder of the eye usually appears normal except for the presence of some retinal edema and folds. All of the symptoms are exaggerated when the head is placed in a dependent position. A trill or bruit is not discernible. Roentgenograms of the skull, orbits, optic foramen, and sinuses are usually normal, although some increased soft tissue density may be apparent on the orbital x-ray films. Arteriograms are usually normal and are notoriously misleading in orbital vascular lesions. Surgical removal of the lesion is indicated. These tumors are not as a rule radiosensitive. Arteriovenous angiomas or vascular malformations of the orbit produce a similar clinical picture, and differentiation is made by biopsy during surgical exploration of the orbit.

Other benign tumors of the orbit include orbital abscesses (Fig. 10), dermoid cysts,

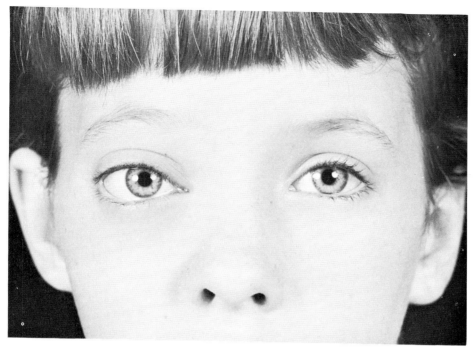

Fig. 7. Right exophthalmos caused by angioma of right orbit.

Fig. 8. Right lateral view showing exophthalmos.

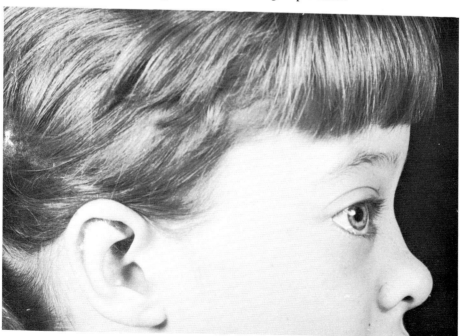

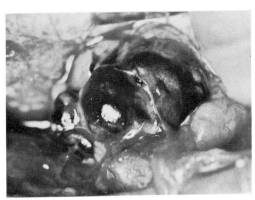

Fig. 9. Demonstrating angioma following unroofing of right orbit.

mucoceles of the frontal sinuses, lymphomas, gliomas of the optic nerve, and osteomas of the orbital wall. The dermoid cysts usually lie in the medial or lateral wall of the orbit and are usually palpable but may extend deeply into the orbit or even into the cranial cavity. They frequently become infected and then produce some deviation of the eyeball, accompanied by tearing and photophobia. Surgical excision must be complete, or recurrence is inevitable.

Mucoceles of the frontal sinus are usually located in the superior medial aspect of the orbit. They frequently become swollen and infected and produce deviation of the eye as well as pain, photophobia, and lacrimation. Roentgenograms frequently reveal some notching of the superior orbital margin. Surgical excision is indicated.

Gliomas of the optic nerve produce exophthalmos, associated with pallor of the optic nerve head, loss of vision, and enlargement of the ipsilateral optic foramen. This tumor may be one of the manifestations of Recklinghausen's disease. Excision is recommended using a transfrontal approach to unroof the orbit.

Osteomas usually affect the superior temporal margin of the orbit; they exhibit characteristic roentgenological changes, and they can be easily excised if they give rise to significant ocular symptoms.

Benign lymphomas (pseudotumor of the orbit or inflammatory orbital tumor) give rise to a bilateral exophthalmos, with multiple orbital tumors usually being palpable in

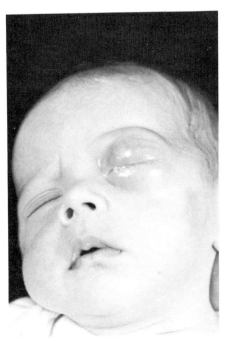

Fig. 10. Left exophthalmos caused by an orbital abscess resulting from ethmoiditis.

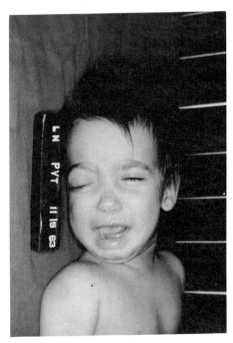

Fig. 11. Left exophthalmos caused by angiosarcoma of the orbit.

both orbits. The eyes are frequently divergent, and there is some edema of the lids and conjunctivas. Roentgenograms of the orbit may reveal some increased soft tissue density. The peripheral blood smear is usually normal. Biopsy is necessary to establish the diagnosis, and the condition is sensitive to radiation and steroid therapy.

The most common malignant tumor of the orbit is a sarcoma (Figs. 11 and 12). The condition develops quite rapidly, giving rise to a marked unilateral exophthalmos. These lesions tend to push the eye down and out. There is usually some congestion of the eye and eyelids, and there may be some edema of the posterior pole of the fundus. Roentgenograms of the orbit may reveal an increased soft tissue density. Arteriograms are usually noncontributory, although if the le-

sion should prove to be an angiosarcoma, it could well be outlined by the arteriogram.

Diagnosis is confirmed by an orbital biopsy. Histological differentiation between embryonal sarcoma and metastatic neuroblastoma is often difficult. The presence of other lesions, particularly in the long bones, strongly favors a diagnosis of neuroblastoma.

Metastatic malignant tumors to the orbit include neuroblastoma (Fig. 13), leukemia, and malignant lymphomas. Surgery is not indicated for the metastatic neuroblastomas, since satisfactory palliation is possible with radiation.

The orbital tumors associated with leukemia and malignant lymphomas are usually associated with systemic evidence of the diseases, and the orbital tumors are a coincidental finding.

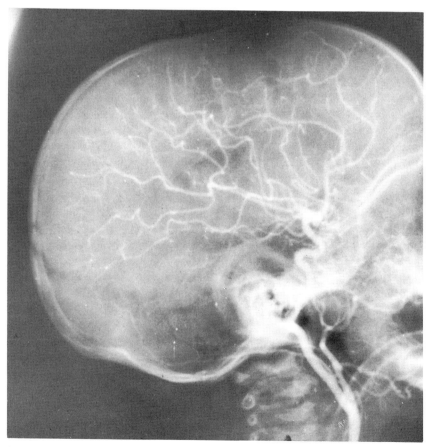

Fig. 12. Arteriogram of the left internal carotid artery demonstrating left orbital angiosarcoma.

OPHTHALMIA NEONATORUM

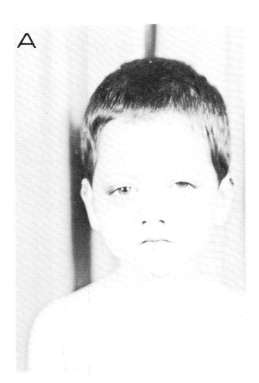

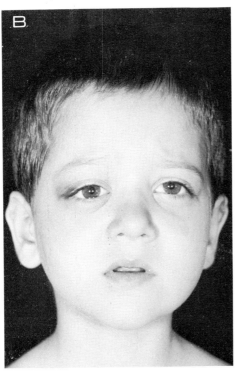

Fig. 13. Right exophthalmos resulting from metastatic neuroblastoma to the right orbit.

Inflammation of the conjunctiva, occurring in the first postpartum week is referred to as ophthalmia neonatorum. These inflammations generally may be divided into three groups; those occurring during the first two postnatal days; those occurring between the second and the fifth days; and those occurring after the fifth day.

Those infections occurring during the first two days are generally caused by silver nitrate or one of the soaps or detergents used to bathe the child. They may give rise to a mild or moderate conjunctival inflammation with moderate photophobia with moderate secretion and with edema of the lids. In addition the detergents may produce punctate erosions of the cornea. Conjunctival smears and cultures are not required, and isolation of the infant is not indicated. Spontaneous resolution generally occurs.

Those conjunctival inflammations occurring from the second to the fifth days usually result from mixed infections, frequently from birth canal contamination. Cultures of the conjunctiva reveal staphylococcus, streptococcus, or colon bacilli and produce moderate to severe conjunctivitis with some secretion, lacrimation, and photophobia. It is helpful to take conjunctival smears and cultures. Local antibiotic treatment should be guided by sensitivity determinations. Those inflammations occurring after the fifth day are frequently of gonococcal origin and give rise to severe fulminating conjunctival infections with corneal ulceration. If left untreated the cornea may perforate, leading to the loss of the eye. There is a marked conjunctival hyperemia with edema and swelling of the lids and profuse secretions. Smears and cultures of the conjunctivas must be made, and isolation of the patient is mandatory. Treatment consists of local and systemic antibiotics, local atropine drops, and frequent profuse saline irrigation of the conjunctival sacs. Occasionally a conjunctival flap will have to be made as an emergency procedure to cover an impending corneal perforation.

STRABISMUS

Strabismus may be of two varieties, that resulting from a paralyzed ocular muscle (paralytic) and that in which no paralyzed ocular muscle is present (nonparalytic, or accommodative). In clinical practice, the paralytic variety is much less common than the nonparalytic. The most common paralytic eye muscle is the external rectus muscle. In these cases, the eye may deviate inward (convergent strabismus), although it may not be crossed at all. Patients with this condition are unable to abduct the eye with the paralyzed external rectus muscle. In this regard, however, it should be remembered that many infants and some children will not turn the eyes outward when following a light or an object. This does not necessarily mean that the external rectus muscle is paralyzed, for the abducted position of gaze is seldom used or required by infants or young children, and as these children develop they are able to move their eyes normally. Another eye muscle which may be paralyzed is the medial rectus. Paralysis of this muscle usually but not invariably causes the eye to deviate outward (divergent strabismus), and the patient will be unable to adduct the eye with the paretic muscle. Paralysis of this muscle is not commonly seen in ordinary clinical practice. Paralysis of the vertically acting muscles is also seen on occasion. Paralysis of the superior rectus muscle manifests itself by an inability on the part of the patient to elevate the globe when the eye is abducted. When the inferior rectus muscle is paralyzed the patient is unable to depress the globe when the eye is abducted. A paralysis of the inferior oblique muscle is indicated when the patient is unable to elevate his eye when the eye is adducted. A paralysis of the superior oblique muscle should be considered when the patient is unable to depress the globe when the eye is adducted. Patients with a paralysis of the superior oblique muscle frequently demonstrate a head tilt to the side opposite the eye with the paralyzed superior oblique muscle.

Much more common than these, however, are those cases of strabismus in which there is no paralysis of one of the extraocular muscles. These may be grouped into two categories: those in which one eye turns inward (esotropia), or convergent strabismus, and those in which one eye turns outward (exotropia), or divergent strabismus.

The age of onset of convergent strabismus is at two and a half years. Frequently the mother will say that the strabismus followed a fall or a febrile illness or a fright. However, this is usually coincidence.

In the early stages the mother will often relate that the crossing will appear only at the supper table or when the child is upset or nervous or has recently been scolded. In many instances some other member of the family, such as a brother, sister, parent, or grandparent, will be mentioned as having had one eye which was crossed. Most of these children reveal a hyperopic (farsighted) refractive error, and proper lenses will frequently help to correct the strabismus. In some instances one eye will become lazy (amblyopic), and this will necessitate the covering of the good eye with an elastoplast eye occluder. The occluder is worn from morning to night, and the child's vision is checked at periodic intervals. Occlusion should be continued until the vision in the unoccluded eye returns to normal or until it is established that vision cannot be improved. If the crossing is corrected by glasses, then the spectacles should be worn continuously and should be checked at periodic intervals. The child may have to wear glasses throughout his life, but in some cases the power of the corrective lenses may be reduced in succeeding years until a stage is reached at which the eyes remain straight without the aid of glasses. If the eyes are not straight after glasses have been worn for a period of one to two years, then surgery is indicated. This may be performed at about the age of three and a half to five years. The operation is performed under general anesthesia. The procedure consists of recessing (weakening) one or both of the medial rectus muscles in combination with a resection (strengthening) of one or both of the external rectus muscles. The patients are discharged on the second or third postoperative day.

The onset of a divergent strabismus most often occurs at about the age of four or five years. Some of the cases may be associated with a hyperactive divergence center that tends to drive the eyes outward. There is usually an associated degree of myopia. Because these children use either eye alternately, neither eye becomes lazy (amblyopic). Therefore occlusion of one eye is not required. Treatment in the early stages consists of prescription lenses for the correction of myopia and convergence exercises. If after a year or two of this regimen the divergent strabismus is cosmetically unacceptable, sur-

gery may be performed. It should be performed at about the age of five to seven years. The surgery is performed under general anesthesia and consists of recession (weakening) of one or both external (lateral) rectus muscles in combination with a resection (strengthening) of one of the medial (internal) rectus muscles. The patient is discharged on the second postoperative day.

Generally speaking, these surgical procedures are successful, but in some instances a second or even a third operation may be required to achieve adequate correction.

JOSEPH E. ALFANO

REFERENCES

ADLER, F. H. Physiology of the Eye, Clinical Application. St. Louis, The C. V. Mosby Co., 1950.
——— Gifford's Textbook of Ophthalmology. Philadelphia, W. B. Saunders Co., 1957.
BECKER, B., and SHAFFER, R. N. Diagnosis and Therapy of Glaucoma. St. Louis, The C. V. Mosby Co., 1961.
BENDER, M. B., ed. The Oculomotor System. New York, Hoeber, Harper and Row, 1964.
BONIUK, M., ed. Ocular and Adnexal Tumors. St. Louis, The C. V. Mosby Co., 1964.
BOYD, B. Highlights of Ophthalmology. Panama City, Starr and Herald Co., 1960.
DUKE-ELDER, S. Textbook of Ophthalmology. St. Louis, The C. V. Mosby Co., 1949.

FASANELLA, R. M., ed. Complications in Eye Surgery. Philadelphia, The W. B. Saunders Co., 1965.
GARNER, L. L. Toography and the Glaucomas. Springfield, Ill., Charles C Thomas, 1965.
HUBER, A. Eye Symptoms in Brain Tumors. St. Louis, The C. V. Mosby Co., 1961.
NELSON, W. F. Textbook of Pediatrics, 8th ed. Philadelphia, W. B. Saunders Co., 1964.
SMITH, L. L., ed. The University of Miami Neuro-ophthalmology Symposium. Springfield, Ill., Charles C Thomas, 1964.
VAIL, D., ed. International Ophthalmology Clinics. Boston, Little, Brown and Company, 1961.

13

The Nose

EMBRYOLOGY AND CONGENITAL LESIONS

Olfactory epithelium first appears in the human embryo when it is about 4 mm long. The nose develops in a medial relationship to the two halves of the first branchial arch (the maxillary and mandibular processes). As the oral cavity appears it is at first common with the nasal space, but in the eighth to twelfth week of fetal life the halves of the hard and soft palates advance toward each other across this space and fuse, separating the two cavities. The thin membrane that covers the anterior nares very rarely fails to rupture, but the one that closes the posterior nares at the posterior margin of the hard palate does occasionally fail to open, producing the choanal atresia which is sometimes encountered at birth. This may be only a web of mucous membrane, but it can also contain a fairly heavy mass of bone between the epithelial layers.

The treatment of choanal atresia is difficult, particularly if bone is present in the occluding membrane. It is usually difficult to resect the bone without damaging the covering mucosa. If much of the covering mucosa is destroyed, the posterior naris will be closed by scar tissue unless skin graft coverage can be obtained here—which again is very difficult to maintain as an open cavity unless the patient wears a hollow prosthesis for a long time. A simple web of mucosa across the posterior naris may be readily punctured but quite as readily closes again.

The author has used the transpalatal approach to the resection of the web but believes that it is better to achieve aeration of the affected nasal cavity in the unilateral case by the resection of a large hole in the posterior portion of the nasal septum. This can usually be accomplished through the anterior naris or may be done transpalatally if necessary.

Dermoid cysts and sinuses are also thought to result from abnormal embryonic development, although it is difficult to document accurately just why these structures should occur where they do occur. It is presumed that in the invagination of ectoderm in the formation of the central nervous system some epithelial cells may be trapped in the area between the root of the nose and the inside of the skull. Figure 1 indicates most of the area in which dermoids of the nose may be found. Any single cyst or sinus will usually occupy only a small portion of this indicated area. The diagnosis of dermoid cyst of the nose is usually based on the presence of a draining sinus somewhere along the bridge of the nose, often with a few hairs projecting from the opening. Some secretion, clear to milky or purulent, can usually be expressed by pressure. Often the contour of the nose is quite normal. However, there may be external swelling, and if it is located just at the junction of the nose with the forehead, an encephalocele might possibly be present. If the encephalocele is of an

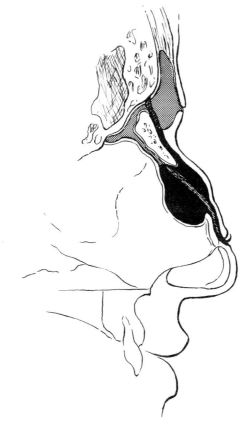

Fig. 1. A composite of the areas found involved in a dermoid cyst of the nose in the 14 cases. No one cyst was found to involve all of this area but the drawing emphasizes the fact that one must be *prepared* for an extensive procedure when removing the cyst. (Redrawn from Crawford and Webster. Plast. Reconstr. Surg., 9: 235, 1952.)

appreciable size (greater than 1 cm), then pulsation may be observed and the bony defect in the skull palpated.

Hemangiomas, both capillary and cavernous, are common in the midforehead and at the root of the nose. They can be present with or without a dermoid cyst or an encephalocele. It is important that one look beyond the swollen or discolored hemangiomatous lesion to be sure nothing else is present.

Sebaceous cysts and lipomas can also be present in this part of the nose and present further diagnostic possibilities.

The treatment of dermoid cysts is complete removal. As indicated in Figure 1, this

can be a very extensive operative procedure. If there is any hint from the physical examination (widened nasal septum, reduced nasal space, repeated deep-seated nasal infections) that the patient has an extensive lesion, then x-ray studies with radiopaque material in the draining sinus can be very helpful in defining its limits before going to the operating room. One is therefore better prepared, as suggested by Crawford and Webster (1952), both to remove the cyst completely and, if a large dead space is thus created, to fill it with autogenous bone or cartilage, preferably the former.

The treatment of encephalocele may come within the purview of the neurosurgeon, but this defect can often be readily repaired in a single step by the plastic surgeon. Again, it is important to go into the operating room as fully prepared as possible. Posteroanterior x-ray films of the skull will show the bony defect if it is of appreciable size. A defect in the skull 1 cm in diameter or larger usually allows a visible pulsation of the mass at the root of the nose—that is, visible *if* one thinks to look for it. Often there is an associated hemangioma of the overlying skin, and the surgeon may see only the blood vessel lesion and miss the fact that he is also dealing with an encephalocele. Hypertelorism is also present with most encephaloceles but again may be missed because one's attention is focused on the swelling.

In the repair of the encephalocele it is worthwhile to design a skin flap with its base upward on the forehead which will reach below the level of the bony defect. The flap is lifted up, and the dura is exposed and freed all about the margin of the bony defect in the skull and also pushed away from the *inside* of the skull for about 1 cm. The dura is then opened. If brain tissue is present in the sac, it is amputated, since it has no function. Enough of the dura is spared to make a good closure that is level with the inside of the skull. For repair of the bony defect it is best to use a section of bony rib (Longacre and de Stefano, 1957; see also Figure 2). The rib section can be removed

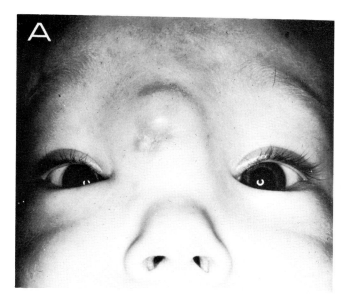

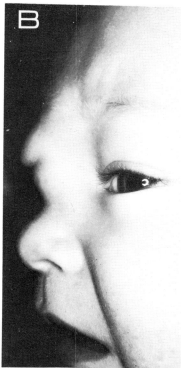

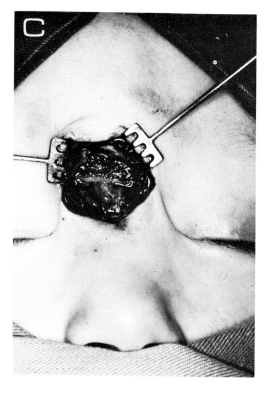

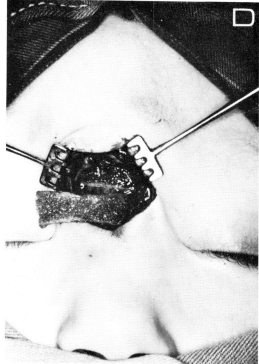

Fig. 2. A and B. Preoperative views of encephalocele. C and D. Operative repair with split rib grafts to close the bony defect, as described in the text.

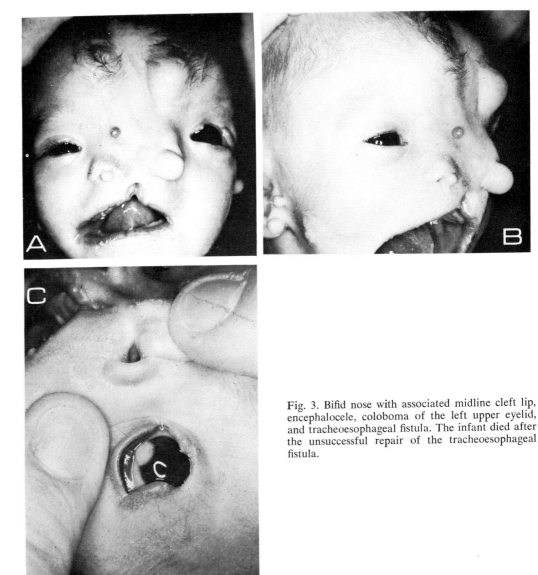

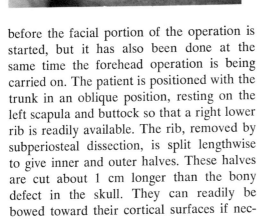

Fig. 3. Bifid nose with associated midline cleft lip, encephalocele, coloboma of the left upper eyelid, and tracheoesophageal fistula. The infant died after the unsuccessful repair of the tracheoesophageal fistula.

before the facial portion of the operation is started, but it has also been done at the same time the forehead operation is being carried on. The patient is positioned with the trunk in an oblique position, resting on the left scapula and buttock so that a right lower rib is readily available. The rib, removed by subperiosteal dissection, is split lengthwise to give inner and outer halves. These halves are cut about 1 cm longer than the bony defect in the skull. They can readily be bowed toward their cortical surfaces if necessary to fit the contour of the defect. They are then slipped into the space between the skull and dura and locked in place by having about 5 mm of rib extend on each side of the defect. Additional bone chips may be laid over them if desired.

The skin is then closed over the bone graft after it is tailored as required to remove the excess that previously covered the bulge of the encephalocele.

A median cleft of the lip with a bifid nose is an extremely uncommon deformity, and

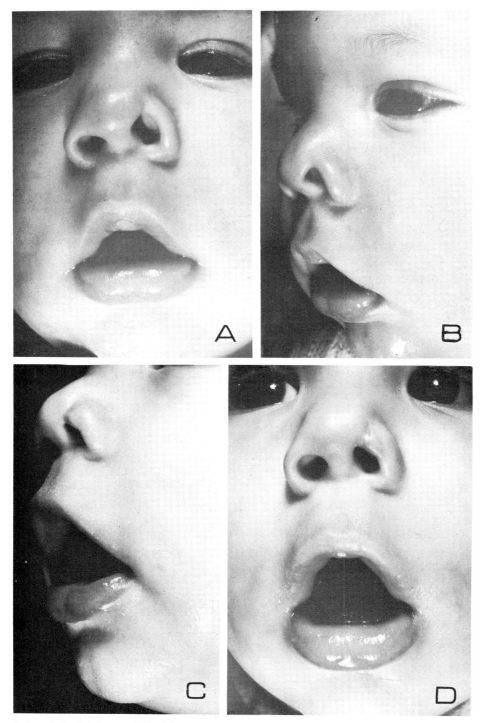

Fig. 4. A and B. Coloboma of the left ala nasi. C and D. Three months after repair with a composite graft from the ear.

its embryological derivation is very difficult to understand. The child shown in Figure 3 at five days of age also suffered from a tracheoesophageal fistula and did not survive repair of the defect. It is to be noted that the infant also had coloboma of the left eye and encephalocele. The left nostril is partially occluded by a large skin polyp.

Nasal deformities associated with cleft lip and palate are discussed in the chapter dealing with cleft lip and palate.

INJURIES

Lacerations of the nose, as of other parts of the body, require anatomical restoration. This means that in dealing with lacerations that pass through to the inside of the nose one should approximate the mucosal lining as accurately as one does the skin on the outside. The rather common practice of simply repairing the external cover often leaves the patient with a severe loss of airway. Often this can be repaired only by reopening the entire wound, and even then scar contracture may have markedly altered the potential for a good result. It is also well in repairing lacerations through the cartilaginous framework to suture the cartilage fragments back together with fine buried dermal or wire suture.

Either congenital or accidental loss of substance of the nose is repaired in children in much the same fashion as in adults. The author has had some success with the use of composite grafts to restore the ala in very small children whose arms can be adequately restrained (Fig. 4). In general, however, this procedure or the construction of tubed pedicle grafts must await adequate maturity on the part of his patient for the surgeon to have his cooperation.

Fractures of the nose, if displaced, should be reduced even in small children. This may occasionally require general anesthesia but most often can be done under local anesthesia with some sedation. If one gently works into the nostrils with a cotton swab soaked in 5 percent cocaine solution or cocaine-epinephrine (half and half), then the shrinking agent will also allow a good look at the lining. After the mucosa is well anesthetized one may insert a small curved clamp into each nostril and lift strongly but briefly to bring the bones and septum back into the midline. This short lift is admittedly painful but often is a better answer than putting to sleep a patient who is not properly prepared for general anesthesia. Such reduction will not prevent the excessive callus formation which gives many people a hump on the upper third of the nasal bridge after an injury. This is inherent in the healing of all bony fractures, since the body always produces more new bone than is essential to repair the break. It is well to warn the parents of this in advance. But straightening the septum and nasal bones at the time of injury can avoid many subsequent problems with the airway.

CLARENCE W. MONROE

REFERENCES

CRAWFORD, J. K., and WEBSTER, J. P. Congenital dermoid cysts of the nose. Plast. Reconstr. Surg., 9: 235, 1952.

LONGACRE, J. J., and DE STEFANO, G. A. Reconstruction of extensive defects of the skull with split rib grafts. Plast. Reconstr. Surg., 19: 186, 1957.

14

Cleft Lip and Palate

EMBRYOLOGY AND ANATOMY

Studies by many investigators have demonstrated that the abnormal pattern of growth which results in a child's being born with a cleft of the lip or palate is fixed in the second month of fetal life. Stark, in his study of six embryos with cleft lip (Stark and Ehrmann, 1958), has further pinpointed this abnormality, showing that clefts of the primary palate—that is, those clefts anterior to the incisive foramen—probably are determined by the fourth to fifth week of fetal life, while clefts of the posterior palate—that is, behind the incisive foramen—probably are not determined until the seventh to twelfth week of fetal life. It appears from the work of Veau (1937–1938) and others that the penetration of mesoderm into the epithelial wall of the lateral lip segments and the premaxilla and prolabium is essential for the development of a normal lip. When mesodermal penetrance is partial or absent the epithelial wall becomes thinned and will rupture (Stark and Ehrmann, 1958), leaving a cleft of the lip or palate or both. The severity of the cleft is measured by the degree to which mesodermal penetrance has been inhibited.

Theories of causation of this arrest in growth come under three general headings: inheritance, disease and drugs, and psychic trauma.

INHERITANCE

Most clinics can readily elicit a history of deformity in 30 to 35 percent of the patients they see. Fraser and his colleagues (1961) state that no simple genetic hypothesis will account for all cases of cleft lip or cleft palate. But they were able to work out a probability curve for the occurrence of subsequent clefts in the same family. When no other individual in the patient's family is affected, there is a 4 percent chance of another child in the family having a cleft lip or palate. If one of the parents has the deformity, there is a 17 percent chance that a second child in the family will also be affected. These percentages are to be compared with an incidence of cleft lip, cleft palate, or both in the general population of 0.1 percent or with an incidence of isolated cleft palate of 0.04 percent.

DISEASE AND DRUGS

The occurrence of congenital deformities eight times more frequently in the offspring of mothers having German measles during the first trimester of pregnancy than in those who are well has made it obvious that disease in the mother can surely have a bearing on the developing fetus. Heart deformities more frequently follow measles than does cleft lip or palate. Thus far no specific disease has been shown to produce more cleft lips and palates than other deformities. The drug thalidomide when taken during the early months of pregnancy produced more abnormalities of extremities than any other type of deformity.

PSYCHIC TRAUMA

Most physicians discount the effect of emotional disturbances on the developing fetus because so many normal children are born of disturbed mothers. Peer and his colleagues (1958) have shown that mice can be made to produce cleft palates in 87 percent of their offspring if the mothers are given cortisone. Efforts at producing the same effect by physical and emotional trauma, which would supposedly increase the normal secretion of cortisone in these animals, was ineffective. However, it is most interesting to note that the clefts caused by cortisone injections could be prevented if the pregnant animal was given folic acid and vitamin B_6 (5 mg folic acid and 10 mg pyridoxine hydrochloride daily). Peer and his colleagues have recommended the prophylactic use of these two substances along with stress formula vitamins from the very earliest sign of pregnancy in mothers who have had children with cleft palates, in the hope of averting deformities. Fraser and Warburton (1964) dispute these recommendations and feel that no proof can be adduced to show a beneficial effect of a nutritional supplement—or even evidence that maternal stress is related to the occurrence of cleft deformities.

CLASSIFICATION

The ordered study of the deformities of cleft lip and palate has been markedly improved by Stark's recent work on the embryology of this disorder. It now seems quite clear that dividing clefts in relationship to the incisive foramen in the palate makes much more sense than any previous classification. On this basis the formation of the

early "primary palate," which includes all tissues anterior to the incisive foramen, permits us to classify clefts in this region as unilateral, bilateral, or median (rare).

The palate posterior to the incisive foramen develops at a somewhat later time in fetal life, and here again a cleft can be classified as unilateral or bilateral, depending upon whether the septum remains united to one horizontal plate of the palate. Midline clefts can, of course, occur along the entire area and often are more apparent when the posterior portion of the septum is exceedingly short or almost nonexistent.

DEALING WITH THE PARENTS AND THE PATIENT

The birth of a baby with a cleft lip is a particularly disturbing experience for any new parents. If the deformity happens to be a severe one, as in a bilateral cleft of the lip and palate with a protruding premaxilla, the parents may undergo a greater psychic shock than they would if the child was found to have a heart deformity. One of the first obligations of the surgeon who proposes to repair such a deformity is to discuss in detail with the parents what they may expect in the way of results from the operative procedure and what will happen to the child over the next several years. The techniques for cleft repair presently available are sufficiently advanced that a large proportion of children can be made to appear essentially normal. If the parents can appreciate this by seeing photographs of other children with similar deformities suitably repaired, they will be greatly assured. Most parents appreciate knowing just how soon the lip is to be repaired and, if the palate is also cleft, at what time that should be repaired. Parents also wish to know how much speech is going to be affected. This question cannot be answered categorically in the newborn, but the surgeon should observe the relative length of the soft palate and should determine whether or not there is good muscular activity in it upon gagging or crying. The long palate with good muscular activity which could conceivably reach the posterior pharyngeal wall has the potentiality for producing good speech. If the parents are told this shortly after the birth of the child it contributes much to their emotional stability.

The recent use of a team of experts to manage the problems of a child with a cleft lip or cleft palate has pointed up the value of having at least one person on this team assume continuing responsibility for the patient. He may not choose to do all the work that needs to be done on the patient, but he should have an adequate knowledge of what is to be done over a period of years and be able to function as the go-between for everything that the child should require in the way of rehabilitative services. The decisions which will be made by the surgeon probably have more far-reaching effects on the growth and development of the patient than those made by the pediatrician, dentist, orthodontist, social worker, or anyone else. Therefore, I think that the surgeon should be willing to assume a continuing responsibility for this patient. If he will volunteer to assume this responsibility at the parents' first visit, they will be much more confident and will not feel that they are left alone in an unfriendly and uncertain world.

Finally, it is important that the parents be assured, as far as possible, about the occurrence of deformities in subsequent children born to them. The data, quoted above, from Fraser's work on the frequency of subsequent deformities in the same family, plus Peer's work on the prophylaxis, as yet unproved, using folic acid and pyridoxine, should be communicated to the parents. It must be stressed, however, that the mother must begin taking folic acid and pyridoxine at the very earliest sign of pregnancy if they are to be of any conceivable benefit because the fourth to twelfth weeks of fetal life constitute the period in which this deformity becomes fixed in the individual.

TREATMENT

CLEFT LIP

AGE OF REPAIR

The age at which repair of the cleft lip is carried out varies quite markedly with the individual surgeon's preference. Some surgeons prefer to undertake the repair within the first few days of life. Others wait as long as three, four, or even six months before carrying it out. There is certainly some merit in having a child's deformity repaired before he leaves the hospital following birth, so that other children in the family will not be subjected to the trauma of seeing a sibling with a severe deformity. However, it is encumbent upon the surgeon who makes a decision for early repair to be quite certain that the child does not have other congenital anomalies which may be even more serious or even threatening to the life of the patient. This decision cannot always be made within 24 to 48 hours after birth.

On the other hand, the change in the size of the lip between birth and three or four months of age is relatively small, and there seems relatively little merit in the prolonged wait in order to have larger tissues with which to work.

The author's own preference is to repair the lip shortly after the child has regained his birth weight and preferably by the use of local anesthesia. Local anesthesia for lip repair is much more readily carried out if the patient weighs between 7 and 10 pounds. If one waits until the child weighs 11 or 12 pounds, lip repair with local anesthesia is rather difficult and may be hazardous to the patient, since the dosage of medication required to obtain a quiet patient gets nearer the dosage that produces sedation for a period of 24 to 48 hours.

All plastic surgical procedures should be done with gentleness, but the surgeon who has always worked under general anesthesia may not realize how gentle he *can* be until he has schooled himself in the niceties of a lip repair under local anesthesia. Here one finds that marked traction on a lip with either fingers or hooks is not always necessary to the competent repair of the deformity. The reduced morbidity seen in patients repaired under local anesthesia, even when very competent pediatric general anesthesia is available, is rather surprising to the surgeon who has just started using local anesthesia.

ANESTHESIA

The preparation of the patient for this type of surgery under local anesthesia must be meticulous, and if it is not carried out properly, it may prove quite unsatisfactory for the repair. The author's technique is based on the description given by Straith and his colleagues (1955) but modified in important respects; for example, premedication by rectal suppository is not done because it is an extremely undependable method of medication. The modified routine is as follows: One hour before the projected surgery the child is given a full feeding. It is important that the child not be fed for at least four hours before this feeding so that he will be hungry and will take the entire feeding. It should be possible to complete this feeding within 15 minutes. Forty-five minutes before the planned surgery the patient is given Nembutal Sodium by intramuscular injection in the following dosage:

Weight in pounds:	7	7.5	8	8.5	9	9.5	10
Milligrams of Nembutal Sodium:	45	50	55	60	65	70	75

The patient is sent to the operating room about 20 minutes before projected surgery. Here all clothing is removed except the diaper. The wrists are wrapped with a plain gauze roller bandage and a 1-inch strip of adhesive tape placed around one wrist, across the back, fastened to the other wrist and then back again to the first wrist (Fig. 1). This holds the arms at the sides loosely enough for the patient to lie flat without lying on his arms but tightly enough to prevent the arms from being able to move far from the sides. A small doughnut is fastened to the back of the head with a strip of adhesive tape that goes completely around the head and is fastened not only to the occipital scalp but also across the forehead. This doughnut should be placed in such a position that with a small roll under the shoulders the head is tipped back slightly in extension, both to increase the visibility of the lip and nose and to improve the patient's airway. The patient is then laid on the operating table with a 2-inch wide strip of adhesive tape going across the thighs and fastened to the side of the table. This permits the table to be turned down in the Trendelenburg position if the surgeon so wishes.

After this much handling of the patient one can see whether or not he is constantly sleepy. If he is, no further medication is given. If the patient responds to this much handling by moderate or severe crying, then an additional bit of sedation with Demerol is given. This also is regulated according to experience, the dose being from 2 to 6 or 8 mg intramuscularly. The Demerol is prepared by drawing 10 mg of the commercially prepared solution into a 1-ml tuberculin syringe. This is diluted to a full ml with sterile water. Each 0.1 ml in the syringe then represents 1 mg of Demerol.

The decision about how much, if any, Demerol is to be given the patient is made by 10 minutes before the operation is to be begun. This amount is administered to the patient, and he is then promptly covered with a warm blanket and left entirely alone for a period of 10 minutes while the surgeon scrubs his hands.

It will then be found that the patient can be handled gently without undue response, and the washing of the face and draping can be carried out and the operation begun.

It is my practice to mark the important points of lip anatomy with methylene blue

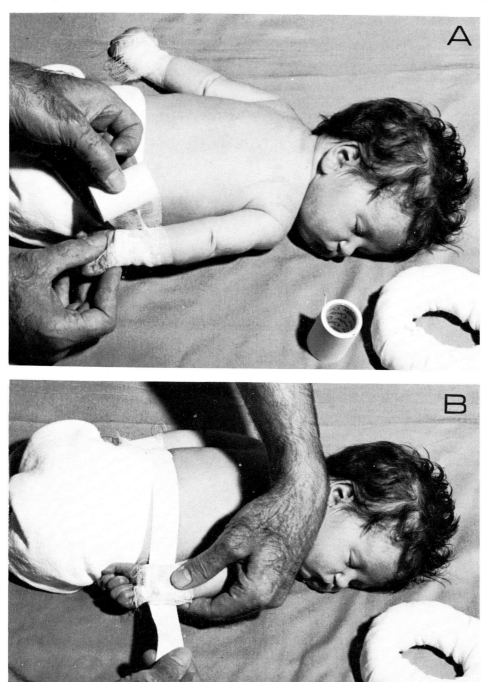

Fig. 1. A and B. A Method of restraining an infant for the repair of a cleft lip under local anesthesia. See text for details.

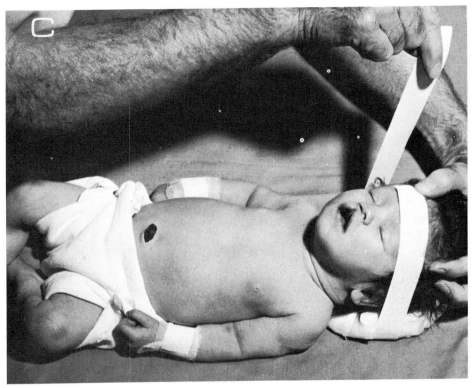

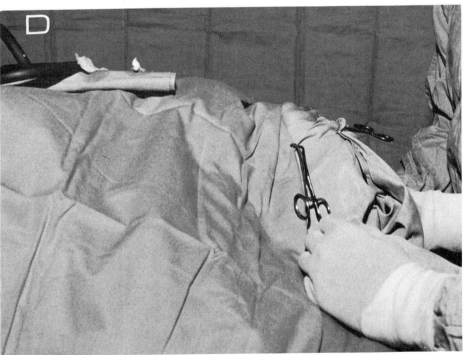

Fig. 1 (cont.). C and D. A method of restraining an infant for the repair of the cleft lip under local anesthesia. See text for details.

before local anesthesia is introduced into the lip. The preferred anesthetic agent is 1 percent lidocaine or procaine with epinephrine, 1:100,000. Not more than 4 ml is required for complete anesthesia of the lip and nose in the ordinary infant when the agent is properly used. The epinephrine effect is also adequate to prevent any appreciable blood loss. Most of these patients are operated on without more than 10 to 20 ml of blood loss.

When the patient is older and larger and it is felt that the procedure cannot be carried out under local anesthesia, it is still the author's practice to use a small amount of local anesthesia containing epinephrine to reduce blood loss even though the repair is done under general anesthesia.

OBJECTIVES OF REPAIR

The objective of the surgical repair of a cleft lip is the production of a normal looking unscarred lip and nose. This objective is at times difficult to achive. The following factors are important in attaining it: A straight contact border of the lip, a well-matched vermilion border, a scar through the upper lip that falls into the normal markings of the lip and can be mistaken for them, a columella that is straight and in the midline, a nostril floor that has the same level as the normal side and a nostril opening that appears symmetrical with its mate from each direction that it may be viewed, and, finally, a nasal tip that is as symmetrical as it is possible to make it at this age.

Most unilateral cleft lips are demonstrably shorter on the cleft side than on the normal side. The correction of this shortening is the basis for the multitudinous techniques which have been described for the repair of a cleft lip. When the shortening is relatively mild and the lip segments are of appropriate fullness, as occasionally occurs, then the straight line or slightly elliptical excision of the cleft itself and immediate suture can often produce a lip with an excellent appearance. However, lips with moderate to severe shortening will not respond adequately to

this technique and therefore require something in addition. The most efficacious means of increasing the length on the cleft side is the use of a Z-plasty in the course of the lip repair. The many types of repair described can be readily divided into those that put the Z-plasty at the nostril border in the upper third of the lip, those that put it at the lower margin of the lip just above the vermilion border, and those that put a Z-plasty only in the contact border of the lip or in conjunction with a Z-plasty above.

TECHNIQUES OF LIP REPAIR

In the execution of any one of the three types of lip repair mentioned above, it is imperative that the normal markings of the lip be properly identified and utilized in the repair. These minimum markings must be made: Point 1, the midpoint of the floor of the nostril on the normal side. This point should be chosen so that it will be possible to find a corresponding point on both the alar and columellar tissues on the cleft side. Point 2, the height of the cupid's bow on the vermilion border on the normal side. Point 3, the depth of the valley of the philtrum (the lowest point to which the philtrum extends) along the vermilion border. Point 4, the height of the cupid's bow on the cleft side of the medial lip segment. This point will be the same distance from point 3 as point 2 is from point 3. Point 5, the height of the cupid's bow on the lateral lip segment. This will be the point at which the fullness of the vermilion border begins to thin out. Points 6 and 7, the symmetrical points on the cleft side to match point 1 on the normal side. Any repair that matches these landmarks in a symmetrical fashion is likely to be a good repair.

In the occasional patient whose lip will respond to closure in a straight line (Fig. 2), the height of the cupid's bow on the cleft side becomes the point of union with the lateral lip segment, and in this instance one of the more important features of the operation is that one actually cuts out the portion of the

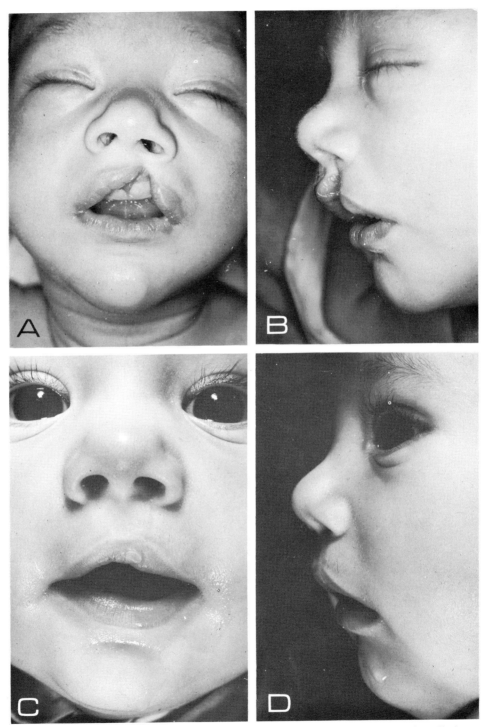

Fig. 2. Illustrating the merit of a straight line closure when the lip deformity is minimal. A Z-plasty was used only across the vermilion. A rotation advancement technique would have narrowed the left nostril. The use of a quadrilateral flap in the lower third would have made the cleft side too long. A and B show the patient preoperatively. C and D show him four months after repair.

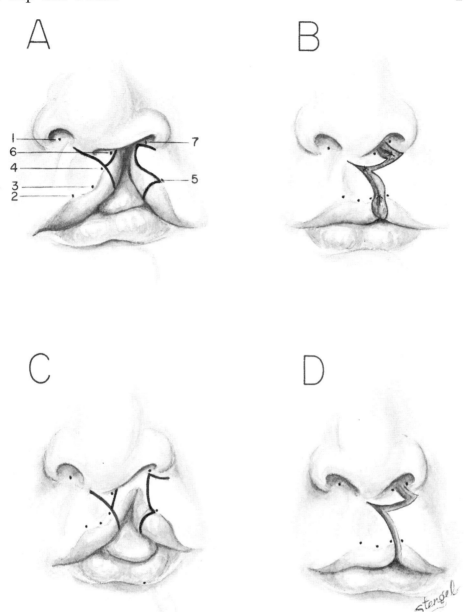

Fig. 3. Redrawn from Millard's rotation advancement technique. In A are marked the anatomical points that must always be identified in any lip repair. A and B show the minimal amount of tissue that is discarded when the cleft is wide and there is a scarcity of material for repair. The great merit of this procedure is that one may extend the incision across the columella if the cleft side is not long enough or close it if it has been made too long. With a partial cleft and abundance of tissue, much more must be sacrificed to make an attractive repair, as shown in C and D. The author believes that practically every lip requires a Z-plasty across the vermilion border. This is not shown in these drawings.

skin in the cleft under which there is no muscle. If the muscle bellies of the lateral and medial lip segments are not properly approximated, an adequate repair will not be made. It should also be noted that in the straight line closure of the lip, the puckering which fairly often accompanies any scar formation is likely to pull the contact border

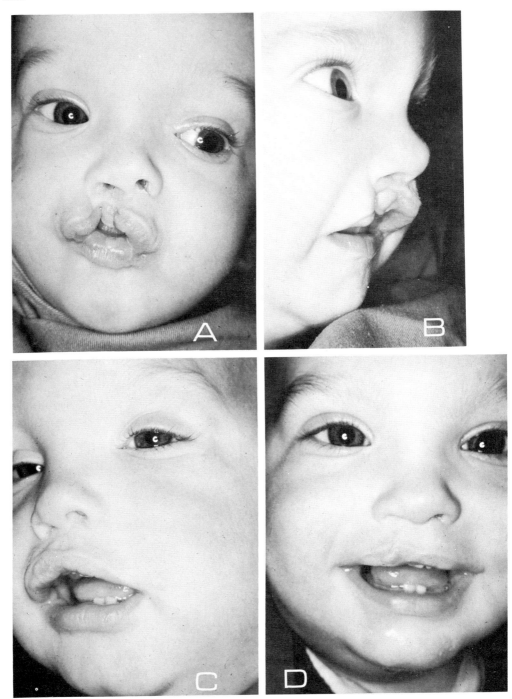

Fig. 4. Millard's technique used in a cleft that is fairly wide but with abundant tissue. The nostril is properly narrowed and the cupid's bow preserved. A and B are preoperative views; C and D show the patient one year after repair.

of the lip into a notch unless a Z-plasty is done across the vermilion border.

When it is obvious that there is appreciable shortening on the cleft side and the defect is not unduly large, then Millard's rotation advancement technique certainly gives most excellent results. In Figure 3A the cardinal points of lip anatomy are marked out as

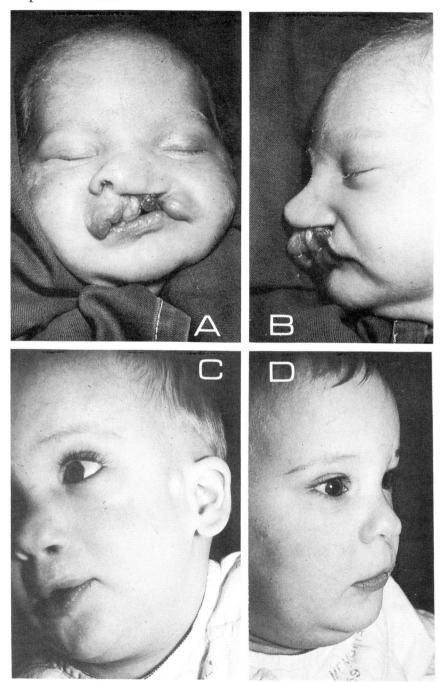

Fig. 5. A and B show an exceedingly wide cleft of the lip (the alveolar ridge was separated by 12 mm) that was closed with a small triangular flap from the cleft side in the lower third of the lip. C and D show the patient one year after repair, when the alveolar ridge had overclosed by 3 mm.

described above. Millard (1964), describing this procedure, refers to it as "cut-as-you-go." In this respect it is different from almost any other lip repair. In the wider cleft one must go up inside the ala to borrow all the skin possible to carry over to the normal side. But once this is done one may divide further and further across the base of the columella until the medial lip segment rotates down far enough for a symmetrical repair to be made

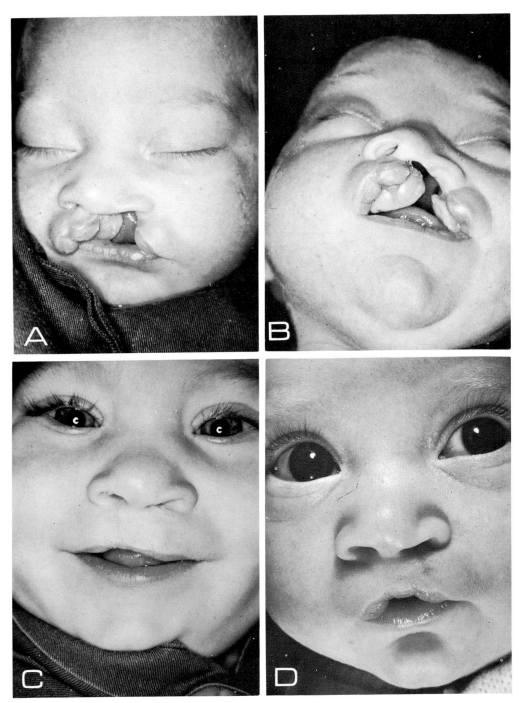

Fig. 6. A and B show a wide cleft of the lip in a month-old child. C shows the patient one month after repair with a small rectangular flap. It is now more apparent that there is a mild partial cleft on the right side. D shows the patient six months after repair.

(Fig. 4). It can be seen in Figure 3C that the partial cleft lip requires a much greater sacrifice of tissue for a good repair to be achieved than must be made in the complete cleft. Millard states that he uses this technique even for very wide clefts. In this author's experience this is not always possible. A Z-plasty in the upper third of the lip repair requires more loose lip than does one done in the lower third of the lip.

Brown's small triangular flap in the lower third of the lip is one answer to this problem (Fig. 5), but it often fails to make the most of whatever cupid's bow the patient has.

The popularity of Le Mesurier's quadrilateral flap lip repair was based, in part at least, on its ability to put a full pleasing border across the lower third of the lip (Fig. 6). However, it frequently distorted the cupid's bow, and it quite often produced too long a lip on the repaired side by the time the child was five or six years old.

The answer to this problem of overgrowth on the repaired side has been suggested by Brauer and Cronin (1966) in their modification of the Tennison lip repair. They have devised a meticulously measured lip repair which is intentionally made 1 mm shorter on the repaired side than on the normal side to allow for growth. The insertion of the triangular flap from the lateral lip segment is offset above the vermilion border by 1 mm so that it may not be mistaken for the vermilion, as sometimes occurred after the original Tennison repair. The method seems so worthwhile that it is reproduced here in detail.

In Figure 7A we see again the seven cardinal points of lip anatomy as shown in Figure 3. The extra points used by Cronin and Brauer in opening the lip are designated by *A, B, C* and *A', B', C'*. To close 4 to 5 and obtain a predictable distance from 4 to 6 equal to 1 mm less than the distance from 1 to 2 requires attention to the following details: The columellar side is marked first. *B* is placed at right angles to the vermilion border and 1 mm away from it. *A* is placed on the vermilion border in such a position that the straight line *ABC* will make the angle *CA*6 slightly more than 90°—perhaps 100° or 105°. Only thus will the vermilion on the medial lip segment rotate down adequately. The line *AC* has been found by experience to be 3.5 to 4 mm long in most cases.

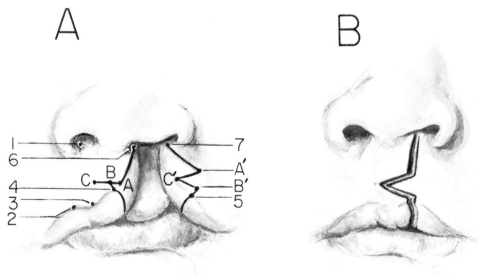

Fig. 7. A and B show Cronin and Brauer's modification of the Tennison lip repair. Redrawn from Croin and Brauer (personal communication but soon to be published in the Cleft Palate Journal).

On the lateral lip segment, B' is again at right angles to the vermilion border and 1 mm away from it. Line $7A'$ must equal line $6A$. Supposing the length 1–2 to be 11 mm, then the cleft side should be repaired 10 mm in length. Further supposing that $6A$ is 5 mm long and $4B$ is 1 mm long, then the base $A'B'$ of the triangular flap $A'C'B'$ will have to be 4 mm to make a total height of 10 mm.

To locate A', one caliper is set for the distance $6A$ (5 mm in the instance above) and one point of the caliper placed at 7. A second caliper is set at the required distance for the base of the flap (4 mm in the instance above) and one point placed at B. The point at which these two calipers intersect will be A'. C' will then be adjusted to make $A'C'$ equal AC and to make $B'C'$ equal BC.

In incising these lip segments accurately it is well to heed the authors' suggestion that the upper buccal incisions be made first. Then the freed lip is placed on a tongue blade for the definitive, accurate incisions.

MAXILLARY ORTHOPEDICS

The use of maxillary orthopedics in recent years has added a new dimension to the care of children with complete clefts of the lip and palate (Brauer et al., 1962; Des Prez et al., 1964; Georgiade, 1964). Some surgeons have used these techniques to secure approximation of the bony segments of the maxilla before repair of the lip. Experience at The Children's Memorial Hospital has shown that this is very seldom required. The more urgent need is that the bony segments not be closed so rapidly that they overclose. In fact, we have been most pleased with the construction of a retainer to fit into the cleft in the hard palate that allows the bones to come more slowly into position and truly shapes the alveolar ridge into a normal upper dental arch. The retainer has been kept in place for as long as six months and occasionally to the time of palate repair.

The technique requires the taking of an impression of the upper jaw and cleft of

the palate (Rosenstein, 1963). This is then made up into an acrylic retainer. It is placed in the mouth at the close of the cleft lip repair. Since it tends to hold the alveolar ridge on the cleft side out, it then permits the premaxilla to rotate back into good alignment.

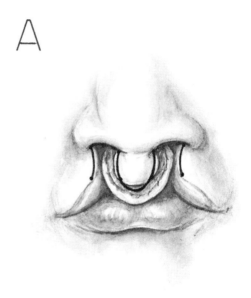

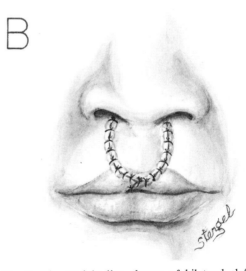

Fig. 8. The straight line closure of bilateral cleft lip. It is most important that a generous flap of mucosa from the medial aspect of the lateral lip segment be turned down with its base on the vermilion border to interdigitate across the lower edge of the prolabial skin, in order to give fullness to the medial third of the lip.

In the small number of patients in whom we have used it, the results have been much more pleasing than in those whose alveolar ridges collapsed.

BILATERAL LIP REPAIR

The literature on the repair of bilateral cleft lip is replete with many different techniques for achieving a full, pleasing lip. Unhappily many of these techniques do not make adequate allowance for the growth factor in the prolabium. When prolabial skin is placed under tension, as it is during integration into the middle third of the upper lip, its growth potential is enormous. Therefore, in the light of experience, it seems that there can be little argument about what should be done in *any* bilateral cleft lip repair: The simplest straight line closure one can achieve is by all odds the preferred method of treatment (Fig. 8). This permits the prolabium to undergo the kind of growth for which it is famous and then permits, from straight line scars, whatever revision may be required by the time the patient is four or five years of age (Fig. 9).

Many but not all bilateral cleft lips have severely shortened columellas. If the tissue of the prolabial skin is unscarred, it provides an excellent source of tissue to lengthen the columella as the child becomes older and the snubbed-down nasal tip presents a real problem in appearance. Of great benefit in the straight line closure of the bilateral lip repair is the turning down of very generous mucosal flaps from the lateral lip segments to interdigitate across the contact border of the middle third of the lip just below the normal mucocutaneous line of the prolabial skin. If these flaps are not made sufficiently large there will, of course, be quite a severe whistle deformity of the middle third of the upper lip. In the patient who has an extremely small prolabium, even with generous mucosal flaps from the lateral lip segments, the middle third of the upper lip will still appear exceedingly small at the primary repair. However, if the surgeon considers

the growth potential in this area he will realize that by the time the child is four or five years of age this middle third of the upper lip will be quite as large as the rest of the lip and that it has within it potential for much greater help for the appearance of the nose.

THE PROTRUDING MAXILLA

In the patient who has had a bilateral cleft of the lip and palate with the premaxilla protruding far ahead of the lateral alveolar segments, additional surgery may be required to achieve a proper repair. While it is true that many of these premaxillas will come back into good relationship with the lateral alveolar ridges following repair of the lip, it is also true that the pressure of the lip repair often closes the lateral alveolar segments against the septum, thus locking the premaxilla out of the upper dental arch.

When a patient is encountered whose lateral lip segments are not loose enough to permit reasonably tension-free repair of the lip, it is the author's preference to recess the premaxilla surgically. Probably not more than half the patients seen with protruding premaxillas have this structure far enough forward to require surgical recession to achieve a competent lip repair. In those whose lip segments can be approximated well, the use of the molded prosthesis described above to prevent closure of the lateral alveolar ridges behind the premaxilla is certainly desirable. The author reported an anatomical study (Monroe, 1959) of fetal heads of infants who died shortly after birth and who had cleft lips and palates and other abnormalities that caused death. These heads were compared with those of normal infants who were stillborn for maternal reasons. It has been determined in both deformed and normal infants that the epiphyseal line between the premaxilla and the septum and vomer occurs immediately behind the bulge of the premaxilla. Therefore, the surgical approach to the vomer and septum made 1 cm or 1.5 cm behind the area of the epiphyseal line does not interfere with the

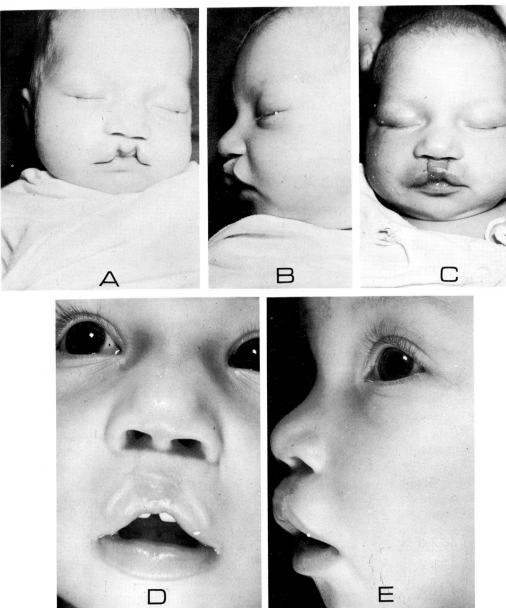

Fig. 9. The procedure described in Figure 8 was used here. This patient and many others show that only prolabial skin should be used for the full height of the upper lip, even when the prolabium seems very short. A and B are preoperative views, C shows the patient one week after repair of the lip under local anesthesia, and D and E show her one year after repair. She appears equally attractive at seven years of age.

growth of the middle third of the upper jaw and does permit the repositioning of the premaxilla to a point where the lip segments can be united in front of it without undue tension.

An eight-year followup on patients who have had this procedure done (Monroe, 1965) has failed to show any significant loss of bone growth in the middle third of the upper jaw. It will be necessary to follow these patients to at least their middle teens before this can be said without any question, but certainly the present data on this group of patients favor the use of this procedure, where it is indicated, to accomplish an adequate repair.

It is the author's preference to recess the premaxilla surgically and to repair the bilateral cleft lip in a single operative procedure. This can be done under general anesthesia from three weeks of age onward. The technique is as follows.

Under endotracheal anesthesia and using 1 percent lidocaine with epinephrine injected into the mucosa of the septum and vomer for hemostasis, a straight incision is made over the lower margin of the septum about midway in its anteroposterior length. The mucoperiosteum and mucoperichondrium (Fig. 10) are elevated from the bone and

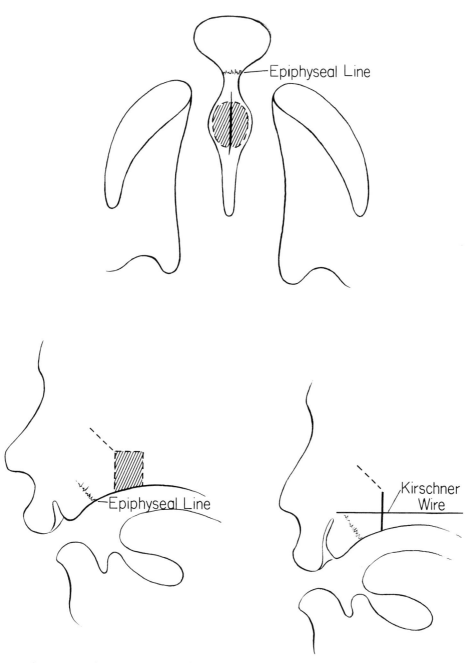

Fig. 10. Technique for accomplishing recession of the premaxilla. See text for details.

cartilage straight up into the upper portion of the nose. The septum is freed over a slightly greater anteroposterior length of septum than it is proposed to sacrifice. When the premaxilla is brought back into the mouth, its lateral and posterior margins will then make good contact with the lateral alveolar ridges.

With a very sharp osteotome the anterior of the two cuts in the septum is first made up to the upper border of the nasal septum. As the posterior cut is made, if the vomer seems unstable, the segment of bone is removed with a rongeur rather than risk a fracture of the vomer from the base of the skull. It is usually necessary to insert a curved scissors into the wound and cut the septum to the

root of the nose so that the entire premaxilla is free to be pushed straight back into the face. It must not swing like a gate on its superior attachment, or the incisor teeth which erupt in it will point backward into the mouth rather than downward.

The premaxilla is fixed to this new position by a Kirschner wire drilled through from just under the prolabium back into the posterior stable portion of the vomer. It has not been found necessary to remove this wire. The wound in the septum is closed with 5-0 chromic catgut and the operative field then carried to the lip (Fig. 11).

A nonoperative repair of the protruding premaxilla is advocated by Brauer and his colleagues (Brauer, 1965).

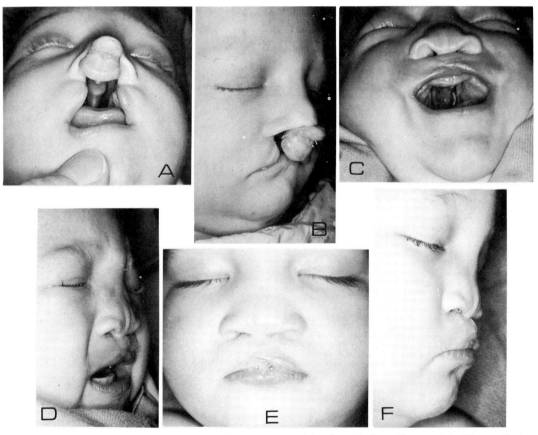

Fig. 11. A and B. The protruding premaxilla was recessed by the technique illustrated in Figure 10 at three months of age and the lip repaired in the same procedure. C and D show the repair two months after surgery. E and F show the repair one year after surgery.

CLEFT PALATE

OBJECTIVES OF REPAIR

The objectives of any repair of the cleft palate is to secure a palate that is long, mobile, and unscarred and that has sufficient motion to be able to reach the posterior pharyngeal wall. By achieving these objectives one hopes to have the patient able to suck and to blow and to speak without nasality. Obviously the anatomical and physiological functions of the palate are not the only factors in the development of adequate speech. The patient who does not have adequate control of the tongue or lips or who is mentally retarded cannot achieve adequate speech no matter how adequate the palate may be. But it is extremely helpful to observe preoperatively how much motion is present in the halves of the soft palate when the patient cries or attempts to phonate. This observation should be made a part of the patient's record. The patient who has very little motion of the soft palate preoperatively is unlikely to have good speech after the repair.

AGE OF REPAIR

The age at which the cleft palate is repaired should be determined largely on the basis of the particular case being considered. An occasional patient is seen who has a cleft of the soft palate only in which the halves of the palate lie almost adjacent to each other. In this instance one need only to trim off the mucosa on the opposing surfaces of the soft palate and unite the nasal mucosa, muscle, and oral mucosa. Such a repair can be carried out even at six months of age without any hazard to the patient and probably with some gain for the patient in that there will be early use of the repaired palate.

In contrast, the patient who has a wide cleft of the palate with relatively narrow horizontal plates of the palate and relatively little tissue out of which a repair may be accomplished should be allowed to grow and develop to the point where the surgeon feels that he can accomplish a repair without undue tension and can secure primary healing. Primary healing of the cleft palate at the first operation is of crucial importance. Anyone who has had to reoperate on a palate which has reopened following the primary repair is well aware of the tremendous scarring which follows even a single operative procedure. If a series of operative procedures has to be done on the palate, it is quite certain to be left as a firm scarred mass which cannot be of any real use in the production of normal speech.

Although it must be observed that the first palatal repair should be the only palatal repair, it is also true that the earlier one can achieve a repair, the more likely the patient is to be able to use his palate.

TECHNIQUES OF REPAIR

Two basic techniques for palate repair have been in use for many years. One is that described by Langenbeck, in which the mucoperiosteum of the hard palate, together with the muscle, fascia, and mucosa of the soft palate, is widely mobilized and brought to the midline for suture. The second technique consists in mobilizing the soft palate, as is done in the Langenbeck procedure, but leaving the mucoperiosteum attached to the horizontal plate of the palate and chiseling this loose from the remainder of the palate to be moved to the midline as a so-called bone flap technique. The majority of surgeons in the United States prefer the Langenbeck technique or a modification of it. I have had no experience with the bone flap technique and will therefore not discuss it.

To conserve time and to minimize blood loss in the repair of the cleft palate it is wise to have a fixed routine of repair of the palate. Thus the surgeon is always aware of what his next step will be, and little or no time is lost in going from one step to the next. My sequence in a Langenbeck-Wardell repair is as follows:

(1) The entire palate area to be operated

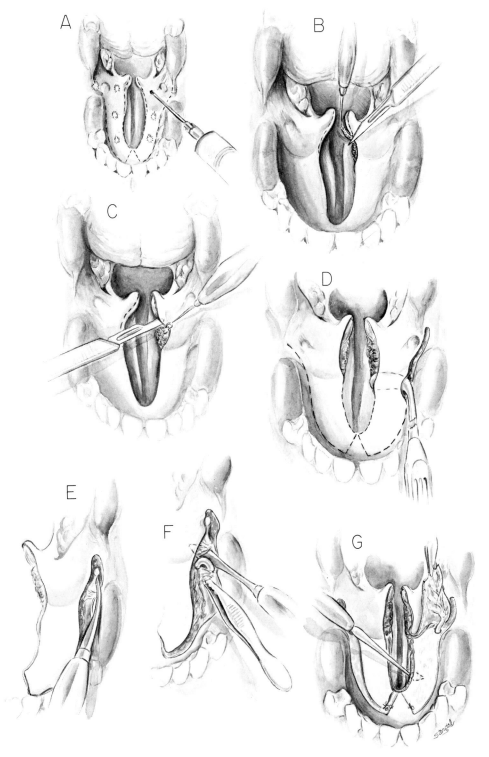

Fig. 12. The modified Langenbeck-Wardell repair of a cleft palate.

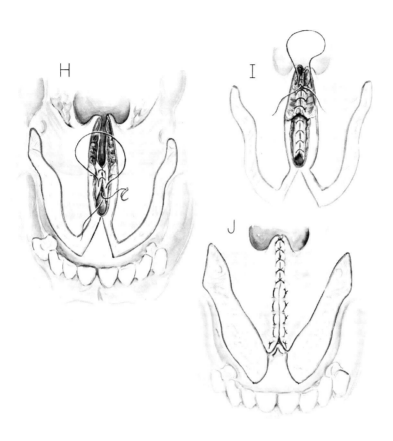

Fig. 12 (cont.). The modified Langenbeck-Wardell repair of a cleft palate. See text for details.

on is infiltrated (Fig. 12A) with 1 percent lidocaine with epinephrine, 1:100,000. A total of not more than 2 or 3 ml is used for this purpose. The operative procedure is not started until the palate has definitely blanched from the use of the vasoconstrictor.

(2) With a one-pronged hook and a # 11 blade the mucosa bordering the medial margin of the cleft in the soft palate area is trimmed away (Fig. 12B). This does sacrifice some mucosa, although the strip should be a very thin one. However, it also completely ensures that no mucosa has been left along the medial margin of the palate, which

could leave the patient with a perforation of the palate. The nasal and oral mucosa are separated from the muscle of the soft palate (Fig. 12C).

(3) With a # 15 blade the incision to mobilize the mucoperiosteal flap is started at the ramus of the mandible and carried up to the posterior tuberosity of the maxilla, around the necks of the teeth, and anteriorly along the palate in the small groove which is always readily apparent between the alveolar mucosa and palatal mucosa.

(4) A curved Blair elevator, right and left for the respective sides of the hard palate

(Fig. 12D), is inserted through this incision in the mucoperiosteum, and the elevation of the palatal mucosa from the bone of the horizontal plate is started. When it is free almost to the midline, the elevator is changed to a Langenbeck and carried through to the raw surface previously opened by excision of the mucosa along the medial margin of the soft palate. At this level the mucosa of the hard palate and that on the nasal side of the hard palate are separated anteriorly for the full length of the cleft (Fig. 12G). When the septum is attached to half of the hard palate, an incision is made at the junction of nasal and oral mucosa. The septal mucosa is mobilized and brought over to the mucosa from the nasal side of the hard palate on the opposite side. This always leaves an area in closure at the junction of the hard and soft palate where it is rarely possible to approximate completely nasal mucosa along the full length of the palate repair. Millard (1962) has described a most ingenious and useful technique for lengthening the palate and reinforcing the repair at the junction of the hard and soft palates by creating an island flap of mucoperiosteum of the anterior hard palate based on the neurovascular bundle which comes through the posterior palatine foramen and courses anteriorly along the undersurface of the palatal flap. This flap of mucosa is turned over to face the nasal space and its pedicle rotated 90° to provide a good blood supply. Edgerton states that children on whom he has done this procedure have referred touching of this nasal flap to the anterior hard palate.

(5) The Langenbeck elevator is then inserted into the wound between the mandible and maxilla. The entire substance of the soft palate is mobilized in a single mass and brought to the midline. In accomplishing this it is necessary to fracture the hamular process medially (Fig. 12E). The mucoperiosteum is dissected off the posterior margin of the hard palate and around the foramen of the posterior palatine artery. When all of the attachments are free here, it is usually possible to pull the vessel out of the foramen (Fig. 12F) by 8 to 10 mm on the side that will not be used for an island flap. This, in the author's experience, permits as much retropositioning of the palate as is accomplished by the Linberg osteotomy (chiseling out the posterior margin of the foramen to permit posterior displacement of the vessels).

(6) The suturing of the repair is then begun, first in the hard palate area, starting at the posterior margin of the hard palate and carried anteriorly (Fig. 12H). The island flap (where it is required) is then sutured to the posterior margin of the nasal mucosa immediately behind the hard palate and the anterior edge of the freed soft palate. Then the nasal mucosa of the soft palate is approximated, with the knots being tied on the nasal side. The muscle of soft palate is brought together with the same type of suture (Fig. 12I), and finally the oral mucosa is closed (Fig. 12J). My preference for suture material in this repair is 5-0 chromic catgut on a small curved cutting needle which is readily bent to take an even smaller curve and thus can be utilized in the narrow space that is commonly available. When Millard's island flap is used it is necessary to make two small drill holes through the posterior edge of the hard palate so that the anterior tip of the mucoperiosteal flap may be securely fastened to the roof of the mouth.

PHARYNGEAL FLAP

The excellent study by Lindsay and others (1962) indicates that even in very competent hands cleft palate repair fails to allow adequate speech in about 20 to 30 percent of patients. Some of the important factors in inadequate speech are shortening, scarring, and immobility of the soft palate or pharyngeal wall. When one or more of these factors is present and precludes the development of an adequate nasopharyngeal valving mechanism, then something else must be done to assist the patient. Many different procedures have been devised to correct this inability of the soft palate and posterior pharyngeal wall to appose each other. However, the one which is most effective in this author's hands and which seems to be most generally accepted in cleft palate clinics is that of the pharyngeal flap. The pharyngeal flap was first described nearly 100 years ago by Trendelenburg. In the intervening years many surgeons used it briefly but gave it up as being ineffective. To Moran (1951) and Conway (1951) belong the credit for popularizing the procedure in the early 1950's.

The function of the pharyngeal flap is to narrow the nasopharynx both by removing

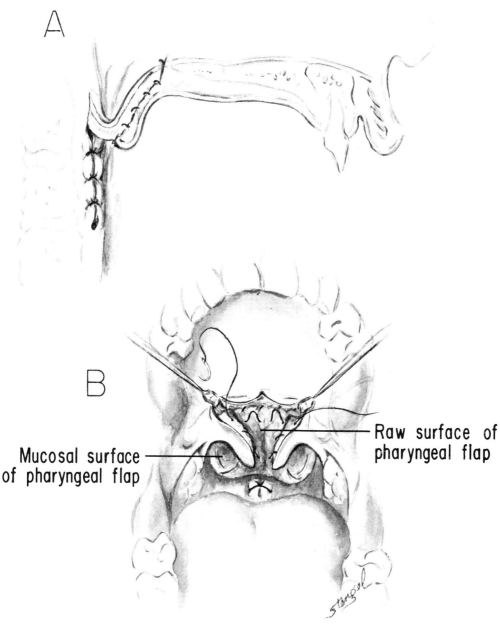

A

B

Mucosal surface
of pharyngeal flap

Raw surface of
pharyngeal flap

Fig. 13. The construction of superiorly based pharyngeal flaps (A and B).

some of its lining and by placing a bridge across this space, which impedes the flow of air through it. It is then hoped that the patient will be able to close the too small nasopharyngeal spaces on either side of the mucosal bridge where he could not previously close the original large open space.

A pharyngeal flap (Fig. 13) is constructed by lifting from three quarters to the full width of the mucosa and muscle of the pos-

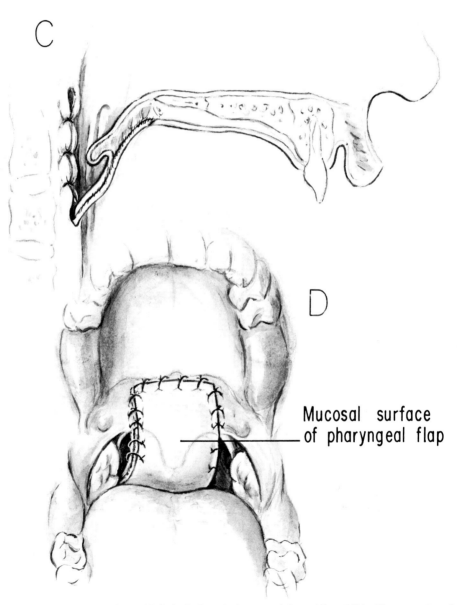

Mucosal surface
of pharyngeal flap

Fig. 13 (cont.). The construction of inferiorly based pharyngeal flaps (C and D). The posterior pharyngeal wall is closed by suture to avoid bleeding.

terior pharyngeal wall away from the pre-vertebral fascia and suturing it to a raw surface created on the soft palate. It must, of course, be left attached to the pharyngeal wall at either its lower or its upper end. With an inferiorly based flap it is attached to the front surface of the soft palate. If a superior base is chosen, one must suture the flap to the dorsal surface of the soft palate—usually by reincising the area of the previous soft palate repair so that the pharyngeal flap may be accurately sutured in place.

Since in speech the normal closure of the soft palate to the posterior pharyngeal wall is upward and backward, it would seem that the superiorly based flap would produce the better results. Both flaps are used at our hospital, and there seems very little evidence thus far that one base produces better speech than the other.

ORONASAL FISTULA

There are many patients in whom a complete closure of the anterior portion of the primary palate or the alveolar ridge is not achieved at the time of the lip repair. Many authors recommend the elevation of a flap of mucosa off the side of the septum to be sutured to the lateral portion of the alveolar ridge in these patients, as described by Veau (1937–1938). This does, obviously, uncover the epiphyseal line which is immediately behind the premaxilla and theoretically, at least, should interfere with bone growth in this area. However, lack of bone growth has

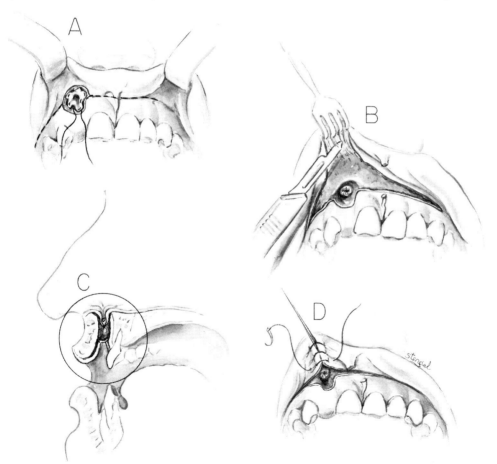

Fig. 14. Technique for closing oronasal fistulas anterior to the alveolar ridge. See text for details.

been observed in this area even when no flap was taken off the septum or vomer and no bony injury caused to the septum or pre-maxillary area. My usual practice is to repair only the lip without making an attempt to close the fistula with a flap off the septum or vomer. Consequently patients do return afterward with a fistula into the nose just in front of the alveolar ridge. However, by this time the bony ridges have practically always moved together.

The closure of these fistulas does not present any major problem, as a rule (Fig. 14). It is necessary only that their margins be completely incised. The mucosa necessary to line the nose is freed and pushed upward into the nose and sutured into this position. Incision is then carried along the upper buccal sulcus on both sides of the fistula and the adjacent mucosa mobilized and brought toward the fistula to provide an adequate oral lining for this area. At the time this is done it is also easy to increase the depth of the upper buccal sulcus if that was not adequately achieved at the primary lip repair. Such deepening of the sulcus is usually fol-

lowed by much more adequate function of the upper lip and a better covering of the incisor teeth.

PERFORATIONS OF THE HARD AND SOFT PALATES

Where primary healing has not occurred after the repair of the cleft of the hard or soft palate or where it has been impossible to close the anterior 3 to 10 mm of the hard palate at the original palate repair, a secondary procedure must be carried out to accomplish this (Fig. 15). Ordinarily it is necessary to completely remobilize the mucoperiosteum from one half of the hard palate. At the same time the lining for the nasal side of this fistula is provided by incising a flap adjacent to the perforation on the side opposite that to which the entire mucoperiosteal flap is to be elevated. The flap for the lining of the nose is turned on the edge of the fistula into the nose and sutured into this position. The large flap from the opposite side of the hard palate is then rotated over it and sutured in position.

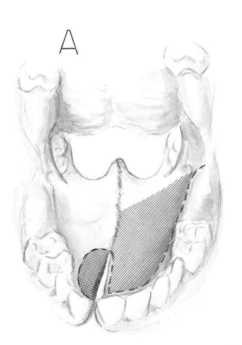 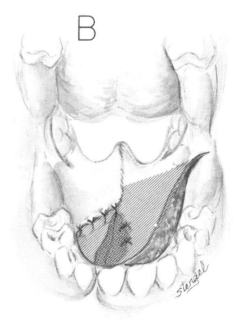

Fig. 15. One means of closing a fistula in the hard palate.

OBTURATORS AND SPEECH BULBS

Several years ago, when the results of cleft palate surgery were not as predictable as they are today, some exceedingly competent dentists and prosthodontists were strongly in favor of having the patient with a cleft palate undergo no surgical procedure but having the cleft in the palate filled by the use of a denture to which a speech bulb was attached. The predictability of adequate repair in a large share of patients with cleft palate in the present day has led to lessened enthusiasm for the use of an artificial appliance. However, these appliances still have a place in the management of a patient with a cleft palate when other factors preclude the child's going through the surgical procedure required for repair in his own tissue. In the occasional case where infection or some other untoward incident has led to the complete dissolution of the surgical repair, a speech bulb may be the only thing that will lead to a reasonably functional repair. When a child has general health problems which preclude a surgical repair, it may be worthwhile to use a speech bulb as a temporary expedient, and occasionally patients are found who do so well with it that they are reluctant to undergo a surgical repair.

SPEECH AND HEARING

It is essential for anyone who is interested in the total rehabilitation of a patient with a cleft palate to be affiliated with someone who does good speech and hearing evaluation and treatment. These two modalities must be in constant use until the patient is really stabilized in the early or middle teens. We find that there can be progressive atrophy of the adenoids with a consequent change to a nasal type of speech in some patients with very short palates. They speak well at an early age but later regress because of the nasopharynx's failure to close.

Middle ear infections are also a threat during the entire childhood and can play havoc with the child who must hear accurately in order to mimic correctly the sounds of normal speech. Many American families have tape recorders. This machine has great value for the speech training of a child with a cleft palate because many of these children do not actually learn to talk well until they hear themselves on the playback. It therefore is very helpful for the parents to recite or read something which the patient immediately repeats after them, both being done into a tape recorder. When the tape is played back the child hears the difference between his own speech and that of his parents.

ORTHODONTIA

Almost 100 percent of children who have any deformity of their palates also have enough deformity of their teeth that orthodontia is required. This is another of the features which must be reckoned with in the total care of the patient with cleft palate. The use of this modality very early in the patient's life has been discussed above. It is important that the surgeon supervising the total care of the patient makes certain that the child sees a good orthodontist at 10 to 12 years of age, when the definitive correction can be started. Before this age the surgeon must constantly emphasize the patient's need for good general dentistry and daily dental care. If he fails, the child gets to the age for orthodontia with no good teeth to straighten.

There are occasional instances where orthodontia on deciduous teeth between $3\frac{1}{2}$ and 5 years of age is rewarding, but most frequently the major orthodontic effort is carried out when the permanent teeth have erupted. A good orthodontist frequently makes the surgeon's efforts look even better than they are, but there are some things which even the orthodontist cannot accomplish without the assistance of the surgeon. Reference is made here to the patient with severe growth problems in the upper jaw which produce a relative prognathism of the lower jaw. With orthodontist and surgeon working together, the Dingman procedure

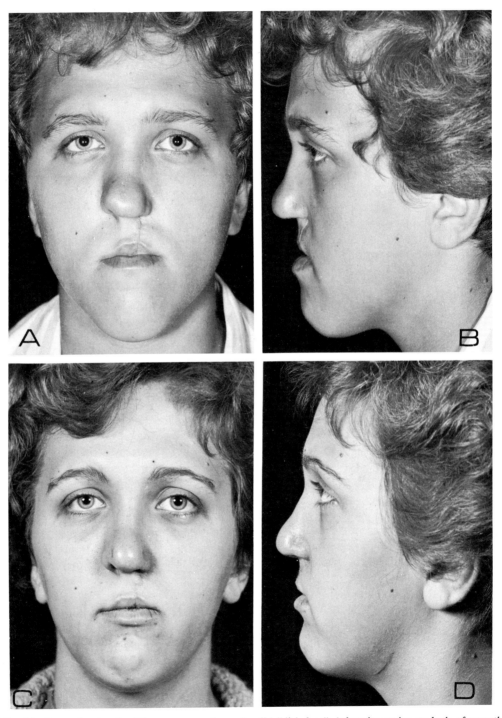

Fig. 16. Correction by the Dingman procedure of mild "dish-face" deformity owing to lack of growth in the upper jaw. After appropriate dental models were taken and studied, one tooth was sacrificed on each side of the lower jaw and a comparable amount of mandible removed to set the lower jaw back. About three months of stabilization is necessary to secure good bony union.

for setback of the mandible (Dingman, 1948) can be accomplished with marked improvement in both appearance and function of the jaws (Fig. 16).

BONE GRAFTING OF THE ALVEOLAR RIDGE

In recent years it has been realized that the upper dental arch does not become a stable structure simply by the premaxilla and the alveolar ridge coming together in good alignment. The bony defect in the region of the cleft may be quite extensive. Filling this defect with a bone graft adds greatly to the stability of the arch. Even more important, it has been found by some Swedish surgeons that the insertion of a bone graft in the upper alveolar ridge will provide a means by which tooth buds may erupt in the area of the cleft, which would never happen as long as there was no bone through which the tooth bud could erupt. The most efficient type of graft here is the inlay-onlay graft, usually with rib bone being used as the grafting material. Small fragments of bone are inserted between the edges of the maxilla, but a somewhat larger onlay graft is laid over the front as well, in order to provide adequate new bone for complete stabilization of the upper arch. This becomes exceedingly important in a patient with a bilateral cleft of the alveolar ridge and palate. Some surgeons do this procedure quite early in life, even at six to eight months of age, if the dental arch is in good alignment.

SECONDARY LIP AND NOSE DEFORMITIES

With the advent, in recent years, of the lip repairs designed to preserve the natural cupid's bow insofar as it is present in the lip, there are fewer and fewer *gross* deformities of repaired cleft lips. However the minutiae which make for perfection can still plague the surgeon who strives to make the patient look as though he had not been born with a deformity. Even with the most careful analysis of the patient's deformity by an experienced plastic surgeon, the selection of the proper matching points on the two sides of the cleft at the original repair is made on the basis of a highly educated guess. One may still err by $\frac{1}{2}$ to 1 mm. When the error is magnified two or three times by growth at age five or six, the disproportion may be quite marked. Other factors, over which the surgeon has even less control, are the position and shape of the cartilages of the nasal tip. It is difficult to determine whether wide dissection and mobilization of the nasal cartilages interfere with their growth. However, the possible hazard of altering growth deters many surgeons from extensive handling of the cartilages at the original lip repair. The child often reaches school age with obvious asymmetry of the nasal tip and perhaps some of the lip as well.

Figure 17 illustrates a severe example of the sort of nasal asymmetry which occurs fairly frequently and is quite difficult to correct. This repair was carried out a few years ago by the use of a "batwing" incision made just inside the ala on each side and carried across the columella to expose completely the cartilages of the tip and match them as well as possible. However, the recent analysis of this deformity by Reynolds and Horton (1965) seems more accurate than anything previously written. I have used their method for repair in only a few recent cases, but the immediate results seem far superior to prior techniques. Their principal diagram and its legend are reproduced here (Fig. 18).

The short or nonexistent columella also requires correction before the child goes to school. Many techniques for this procedure have been described, but the most effective in the author's experience is the use of a forked flap out of the prolabial skin. This requires the bilateral cleft lip to have been repaired originally with a straight line closure using the prolabium for the full height of the lip, so that one has unscarred skin with an adequate blood supply to work with. The operation (Millard, 1958) has the merit not only of making an adequate columella

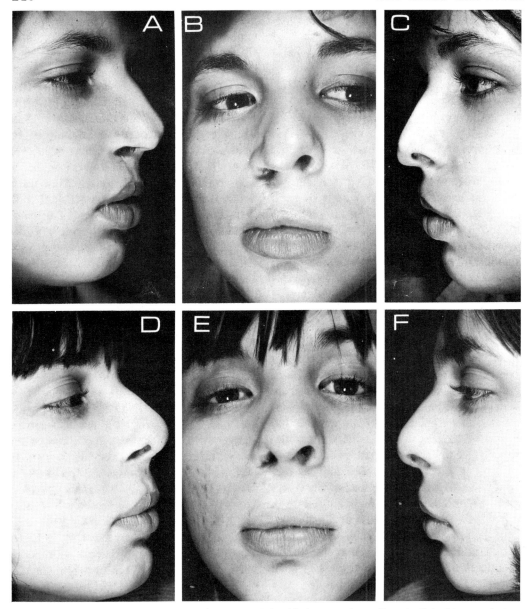

Fig. 17. Typical deformity of the nasal tip corrected in this instance by a "batwing" incision made just inside the nostril rim and passing across the columella. The entire skin of the dorsum was turned back to inspect the cartilages directly. They were altered to make them as symmetrical as possible. A, B, and C are preoperative views; D, E, and F show the patient three years after repair.

but also of narrowing the space between the suture lines on the upper lip to make them resemble the markings of a normal philtrum (Fig. 19).

Another obvious deformity of a repaired cleft lip is the disproportion in size sometimes seen between the upper and lower lips. Most frequently the upper lip is short and flat and perhaps has a shallow buccal sulcus. When the repair has been wrongly planned the upper lip may be long, flat, and tight. Occasionally growth in the upper jaw may be markedly retarded. It is also possible for the patient to have an unrelated prognathism as well as a cleft lip and palate.

In the short, flat lip with an adequate buc-

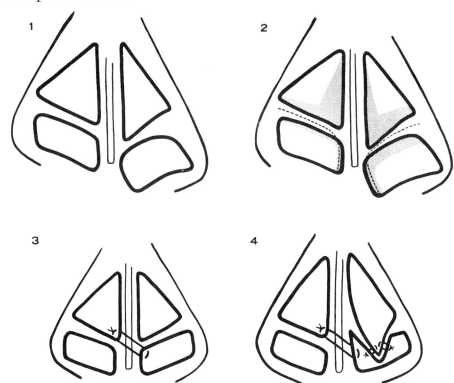

Fig. 18. Nasal asymmetry repair. 1. The usual nasal deformity associated with a unilateral cleft lip. 2. The dotted lines represent intranasal incisions; the shaded area represents a typical amount of cartilage to be removed. Note the limited amount of cartilage that is removed from normal lateral cartilage. 3. Suture to rotate and elevate abnormal lower lateral cartilage, which is then fixed to opposite upper lateral cartilage. 4. After the fixation suture is in place, if the airway is compromised by webbing or deficient mucous membrane, then the redundant inferior tip of the abnormal upper lateral cartilage, with its lining, is not discarded but is inserted into a relaxing incision in the lower lateral cartilage. (From Reynolds and Horton. Plast. Reconstr. Surg., 35: 377, 1965.)

cal sulcus, symmetry may be improved by the construction of a denture which lifts the upper lip forward (Figs. 20A, 20B, and 20C). If the patient has lost the upper front teeth (which is frequently true), an upper denture will be required, in any case. A very short upper lip without an adequate buccal sulcus can be corrected by a free transplant of skin known as a "Stent graft" or "Esser inlay graft."

To accomplish this the mucosa is dissected from the alveolar ridge and a mold of the defect taken in dental molding compound. A thick split skin graft is then sutured about this mold (or Stent—named for the nineteenth century dentist who first described it) with its raw surface outward. The Stent is then inserted into the open wound and the

mucosa sutured over it. After two to four weeks the wound is opened and the mold removed, revealing a cavity lined with skin.

When augmentation with dentures does not correct the asymmetry between the patient's lips, it may be necessary either to sacrifice completely a portion of the lower lip or —more frequently—to transfer its excess to the upper lip by means of a pedicle flap. This procedure, called the Stein-Abbé-Estlander procedure, is carried out as follows: The portion of the lower lip deemed to be excessive is marked (taking into account that the upper lip is to be augmented by this same amount). One side of the wedge in the lower lip is cut completely through. On the other side, which is to be the pedicle, the skin muscle and mucosa are cut through up to

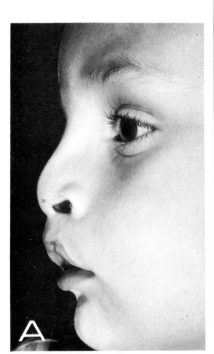

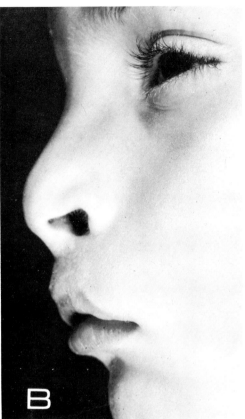

Fig. 19. Snubbed-down nasal tip following bilateral cleft lip repair is released by a forked flap made of prolabial skin. A is a preoperative view, B shows the patient nine months after the operation.

the vermilion border of the lip. The labial artery and vein are spared. The wedge of lower lip is then turned into the defect previously opened in the upper lip. The lips are then sutured together for 10 to 14 days (Figs. 20D, 20E, and 20F), during which time the patient eats and drinks through a straw on either side of the pedicle. The pedicle is divided safely by 10 to 14 days if primary wound healing has taken place. Both operations must be done under local anesthesia. A tracheostomy is required to assure an adequate airway if the operation is done under general anesthesia. This means that most children will have to wait until they are at least 10 or 12 years of age, when they are able to tolerate this much surgery under local anesthesia.

PREOPERATIVE AND POSTOPERATIVE CARE

The infant or child with a cleft lip or palate ready for repair need only be in good health and have a reasonable hemoglobin level (preferably 10.5 to 14 gm). As indicated earlier in this chapter, the use of local anesthesia with epinephrine (1:100,000) makes most of these operations relatively bloodless. The author rarely finds it necessary to give blood to these patients if the hemoglobin is at the level indicated above.

Children with cyanotic heart disease may frighten the surgeon, but, in my experience, when the cardiologist has approved the procedure it has proved to be safe. Since the operation for such individuals is done under

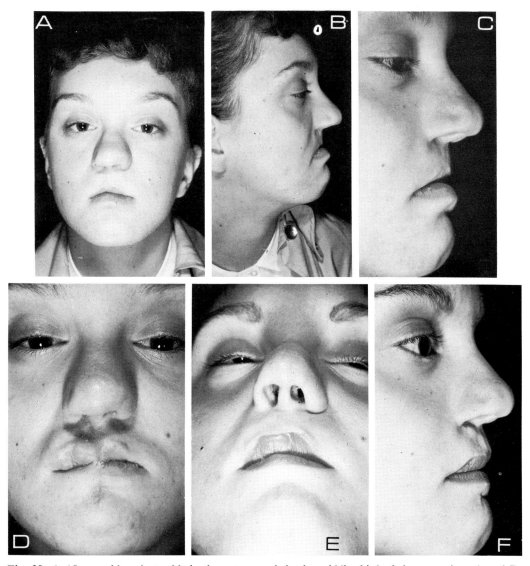

Fig. 20. A 15-year-old patient with inadequate growth in the middle third of the upper jaw. A and B show the patient without a denture. C shows him with a denture but showing major disproportion between upper and lower lips. D shows him with an Abbé flap attached from lower lip. E and F show the patient one year after section of Abbé flap pedicle, and two months after tip rhinoplasty.

endotracheal anesthesia (local is not recommended here), one usually finds that the patient is better aerated during the operation than in the normal state.

Children being prepared for repair of the palate are changed from bottle to cup-and-spoon feedings *before* the operation. Those who suck their thumbs will have to be denied this privilege also, postoperatively.

One gets only one good chance to repair a palate—the first time it is done. For this reason it is wise to deny the operation when there is any real suspicion of a respiratory infection, no matter how mild. Antibiotics can rarely prevent such an infection from causing a dissolution of the repair.

Postoperatively the greatest aid to the healing of the lip and mouth is early oral hydration. Clear liquids are given on the day of operation, nourishing liquids the next day, and, for the cleft palate repair, a mechanical soft diet from the second day on for one month. This includes meats and every other food usual for the child, but all must be fairly finely divided (the so-called junior foods). Infants with cleft lip repairs are fed with a rubber-tipped aseptic syringe. The use of medicine droppers should be abandoned. The infant cannot get an adequate swallow of milk from a dropper and consequently swallows a great deal of air and thus requires much more frequent "burping."

Antibiotics are probably not necessary for cleft lip repair, though they may be used for three days. They are used for five days in cleft palate repair.

The suture line in cleft lip repair must be kept meticulously free of blood clots—nothing but skin and suture material should be visible. Crusts should be removed by cotton-tipped applicator sticks moistened in sterile saline. Admittedly this does not dissolve clots as rapidly as hydrogen peroxide does, but the use of hydrogen peroxide should be condemned; it dissolves the clot not only on the surface but also, as commonly used by the nursing staff, between the skin edges, where one wishes to have a clot. Lips repeatedly bathed in hydrogen peroxide get well in spite of the doctor, not because of him. When the clots are washed away with saline and the lip promptly dried, it will usually be found that from the second day on no new clots form on the lip, whereas when peroxide is used, some areas tend to keep oozing for three or four days.

Of course, some sort of elbow restraint is required for all infants and young children to prevent them from putting their hands in their mouths.

Finally, the uncomfortable infant or child should have some mild sedation. Rectal aspirin and barbiturates, separately or in combination, are used much too infrequently—the surgeon should try harder to put himself in the patient's position and decide whether *he* would like relief from the inevitable discomfort of these procedures.

CLARENCE W. MONROE

REFERENCES

BRAUER, R. O. Observations and measurements of non-operative set-back of premaxilla in double cleft lip patients. Plast. Reconstr. Surg., 35: 148, 1965.

BRAUER, R. O., CRONIN, T. D., and REAVES, E. L. Early maxillary orthopedics, orthodontia and alveolar bone grafting in complete clefts of the palate. Plast. Reconstr. Surg., 29: 625, 1962.

CONWAY, H. Push-back and pharyngeal flap in cleft palate. Plast. Reconstr. Surg., 7: 214, 1951.

CRONIN, T. D. A modification of the Tennison-type lip repair. Cleft Palate J., 3: 376, 1966.

DES PREZ, J. D., KIEHN, C. L., and MAGID, A. Use of a silastic prosthesis for prevention of dental arch collapse in the cleft palate newborn. Plast. Reconstr. Surg., 34: 483, 1964.

DINGMAN, R. O. Surgical correction of developmental deformities of the mandible. Plast. Reconstr. Surg., 3: 124, 1948.

EDGERTON, M. T. The island flap push-back and the suspensory pharyngeal flap in surgical treatment of the cleft palate patient. Plast. Reconstr. Surg., 36: 591, 1965.

FRASER, F. C., CURTIS, E. J., and WARBURTON, D. Congenital cleft lip and palate. Amer. J. Dis. Child., 102: 853, 1961.

—— and WARBURTON, D. Stress and the occurrence of cleft lip and palate. Plast. Reconstr. Surg., 33: 395, 1964.

GEORGIADE, N. Early utilization of prosthetic appliances in cleft palate patients. Plast. Reconstr. Surg., 34: 617, 1964.

LANGENBECK, B. Operation der angeborenen totalen Spaltung des harten Gaumens nach einer neuer Methode. Deutsch. Klin., 8: 231, 1861.

LIMBERG, A. Neue Wege in der radikalen Uranoplastik bei angerboren spalden Deformationen. Chirurg, 54: 1745, 1927.

LINDSAY, W. K., LE MESURIER, A. B., and FARMER, A. W. Speech results in a large series of cleft palate patients. Plast. Reconstr. Surg., 29: 273, 1962.

MILLARD, D. R. Columella lengthening by a forked flap. Plast. Reconstr. Surg., 22: 454, 1958.
————. Wide and/or short cleft palate. Plast. Reconstr. Surg., 29: 40, 1962.
————. Refinements in rotation-advancement cleft lip technique. Plast. Reconstr. Surg., 33: 26, 1964.
MONROE, C. W. The surgical factors influencing bone growth in the middle third of the upper jaw in cleft palate. Plast. Reconstr. Surg., 24: 481, 1959.
————. Recession of the premaxilla—A follow-up study. Plast. Reconstr. Surg., 35: 512, 1965.
MORAN, R. E. The pharyngeal flap operation as a speech aid. Plast. Reconstr. Surg., 7: 202, 1951.
PEER, L. A., STREAN, L. P., WALKER, J. C., BERNHARD, W. G., and PECK, G. C. Study of 100 pregnancies of birth of cleft palate infants: Protective effect of folic acid and vitamin B$_6$ therapy. Plast. Reconstr. Surg., 22: 422, 1958.

REYNOLDS, J. R., and HORTON, C. T. An alar lift procedure in the cleft lip rhinoplasty. Plast. Reconstr. Surg., 35: 377, 1965.
ROSENSTEIN, S. W. Early orthodontic procedures for cleft lip and palate individuals. Angle orthodont., 33: 127, 1963.
STARK, R. B., and EHRMANN, N. A. The development of the center of the face. Plast. Reconstr. Surg., 21: 177, 1958.
STRAITH, R. E., TEASLEY, J. L., and MOORE, L. T. Local anesthesia in the newborn. Plast. Reconstr. Surg., 16: 125, 1955.
VEAU, V. Z. Hasenscharten menschlicher Keimlinge auf der Stufe 21–23 mm S. St. L. Z. Anat. Entwicklungsgesch., 108: 459, 1937–1938.
WARDELL, W. E. M. Cleft palate. Brit. J. Surg., 21: 82, 1933.

15

The Ear

ANATOMY AND EMBRYOLOGY

The ear is normally located on the side of the head, with its upper pole in the same horizontal plane with the outer canthus of the eye. Anteroposteriorly it is in the posterior portion of the middle third of the head. The multiple fine carvings and many peaks and valleys all have names—and with good reason, since it is almost impossible to describe what one may do to an ear without specific reference to these landmarks (Fig. 1). The thin layer of cartilage that gives shape to the ear has a very thin layer of tightly adherent skin covering its anterolateral surface, whereas a much looser skin, with appreciable subcutaneous tissue and muscle, covers the posteromedial surface. The external ear, through its concha or vestibule, gives entrance to the external auditory canal. The lateral one third and lower one half of this canal is made up of fibrocartilage, and the remainder is of bone. The

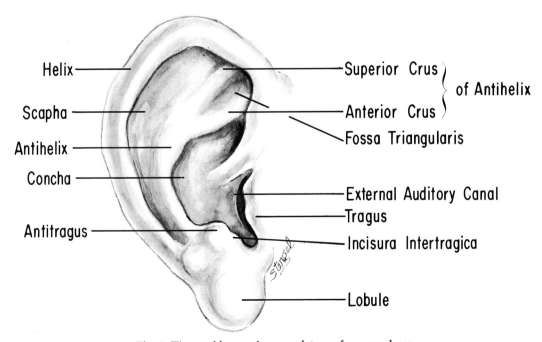

Fig. 1. The markings and nomenclature of a normal ear.

246

epithelial lining of the canal is a thin layer of skin firmly attached to the wall of the canal. It is our inability to reproduce this thin layer of skin on a bony or cartilaginous tube that makes it so difficult to open a closed external auditory canal and keep it open.

The ear develops from the first and second branchial arches and is completed by the fourth month of fetal life. Since it first appears low on the side of the head, gradually moving up as the mandible develops, it is understandable why a large number of the congenital ear deformities are characterized by a low-placed ear. However, the opposite, a high-placed ear, can also occur, as illustrated in Figures 2A and 2B. The patient in these figures stated that her right ear had always been in this superior position. X-ray studies revealed an apparently normal petrous temporal bone and what appeared to be a bony external auditory canal. Dr. B. H. Griffith, my associate, undertook to rotate the auricle downward on a large scalp pedicle and was able to place it over the previously covered external auditory canal (Fig. 2C and 2D). The portion of the external auditory canal that was missing was reconstructed with a free skin graft. For a time it was difficult to keep this canal patent, but since this has been achieved the patient has had her hearing acuity improved materially.

The opposite type of ectopia, in which the ear is low on the head or in the upper neck, is much more frequently encountered. In instances of this the ear is usually over the auditory canal, since the entire picture of maldevelopment is one of an arrest of growth at some point along the ear's usual pathway of migration.

Not only can the position of the ear vary in a vertical direction, but the ear can also be placed farther forward than normal. This variation is not usually so apparent as the difference of the two ears in height but will often be noticed if the patient is looked at from directly above the head.

Except for the case cited above, where the ear was rotated downward on a scalp pedicle, usually nothing is done to alter the position of the low-set ear if it is connected to an external auditory canal. However, many such ectopic ears are likely to have stretched-out lobules, which further accentuates the deformity. Their partial amputation or shortening can often aid in minimizing the deformity.

PROTRUDING EARS

The most common abnormality in the position of the ear is not that related to its anterior, posterior, superior, or inferior position on the head but that related to the partial or complete lack of an acute auriculocephalic curve at the usual site of the antihelix. The lack or essential lack of an antihelical curve causes the helix to stand straight out from the side of the head rather than lying from 1 to 1.5 cm from the mastoid process, and this deformity is known as protruding ears, outstanding ears, or lop ears. In small children this position of the ears is often regarded as "cute." In some ethnic groups (e.g., Koreans) it is so common that it is regarded as the normal, and people are more likely to call attention to the individual whose ears lie quite flat against the head.

In American society such protruding ears are certainly not uncommon, but they are so obviously different from the usual kind that they frequently excite comment, especially by children to other children. The reactions of children being teased about their ears vary widely. Some children enjoy being noticed even in this negative way and could even be made unhappy by the surgical correction of such ears. Others may try to hide their ears by always wearing caps or scarves, and a third group may become extremely belligerent. The last often occurs without either teachers or parents realizing what motivates the child until leading questions are asked. It is most gratifying after carrying out a surgical correction of a child's ears to have the parents say, "We hardly know our boy

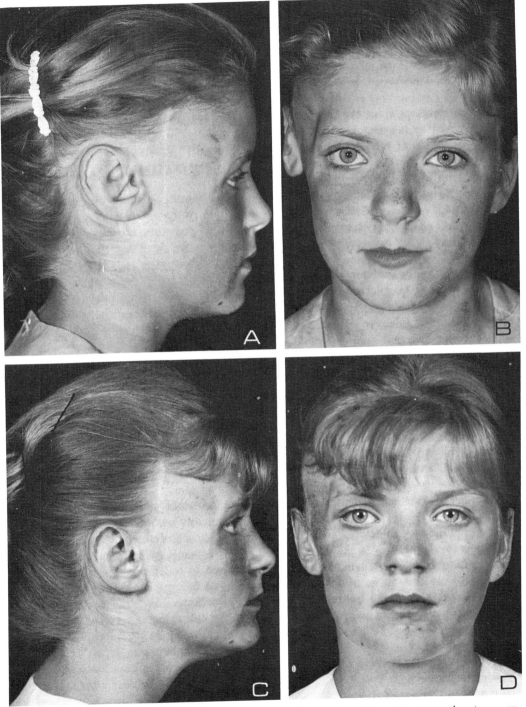

Fig. 2. This patient was born with her ear in this unusual ectopic position. No connection to an external auditory canal exists. By utilizing a very large scalp flap to carry the ear, it was rotated downward until it could be connected to the previously hidden external auditory canal. (Courtesy of Dr. B. H. Griffith.)

since you operated on him. He's the happiest boy on the block. Before, he was always fighting with everyone at school and a great deal with his own brothers and sisters."

OPERATIVE TECHNIQUE
OF OTOPLASTY

In view of the pathological anatomy of protruding ears it is obvious that the surgical procedure must create a new or more adequate antihelix. Since the antihelix is a fold of cartilage, the procedure should aim at making such a fold that will be permanent. The site of this antihelix is marked on the front of the ear (Fig. 3A) by pushing a straight pin through to the back of the ear where the high point of the antihelical curve is to be made. This point is picked out by pushing the helix back against the mastoid to demonstrate where the curve will occur. The first pin is inserted at the lower margin of the concha. Many protruding ears have conchas that are too deep, and, to achieve a good result without having the antihelix much farther from the head than the helix in the corrected position, it is necessary to reduce the height of the concha by turning a portion of it into the scapha. Successive pins (usually four or five) are inserted along the course of the proposed antihelix, and the last pin is inserted in the superior crus of the antihelix close to the anterior rim of the helix. Usually the succession of pins describes an arc of between 70° and 90°. The upper margin of the arc should be in the horizontal plane (with the patient in the anatomical position).

The ear is then turned forward and an ellipse of skin and subcutaneous tissue incised (Fig. 3B) on the back of the ear embracing the points of the needles. The assistant retracts the ellipse enough to show the needles as they come through the cartilage, while the surgeon exerts enough pressure with his fingers on the front of the ear to slow the copious bleeding. As soon as the cartilage is partially incised between the needles, they are removed, as is the ellipse

of skin and subcutaneous tissue. Bleeders are ligated at this point.

Three parallel incisions (Fig. 3C) are then made in the cartilage 1.5 to 2 mm apart—one on either side of the first marked incision. These are started with a knife but completed with a Freer elevator, to be sure that they go all the way through to the skin of the front of the ear and also to be certain no damage is done to the anterior skin. In the lower portion of the conchal area the cartilage must be completely divided into the soft tissue just lateral to the antitragus. Superiorly the final cuts in the cartilage should be directed toward the outer canthus of the eye and should go up to, but not through, the rim of the helix.

The ear is then turned back into the new position, and it is observed whether it still strongly tends to spring back to its former position. If it does, one should check again to be certain the cartilage has been completely divided along the entire course of the three incisions.

To hold the ear in the new position mattress sutures (Fig. 3D) of 5-0 monofilament suture are placed along the cartilage edge (usually five to seven sutures are sufficient). After all are in place, they are tied from the bottom up, with the assistant holding the two cartilage surfaces back to back (Fig. 9E) as each succeeding knot is tied. If the uppermost suture tends to make a notch in the rim of the helix, it is removed. Then, with a running suture of the same material, the skin is closed very loosely, so that should any bleeding occur, the blood readily escapes from the wound and does not produce a hematoma.

In some patients the lobule of the ear continues to stand straight out from the head even when the entire helix moves back satisfactorily. The only way to correct this, in this author's experience, is to extend the original incision down into the area of the lobule, sacrificing a large ellipse of skin but also inserting two or three sutures in the upper portion of the lobule adjacent to the antitragus and carrying this back to the con-

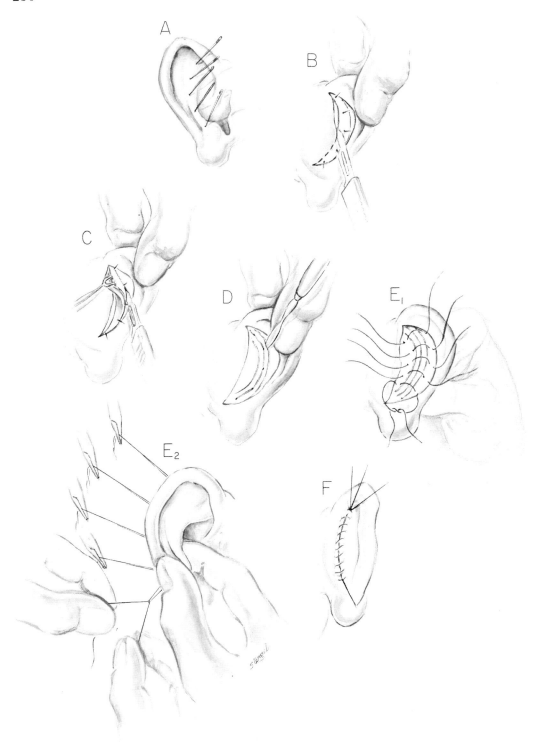

Fig. 3. Operative steps in otoplasty for protruding ears, as described in the text.

chal cartilage. Sutures in the lobule itself always leave unsightly dimpling, but the antitragus is usually heavy enough to be moved back without dimpling.

The dressing for this operation is as important as the operation itself (Fig. 3). It is applied as follows: A sheet of fine-mesh rayon fabric is laid over the ear. A single 4 × 4 gauze dressing, folded to 2 × 4 (and with one margin cut out to fit the back of the ear), pushes the rayon fabric between the ear and the mastoid process. A piece of absorbent cotton (Fig. 4C) the size of the little finger is wet and rolled into a rod that will fit the entire length of the cleft between the helix and the antihelix. The water is squeezed out *on* the ear so that the cotton fits the rayon into the contours of the ear. A similar but larger piece of moist cotton fills the concha of the ear (again over the top of the rayon fabric). The sucker is inserted into the lower margin of the auditory canal so that the ear is not left filled with water. A smooth, flat gauze dressing (Fig. 4D) is then laid over the ear. A doughnut of fluffed gauze (Fig. 4E) is made for the ear, thick enough that the flat hand can barely feel the ear filling up the center of the doughnut.

In order to hold the wraparound dressing in place on a child it is well to put a 2-inch strip of plain gauze bandage across the crown of the head from ear to ear and then two long pieces of the same bandage from in front of one eye back across the opposite occiput (Figs. 4F and 4G). These are short in front and long in back. A Kling or other cotton elastic bandage (Fig. 4H) is then wrapped around the head, holding the ear dressing in place. The long strings of bandage are then brought forward and tied to the piece in front of the eye just tightly enough to keep the dressing out of the eye (Fig. 4I). A piece of adhesive tape is placed across the crown of the head (Fig. 4J) from ear to ear on the strips of bandage there to keep them from slipping off the top of the head and dislodging the dressing downward. A second

strip of adhesive is placed over the ear, carried *loosely* under the chin (Fig. 4K), and carried up onto the other ear to keep the dressing from slipping up. In very small children it may be well to augment this dressing with a head cap made of 4-inch stockinette, with bandage inserted to tie under the chin (Figs. 4L and 4M).

Postoperatively, children rarely complain of much pain from the procedure, especially if the dressing is properly applied. They do not require antibiotics. They are sent home the day after operation and report to the office in one week. At t time all dressings are removed. Removal of the sutures is easy if the child rolls his nose into the pillow on the examining table. No dressings are replaced. However, it is wise for the child to wear a snug-fitting skullcap at night for two months until the new cartilage has become firm. Such a cap is easily made from the top of a woman's stocking, with attached ties that go under the chin. After two months of wearing the cap at night the child returns to the office for final inspection and postoperative photographs. Figures 5A, 5B, and 5C show preoperative views and 5D, 5E, and 5F postoperative views of a patient repaired by the above technique.

OTHER EAR DEFORMITIES

DARWINIAN TUBERCLE

A Darwinian tubercle is an excessive area of skin and cartilage on the rim of the helix located at about the junction of the upper and middle thirds of the helix on its lateral aspect. It is so named because it is usually very prominent about the sixth month of fetal life and at that time makes the fetal ear strongly resemble the ear of an adult monkey. If it is large enough to cause a cosmetic problem (Fig. 6), it is usually readily dealt with by simple amputation of the excessive skin and cartilage.

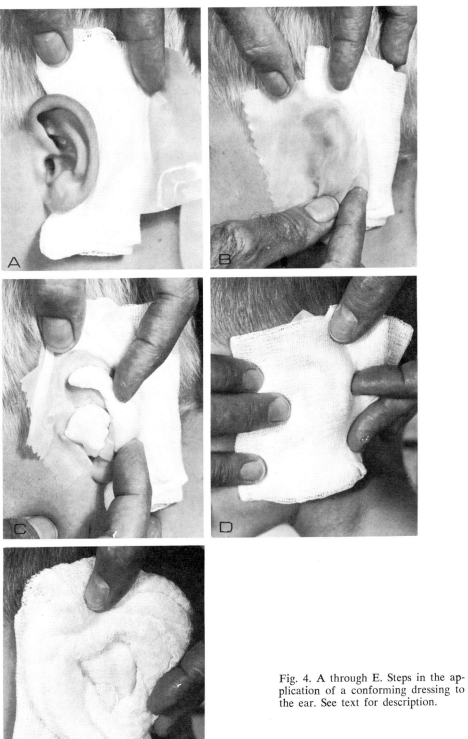

Fig. 4. A through E. Steps in the application of a conforming dressing to the ear. See text for description.

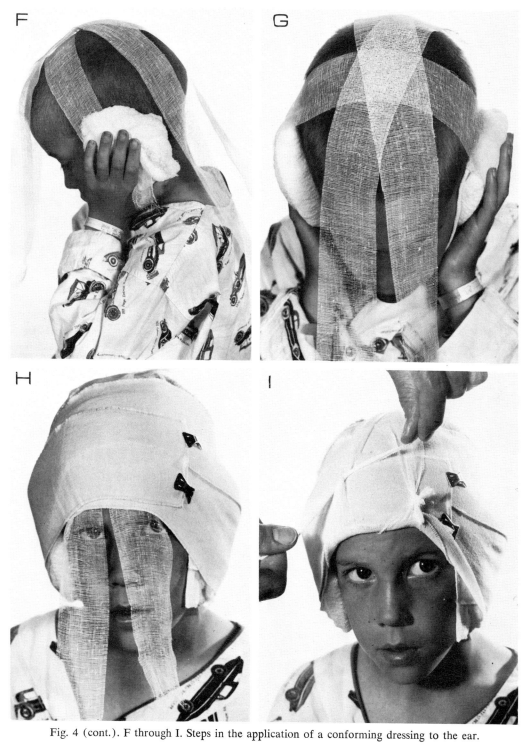

Fig. 4 (cont.). F through I. Steps in the application of a conforming dressing to the ear.

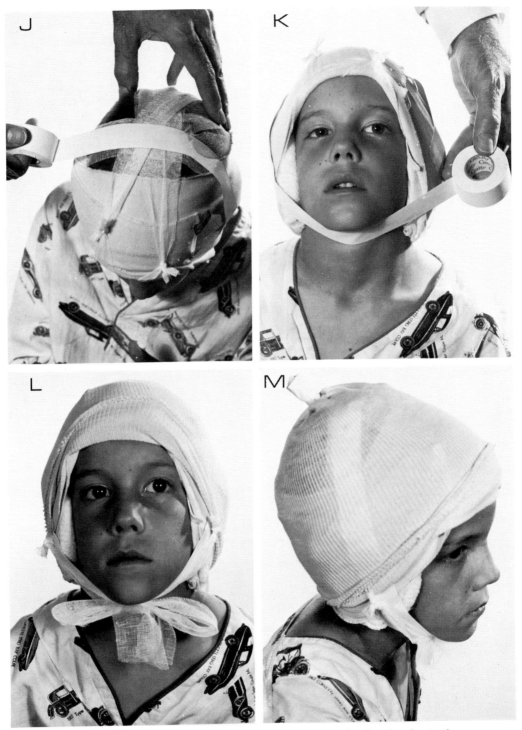

Fig. 4 (cont.). J through M. Steps in the application of a conforming dressing to the ear.

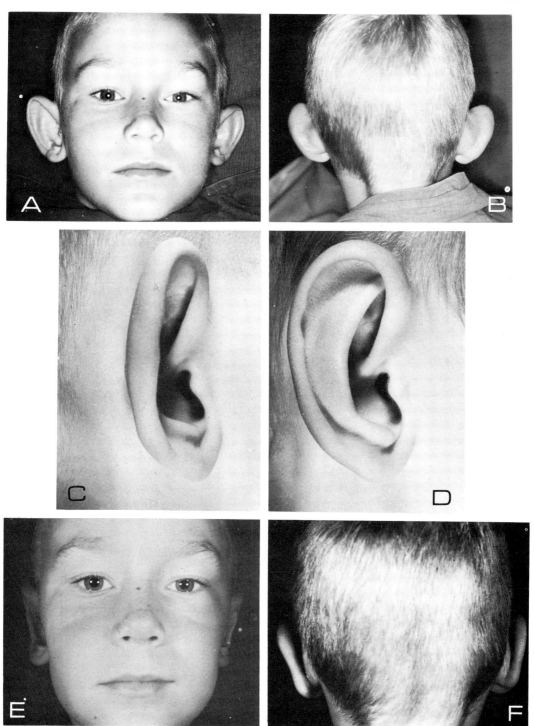

Fig. 5. Preoperative and postoperative views of child whose protruding ears were corrected by the technique shown in Figure 4.

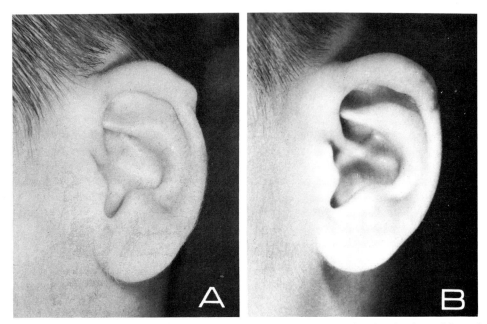

Fig. 6. This patient demonstrates the Darwinian tubercle and its correction by simple excision of the excess skin and cartilage.

EXCESSIVE HELIX

Excessive helix often gives an appearance suggesting the presence of a Darwinian tubercle along the whole upper half of the rim of the helix. In some instances this almost suggests a short curtain hanging over the ear. Again, its correction can be achieved by simple excision of the excess skin and cartilage.

CUPPED EARS

Cupped ears are a variety of protruding ears but with the significant difference that the ears do not simply stand straight from the head but actually incline forward. They are usually smaller than normal ears. When one attempts to push the rim of the helix back in a normal position it is found to be too short to permit the ear to stay in this position even when a new antihelix is constructed as described above. J. K. Grotting (1958) has described an excellent method for correcting this deformity that involves swinging a pedicled flap of postauricular skin to the

lateral aspect to relieve this tightness of skin cover and permit the ear to assume a normal position (Fig. 7).

PREAURICULAR SINUSES AND TABS

Preauricular sinuses and tabs are two discrete entities, both of which commonly appear along the anterior margin of the ear. The first is a sinus tract with its opening located in or very near the root of the helix where it joins the cheek at the upper margin of the ear. Occasionally a hair will protrude from it. More frequently there is only serous or somewhat thicker secretion—unless infection should occur. A narrow opening of the sinus predisposes to infection (Figs. 8A and 8B).

The sinus tracts may be very short, but they can also be very extensive and difficult to follow. Recurrence after surgical removal is the rule unless the operator has carefully dissected out the entire sinus. The tracts can lead to various areas of the cartilage of the root of the ear and can even pass deeply

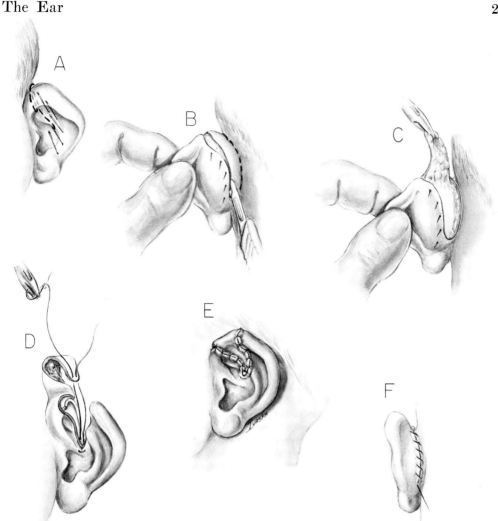

Fig. 7. Technique for correcting cupped ears. (From Grotting. Plast. Reconstr. Surg., 22: 164, 1958.)

along the external auditory canal and enter it near the drum. Wherever it goes, it is necessary to remove it. Gentle injection of the tract with methylene blue before the procedure is begun and injection of local anesthesia with epinephrine in the operative field to reduce the bleeding are particular aids to effective surgery.

Tabs are skin-covered masses of excessive and unnecessary cartilage usually located near the site of the tragus of the ear. They are not, as a rule, related to the sinuses, except that they usually occur in the same areas (Fig. 9). Their surgical removal is simple if the lines of excision are placed in normal skin folds and the cartilage contained in the tab is amputated far enough below the skin to prevent its sticking up under the skin scar.

MICROTIA

Microtia is the term for any ear that is smaller than one would expect in a person of a given size and age. The pathology may vary from a small but well-formed ear to a virtual absence of the external ear. Most such deformed ears do not have external auditory canals open on the surface. Occasionally a canal is present but is quite nar-

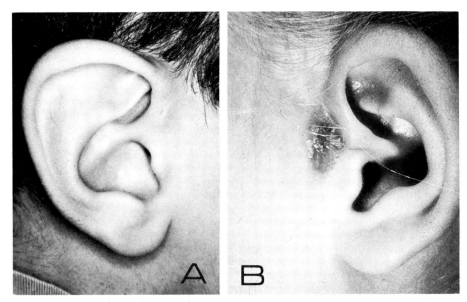

Fig. 8. Preauricular sinuses. A. Uninfected sinus at the root of the helix. B. Infected and repeatedly operated on preauricular sinus.

row. Hearing acuity by air conduction is usually markedly reduced in such ears, but bone conduction is normal, indicating an intact middle and inner ear.

The management of such problems is complex. It is desirable not only to correct the size and shape of the external ear but also to open the external auditory canal to restore binaural hearing. Both procedures are difficult. First, in the present state of our knowledge we do not know how to make a thin layer of skin grow on a thin layer of cartilage—even if both of these items were available to us in the necessary amount and shape. Second, the patient who has a markedly deformed external ear commonly has an abnormal course of the facial nerve, making dissection in the region in which the canal should be opened a procedure fraught with the hazard of injury to the facial nerve. In fact, some patients born with the ear deformity also have accompanying facial weakness or paralysis. However, the area can be dissected safely if the operator is willing to proceed cautiously and with the constant use of a nerve stimulator to identify and preserve the facial nerve.

Most surgeons feel that if the patient has good hearing in the other ear, then opening the deformed canal is not justified. When it is done there is also the difficulty of maintaining its patency unless a canal appreciably larger than the normal is constructed. This difficulty is related to the problem cited

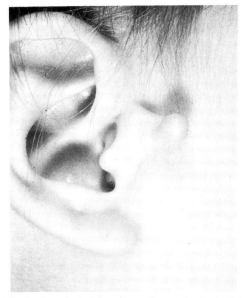

Fig. 9. A typical skin and cartilage tab attached to the tragus of the ear.

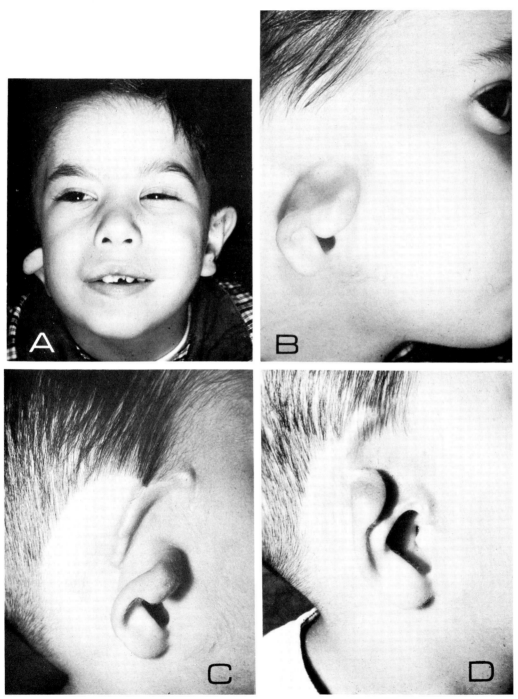

Fig. 10. Reconstruction of the external ear. A and B. Microtia with mild upper facial nerve weakness. C. Implantation of rib cartilage to support upper portion of the helix. D. Curled-up superior border of the ear turned upward to join the transplanted cartilage graft.

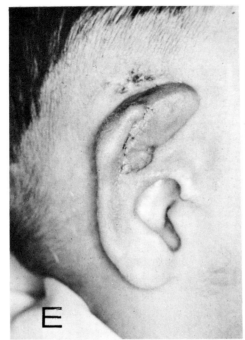
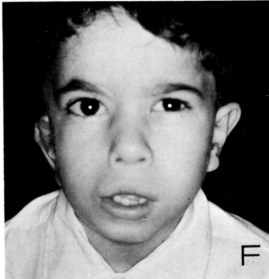

Fig. 10 (cont.). Reconstruction of the external ear. E and F. Results of lifting cartilage graft from mastoid area with a free skin graft.. Note: the entire right ear sits lower on the head than the left one.

above of our inability to graft skin onto a cartilage surface (which is how a normal ear canal is constructed and why its patency is maintained). One usually ends up placing a plastic tube inside the reconstructed canal, and the patient wears this tube indefinitely.

Reconstruction of the external ear was a very difficult and unsatisfactory procedure in most instances until the publication of an excellent article by Tanzer (1963). Although his method requires six or seven steps and an elapsed time of almost two years, the results are far superior to those achieved by any other method. It is strongly urged that the surgeon wishing to do this procedure read and reread the original article. The multitudinous details that are significant to the end result will not be reproduced here.

Tanzer employs autogenous cartilage of three different ribs from the side of the chest opposite to the deformed ear for the framework. It is carefully carved and inserted through a *tragal* incision so that all the mastoid skin can be loosely draped over the new

cartilage framework. The concha is then constructed in a series of three steps which involve lifting the lower portion of the skin-covered cartilage framework away from the head to form a "suitcase handle" and then subsequently reclosing the ear to the head but leaving a depression suggesting a concha. Finally, the tragus is constructed with skin borrowed from the floor of the concha folded on itself at the front of the ear, and the defect in the concha is closed with a free graft (Fig. 10).

It should be stated at this point that the development of Silastic rubber prostheses is progressing so rapidly and that Silastic is so well tolerated by the body that we may, within the next few years, find it feasible to use this material instead of autogenous cartilage as a framework for the construction of an ear. This would materially shorten the time required to construct an ear and would save the patient a significant operation on the chest. Certainly the Silastic prostheses can be more accurately fashioned than the rib cartilage can be by even the most artistic of plastic surgeons.

Hematoma of the ear producing "cauliflower" ear has long been known as a difficult problem to treat. The basic problem, of course, is to find a way to prevent the elevation of the perichondrium from the cartilage, which leads to the growth of new and heavier cartilage on the underside of the elevated perichondrium. This means that the patient must be seen at least within two weeks after the injury. If the patient is seen in the first day or two following injury, the blood separating the cartilage and perichondrium will be clotted and cannot be removed except by incision and extraction of clots. It is probably best to await liquefaction of the clot and then gently aspirate the serum collection. Often it is possible to give the skin an essentially normal contour with this aspiration, but there is a marked tendency for serum to collect again unless adequate pressure can be provided to prevent it. When a large area of the ear is involved the application of an accurately contoured dressing, such as that described on page 251 for dressing the ears after otoplasty, is most likely to succeed. For this dressing to be tolerable for the patient, the pressure on the ear can be no greater than that on the side of the head. This means that a large fluffed mass of dressing placed over the ear is inadequate to achieve contour. The "doughnut" with the ear sticking through equalizes the pressure so that it is no greater on the ear than on the head.

For the small area of hematoma involvement, aspiration followed by an accurate collodion dressing has often succeeded.

KELOIDS

Keloids of the ear are quite common, especially among Negro girls whose mothers or friends have pierced their ears. These keloids require excision and reclosure. However, recurrence is very likely unless triamcinolone acetonide (Kenalog), 0.25 to 0.5 ml, is injected into the margins of the wound at the close of the scar revision (Fig. 11). It is sometimes wise to add prophylactic x-radiation to the above procedures. Larger keloids may occur anywhere about the ear and can present very major problems in reconstruction, as shown in Figure 12. However, the most serious problem is the prevention of the regrowth of the keloid. Until the advent, in 1963, of triamcinolone acetonide for topical injection, the outlook was quite grim. X-radiation was sometimes effective in preventing recurrence, but often it was not. It is now apparent that repeated injections of the corticosteroid can be given,

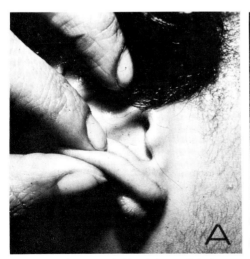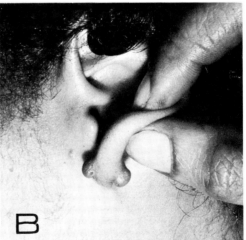

Fig. 11. Keloids of the ear lobules secondary to piercing of the ears for earrings.

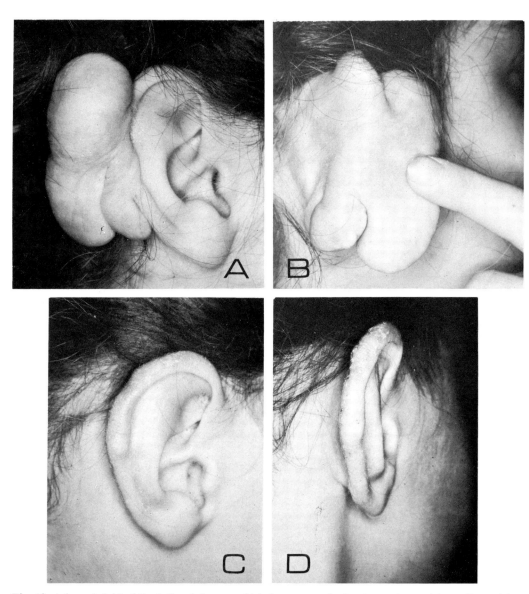

Fig. 12. A large keloid of the helix of the ear which has recurred after two prior excisions. On excision the skin overlying the base of the lesion was spared for primary closure of the wound, but as much of the underlying scar was sacrified as was possible to do without interfering unduly with the blood supply. After the skin was closed, triamcinolone acetonide (Kenalog) was injected into the wound edges completely about the periphery of the wound. The patient was also given irradiation (600 rads) on the same day. The patient has been observed at frequent intervals, but no other treatment has been required in a nine-month followup.

and if one is persistent the overgrowth of fibrous tissue can be prevented.

Injections of triamcinolone acetonide are painful and difficult to give in an old, hard, fibrous keloid or a hypertrophic scar. The drug is most effective if one can spread it through the scar by using a 22-gauge needle and injecting along the tract as the needle is withdrawn. Usually after one or two injections the lesion becomes somewhat softer, and it is then possible to get more of the drug into it. Injections may be given as often as every week or two. The writer has usually given not more than 2 ml at a time, but

Maguire (1965) reports giving up to 6 ml at one time to a nine-year-old child.

Whenever feasible the surgeon should excise the bulk of the keloid, inject the wound edges with triamcinolone acetonide after closure, and then observe the patient closely in the postoperative period. At the first sign of regrowth of the keloid, the scar should be injected with more of the drug. At this time the scar is soft, immature, fibrous tissue and is much more easily distended with the drug. Also, in the immediate postoperative period the scar is relatively anesthetic, and the injections are much less painful than they will be later. One can probably avoid excessive widening of the new scar if one distends it very little with the drug but rather scatters the drug evenly through the scar with a 25- or 27-gauge needle. The heavier needle is not required in a relatively fresh scar.

LACERATIONS

Lacerations of the ear are cared for as elsewhere on the body, utilizing anatomical restoration. It often is valuable to place one or two fine dermal or wire sutures in the cartilage to stabilize the framework. The greatest debate here is whether it is wise to suture on a piece of completely detached lobule or helix. As a rule of thumb, one should not exceed the dictates for using composite grafts from the ear to other portions of the body—that is, if any portion of the free graft is going to be more than 1 cm away from its blood supply, then resuturing the part is valueless. Obviously the condition of both the remaining ear and the detached part in regard to cleanliness, length of period of detachment, and evidences of contusion and disorganization of the tissues plays a real part in making the decision.

On the other hand, the ear laceration which has even a very small pedicle of attachment for a fairly large piece of tissue is practically always a good candidate for successful suture. Again, the application of the conforming dressing as discussed under otoplasty and hematoma may well spell the difference between success and failure.

A fairly common laceration of the ear is the tearing of the earlobe into two pieces by pull on earrings which have been placed through the pierced lobule. The repair is usually better if one adds a Z-plasty to the lower edge of the lobule as well as reattaching the two sides of the lobule to each other.

CLARENCE W. MONROE

REFERENCES

GROTTING, J. K. Otoplasty for cupped ears using a postauricular flap. Plast. Reconstr. Surg., 22: 164, 1958.

MAGUIRE, H. C., Jr. Treatment of keloids with triamcinolone acetonide injected intralesionally. J.A.M.A., 192: 325, 1965.

MURRAY, R. D. Kenalog in treatment of keloids and scars. Plast. Reconstr. Surg., 31: 275, 1963.

TANZER, R. C. An analysis of ear reconstruction. Plast. Reconstr. Surg., 31: 16, 1963.

16

Surgical Treatment of Ear Infections

Purulent ear infections followed by scarring of the eardrum and damage to the middle ear contents used to be common. Today such lesions are rare and have been replaced by an otitis manifested primarily by myringitis, serous effusion, usually without the formation of pus, and accumulation of fluid between the layers of the drum. Loss of drum substance and persistent perforations following infections are rare in properly treated ear infections, for antibiotics quickly eradicate bacterial ear infection. Any hearing loss following otitis media is usually the result of incomplete treatment.

Surgical advances have made possible the replacement of ear ossicles by prostheses. Skin grafts are used to replace damaged tissue and to help restore hearing. Careful selection of patients to be treated with these new techniques is important to secure optimum results.

TYMPANOTOMY

It has long been held that "when in doubt, open the eardrum." This is still valid for acute otitis accompanied by severe pain, temperature elevation, and bulging drum. The pain is usually paroxysmal, occurring every 30 to 90 seconds. Treatment is tympanotomy and the opening of any blebs or fluid-filled bullas. This can be accomplished with a tympanotomy knife, straight bistoury,

diamond-shaped blade, or small gauge needle. Tympanotomy with a knife has the advantage of leaving an opening, the edges of which are opposed and which will seal off as soon as drainage from the acute infection has subsided. A circular opening, produced by a needle, will remain open for a longer period, and at times this may be desirable. Openings made in the lower half of the drum do not endanger middle ear structures.

The second indication for tympanotomy is acute barotrauma associated with a change in altitude such as may be experienced during air travel. Air readily escapes through the eustachian tube into the nasopharynx when pressure is decreased. Because of its anatomy the eustachian tube does not admit air easily from the nasopharynx. Consequently, pressure in the external canal may be sufficiently greater than that in the middle ear to produce pain. Tympanotomy equalizes the pressure, relieves the pain, and restores eustachian tube function.

A third indication is the presence of cerebrospinal fluid in the middle ear following head trauma. Before tympanotomy it is important to establish the diagnosis by hearing tests, skull x-rays, and neurological examination. Infection following tympanotomy is rare, probably because the fluid flows out of the ear rather than back through the drum. Tympanotomy for diagnostic purposes should be done with a tympanotomy knife. A minimal opening encourages healing and prevents the spread of infection into the middle ear and thence through the fistula to the subarachnoid space.

The fourth and commonest reason for tympanotomy is chronic serous effusion in the middle ear. This fluid, which resembles blood serum in its composition, remains in the ear following obstruction of the eustachian tube. Eustachian tube obstruction, which occurs regularly with upper respiratory infections and otitis media, separates the middle ear space from the outside world. Oxygen and nitrogen are absorbed from the middle ear, leaving a greater pressure on the outside of the eardrum. Retraction and brownish discoloration of the drum, with foreshortening of the malleus because of its rotation around the malleolar ligaments, occurs. If the pressure differential is great enough, blood serum will transude into the middle ear space. Fluid may also appear in the ear in response to bacterial infection, and if the virulence of the infecting organism is low or if antibiotics are used and the bacteria are destroyed, then the fluid will often remain and be absorbed slowly. In the normal progress of an otitis or eustachian tube obstruction associated with upper respiratory infections, the tube will eventually regain function and admit air, equalizing pressure and permitting absorption of transudate.

Consequently, restoring eustachian tube function is the single most important factor in the successful treatment of serous otitis. If restoration of function of the tube is not possible or is delayed because of the child's inability to cooperate, tympanotomy is mandatory. This is proper despite long-standing infection and a thickened, leathery drum. Tympanotomy brings air into the middle ear cavity and displacement of fluid either down the eustachian tube or out through the perforation.

Chronic serous effusion in the middle ear produces a thick eardrum. Tympanotomy often fails to produce satisfactory drainage, and insertion of a medium bore needle and aspiration of the middle ear may be required.

This can be done without danger or discomfort as long as the area aspirated is in the inferior half of the drum.

SIMPLE MASTOIDECTOMY

Otitis media is often treated with antibiotics, and the response is usually dramatic, with a drop in temperature and relief of pain. Under certain circumstances the middle ear remains filled with a sterile transudate. This can often be identified by a dull red drum, occasionally bulging. A fluid level may be detected on otoscopy, and inflation of the eustachian tube is usually difficult. If it can be accomplished, there is a momentary improvement of the hearing, which will continue to improve provided repeated aeration of the eustachian tube can be accomplished.

This process may be repeated, and in subsequent infections bacteria may reach the ear either through the eustachian tube or through the general circulation. Bacteria lodging in this sterile transudate multiply rapidly, and within as short a time as half an hour there may be severe pain. If tympanotomy is not done and antibiotics are administered, the transudate will become sterile.

Repetition promotes a gradual buildup of granulation tissue in the middle ear and mastoid. As granulations increase in size around the ossicles, the aditus and antrum tend to close. The separation of the mastoid cavity from the middle ear may be functionally complete in the presence of excess granulations. Posteriorly a thin layer of bone separates the infected material in the mastoid from the jugular bulb. Over the posterior fossa there is usually more bone and less aeration, so that infection inward is not common. The external cortex is often thin, and penetration occurs easily. This is fortunate, for if it occurs the exudate can escape beneath the periosteum and reduce the pressure in the mastoid antrum.

The usual physical finding is swelling behind and above the ear, producing a downward and forward protrusion of the external

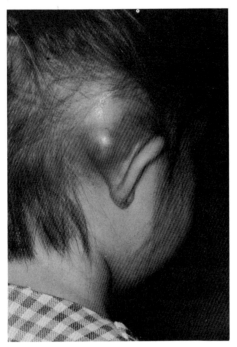

Fig. 1. A patient with acute mastoiditis.

ear (Fig. 1). When first seen, this may be mistaken for cellulitis or an extension of cervical lymphadenitis. This is pathognomonic of acute mastoiditis, yet it is seen so infrequently that it is often unrecognized. The infection may spread forward into the zygomatic root, producing considerable swelling over the temple to the forehead.

Often the infection will have separated itself almost completely from the middle ear and remains as an abscess cavity beneath the periosteum. In some instances the fistula through which the infection spreads to the subperiosteal space has healed so completely that it cannot be identified. In addition, the granulations in the attic region have separated the middle ear from the mastoid, further blocking communication with the abscess cavity. The middle ear space proper may contain no exudate, and consequently the diagnosis of mastoiditis is often delayed until the obvious periosteal abscess has appeared.

Treatment of such an abscess is primarily surgical. Although it is possible to eradicate such an infection with antibiotics, one is always faced with the question whether the infection has spread to the lateral sinus area and become extradural. Even in small children it is possible for complications of mastoiditis to occur, and for this reason it is not entirely safe to use medical treatment alone, especially if x-rays depict definite cloudiness and bone destruction around the mastoid antrum.

Wilde's incisions have long been advocated and certainly merit consideration here; they allow drainage of the subperiosteal abscess. It is assumed that the remaining infection in the mastoid will resolve spontaneously.

However, one cannot know how far the infection has spread until the lateral sinus area and the tegmen tympani have been exposed. This, along with adequate external exposure, is necessary to eliminate possible complications resulting from infections.

Simple mastoidectomy is ordinarily accomplished with a postauricular incision, placed close to the posterior skin fold. The periosteum should be elevated carefully and completely and should be closed at the conclusion of the operation. If the periosteum is closed and a clot is allowed to form in the mastoid cavity, retraction and depression behind the ear accompanying healing will be minimal. Large amounts of bony cortex may be removed without impairment of function. Exenteration of all the infected air cells and removal of all granulation tissue is mandatory. The lateral sinus and dura of the middle fossa should be exposed. Care should be taken to preserve the external bony canal and not to dislodge the incus or to damage the facial nerve. Attention, however, must be paid to the attic area and the area around the incus, to remove granulations and any other tissue obstructing drainage. In recent years it has been possible to close such a cavity without drainage. This allows for formation of a blood clot and for the replacement by scar tissue of the air cells and mastoid space. If there has been no direct damage to the ossicles either by infection or by surgery, then one can expect the patient to have normal hearing. There should also be little or no stenosis of the external membranous canal wall.

CHOLESTEATOMA AND CHRONIC OTITIS MEDIA

The term cholesteatoma has come to mean marginal perforations of the eardrum —that is, those involving the drum at the edge and thereby removing the epithelial barrier at the tympanic annulus, whether in the pars tensa or in the pars flaccida. Because of the invasive tendencies and vigorous growth of the squamous epithelium in the ear canal, there is constantly a tendency for this epithelium to invade adjacent denuded areas or those in which there is a less rapidly growing and less viable epithelium. With the entry of squamous epithelium into the mucus-lined cavity of the middle ear, there may be rapid replacement or crowding out of the cuboidal epithelium and its very delicate underlying connective tissue layer. With the usual desquamation of squamous epithelium, a retained mass of epithelial debris tends to build up in the middle ear, which produces erosion. Low grade infection is common in the deep layers of the epithelium, but, even without this, pressure alone may produce erosion of bone and destruction of mastoid cells, including parts of the labyrinthine capsule. The matrix, or the developing layer from which all the debris is formed, is the significant and active part of the disease, and all the surgery and medical treatment is aimed at controlling the presence or activity of this layer.

It is now being appreciated that the squamous epithelium in the inner half of the external canal is overactive. In this area the epithelium lies on a thin periosteal layer and thus is almost in direct contact with the bone. This epithelium may desquamate and form rather thick crusts in the inner half of the canal and even involve the eardrum. Over a period of time there seems to be some mechanical pressure exerted against these crusts, with some tendency for cavitation of

the canal walls to occur. When these heavy crusts of wax and dead skin are removed, the layer beneath is red and usually without any moisture to indicate active infection. If these crusts and accumulations have been present for a fairly long time, there is a greater tendency to cavitation and to accumulation of infected material beneath the crust. This in turn produces more pressure against the drum, which often becomes thin and atrophic, and there tends to be considerable retraction, particularly in the posterior half of the drum. If the debris is removed when it accumulates and the base is kept dry, the epithelium will often be relatively normal. Even after there has been considerable retraction of the drum and considerable tendency to pocket in the posterior-superior quadrant, an ear such as this can often be cleaned up and will return to normal function. However, the skin does tend to accumulate debris periodically and must be carefully kept clean and free of debris. Many times on initial examination the odor of debris, the retraction of the drum, and the tendency for the posterior-superior quadrant to be pocketed give all the appearances of a secondary perforation and cholesteatoma. Polyps of granulation tissue may even be present, originating from the canal wall. It must be emphasized that in many instances cholesteatomas do appear this way, and this may be visualized even in the same patient in both ears, usually one ear exhibiting greater progress of the disease than the other. Here medical management rather than surgical treatment is the ideal course, unless a frank perforation of the drum and invasion of the mastoid air cells have already occurred.

In deciding whether or not the eardrum is perforated and active mastoid invasion has occurred, these points are helpful:

(1) If movement of the tympanic membrane does not occur with pneumomassage, this indicates that the middle ear space communicates with the external canal and that an actual perforation is present.

(2) If debris is removed from blind areas

in a perforation—that is, if it has accumulated out of view, where it is not directly accessible to swab from the external canal—then one must always suspect invasion of the mastoid air cells.

(3) If repeated cleaning and appropriate medical treatment fail to control purulent drainage, one must use not only conventional drops with and without antibiotics but also powder, irrigations with alcohol, antibotic and enzyme ointments, systemic antibiotics, and so on. If these fail to control infection, one must strongly suspect perforation involving the middle ear space and bone involvement. Careful x-ray examination may in some instances reveal a larger area of mastoid involvement than was suggested by clinical examination.

(4) If there is inadequate drainage to the outside and repeated accumulations of debris in spite of treatment, then there is probably a cavity which is enlarging and which will involve the ossicles or other vital parts of the sound-conducting mechanism, if it has not done so already. This is probably the greatest danger from an incompletely treated perforation and accumulation of cholesteatoma debris. Frequently burrowing behind the drum occurs along with involvement of the ossicles, and there may be a great deal of damage to the sound mechanism without any evidence except that of a thickened drum and, possibly, recurrent drainage and some x-ray changes. The hearing loss is usually moderate in cases such as this because the mass of granulation in cholesteatoma often acts as a sound-conducting mechanism, transmitting the sound to the oval window and maintaining at least a moderate degree of hearing.

RADICAL MASTOID SURGERY

PURPOSES

The first and most important aim in radical mastoid surgery is to eliminate disease, particularly progressive disease. In order to accomplish this, the mastoid is literally "exteriorized." This means that the external canal is opened and the entire mastoid cavity made accessible to the external ear canal. This means removing the posterior and superior canal walls, exenterating mastoid air cells as they are involved, and creating a treatable cavity.

The second aim is to preserve as much as possible the remaining salvable middle ear structures, including the eardrum and the ossicles.

The third purpose is to restore as much as possible of the sound-conducting mechanism to the inner ear. This last, but by no means least important, aim of radical surgery is in part dependent on the adequate accomplishment of the first two aims.

OPERATIVE PROCEDURE

Endaural incisions are used as practiced by Lempert. These give access to the mastoid cortex through the external canal and allow adequate exposure for the uncomplicated radical mastoid approach. The entry into the mastoid is made either through the external canal deep toward the attic or through the cortex beginning in Macewen's triangle and between the linea temporalis above Henle's spine and the posterior canal wall, and a line is drawn vertically from the posterior canal wall. In this triangle and in the area immediately adjacent to it one can enter the mastoid with safety and not be concerned about entering the middle fossa or the lateral sinus. Removal of the mastoid cortex is accomplished either with burrs and drill or with mallet and gouge or, in the case of very small children, even with a sharp curette. The mastoid cells are then excised, including those over the tegmen tympani, over the sinus plate, and into the posterior-superior angle. After the removal of bone and cells along the tegmen tympani forward over the roof of the ear canal is accomplished, the curetting of cells and the removal of infected material is carried down as far as necessary into the mastoid tip, and the posterior and superior canal walls are thinned out. This area, the dura of the middle fossa, may be quite low and very close to the external canal. This will at times create some problems of exposure of the middle ear structures. After the careful removal of bone over the superior canal wall and the thinning of the canal, the mastoid antrum is exposed and the superior and lateral walls of the middle ear are removed. This exposes the incus and the head of the malleus, and all the infected debris in this area is removed. Dissection of the granulation tissue from the ossicles should be carried out using microscopic magnification and the usual tympanoplasty and stapes instruments.

The most important principle in this part of the operation is the complete removal of all infected material. It is extremely important to remove all the matrix of the cholesteatoma in the middle ear space, especially if any skin grafting is to be done or if the middle ear cavity is to be closed, utilizing a skin, vein, muscle, or other type of graft. If the middle ear behind the eardrum has remained free of cholesteatoma or can be thoroughly and completely cleared, then grafting may be done to recreate a middle ear space continuous with the eustachian tube. However, it must be emphasized that surgery must be complete in regard to removing infection and granulation; otherwise, trapped skin beneath the graft will again form a cholesteatoma. If it is not possible to save the ossicles because of partial or complete destruction or because of scarring and impenetrable granulations, then removal of the ossicles will be necessary. Reconstruction of the area, however, can be done if adequate remnants of drum remain. Some protection for the round window can be accomplished quite easily if any drum remains at all, and with grafts of vein, fascia, or skin it may be possible to reconstruct a sound conducting mechanism to the oval window, utilizing polyethylene struts, wire and fat or Gelfoam, or similar prosthetic material. Packing and postoperative care are extremely important, and generally a nonadherent, fine mesh dressing is used over the graft, along with the liberal use of antibiotics in the cavity. After the usual mastoid dressings are in place there will be no need to change the packing until it is removed on the seventh to the twelfth day. Meticulous antisepsis in the followup care is important in keeping the ear free of infection and in promoting healing. Modifications of this procedure that should be mentioned include (1) the use of a temporal muscle flap, swung down from the temporalis muscle at the upper edge of the incision, to obliterate the middle ear space where infection has been so severe that reconstruction is impossible, (2) the closed mastoid technique, in which all of the infection is removed and the ear restored to normal without the removal of the canal wall, and (3) the atticotomy approach, which involves entering the external canal, removing the cells in the posterior-superior quadrant, and opening directly into the mastoid antrum; this last approach is quite satisfactory when disease in the middle ear is limited to a small area.

TYMPANOPLASTY

With the advent of the operating microscope, antibiotics, continuous irrigation during surgery, steroids, and advanced techniques of anesthesia, many new procedures have become possible for restoring function in ears in which perforation has occurred, particularly central perforations of the drum and other instances in which residual hearing loss has occurred because of the anatomical loss of parts of the middle ear.

Where loss of substance of the eardrum has occurred but there is no disease in the middle ear, restoration of function of the eardrum can be accomplished by myringoplasty. The term myringoplasty is used, for instance, in situations in which the eardrum alone is replaced. This can be done in a variety of ways, with either a split skin graft or a full thickness skin graft used externally after proper denudation and preparation of the drum or with a graft placed in the middle ear cavity against the middle ear surface of the drum, held in place with absorbable materials until healing has occurred. The combined use of grafts both on the inside and on the outside of the drum may be desirable. Vein grafts have been used extensively and are very helpful, particularly on the middle ear side of the eardrum. These are effective whether the intimal or adventitious surface of the vein is used against the drum. Temporal fascia and fascia lata have also been used with good results.

Larger defects, which may include loss of the ossicles, either completely or in part, may require the creation of a mechanism for the projection of sound to the round window. If the stapes is gone, a prosthesis may be used, and many of these are available, made of such materials as Teflon, polyethylene, and wire. All depend on a mechanical means of transmitting vibrations received in a skin graft or in what remains of the normal drum to the oval window. In cases of partial obliteration, reaeration of the middle ear may occur, and this is often accompanied by increased hearing, primarily because the normal relationships with the round window are reestablished. Again it must be emphasized that all viable parts of the sound-conducting apparatus are used when possible, not destroyed.

JOHN ELSEN

17

Oral Surgery

ANATOMY OF TONSILS AND ADENOIDS

The lymphoid tissue of Waldeyer's ring is basically divided into two types by the relation to the underlying structures. The first is that of the lingual tonsil, which is composed of single branched crypts and lymph follicles lying directly on muscle tissue of the base of the tongue. This provides a very adequate blood supply associated with frequent movement—swallowing, contraction and expansion of the lymphoid tissue lying on the surface, and so on. The lingual tonsil is very infrequently involved in infection compared to the palatine and pharyngeal tonsils. This may be because of its different arrangement of lymphatics and its close relation to muscular tissue.

The second part of Waldeyer's ring comprises the pharyngeal and palatine tonsils as well as the intermediate mass of lymphoid tissue located in the lateral pharyngeal wall between the tonsils and adenoids, often called the lateral band. These lymphoid structures lie directly on the areolar bed of connective tissue separating them from the surrounding muscle and fascial layers. It is this areolar tissue which appears to make the functional difference between the parts of Waldeyer's ring and explains the frequent spread of infection from the palatine pharyngeal tonsils to the lymphatics, to the lymph nodes, and into the general circulation. This is dramatically demonstrated in persons who have tiny residual lymphoid follicles in the tonsil bed and who have all the symptoms of recurrent tonsillitis until such follicles are removed.

The pharyngeal tonsil is noted for its vertical folds and for its tendency to retain nasal secretions between the folds, and this may be a consideration in tonsillar infection. Infection here is followed by swelling and frequently by obstruction of the eustachian tube by lateral pressure of the adenoid folds against the posterior lip of the torus tubarius. The palatine tonsil is composed primarily of deep, branched crypts surrounded by many lymphoid follicles with germinal centers. These crypts reach into the depths of the tonsil and are confluent in the upper pole in what is called the supratonsillar fossa, reaching to the connective tissue capsule of the tonsil and frequently allowing infection to enter the peritonsillar space by penetration in this area. Infection beginning deep in the tonsils may produce fever, local lymph node swelling, and other signs of sepsis long before redness and exudate are apparent on the surface of the tonsil. The lateral band or lateral tonsil is composed primarily of individual follicles and occasionally has some compound branched crypts. It is located beneath the eustachian tube and on the superior and middle constrictor of the pharynx. It may be very extensive and may produce all the symptoms of tonsillitis when infected. Deep to it lie strands of the styloglossus and stylopharyngeus muscles, which may be removed or damaged during removal of the lateral tonsil.

TONSILLECTOMY

Tonsillectomy and circumcision vie for first place as the most frequently performed operation in children. It is estimated that as many as two million tonsillectomies are performed each year in the United States, and fatalities have been estimated to be approximately three hundred per year in the United States. An operation of this frequency and this mortality certainly deserves thorough and careful consideration by pediatrician, surgeon, and anesthesiologist.

INDICATIONS

In a large series of cases, repeated infections involving the tonsils and adenoids were the indication for operation in approximately 95 percent of the cases. Repeated ear infections and adenoid obstruction were additional indications. These three basic indications are related to all the others listed here —hemorrhagic nephritis, chronic glomerulonephritis with exacerbations following upper respiratory infections, rheumatic fever, failure to gain weight, cervical lymphadenitis, scrofula, mouth breathing, orthodontia problems, adenoid facies, recurrent otitis, conductive hearing loss, and malfunction of the eustachian tubes. The careful examiner will often note infections in the tonsils, and careful history taking will elicit abundant evidence of repeated infections.

Medical opinion concerning the advisability of removing tonsils and adenoids has undergone considerable change. In the 1920's and 1930's it was a popular operation, and entire families were subjected to it. It is claimed, but impossible to prove, that the relatively low incidence of rheumatic fever, rheumatic carditis, and rheumatoid arthritis in individuals who had their tonsils and adenoids removed in the years before antibiotics were available is related to the absence of

the tonsils and adenoids. Early in the 1940's it was generally believed that many people had their tonsils removed unnecessarily, and this is believed by many doctors today. In a community where large numbers of people are seen by the physician on repeated visits, it should be possible to find children who have not improved following tonsillectomy or who have had more infections, but in my experience such children are rare.

Age has often been used as a criterion for tonsillectomy, and the age of five years has often been given as the optimum time for removing the tonsils or as the age before which surgery is not advisable. Tonsillectomy, like any therapeutic operation, is performed when indications exist. No statistics are available concerning the earliest age for tonsillectomy and adenoidectomy, but these operations may be performed before one year of age when sufficient indications are available. Likewise, tonsillectomy may be done in adulthood and even in old age when required. But at the age of five the lymphoid tissues of the body reach their maximum size relative to the total body mass and thereafter constitute a smaller percentage of total body mass.

Another question often raised concerning tonsillectomy is whether the tonsils have any specific function. Tonsillar function is no different from that of the lymphoid tissue in the remainder of the gastrointestinal tract, where lymphoid tissue covered with epithelium of any sort is in close contact with the contents of the alimentary canal. The tonsils constitute a very small amount of the total weight of this tissue, some of the largest amounts being found in the stomach and intestines and even in the colon. If one assumes an immunological function for the tonsils, then that function can undoubtedly be taken over by the lymphoid tissue in the remainder of the gastrointestinal tract.

CONTRAINDICATIONS

The first contraindication to tonsillectomy is active infection, whether it be pulmonary tuberculosis, acute tonsillitis, exanthema, or any other acute disease. The second contraindication is a blood clotting defect.

PREPARATION OF THE PATIENT

Many books, records, and pamphlets are now available to explain the procedure of tonsillectomy and adenoidectomy to the child and to condition him for them. These can be used with great effectiveness to allay fear and to explain to the child exactly what will happen. In many instances it is the unknown that prompts fear reactions in children, and when a matter-of-fact presentation of the actual procedure is made, not once but several times, the child becomes familiar with what will happen. If this is then followed by a sympathetic and understanding approach on the part of the surgeon, the anesthesiologist, the orderlies, and the operating room and floor nurses, the experience of tonsillectomy can be free of apprehension and fear.

ANESTHESIA

In almost every progressive institution anesthesia is conducted by endotracheal tube and with one of a number of satisfactory agents. Ether, ethyl chloride, and other anesthetic agents have been replaced to a considerable extent by halothane anesthesia with or without the use of muscle-relaxant drugs. The use of the endotracheal tube has assured the surgeon of an adequate airway. The endotracheal tube can be easily manipulated so that it is out of the operative field. The depth of anesthesia plays an important part in the ease of surgery and in the amount of bleeding.

TECHNIQUE

The objective of removing the tonsils and adenoids is to eliminate as much as possible the association of lymphoid tissue with the areolar connective tissue in the tonsil and adenoid fossa. There are two general techniques: dissection and mechanical methods. It may well be objected that dissection is an old-fashioned technique and has been supplanted by newer mechanical methods of surgery. When the dissection technique is used the objective is to reach the connective tissue space immediately deep to the tonsil capsule and to free the tonsil from the surrounding connective tissue by sharp dissection. Although there are a multitude of variations in technique and a multitude of small details which facilitate the ease of this procedure, two important principles are outstanding. The first is that the lymphoid tissue alone be removed. This means that the dissection must be kept close to the cleavage plane separating the tonsil from the areolar tissue around it and that excess mucous membrane and other tissue not containing lymph follicles must not be removed. The second principle is to remove as completely as possible all lymphoid follicles from the tonsil bed, as well as from the adjacent base of the tongue, pillars, and supratonsillar fossa, particularly that portion about the uvula. Even a few small follicles growing into the tonsillar fossa may behave like an entire tonsil in allowing susceptibility to infection.

In the mechanical techniques of tonsillectomy the dissection of the cleavage plane ordinarily carried out with sharp or blunt instruments, or both, is accomplished by a wire loop (Beck type) or by a sharp blade (Sluder type) (Fig. 1). The technique is basically the same. The tonsil is everted from its fossa, and the ring of the instrument is placed in such a way that the cutting force is directed between the tonsil proper and the fossa in which it lies. This method misses solitary follicles on the pillars and may leave lymph follicles in the plica triangularis between the tonsil, the pillars, and the base of the tongue. Removal of these lymph follicles is mandatory. Except for the surface blood vessels and those entering the hilus of the tonsil, other adjacent blood vessels pass close to the tonsil but not into it.

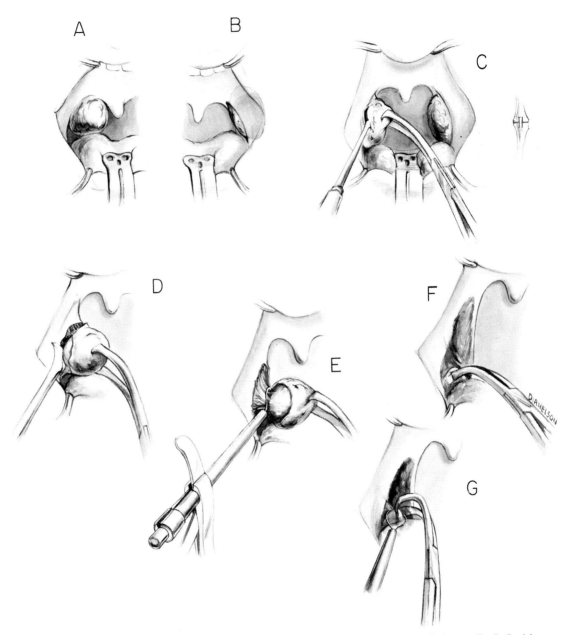

Fig. 1. Tonsillectomy. A. Everted, or pedunculated, tonsil. B. Inverted, or "buried," tonsil. C. Incision through the mucosa anteriorly, superiorly, and posteriorly. D. Blunt or sharp dissection or both, separating the tonsil from its muscular bed. E. Snare used at the lower pole to separate connective tissue from the tonsil. F. Grasping the plica triangularis at the base of the tongue. G. Removing the plica with a snare.

Removal of the lateral tonsil is most frequently accomplished with retractors and the use of punch forceps of various kinds. Because of the elusive nature of the follicles, the retracting technique is most important, and without satisfactory retraction it is impossible to remove all the follicles. Since the lateral tonsil lies over the junction of the middle and superior constrictors, commonly called Passavant's cushion, it is important to remove follicles in this area with great care to avoid damaging the constrictor function of the pharynx. Also, it is quite easy to go too deep and to reach vertical muscle fibers from the styloid muscles. The lateral tonsil actually lies in something of a fossa beneath the eustachian tube, and if care is not exercised, one may damage the tube itself by injudicious removal of tissue high on the lateral wall.

Removing the adenoid is at one and the same time the easiest and the most poorly performed part of the procedure (Fig. 2). Unfortunately, the adenoid is not as well encapsulated as the tonsil. Commonly there is a large adenoid mass in the center and often high in the nasopharynx, with lesser amounts being located laterally around the eustachian tubes. It should be emphasized that both adenotome and curettes should be

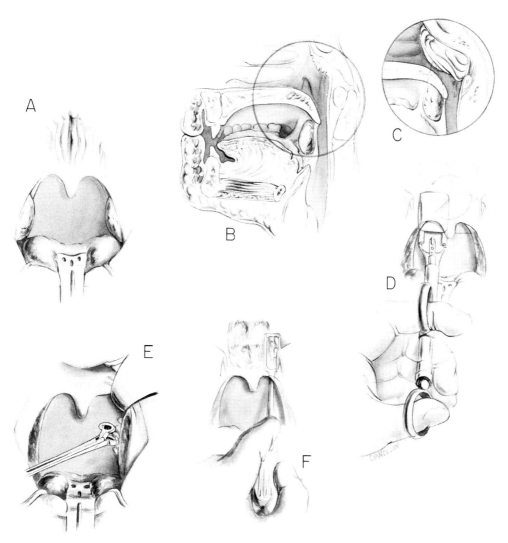

Fig. 2. Adenoidectomy. A. Relation of the adenoid to the palate and the eustachian tube opening in an older child. B. Adult adenoid and nasopharynx. C. Child's adenoid and nasopharynx. D. An adenotome being used to assure removal of all central adenoid tissue. E. Follicles (lateral band) behind the posterior pillar being removed with a punch forceps. F. A curette being used to remove follicles behind the eustachian tube.

used carefully to remove all lymphoid tissue. The most frequent reason for adenoid recurrence is incomplete removal, and this in turn comes from a failure to remove the uppermost part of the adenoid proper. In some instances either the curette or the adenotome, or both, is forced up along the posterior wall and underneath the uppermost portion of the adenoid rather than being brought first forward against the soft palate and then upward into the roof of the nasopharynx and down on the remaining mass of adenoid tissue.

One other common mistake in using the adenotome is a failure to appreciate the contour of the nasopharynx. It is essentially a vault and curves forward from the first cervical vertebra into the back of the nose at the rostrum of the sphenoid. It takes on the curve of the bodies of the cervical vertebra, and injudicious angling or twisting of the adenotome may allow the blades to engage the eustachian tube on either side.

Careful removal of the lymphoid tissue behind the eustachian tubes is most important. Visualization of the nasopharynx can be accomplished in part by the use of Yankauer or Love type retractors or by the use of catheters through the nose and out through the mouth with retraction against the soft palate. Since it is impossible to see the vault of the nasopharynx, palpation is important.

CONTROL OF BLEEDING

There are almost as many ways to control primary bleeding as there are techniques and variations in the removal of the tonsils and adenoids. In primary bleeding, that occurring during the first 24 hours immediately following surgery, it is usually possible to visualize the palatine tonsil fossa so that bleeding can be controlled directly by ligature suture placed through the bleeding point. This applies in the case of the lateral tonsil as well as in that of the lower portion of the pharyngeal tonsil. If bleeding persists from the adenoid area, then the surgeon

should consider a postnasal pack before the patient leaves the operating room. Controlled hypotension during anesthesia or a somewhat deeper plane of anesthesia will often ensure hemostasis long enough for adequate clotting to occur.

The control of bleeding following surgery is a test of the surgeon's skill. The following points are important. The child should be lying on his back with his arms over his head, so that head movements can be controlled by restraining his arms. Suction may or may not be required. The most important factor is the use of local anesthesia. While there may be some exceptions to this, it is a rule that is followed almost universally that no child should be put to sleep a second time for tonsil hemorrhage. The reason for this rule is the amount of blood loss has often been underestimated and the child is very close to a state of shock and often has a stomach full of blood. Injudicious anesthesia may result in vomiting, aspirations, and other disasters. Local anesthesia removes these dangers. Small amounts of adrenalin (1:100,000 or less) with local anesthesia prompt hemostasis as well as relieve the pain and discomfort of manipulation of the throat. Local anesthesia permits one to examine the throat and place sutures for control of bleeding. Astringents, applications of caustics, etc., should not be the primary method of dealing with bleeding but may be used after hemostasis to ensure a firm coagulum over the raw surface. Bleeding from the adenoid fossa also can very often be controlled by injection of anesthetic vasoconstrictor combinations, and, if it cannot, then a postnasal pack is required. There are conflicting reports on the efficacy of various injectable agents for the control of bleeding. It must be emphasized that in the presence of active bleeding, whether primary or secondary, the direct control of the bleeding point by suture or other local means is of prime importance, and other methods should be relied upon only as adjuvants. The one exception to this is the occasional patient in whom the usual membrane does not form over the exposed surface of tonsil and adenoid bed. This is an inherited characteristic, and when the patient having it is seen, usually several hours after surgery, there is complete absence of the usual formation of membrane composed of fibrin and red cells. The tonsil fossa looks as fresh as though dissection had just been completed. In such instances it is necessary to create a coagulum with the use of caustics of one sort or another. When this is done, there is usually complete cessation of bleeding, and healing is not delayed.

HEALING AND RECOVERY

In general, once a firm membrane has formed over the raw surface, there is no danger of bleeding until the sloughing off of the membrane during the healing process. No figures are available on the incidence of delayed primary bleeding (beginning 8–24 hours after surgery), but in my experience it occurs in less than 1 in 1,000 cases. For this reason, children are allowed to return home 8 hours after surgery. Recovery is usually most rapid in children who begin to take fluids and eat food early in their convalescence. When this is encouraged, it is not uncommon to see a child go home after tonsillectomy in the morning and have a part of a meal in the evening and begin eating the next day as though nothing had occurred. The most important factor is the maintenance of fluid intake. The child has usually been without fluids since the night before surgery and may have vomited one or more times after surgery, losing more fluid and chlorides. For this reason, it is common for children following surgery to replenish their chlorides with salty foods by their own volition, which does no harm to the exposed tonsillar fossas. Solid foods are usually chewed, brought to the center of the mouth, and injected into the esophagus without reaching the tonsil fossas at all. Liquids and such solids as gelatin and ice cream do reach the lateral parts of the throat and for this reason often

produce discomfort when taken immediately after surgery.

Bleeding from the fourth to the eighth day occurs as often as 1 in 50 patients and is almost always the result of separation of the tonsillar membrane before healing is complete. The bleeding is usually minor, and caustics are indicated rather than injection of local anesthetic and placement of sutures. While one might expect that infections following tonsil and adenoid surgery would be rather frequent because of the large number of bacteria in the mouth and the infected nature of the tonsils and adenoids themselves, this is an infrequent occurrence. About 25 percent of patients have bacteremia following tonsillectomy. This complication is transient and seldom of any consequence. However, one should not ignore temperatures above the usual 100°–101° F by rectum in the afternoon, and the patient should be treated with antibiotics. Local treatment with antibiotic lozenges is of some value. Local antibiotics do reduce the frequency of infection in the throat as well as bleeding and may be used at the discretion of the surgeon. However, Rhoads has also shown that prolonged use of antibiotics, particularly penicillin, may allow the appearance of pathogens in the throat which would not normally be found there and may create the hazard of a more serious infection.

TONSILLECTOMY AND ADENOIDECTOMY IN CLEFT PALATE PATIENTS

The intimate relationship of the palatine tonsil to the palate musculature and to the bulk and movement of the soft palate can be readily appreciated in the normal individual. It becomes of critical importance in the patient who has poor or impaired palate function following cleft palate surgical repair and in the patient whose palate musculature is inadequate to accomplish velopharyngeal closure. For this reason, any surgery on the tonsils and adenoids must be very carefully studied in relation to any palate function that is present and to what may be expected to remain following surgery.

It is well-known that children with palate abnormalities have more than the usual number of throat infections and very frequently have poorly functioning eustachian tubes and conductive hearing loss. Although each case of this type must be evaluated individually, the benefits to be derived from removing the tonsils and adenoids being weighed against the adverse effects of leaving them in, there are certain guidelines that may be followed. The first is the relationship of the tonsils to the musculature of the pillar. In many instances the tonsils are quite large and deeply buried between the muscles of the anterior and posterior pillars and rest firmly on the lateral pharyngeal musculature. In cases such as this, one can expect, even with careful dissection, that there will be some atrophy and scarring as well as lateral retraction of both the anterior and the posterior pillars following surgery. If the function of these muscles is poor or inadequate to begin with, one may expect that with additional scarring there will be still further impairment of function. On the other hand, if the tonsil is largely everted and attached in a relatively small area, with reasonably good function of the pillars, one may expect to remove it with little or no disability following the procedure. The reason for this is that scarring will be minimal, and loss of muscle function will likewise be very slight if it occurs at all. A second consideration is the amount of closure that is accomplished by the tonsils themselves. In some individuals with large tonsils that fill up the fossa, there may be a very considerable bulk effect, and this may significantly contribute to the closure of the soft palate and to the maintenance of satisfactory speech. In such cases one is reticent to remove tonsils unless the infections are of sufficiently serious consequence to outweigh any adverse effect on speech following surgery. If, on the other hand, the tonsils do not contribute bulk to the closure of the pharynx and to the func-

tion of the palate and speech, then one can remove them with little likelihood of consequent difficulty in speaking.

The second and perhaps more important problem in relation to the function of adenoid tissue is velopharyngeal closure. The large adenoid mass which is often present in children with cleft palates provides an excellent pad against which the poorly functioning or weak soft palate may elevate and form closure with a minimum of muscular effort. If this large pad of tissue is removed, a much greater movement on the part of the palate is required to accomplish the same functional closure. This is often impossible in the child with a cleft palate. For this reason it is often advisable, even in badly infected cases, to remove only a portion of the adenoid. This can be very easily accomplished by the simple expedient of removing only the lateral portions of adenoid tissue. By direct vision and with the examining finger it is possible to determine how much tissue must be removed in order to allow for adequate aeration of the eustachian tube and to eliminate pressure against its surface. Often just removing the lymphoid tissue posterior to the tube, with a sharp curette carefully delineating the area from the central portion of the adenoid, will allow satisfactory function on each side. The torus tubarius and the eustachian tube opening then lie free in an island position in the lateral wall of the nasopharynx, and secretion from the nose may then course easily down each side of the tube, rather than bathing its entire surface in thick and often infected secretion. Posterior contraction of the palate against the central adenoid mass may cause some spread of this mass laterally toward the tubes on each side, but this is seldom of any serious consequence. It continues to accomplish closure at least in the central area, which allows for only a small escape of air on each side. This, then, in effect accomplishes the same thing as a pharyngeal flap in providing functional closure of the nasopharynx for speech purposes while allowing adequate ventilation and drainage of secretion from the nose when the child is not speaking. Again it must be emphasized that in all the decisions concerning tonsil and adenoid surgery in cleft palate cases there must be a careful evaluation of the expected functional result in terms of the child's speech. This is not to say that infection is not as important in these children as it is in others, but one is sometimes faced with a decision about which defect will ultimately have the least adverse effect on the life of the individual. Since antibiotics, gamma globulin, vitamin therapy, autogenous vaccine, and many other means are available for the control of infection, the surgeon is not faced with such narrow alternatives in his decision.

PARAPHARYNGEAL ABSCESS

Parapharyngeal abscess has not been common since the improvement in the general health of the pediatric population brought about by better nutrition and the use of antibiotics. There still remain, however, occasional instances in which sepsis of particular virulence in an individual of less than usual resistance results in a retropharyngeal or parapharyngeal abscess. It is extremely important that such an individual be handled properly, so that systemic effects of sepsis as well as the complications of surgical drainage can be avoided.

For practical reasons one may group parapharyngeal and retropharyngeal abscesses together, since they both represent collections of pus external but adjacent to pharyngeal constrictors. In the case of the retropharyngeal abscess, it is usually seen before the age of two or three years and represents suppuration in the retropharyngeal lymph nodes that are commonly found up to the age of two or three years. After this age there is considerable atrophy of the nodes, and infection seldom occurs in this area. The parapharyngeal abscesses or lateral pharyngeal abscesses are also commonly the result of virulent infection involving the pharynx itself that spreads to and penetrates the mu-

cous membrane and involves the surrounding connective tissue. The infection of these spaces is limited very definitely by facial cleavage planes, and these also make it easy for the surgeon to determine the method of drainage.

The most important consideration in the drainage is to have the child's upper respiratory tract under complete control at all times. There is often a temptation to open an abscess under less than optimum conditions, but this is to be avoided. Optimum conditions are basically as follows:

(1) Drainage or aspiration of abscesses should be done in the operating room or in a place where full anesthetic and cardiac resuscitation equipment is available as well as adequate suction and oxygen.

(2) The child must always be positioned so that his head is lower than any part of the respiratory tract. This allows for drainage of pus out of the airway, eliminates problems of aspiration, and so forth.

(3) Aspiration of all suspected areas should be done first with a needle and syringe or suction so that it can be determined whether pus is present before incision is carried out. Needle aspiration is seldom accompanied by any complication and is a most satisfactory way to determine just where the pus is and how much one may expect to remove by aspiration. After the pus has been located, incision and drainage may be carried out. This must always be done in a vertical fashion so that large blood vessels are not cut across. Even though the circular muscle fibers of the pharynx are cut across, this is the only safe method of incision and drainage. Most surgeons prefer to make a relatively small incision and to spread it with forceps or scissors to provide further exposure. The use of drains in such incisions depends entirely on the amount of pus found, its depth, and the surgeon's estimate of the need for drainage.

(4) The monitoring of the heart beat either by stethoscope or by continual palpation of the pulse is most important during the operative procedure. It is very easy for

a vagal reflex to occur and to affect the pulse rate markedly.

(5) Equipment for intubation of the larynx should be immediately at hand for instances of aspiration of purulent material or in case of cardiac arrest.

LACERATIONS OF THE MOUTH

The most frequent mouth injury is that which results when a child falls on a blunt object that is already in his mouth. Lollipop sticks, pencils, and rods of various kinds, toys, spoons, and other utensils are very frequent offenders. They produce lacerations of all sizes and shapes, many of which are everted and which present areolar tissue and occasionally adipose tissue through the wound area. In general, these need be sutured only if the edges of the wound gape more than $\frac{1}{2}$ to 1 cm. In most instances the laceration will be partially closed by blood that has coagulated in the wound edges. When laceration is extensive, closure with interrupted catgut in the usual fashion is in order. One must always remember to provide adequate drainage for infection to any wound in the mouth.

Lacerations of the tongue are sometimes quite severe and often accompanied by a large amount of bleeding. This is because of the large blood vessels running in the substance of the tongue muscle and the ease with which the teeth cause penetrating wounds to the tongue. The teeth, of course, carry many virulent pathogenic and saprophytic organisms deep into the wound, and this creates some problem with regard to antisepsis. If the laceration of the tongue is sufficiently large, then silk or buried catgut provides the best suture. Through and through suture exposed on the surface of the tongue is seldom satisfactory, and an inverted suture is usually best, with a knot buried deep in the tongue. Large sutures are seldom required even though muscle tissue is quite friable and not easy to work with. Hydrogen peroxide and local antiseptics are frequently used following surgery. These

may delay healing but are advantageous in keeping the area clean.

FRENULECTOMY

Frenulectomy is most commonly done at the parents' behest for fear of some impairment of movement of the tongue and some deficiency in speech development. A considerable number of children with short frenula will develop normal speech without any special attention or care. The only instance in which there may be a definite speech impairment is when the frenulum is so short that the tongue cannot be protruded between the upper and lower teeth. Without this ability, the *th* sound is often affected. Since the great majority of tight frenula are not this severe, correction may be done at any time. The simplest and most accepted method is simple clamping of the frenulum immediately beneath the tongue so that there is no disturbance in the area of the openings to Wharton's duct. After clamping and cutting through the clamped area, a single suture is put at the apex of the incision in order to prevent the mucous membrane edges from spreading at this point. This will usually allow for satisfactory healing in a very short period of time with no disability.

THE NOSE

There has been a tremendous change in thinking concerning nasal infections and surgery in children in the past 25 years, particularly because of the emphasis placed by A. J. Proetz on the functional evaluation of the nose. The physiology of the nose has been taught to more than a generation of otolaryngologists, and for this reason there has been marked improvement in understanding of the nose, what makes it work and what will help when its function is not normal. Generally speaking, the indications for surgery are much more stringent now than at any other time, and this has resulted in much better rehabilitation of function in those individuals who have nasal problems.

Whereas allergy is not a surgical condition, it is such a frequent cause of nasal congestion that one must consider it present until the contrary is proved. The presence or absence of allergic reaction is suggested by a carefully obtained history, followed by a careful search of the nasal secretion for the presence of eosinophils. Even a small number of eosinophils in the nasal secretion is significant, particularly when they are found closely spaced. This is a very strong indication of active nasal allergy.

NASAL TRAUMA

In infants the nasal bones are extremely small and are protected by the overlying frontal bone as well as by the soft tissue of the face, maxilla, and mandible. Even with direct trauma caused by falling flat on the face, there is seldom sufficient nasal bone present for an injury to be sustained. If one draws a line on the lateral x-ray of the skull from the frontal boss down to the chin, one does not very often encounter even the tip of the nasal bone in the newborn. This condition continues to a greater or lesser extent through childhood, up to adolescence. During adolescence the nose usually increases markedly in size and may double its dimensions in a few years.

The most common injury to the nose is deviation of the nasal septum, with or without fracture. Septal deviations are best understood in the light of the development of the septum. The nasal septum is composed of three parts, the first and most obvious one being the quadrilateral cartilage. This is located in an angle of 90° or less between the perpendicular plate of the ethmoid, the vomer, and the maxillary crest. The cartilage sometimes extends back between these two bones almost to the rostrum of the sphenoid, particularly in infants. However, in most adults the perpendicular plate and vomer join directly together, and with the quadrilateral cartilage join in a so-called three-cornered hat. Because the rate of growth of the bones and the cartilage may differ, it is possible to have a marked overgrowth or undergrowth of the cartilage, with a result-

ant internal septal deformity. This differential rate of growth is the most frequent cause of septal deviations and is seen in many children and adults in whom there is no history or evidence of trauma to the nose. The degree of variation may vary from a very minute amount to almost complete obstruction of one or both nostrils.

Traumatic deviation of the nasal septum most commonly involves the quadrilateral cartilage and consists primarily of dislocation of the cartilage out of the shallow groove in the maxillary crest and vomer in which it normally lies. If there is already a differential rate of growth and the septum is somewhat larger than the space in which it lies, there will be an immediate release of tension, and the dislocated portion will be difficult, if not impossible, to return to its previous position. In addition to the lateral dislocation, there is very frequently a posterior dislocation. This tends to push the cartilage at the tip of the nose downward and backward, producing a buckling effect. Often there is a fracture of the cartilage and an overlapping of the fragments. This produces not only deviation but also duplication of the septal cartilages at the point of fracture and reduces the amount of space available for air passage.

Treatment of the acute dislocation is perhaps one of the most controversial subjects in nasal surgery. Rhinoplastic surgeons debate this matter and write prolifically about it. To operate on a freshly fractured nose where considerable hematoma and swelling is already present in addition to softening of the tissues is at best very difficult. It is no wonder that even the experienced nasal surgeon sometimes cannot produce a thoroughly satisfactory result. In many instances it is wisest to let the nose heal and then operate on the nose when known and predictable qualities of mucous membrane, cartilage, bones, and scar tissue can be identified. This is commonly done with tendon lacerations, with good results, and a similar procedure may often be best in the nose. There is a reasonable chance that a good result will occur. The packing of the nose after reduction, along with the use of external splints of metal or molding compound, is in order, probably the most important factor being the packing within the nose, which maintains the fragments as close to normal position as possible.

FRACTURES OF THE NASAL BONE

Nasal bone fractures usually involve the distal half of the nasal bone in its thinnest and most delicate part and also involve the adjacent membranes, which may be in the process of beginning ossification. Depression is the most common result, accompanied by deviation. Only in very severe injuries may one expect zygomatic involvement or involvement of the orbital rim or upper teeth. The upper lateral cartilages underlie the nasal bones for as much as half of their length and provide quite an adequate splint for most simple fractures on the nasal bones. When the cartilages have been dislocated from the bones or are themselves markedly deformed or depressed, then one must rely heavily on intranasal packing after reduction to maintain the position of the nose. With realignment of the fragments in their normal position there is often a "leveling" in place, and no fixation is required. External splints are quite commonly used and are probably as effective in reminding the child not to touch his nose as they are in protecting it from further trauma. In most children healing will have progressed quite satisfactorily in 14 days, and even earlier in very small children. After three weeks the nose is almost as solid as at any previous time, and bandages or dressings are rarely required this long.

ETHMOIDITIS

The most frequent infection in children is that involving the ethmoid sinuses. It is usually manifested by simple purulent drainage from the upper straits of the nose and will often clear without difficulty if adequate nasal ventilation and drainage are provided.

The first sign of acute ethmoiditis is swelling over or under the inner canthus, or both. It progresses rapidly, with marked edema, often closing the eye and accompanied by a slight fever and considerable leukocytosis. The reason for this is apparent from the anatomy of the ethmoid capsule. The orbital wall of the ethmoid is extremely thin and is traversed by a number of small blood vessels. Infection both directly and through retrograde thrombophlebitis may occur on the orbital side of the ethmoid capsule, and this immediately produces a tissue response.

There is a great temptation to look for pus in the ethmoid sinuses. Although pus is occasionally found, it is most frequently not the case. For this reason, it is strongly urged that needling or opening of ethmoid cells not be done unless there is a pointing abscess. The three cardinal points of treatment are (1) adequate use of antibiotics, (2) maintenance of ventilation of the nasal fossa, and (3) provision for adequate drainage from the nasal area. If these three things are done, improvement may be expected, although it may be slow. Differentiation from streptococcus cellulitis of the eyelids, cavernous sinus thrombosis, maxillary osteomyelitis, and so on, must be made.

Infections of the other sinuses are extremely rare in children and should be dealt with in a somewhat different way. The first is that of acute maxillary sinusitis, which sometimes occurs in swimmers. It is not usually found in small children and is more common in adolescence. It is a definite osteomyelitis of the superior maxilla. The edema is severe, often producing serious effects on the contents of the orbit, even leading to blindness. Here again there is a great temptation to approach the problem surgically, but the only manipulative procedure that should be done is drainage by antrum puncture and irrigation or displacement of pus from the ethmoids and sphenoids. One must always remember that the lateral walls of the maxillary sinuses contain the unerupted permanent teeth.

JOHN ELSEN

18

Endoscopic Techniques in Children

Pediatric endoscopy requires a well-coordinated team that includes the endoscopist, the head holder, the scrub nurse, and the circulating nurse. The technique of peroral endoscopy in children varies somewhat from that used in the adult, because of the patient's small size and his lack of cooperation, and because of anatomical variations in the proportions of the endoscopic field. In adults the procedures are usually done under topical or general anesthesia, general anesthesia being reserved for anatomically, technically, or psychologically difficult cases. In contrast, in infants and children many of these examinations are done without anesthesia, and in older children with minimal amounts of topical anesthesia. With the newer, safer general anesthetics now available, however, a shift toward the more frequent use of general anesthesia is apparent. Preoperative sedation with morphine sulfate is given to children two years old and older in amounts varying with the child's size and with the amount of respiratory obstruction present. In addition, when the collection of secretions for laboratory study is not necessary, atropine is added to the preoperative sedation to minimize the amount of secretion. With the infant or child well wrapped in a restraining sheet, brief procedures need no anesthesia. For longer procedures, such as the removal of extensive papillomatous obstructions of the larynx, however, general anesthesia is an advantage, provided an adequate airway can be maintained. General anesthesia also is helpful during the removal of difficult esophageal foreign bodies, where relaxation of the patient is necessary in solving the mechanical problems which may be encountered.

THE LARYNX

LARYNGOSCOPY

For laryngoscopy in children, several types of laryngoscopes are available, with a range of sizes for each type. The most commonly used laryngoscope is tubular, with a spatula which is slightly curled at its distal end. A proximal removable section is provided to facilitate the introduction of a bronchoscope or the use of instruments. This type is most useful for a general overall view of the pharynx, the base of tongue, and the larynx because a wide visual field is obtained when the blade is inserted into the vallecula. The size and shape of the epiglottis and the motility of the cords can be evaluated prior to viewing the arytenoepiglottic folds, arytenoids, and interior structures of the larynx. This overall survey is most important in children with laryngomalacia, since the curled epiglottis and inspiratory fluttering of the arytenoids are more easily evaluated if the epiglottis is not freed under the blade of the laryngoscope. At the same time, the motility of the vocal cords can be more easily studied when the epiglottis or aryepiglottic folds are not fixed by the blade. Poor motility of the cords may give a false impression of a vocal cord paralysis if these extrinsic fixations are not carefully avoided. The disadvantage of the standard laryngoscope is that visualization of the anterior commissure may be impossible, since soft tissue structures usually slide into the field of vision anteriorly. Special anterior commissure laryngoscopes are available which are tubular in shape and somewhat pointed anteriorly to overcome this difficulty. A smooth-tipped anterior commissure laryngoscope has a light carrier slanted into the tube so that this laryngoscope can, in certain instances, be passed between the cords without soft tissue trauma, allowing observation of the immediate subglottic or proximal trachea. The flare-tip anterior commissure scope is also a tubular instrument, with the distal tip of the scope widened to increase its field of vision. Because of this widening, examination with this type of laryngoscope is limited to the area above the level of the vocal cords and to the cords themselves.

TECHNIQUE OF LARYNGOSCOPY

All of the laryngoscopes mentioned above are introduced into the larynx with the same basic motions. The child is held firmly by the head holder, with the neck flexed slightly on the chest and the head extended on the neck. A bite block is placed between the jaws on the left side and held in place by the head holder, whose right arm passes under the neck of the child and whose left hand lifts the occiput. The endoscopist then introduces the scope on the right side of the mouth, and the instrument is passed laterally to the tongue and advanced to the vallecula. The epiglottis is then easily identified. In very small children the tongue is lifted forward at approximately 45° from the horizontal. It is important to avoid all leverage back against the upper gum, which produces severe dis-

comfort. In older infants and children, in whom the epiglottis has become flatter than the omega-shaped infant epiglottis, the lip of the laryngoscope must be passed behind the epiglottis in order to visualize completely the interior of the larynx. With firm anterior lifting of the larynx, the entire structure is raised above the secretions that frequently accumulate on the posterior pharyngeal wall and often obstruct all visualization of the larynx. After the mouth and pharynx are aspirated, the base of the tongue, vallecula, epiglottis, true and false cords, aryepiglottic folds, and arytenoids are observed and evaluated in terms of their mobility and shape and the character of the mucous membranes. The subglottic regions must also be evaluated, particularly if no abnormality is seen at a higher level.

TRACHEA AND BRONCHI

BRONCHOSCOPY

Bronchoscopy in infants and children begins with the technique used for laryngoscopy. It is necessary to stabilize the larynx with the standard laryngoscope while the bronchoscope is introduced between the vocal cords into the trachea, particularly when no anesthesia is used. With the bronchoscope in the trachea, the slide of the laryngoscope is withdrawn so that the main portion of the laryngoscope itself can be removed before the bronchoscopic evaluation is begun. A variety of bronchoscopes are available. Which one is chosen depends on the size of the child and whether or not continuous aspiration of the bronchial secretions is necessary. Most bronchoscopes have an aspirating channel as well as the usual side channel for insufflating oxygen if it should be needed. Scopes modified with extra small light carriers in diameters of 3 mm, 3.5 mm, 4 mm, and 5 mm give a much needed increase in the interior diameter of the child's size bronchoscope.* For the intermittent removal

* Available from George Pilling & Sons, Philadelphia, Pa.

of secretions, independent aspirators of appropriate length are used. Flexible aspirators are available for obtaining secretions from the upper lobes. The tubing is attached to a trap for collecting sputum specimens for bacteriological study or chemical analysis.

Once the bronchoscope is introduced into the trachea and the laryngoscope has been removed, the bronchoscope is supported in place with the fingers of the left hand, which rest lightly on and protect the lips, the upper teeth, and the gums. The general pattern for inspection of the tracheobronchial tree is the same as it is in the adult. There are some noticeable differences, however, in the appearance of the various structures in the pediatric age group. Mucous membranes seem slightly pinker and more velvety-looking than those seen in adults, and the movement of the tracheobronchial tree is much more noticeable. Some of this movement, of course, is a result of the restlessness of the unanesthetized child, but the whole appearance always has much more flexibility than it has in the adult. This is especially apparent in tracheomalacia or bronchomalacia. The carina appears somewhat broader in the child than in the adult, a reflection of the shorter, broader chest of the infant and young child.

After the trachea and the carina have been aspirated, the scope is directed into the right main bronchus, and the orifices of the right upper, middle, and lower lobes are inspected individually. Secretions are aspirated as they collect, and the configuration, motility, and mucosa are noted in all of the bronchial segmental orifices. The left side is similarly examined. In order to facilitate passage of the bronchoscope into the left bronchus the patient's shoulders must remain in the midline, and the head must be brought far to the right in a slightly flexed position.

BRONCHOGRAPHY

Bronchography in children is frequently done in association with or subsequent to a bronchoscopic examination. A small catheter is placed into the trachea, either through the nose or directly through the mouth. Cinefluoroscopy and spot films are taken during the addition of contrast media, to record the findings the fluoroscopy indicates. In very young children bronchography is done without anesthesia, either general or topical; however, in larger children bronchograms can conveniently be performed under general anesthesia with an endotracheal tube in place. This permits control of the child's respiration, allowing rapid introduction of the small catheter for installation of the contrast material. Cinefluorography has been an extremely valuable addition to bronchographic techniques, allowing for subsequent repeated examination of the flow of oil and the outline of the bronchial system.

REMOVAL OF FOREIGN BODIES

In addition to the inspection of the tracheobronchial tree for gross abnormalities and the aspiration of secretions for laboratory studies, the most frequent use of bronchoscopy in children is in the removal of a foreign body. The most common foreign body in the tracheobronchial tree in children is the peanut. Other vegetable products and small hard objects are also frequently aspirated in the one-to-three-year age group. Since the right main bronchus is most closely in alignment with the trachea, these foreign objects have a tendency to lodge on the right side.

Forceps have been designed in various sizes and of various types to solve the specific mechanical problems involved in the extraction of different objects from any of the major bronchi. The more commonly used types include forward-grasping, peanut, globular object, side-curve, and rotation forceps, and numerous others have been devised for special problems. The forceps chosen must be of the proper length and of a size to fit through the bronchoscope that is being used. It is important to adjust them immediately before each use so that the blades and handles close simultaneously. This closure ensures that when the blades of the forceps have grasped the foreign body and can be closed no further, the operator can obtain a direct indication of the grasp of the forceps by palpating the handle with his index finger. Small objects are withdrawn directly through the scope. Objects too large for this maneuver are fixed, along with the forceps, against the scope and are withdrawn as one with it. Sharp or pointed objects must be maneuvered so that the points either are protected by the forceps or the bronchoscope or are so rotated that they are trailed as they are removed with the scope. The details of removal of many different types of foreign objects have been fully considered in Jackson and Jackson's classic textbook (1936).

ESOPHAGOSCOPY

Esophagoscopy requires a somewhat different technique, and a slightly different instrument, from that required for bronchoscopy. The esophagoscope is similar to the bronchoscope but utilizes constant suction at the distal end through a separate aspirating channel running the full length of the esophagoscope. In addition, the esophagoscope is built without the distal perforations needed for aeration of the contralateral lung during bronchoscopy. The instrument is introduced, without the aid of the laryngoscope, down the right side of the mouth and pharynx. The lip of the scope is then advanced along the right lateral border of the tongue until the epiglottis is identified, following which it is passed laterally to the epiglottis and to the right of the aryepiglottic fold into the right pyriform sinus. At this point a woven silk esophageal bougie may be inserted through the cricopharyngeus into the cervical esophagus so that the esophagoscope can be advanced over it, using the bougie as a guide. In children who are breathing deeply and crying frequently, the cricopharyngeus often relaxes sufficiently with each deep inspiration to allow direct entry of the scope into the cervical esophagus, making identification of the lumen with a "lumen finder" bougie unnecessary.

With each inspiration, the esophagus expands and shows an open lumen; with each expiration, the walls of the esophagus collapse and the lumen disappears. Therefore, the best time for inspection of the esophageal walls and for advancement of the esophagoscope is during inspiration. The configuration, motility, and mucosal pattern should be observed. The scope is advanced to the cardia, which usually appears as a closed sphincter, but which may also open during inspiration. To complete the examination, the esophagoscope is advanced into the stomach. Here motion with respiration ceases, although gastric rugae will be seen to roll in front of the open tube. If gastric mucosa is seen above the level of the diaphragm, the amount of herniation should be measured, and any extent of associated esophagitis should be noted.

It must be remembered that there are three areas of physiological narrowing in the esophagus. These are at the cricopharyngeus, at the point of crossing of the aorta and left main bronchus, and at the cardia. The narrowing of the midesophagus is not quite as pronounced as in the other two areas, except in congenital vascular anomalies. These three areas are actual barriers to the passage of ingested materials, and for this reason they are frequently the sites of caustic strictures or of foreign body lodgment. When strictures are present, either in these areas or elsewhere, because of congenital, caustic, or postoperative problems, the technique of esophagoscopy becomes more difficult. The stricture is aligned with the lumen of the esophagoscope, and a small bougie is passed distally to the area of stricture. With a steady forward pressure, associated occasionally with rotation of the scope in one uniform direction, the esophagoscope is advanced over the bougie and through the stricture as a means of active dilatation. In all cases of stricture dilatation, the lumen beyond the stricture must be positively identified so that the lumen of the distal esophagus may be oriented with that of the esophagoscope in order to minimize the danger of perforation.

INDICATIONS FOR ESOPHAGOSCOPY

Esophagoscopy may be performed in infants or children of any age. The indications are inability to swallow, incoordination of swallowing, dysphagia, pain on swallowing, regurgitation, and, in certain instances, hematemesis. A prolonged feeding time in an infant and "feeding problems" in older children are additional indications for esophagoscopy. In every instance the esophagoscopy should be preceded by careful fluoroscopic and cinefluoroscopic studies, and the findings, even if negative, should be recorded on films.

Both mechanical and neurogenic lesions affect the esophagus of infants and children and necessitate esophagoscopy for diagnosis or treatment. The mechanical lesions consist of congenital or acquired webs, stenoses, fistulas, inflammatory conditions, and, rarely, benign or malignant neoplasms and external compression. Strictures caused by ingested caustics or corrosives constitute the largest series in this category of mechanical lesions. Varices are examples of nonobstructing pathology that necessitates esophagoscopy for diagnostic purposes, since as many as 20 percent of varices are not demonstrable by x-ray means. Of the neurogenic lesions, the commonest are the disorders of deglutition owing to central nervous system damage: birth injuries, massive cerebral trauma, polio, and cerebral agenesis. Cardiospasm, reflux peristalsis, and nasopharyngeal incoordination resulting from peripheral nerve defects are occasionally encountered. These conditions are all considered in more detail in Chapter 29.

The diagnosis and management of strictures of the esophagus constitute the most common use of esophagoscopy in infants and children. Congenital strictures may be single or multiple webs or a fibrous stenosis involving portions of the distal half of the esopha-

gus up to 10 cm in length. Webs often respond to a single passage of the rigid esophagoscope through the lumen, followed by maintenance of the lumen site by the passage, without anesthesia, of soft rubber, mercury-filled Hurst bougies. The fibrous segments of congenital strictures may be dilated with esophagoscopes guided over an esophageal

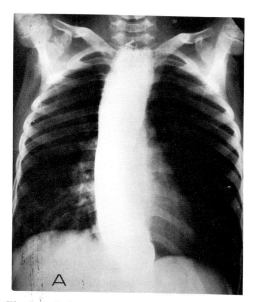

Fig. 1. A. Strictures at the cardia and of the esophagus. B. A Plummer bougie in place.

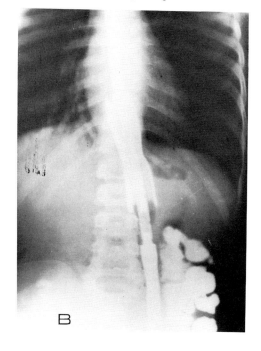

bougie or over a previously swallowed thread, such as # 14 surgically braided silk, which is strong enough to serve as a rigid guide. When a gastrostomy has become necessary for feeding purposes because of the severity of the stricture, dilatations are facilitated by recovery of a small (6-0 silk) thread from the gastrostomy after it has been swallowed. With this thread being used to draw a larger one through the esophagus, retrograde or prograde dilatations with rubber Tucker dilators or olive-tipped metal Plummer bougies (Fig. 1) can be more safely accomplished.

Caustic burns of the esophagus are best treated by early systematic dilatation with graduated mercury-filled bougies. Beginning within the first 24 hours after the ingestion of the alkali or acid, the esophagus is dilated daily for the first few days. The interval between dilatations is increased to once or twice a week and later to once a month, lengthening the interval as the symptoms and fluoroscopic observation indicate that the lumen is adequate. Antibiotics are used routinely in the early postburn period, but steroids are avoided because of the increased incidence of perforation, either spontaneous or during dilatations, when they are administered. The management of late stricture formation consists of dilatation by means of the esophagoscope or by the performance of a gastrostomy with a subsequent bouginage over a thread. When a moderate lumen has been attained, the enlargement of the opening is maintained by means of Hurst or tapered Maloney mercury-filled bougies.

Cardiospasm, which is relatively rare in infants and children, responds favorably to dilatation in the majority of instances. Dilatation with Hurst bougies may be done without anesthesia. More active dilatation with pneumatic bougies is best performed under general anesthesia with fluoroscopic guidance, to ensure proper placement of the pneumatic bag in the stricture.

Stenoses developing at the point of anastomosis in esophageal replacements, or those following repair of an esophageal atresia or a severe caustic burn, present an increasingly complicated series of problems in endoscopy. It should be stressed that the maintenance of a lumen through the anastomotic site is easier than reestablishing it or even dilating it once a stricture is firmly established. Early postsurgical fluoroscopy is advocated after the repair of an esophageal atresia with a tracheoesophageal fistula, to be followed by dilatations with soft rubber bougies or Tucker dilators if stenosis is apparent. The frequency of foreign body problems complicating postsurgical strictures of the esophagus is reason enough for advocating this type of early dilatation.

ESOPHAGEAL FOREIGN BODIES

Foreign bodies in the esophagus constitute a never-ending challenge. Any object small enough to enter the mouth of an infant or child may become lodged and fixed, necessitating endoscopic removal. Esophageal foreign bodies are usually larger than aspirated foreign bodies, and forceps appropriate for the size, shape, and depth of the object are needed. Initial symptoms of coughing, gagging, choking, and excessive salivation suggest the presence of a foreign body in the esophagus. However, these symptoms may quickly disappear if the object, such as an open safety pin, does not actually obstruct the lumen. Careful x-ray studies should be made to demonstrate the location of the object whenever these initial symptoms are noted. The possibility that the swallowed object may be made of a nonradiopaque plastic must be kept in mind. Successful esophagoscopic removal is dependent on the knowledge of the mechanical problem likely to be presented by the foreign body to be encountered, an adequate instrumentation, and an experienced endoscopic team. The complications consist of esophageal perforation from the foreign body itself or from laceration of the wall incurred by efforts to remove it, or respiratory obstruction due to tracheal compression by the foreign body of the endoscope. This last complication is best avoided by the use of an endotracheal tube with general anesthesia. Perforation necessitates prompt and adequate surgical drainage of the mediastinum by the supraclavicular or posterior routes.

PAUL H. HOLINGER
JOYCE A. SCHILD

REFERENCE

JACKSON, C., and JACKSON, C. L. Diseases of the Air Passages of Foreign-Body Origin. Philadelphia, W. B. Saunders, 1936.

19

Abnormalities of the Larynx and Tracheobronchial Tree

Abnormalities of the airway are among the most frequent causes of serious morbidity and death during infancy and early childhood. They may assume direct importance at birth, as in the case of choanal atresia or an obstructing laryngeal web, or they may produce difficulties later in childhood as the result of chronic obstruction or infection. Acute inflammatory processes of the upper airway are very serious in children because of the smallness of the passages. Even moderate mucosal edema may lead to almost complete cessation of air exchange, with consequent anoxia, acidosis, and cardiac arrest. It is of the greatest importance for all physicians engaged in the care of children to be aware of the various types of congenital and acquired abnormalities of the air passages that may lead to acute airway obstruction or to chronic debilitating pulmonary infection.

THE LARYNX

ANATOMICAL CONSIDERATIONS

The infant larynx differs from that of the adult in more ways than size alone. In the newborn the dimensions of the triangular aperture are approximately 7 mm in the anteroposterior direction by 4 mm across the posterior commissure. Considering the glottic chink to have an area of 14 sq mm, an edema of 1 mm of the mucosal surfaces will reduce the aperture to 5 sq mm, or only 35 percent of the normal glottis. (Figure 1 shows the normal infant larynx.) Mucosa is rigidly adherent to the posterior surface of the epiglottis and loosely attached to its anterior surface and along the aryepiglottic folds. Thus, edema of the epiglottis forces it to curl and often to assume a tubular shape, thus obstructing the airway. Similarly, soft areolar tissue of the subglottic conus elasticus encased in the rigid cricoid ring rapidly swells with trauma or infection, at the expense of the airway. Distress may be relieved temporarily by intubation, which occasionally obviates a tracheostomy. Prolonged intubation, however, results in ulceration of the mucosa, perichondritis, and, finally, destruction of the cricoid cartilage. Therefore, acute inflammatory, traumatic, or neurogenic obstruction, particularly of the subglottic tissues, should be relieved by a tracheostomy unless the condition is expected to resolve in a reasonably short period.

CONGENITAL ANOMALIES

LARYNGOMALACIA

Laryngomalacia is characterized by an inspiratory laryngeal stridor, often crowing in

WEBS

Webs of the larynx are found supraglottically, across the glottis, or in the subglottic area. *Supraglottic webs* consist of portions of the false cords that remain sealed together in development. They cause serious respiratory obstruction and an absent cry in the newborn infant (Fig. 2). *Glottic webs* may be thin or thick membranes between the anterior half to two thirds of the true cords, or they may consist of a fusion of the membranous portions of the cords (Fig. 3). *Subglottic webs* usually are deformities of the cricoid cartilage (Fig. 4). Congenital subglottic stenosis consists of an infiltration of the subglottic areolar tissues. This abnormality is often seen in mongols, in infants with Pierre Robin syndrome, and in infants with hemangiomas of the face and neck. Webs sometimes may simply be incised under direct laryngoscopy and repeatedly dilated to prevent reforming. If the webs are thick, they may respond to incision and the placement of a polyethylene tube between the cords to maintain the patency of the glottis while the cut edges are

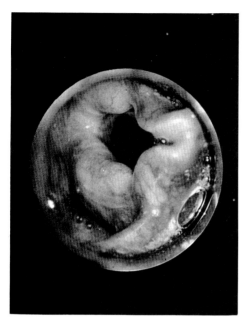

Fig. 1. The normal infant larynx seen through the direct laryngoscope. The tip of the laryngoscope is in the vallecula, exposing the larynx from slightly to the right of the midline. The omega-shaped epiglottis is seen in the anterior half of the field, and the arytenoids and the entrance to the esophagus are seen posteriorly. The glottis is partially covered by the epiglottis and the somewhat flaccid arytenoids.

nature, which is accentuated when the infant lies on its back. The symptoms are noted at birth, increase for the first six to eight months, and then gradually disappear. Since any laryngeal obstruction creates a stridor, direct laryngoscopy is necessary to establish the diagnosis and rule out other causes of blockage of the airway. The condition is best observed with the tip of the laryngoscope in the vallecula. Direct laryngoscopy reveals a loose, flabby epiglottis and arytenoids which flutter back and forth with respiration. Infants with severe congenital laryngomalacia become breathless and even cyanotic during feedings, necessitating frequent interruptions to regain color during breast or bottle feedings.

Treatment is rarely necessary, since the condition corrects itself by growth during the first $1\frac{1}{2}$ to 2 years of life.

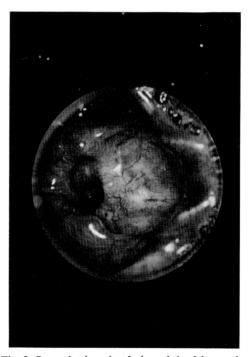

Fig. 2. Supraglottic web—fusion of the false cords.

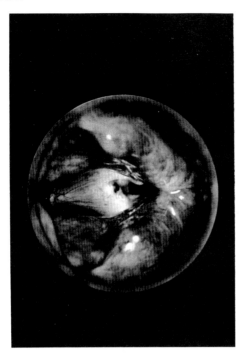

Fig. 3. Congenital glottic web with an almost complete fusion of the membranous portion of the cords.

epithelialized. A thyrotomy with the insertion of a tantalum plate after incision of the midline of the glottis may be required occasionally.

CYSTS

Cysts of the larynx in infants are usually laryngoceles (Fig. 5). They originate from the utricle, on the anterior-inferior surface of the false cords in the laryngeal ventricle. They may involve one of the aryepiglottic folds and occlude the airway, or they may protrude from the ventricle into the glottis. Respiratory obstruction is severe, and the voice is almost absent (Fig. 6). The diagnosis may be suspected when dyspnea and an absent or a muffled cry are the presenting neonatal respiratory symptoms and the infant is obviously expending great effort in breathing. A lateral x-ray of the neck taken with the infant's arms down and back and the head extended often shows the outline of the cyst. The differential diagnosis is established

by direct laryngoscopy. Cysts between the false and true cords may be incised under direct laryngoscopy and the edges removed with cup forceps. Laryngoceles involving the aryepiglottic folds should be aspirated with a large bore needle through the direct laryngoscope. After repeated aspiration they eventually resorb. If they do not do so, external resection is required.

PARALYSIS OF THE LARYNX

Paralysis of the larynx in infants may be unilateral or bilateral. The cry in unilateral paralysis is weak and breathy; in bilateral paralysis it is generally more normal in quality, but stridor is extreme. In unilateral paralysis the affected cord lies flaccid in the midline, and breathing takes place through slightly more than one half of the glottic chink. In unilateral right cord paralysis the etiology is often an Erb's palsy, whereas in left cord paralysis a cardiovascular anomaly, a mediastinal tumor, or an injury to the re-

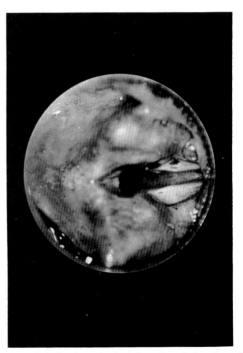

Fig. 4. Subglottic web. A deformity of the ring of the cricoid cartilage obstructs the airway, leaving only a small opening posteriorly.

current nerve during correction of an esophageal or a cardiovascular anomaly is usually responsible. Bilateral paralyses are of central nervous system origin. They are seen in connection with cerebral agenesis, a birth injury, or a meningomyelocele. In bilateral paralysis both cords lie flaccid in the midline, and so the cry is clear.

The possibility of laryngeal paralysis is frequently overlooked. It can be recognized only by direct laryngoscopy, without anesthesia, the cord action being observed during phonation (crying), and particularly during inspiration. Delays in diagnosis result from the clinical impression that cyanosis or a weak, breathy cry are the result of postoperative weakness or the heart lesion in a cardiac patient, rather than obstruction produced by the laryngeal paralysis. The recognition of a vocal cord paralysis pre- or postoperatively should be a warning that postoperative problems of retention of secretions owing to an ineffectual cough and poor deglutition may occur. In the treatment of

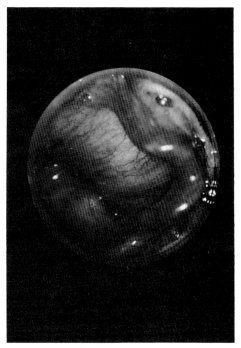

Fig. 6. A laryngocele protruding from under the left false cord and causing severe respiratory obstruction at birth.

unilateral paralysis, tracheostomy is rarely indicated except following prolonged intratracheal anesthesia or in association with inflammatory laryngeal edema, since the glottic chink is usually adequate. In bilateral paralysis a tracheostomy is mandatory, for serious obstruction is the rule. The laryngeal obstruction is corrected later by an arytenoid transposition or partial cordectomy.

INFLAMMATORY LESIONS

The infant larynx is susceptible to inflammatory changes that rapidly develop life-threatening proportions. *Hemophilus influenza* infection may cause extreme edema of the epiglottis and a consequent obstruction requiring tracheostomy. The epiglottis in this situation is cherry red in color. Acute laryngotracheobronchitis is generally of streptococcal origin and descends into the trachea and bronchi to destroy the mucosa. Obstruction results from edema and the cellular

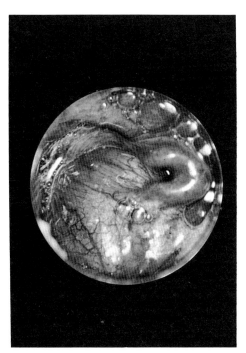

Fig. 5. A large laryngocele involving the entire right half of the larynx and totally obstructing the airway.

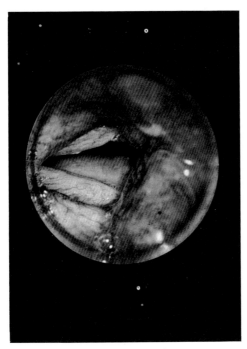

Fig. 7. Subglottic edema. The laryngoscope exposes the glottis from the right, thus showing the edematous subglottic tissue most prominently under the left true cord.

products of the inflammation (Fig. 7). Gentle aspiration as an emergency procedure or the temporary use of an endotracheal airway for no longer than 48 hours may relieve obstruction long enough for humidity and antibiotics to be effective. If not, tracheostomy over an intubation tube or a bronchoscope may be necessary.

In reviewing the etiology of tracheostomy in infants over a 30-year period, it is apparent that the incidence of tracheostomy necessitated by inflammatory lesions is decreasing. Tracheotomy for lesions associated with congenital anomalies, however, is rising, not only for congenital laryngeal anomalies but also in association with or following surgery for anomalies of other systems, particularly the cardiovascular, gastrointestinal, and central nervous systems.

NEOPLASMS

Neoplasms of the larynx in infants are relatively rare, with the exception of the laryngeal papillomas. These are warty tumors usually originating on the vocal cords, which sometimes grow rather rapidly to occlude the airway as the result of multiple, tiny tumors or, more rarely, because of the presence of a solitary pedunculated mass. They may extend onto the pharyngeal walls or grow downward into the trachea and bronchi. Laryngeal papillomas frequently require laryngoscopic forceps removal or tracheostomy. Maintenance of the airway during anesthesia is critical. Preliminary removal of major obstructing papillomas without anesthesia may obviate a tracheotomy, the residual papillomas then being removed under general anesthesia.

Hemangiomas or lymphangiomas may involve the pharyngeal or laryngeal airway as a direct continuation of mucous membrane involvement of the oral cavity, and tracheostomy may be required in early life as the lesions increase in size and extent. Their irradiation is to be avoided. Subglottic stenosis may affect the airway even in the absence of

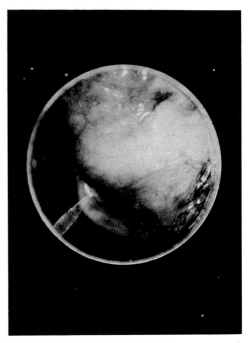

Fig. 8. Direct view through the laryngoscope of a large thyroglossal duct cyst at the base of the tongue protruding posteriorly and pushing the epiglottis downward and obstructing the glottis.

direct involvement by the hemangioma. Sarcomas occasionally involve the larynx of infants or children. An aggressive approach, including a laryngectomy, may be necessary following confirmation of the diagnosis by biopsy. Lesions, such as a thyroglossal duct cyst at the base of the tongue must be differentiated from laryngeal lesions (Fig. 8).

THE TRACHEOBRONCHIAL TREE

Congenital anomalies of the tracheobronchial tree can be responsible for serious respiratory problems in the first days or weeks of life. They manifest themselves by evidences of tracheal or bronchial obstruction

TABLE 1.   CLASSIFICATION OF CONGENITAL ANOMALIES OF THE TRACHEO-
BRONCHIAL TREE

ANOMALIES OF THE TRACHEA

    Agenesis or atresia
    Constriction
      Fibrous strictures
        Webs
        Fibrous stenosis of tracheal segments
        Stenoses associated with a tracheoesophageal fistula
      Absence or deformity of tracheal cartilages
        Tracheomalacia
        Deformity owing to vascular anomalies
        Individual cartilage deformity
        Tracheopathia osteoplastica
    Congenital tracheal enlargement (trachiectasis)
    Tracheal evaginations or outgrowths
      Tracheoceles, diverticula, and cysts
      Fistulas
      Tracheal lobe
    Abnormal bifurcation or deviation
    Other anomalies of gross morphology

ANOMALIES OF THE BRONCHI AND LUNGS

    Agenesis or atresia
    Constriction
      Fibrous strictures
        Webs
        Fibrous stenoses of bronchial segments
      Absence or deformity of bronchial cartilages
        Bronchomalacia
        Cartilage deformity or compression owing to cardiovascular anomalies
    Congenital bronchial enlargement (bronchiectasis)
      Kartagener's syndrome
    Bronchial evaginations or outgrowths
      Bronchoceles, diverticula, and cysts
      Fistulas
    Subnumerary bronchi, lobes, and fissures
    Supernumerary bronchi, lobes, and fissures
    Anomalous bronchial and lung tissue attached to some part of the respiratory system
    Anomalous bronchial and lung tissue attached to tissues other than those of the respiratory system

with wheezing or stridor, obstructive emphysema of one or both lungs, or atelectasis of a segment, a lobe, or the entire lung. A classification of congenital tracheobronchial anomalies is given in Table 1.

TRACHEAL ANOMALIES

Tracheal anomalies must be considered in any newborn with bilateral respiratory obstruction; a clear voice assists in differentiating a tracheal from a laryngeal obstruction, except in the rare case of bilateral recurrent laryngeal nerve paralysis. Agenesis and atresia of the trachea are obviously incompatible with life. Membranous webs and an hourglass-shaped constriction of the trachea are best demonstrated on lateral chest roentgenograms taken with the patient's arms held down and back to delineate both the laryngeal and the tracheal airway. Long, fibrous constrictions of tracheal segments without cartilage deformity are rare. Fibrous stenosis associated with a tracheoesophageal fistula is not common and is seen as a narrowing around the entrance to the lower esophageal segment. A narrowing of the tracheal lumen at the level of an "H" fistula may suggest the presence of this anomaly. Tracheal webs are treated by simple dilatation with bougies or with the tip of a bronchoscope. Longer fibrous strictures may require extensive surgical procedures, including tracheostomy, and advancement of the tracheostomy tube through the area of the constriction.

Anomalies involving the absence or deformity of tracheal cartilages are not common. Symptoms are primarily associated with respiratory obstruction. True tracheomalacia may involve several tracheal rings, but cases have been observed in which all of the supporting cartilages were absent, including those of the bronchi. Cinefluoroscopy is a valuable diagnostic aid, demonstrating the expansion and collapse of the flaccid trachea.

The absence of tracheal or bronchial rings at the site of a compressing vascular anomaly has been demonstrated repeatedly (Fig. 9). The symptoms include progressive

dyspnea, which often reaches an alarming degree by four or five months of age. In addition, dysphagia and cyanosis associated with feeding are characteristic, and in some cases dyspnea and dsyphagia are present at birth

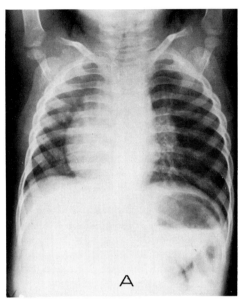

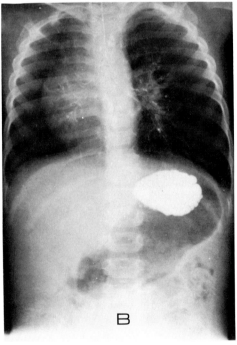

Fig. 9. A. Dextrocardia with the right aortic arch causing anomalous elongation of the right main bronchus. B. A bronchogram showing the unusually long right main bronchus and the displaced origin of the right upper lobe bronchus.

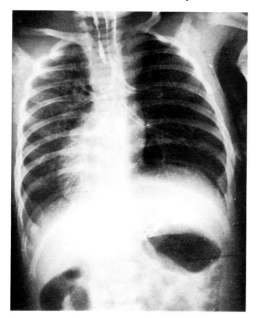

Fig. 10. Dextrocardia with multiple tracheobronchial anomalies. The right and left upper lobe bronchi originate from the trachea, which then continues inferiorly to divide into right and left middle and lower lobe bronchi.

(Fig. 10). The constriction apparently is not a compression stenosis alone but a developmental anatomical constriction of the tracheal or bronchial cartilages, resulting from vascular compression in fetal life. It is significant that persistence of the deformity will be demonstrable on bronchograms taken after severance of a vascular ring.

Tracheal obstruction produced by deformity of individual cartilages is often indistinguishable from true stenosis except by postmortem and histological examinations. Tracheal cartilages in infants are deflected with ease by an advancing bronchoscope, making the differentiation difficult in infancy. Deformities of individual cartilages are most often encountered either in the cervical segment of the trachea or close to the carina. They consist of thickened or distorted cartilaginous rings or solid cartilaginous plaques replacing the normal horseshoe-shaped rings. Similar deformities may involve the bronchial cartilages, causing lobar or segmental atelectasis.

Congenital tracheal enlargement or tra-

chiectasia is rarely seen in infants, although it has been described as an associated finding in fibrocystic disease of the pancreas. The trachea as well as the major bronchi are increased in diameter, and tracheal diverticula may be present. It is not established whether these are the result of acquired inflammatory changes or a congenital defect of elastic and muscular tracheal fibers.

Tracheal evaginations or outgrowths may develop as diverticula lined by secreting tracheal mucosa. They may become isolated from the lumen, forming tracheoceles. As they enlarge, these cystic structures compress the trachea and give rise to wheezing, a brassy cough, and respiratory obstruction that becomes progressively more severe (Fig. 11). Frequently they compress the esophagus as well, causing dysphagia and an accentuation of respiratory obstruction during feedings. It may be difficult to distinguish between a tracheocele and a vascular ring because of the similarity of the symptoms. Treatment in either case is surgical, but a preoperative diagnosis should be established by angiography if it is uncertain which lesion is present. Similar cysts are found adjacent to major bronchi, where they produce severe bronchial compression. Again, the treatment is surgical removal. The cysts generally contain a thick, clear, viscid mucous secretion. Histological examination of their walls demonstrates respiratory epithelium.

Another anomalous outpouching, a tra-

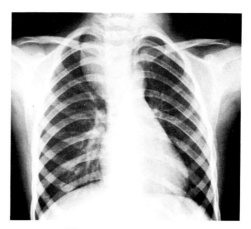

Fig. 11. Tracheogenic cyst.

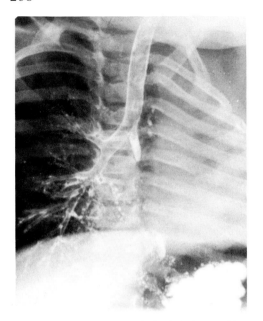

Fig. 12. Total agenesis of the left lung with an anomalous stump of the left main bronchus.

cheal lobe, is probably more common than one would surmise from a review of the literature. Numerous variations of the anomaly exist. Many are associated with abnormal development of the upper lobe of the right lung. In the simplest form, an otherwise normal upper lobe bronchus originates above the level of the tracheal bifurcation and gives rise to three normal divisions. In another form of the anomaly a complete duplication of the bronchus and lobe is seen, with a normal right upper lobe bronchus originating just beyond the bifurcation and an abnormal second identical bronchus originating in the trachea. More commonly the tracheal evagination consists of only the apical segment, with the anterior and posterior bronchi and segments arising together beyond the bifurcation. Demonstration of a tracheal lobe is usually an incidental finding on bronchoscopic or bronchographic examination. However, if the anomalous lobe or segment is associated with a pulmonary anomaly, such as a cyst, this may lead to discovery of the tracheal evagination.

The most common congenital fistulas of the trachea are those associated with esopha-

geal anomalies. These are discussed elsewhere in the book.

BRONCHIAL ANOMALIES

Abnormal tracheal bifurcations are numerous, associated with either agenesis, stenosis, or duplication of the main bronchi. Agenesis of an entire lung is not uncommon. Schneider (1950) divided these anomalies into three classes. In Class I there is no trace of a bronchus or lung on the affected side. In Class II lung tissue is absent, but there is some trace of a bronchus (Fig. 12). In Class III the main bronchus is partially or completely developed, but there is marked hypoplasia of one or both lungs. Clinically, bronchopulmonary agenesis must be distinguished from atelectasis produced by bronchial compression or mucous obstruction. Bronchoscopic and bronchographic studies are essential. Although the agenesis per se is not incompatible with life, frequently the infant has other anomalies of major systems, which makes the prognosis guarded.

Constrictions or enlargements of the bronchi are produced by processes similar to

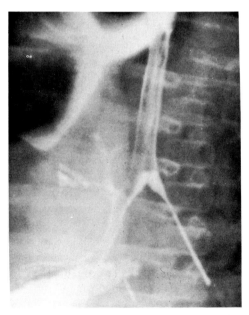

Fig. 13. Congenital stenosis of the left main bronchus.

those which constrict or enlarge the trachea (Fig. 13). Webs or congenital fibrous stenoses may account for severe obstruction emphysema or atelectasis of a segment, a lobe, or an entire lung. Bronchoscopic dilatation may relieve the obstruction caused by a bronchial web, but fibrous stenoses of bronchial segments do not readily respond to this procedure. Stenoses must be carefully differentiated from the bronchial compression, whether partial or complete, which is produced by anomalies of the heart or great vessels or by bronchogenic cysts. Angiography is important in making the diagnosis. Cardiac anomalies may compress the left bronchus or increase the angle of the tracheal bifurcation to such an extent that both main bronchi are seriously obstructed. Anomalies of the great vessels may affect the right or the left bronchus, in addition to obstructing the trachea. Right-sided obstructive emphysema can result from partial obstruction of the right main bronchus by a right-sided aortic arch or by an anomalous left pulmonary artery curving laterally around the right main bronchus before coursing to the left lung. Since both these anomalies are proximal to the right upper lobe orifice, the diagnosis may be suspected if the right upper lobe bronchus originates at an unusual distance beyond the carina. Neither anomaly affects the esophagus.

Bronchial obstructions associated with vascular anomalies, like similar conditions in the trachea, are marked by gross deformity or absence of the bronchial cartilages at the site of the compression. As in the trachea, the obstruction may persist to some degree after the constricting vessel is severed. This persistence accounts for the failure of surgical treatment to relieve symptoms completely in some of the cases, but growth usually results in complete disappearance of the obstruction.

Bronchomalacia affecting a portion of a bronchus is similar to the corresponding tracheal entity. Rapidly progressive respiratory distress resulting from obstructive emphysema may necessitate emergency thoracot-

omy and lobectomy in some of the extreme cases. Prior to surgical intervention, one should rule out a bronchial web by bronchoscopy. Subsequent histological examination of the excised bronchial and pulmonary tissues will be required to distinguish the condition known as idiopathic congenital pulmonary emphysema, which is marked by signifi-

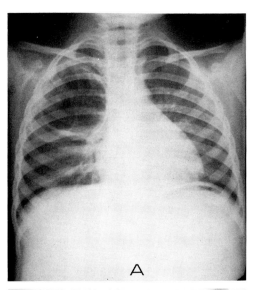

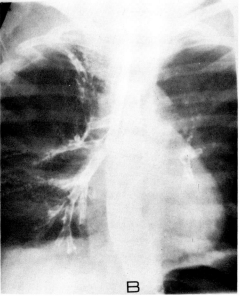

Fig. 14. A. Congenital bronchogenic cyst, right upper lobe. B. Bronchogram showing an anomalous duplication of the right upper lobe bronchus. The anomalous bronchus (tracheal bronchus) leads to the congenital cyst.

cant changes in the elastic tissue of the lungs.

Evaginations or outgrowths of bronchi consist primarily of fistulas, bronchogenic cysts, diverticula, and bronchoceles. A fistula between a bronchus and the pleural cavity resulting in severe tension pneumothorax has been described. A more unusual anomaly, difficult to explain embryologically, consists of a bronchobiliary fistula that arises from the medial aspect of the right main bronchus opposite the right upper lobe orifice and passes through the diaphragm to connect with a bile duct. Bronchogenic cysts manifest their presence by varying degrees of localized bronchial obstruction. (Fig. 14). Like tracheal cysts, they are usually found in the posterior mediastinum and contain a clear, thick, viscid fluid and exert pressure on both the airway and the esophagus. The walls are lined with ciliated, pseudostratified columnar epithelium containing mucus glands and occasional plaques of cartilage. Definitive diagnosis of a bronchogenic cyst rests on histological study of the cyst wall following its resection.

Subnumerary bronchi, lobes, and fissures are common, but they seldom coincide with bronchial variations. Most frequently seen on surgical exploration is a single large fissure on the right side or a total absence of fissures. Hypoplasia of the lung is usually as-sociated with a bronchial abnormality. The bronchial pattern may be entirely normal, however, in spite of a total absence of fissures. Supernumerary bronchi, lobes, and fissures may be grouped in two categories, tracheal lobes and lower accessory lobes. About 10 percent of normal persons have accessory third lobes of the left lung, usually the medial division of the lower lobe. Supernumerary fissures without additional lobes are commonly observed during thoracic surgical procedures and are of little practical significance. The lateral divisions of the right upper lobe, which are present in about 10 percent of persons, and the subsuperior (subapical) divisions of the lower lobes, which are present in about 25 percent, are considered to be normal variants and not regarded as accessory lobes. Supernumerary fissures in the right lower lobe, with normal bronchi, may be accompanied by numerous anomalous vessels, some arising directly from the aorta and some even originating below the diaphragm. As many as five lobes on the right side have been reported in addition to an azygous lobe. An azygous lobe formed as the result of azygous venous constriction of the right upper lobe is not a true supernumerary structure.

PAUL H. HOLINGER

REFERENCE

SCHNEIDER, L. Upper bronchial abnormalities simulating significant pulmonary tuberculosis (with seven illustrative cases). Radiology, 55: 390, 1950.

20

Tracheostomy

A tracheostomy is a surgical procedure that establishes direct access to the airway at its most superficial point in the neck. Although the tracheostomy was originally used exclusively to relieve laryngeal obstruction, it is now recognized that it also provides ready entry to the tracheobronchial tree for the frequent aspiration of secretions and an easy path for the introduction of a tube for establishing and maintaining positive pressure respiration. Thus, the indications for tracheostomy are related to three major disease processes: (1) acute or chronic progressive laryngeal obstruction caused by inflammatory, traumatic, paralytic, or neoplastic diseases of the larynx or trachea; (2) repeated and persistent retention of tracheobronchial secretions in paralytic, traumatic, or postoperative states in which the formation and stagnation of secretions is accentuated; and (3) failure of the central nervous system respiratory center, necessitating prolonged artificial respiration.

Normally the trachea lies in the midline of the neck and descends from the cricoid cartilage caudally and somewhat dorsally to its entrance into the thorax at the suprasternal notch. The cricoid cartilage lies at the level of the fourth cervical vertebra in the infant, the fifth in the child, and the seventh in the adult. The length of the cervical trachea is approximately 3 cm in the newborn, 4 cm in the five-year-old, and 6 cm in the ten-year-old. However, these figures vary considerably. It is this variation which is responsible for many of the complications of the operation. In some short, thick-necked infants or children, for example, the cricoid cartilage seems to lie almost within the suprasternal notch, whereas in others the thyroid isthmus, the caput of the lungs, a large pad of fat, or major vessels from the aortic arch may rise high to shorten the amount of trachea in the neck.

TECHNIQUE

Three procedures for securing a reliable airway are available to the surgeon when a tracheostomy is indicated for respiratory obstruction. These are intubation, cricothyroidotomy (emergency tracheostomy), and the standard type of tracheostomy. It is increasingly apparent that tracheostomy under emergency conditions without the previous establishment of an airway is not only hazardous to the patient but also unnecessarily difficult for the surgeon. For this reason it is the practice of experienced surgeons, as a preliminary measure, to intubate all patients requiring tracheostomy. Through the use of oxygen and positive pressure breathing, the anoxia (which is the primary indication for the procedure) can be reversed, acidosis corrected, and the heart function restored. The result of such preliminary oxygenation is that the patient usually goes to sleep, the distension of the neck veins subsides, and a tranquil surgical procedure can be accomplished.

ENDOTRACHEAL INTUBATION

Exposure of the larynx with a laryngoscope and insertion of an endotracheal tube or a bronchoscope between the cords is the simplest way to establish an airway. The advantage of this procedure is that it is rapid, permits aspiration of secretions to clear the airway, and allows instantaneous positive pressure assistance in initiating or maintaining respiration. It also permits the completion of a tranquil, routine tracheostomy under local or general anesthesia as a planned surgical procedure with adequate time for establishing aseptic conditions. The disadvantage is, obviously, that it depends on the availability of the laryngoscope and endotracheal tube of the appropriate sizes. However, these are—or should be—standard equipment in emergency rooms, in post-surgical recovery rooms, and on the wards in which seriously ill infants or children are being cared for. One real disadvantage of this procedure is that occasionally the laryngeal pathology has so distorted or obstructed the glottis that the airway cannot easily be identified, and critical time is lost in searching for it. In addition, sometimes it is impossible to open the mouth of a patient who is in the agonal, terminal stage of asphyxia. Nevertheless, in spite of these serious objections, the use of an endotracheal tube or a bronchoscope is the safest, most commonly used procedure for rapid relief of laryngeal obstruction. All physicians caring for infants and children should learn how to use these instruments efficiently and safely.

CRICOTHYROIDOTOMY (EMERGENCY TRACHEOSTOMY)

In an extreme emergency, in the absence of the equipment described above and when time does not permit the establishment of an opening into the trachea itself, the airway can be reached most quickly between the thyroid and cricoid cartilages. A transverse stab incision is made between these two cartilages. They are easily palpated as the patient's head is extended, and they lie above the thyroid isthmus, which is also an advantage. Respiratory obstruction is increased in the extended position, but the landmarks are more easily identified and access to the point of incision is better than if the head is flexed. The ideal position in the recumbent patient is with the angle of the jaw lifted and the chin pointed upward. After the knife is inserted through the cricothyroid membrane the blade should be rotated to a midline position to separate cricoid and thyroid cartilages and improve the airway through the opening just established. Care is necessary to avoid perforation into the esophagus posteriorly. Such perforation has been observed in a few cases in which a tracheoesophageal fistula has developed as a complication. Hemorrhage is very likely to occur during this emergency procedure from the two small cricothyroid arteries which enter the membrane laterally. The bleeding can usually be controlled by pressure or, if they are available, by hemostats placed in the lateral aspects of the incision through the membrane.

The use of trocars sheathed with a tracheostomy tube, or even simply a heavy gauge needle, to enter the airway through the cricothyroid membrane has gained considerable popularity. This again necessitates the availability of an instrument of the appropriate size. The method also increases the risk of perforation into the esophagus, mediastinum, or pleural cavity, especially in infants and children, where the trachea is small, soft, and often difficult to palpate. The opening in the cricothyroid membrane should be abandoned as soon as the patient's condition permits. A terminal tracheostomy through the second, third, and fourth tracheal rings is done to avoid permanent injury to the cricoid or thyroid cartilages by infection or pressure necrosis, since these often result in chronic laryngeal stenosis or de-

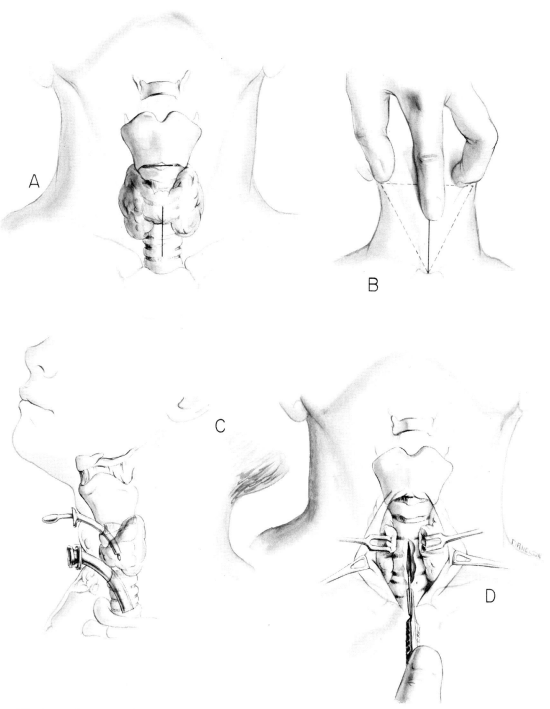

Fig. 1. Tracheostomy. A. The position of the tracheostomy incision in relation to anatomical structures. B. Palpation to ensure the proper placement of the incision. C. Lateral view indicating the position of the tube for cricothyroidotomy and standard tracheostomy. D. Two tracheal rings are divided one or two rings below the larynx.

struction of the subglottic structures and in injury to the vocal cords.

STANDARD, OR CONVENTIONAL, TRACHEOSTOMY

A tracheostomy, particularly in a small child or an infant, is greatly facilitated by the insertion of a bronchoscope or an endotracheal tube. This maintains the midline position of the trachea and provides a constant, rigid tracheal support that is easily identified as the dissection proceeds. Local anesthesia infiltration into the anterior surface of the neck is usually employed. General anesthesia may be used if the operator desires, but this is safe only if an adequate airway has first been established by an endotracheal tube. A right-handed operator stands to the patient's right and, with his thumb and middle fingers of the left hand on the anterior surface of the neck, identifies the medial borders of the sternomastoid muscles while his index finger palpates the cricoid cartilage. An adequate midline incision

is made from the tip of the operator's index finger toward the suprasternal notch (Fig. 1). Although it is taught that the transverse incision produces a much better scar after tracheostomy, this is not true in infants and small children. In addition, the smallness of the structures makes the positioning of the skin incision over the tracheal stoma a very important consideration. Too high a skin incision will cause rotation of the tip of the tracheostomy tube anteriorly, and too low an incision will rotate it posteriorly. Constant pressure by the tube tip may result in erosions of the tracheal mucosa, with a resulting troublesome and possibly fatal granuloma formation. It is far easier to adjust the skin opening to the tracheostomy and to prevent this complication when a vertical incision is made.

The paired sternohyoid and sternothyroid muscles are separated in the midline to expose the thyroid isthmus at the upper end of the incision. This may be clamped, divided, and ligated to expose the trachea from the first to the fourth tracheal rings, or the isthmus may be retracted upward or down-

TABLE 1.   SUGGESTED BRONCHOSCOPE AND TRACHEOSTOMY TUBE SIZES
FOR INFANTS AND CHILDREN

AGE OF CHILD	LARYNGOSCOPE			BRONCHOSCOPES	TRACHEOSTOMY TUBES	
	Working length cm	*Internal diameter mm*	*Jackson number*	*(With Infant's-size Light and Carrier)*	*Routine*	*Respirator*
Premature	6	9	newborn	3 mm × 20 cm	00	0
Newborn–3 months	6	9	infant	3 mm × 20 cm or 3.5 mm × 25 cm	00 or 0	0 or 1
3–6 months	7.5	10	9	3.5 mm × 25 cm	0 or 1	1
6–12 months	7.5	10	9	3.5 mm × 30 cm or 4 mm × 30 cm	0 or 1	1 or 2
1–2 years	9	10	11	3.5 mm × 30 cm or 4 mm × 30 cm	1 or 2	1 or 2
3 years	9	10	11	4 mm × 30 cm	1 or 2	2 or 3
4 years	10.2	11.5	12	4 mm × 35 cm or 5 mm × 30 cm	2	2 or 3
5–7 years	10.2	11.5	12	5 mm × 35 cm	2 or 3	3 or 4
8–12 years	13.6	12	16	5 mm × 35 cm or 6 mm × 35 cm or 7 mm × 40 cm	3 or 4	4 or 5 or 4 cuff

ward, depending on its configuration and position relative to the cricoid cartilage. The trachea is then grasped securely with a thyroid hook to stabilize it, and the second, third, and fourth rings are cut vertically in the midline. Accuracy in the positioning of the tracheal opening is exceedingly important: too high an incision results in trauma to the cricoid cartilage by the actual severance or necrosis caused by the pressure of the tube; too low an incision results in a pneumothorax or pneumomediastinum as the head is flexed and the tracheal opening slides into the thorax at completion of the operation. The edges of the tracheal incision are separated with a Trousseau dilator or curved hemostat and the tracheostomy tube inserted. Some prefer to hold the edges of the tracheal opening apart with two small silk sutures that are left dangling out of the incision in order to separate the tracheal opening in case the tube inadvertently is allowed to come out of the trachea.

After ligation of bleeding points and suture ligation of the divided thyroid isthmus, one or two skin sutures may be used to approximate the edges of the incision above the tube. The wound is left open inferiorly to permit drainage and avoid the development of subcutaneous and mediastinal emphysema, which will invariably occur if the wound edges are tightly approximated. The tracheal tube is held in place by twill tape tied firmly with a square knot, to prevent its being untied by mistake when the patient's gown is being changed.

The choice of tracheostomy tubes is dependent upon many factors (Table 1). No size, shape of curve, length of tube, design of plate, or even design of material used in the manufacture of the tube can be considered universal. The tube with a small plate rigidly attached to the outer tube at a 65° angle serves best for infants and children, and it varies in size from # 00 to # 4 or # 5, depending on the size of the trachea. Proportionately larger tubes are necessary if the tube is to be used with a respirator. Length and angle of curve have to be ad-

justed individually to avoid pressure on either the anterior or the posterior tracheal wall or on the carina. Tubes made of various soft plastics now offer some advantages over rigid silver tubes. Variations in the design of the plates may assist in positioning the tube so that complications do not occur.

POSTOPERATIVE CARE

The postoperative care of the infant or child with a tracheostomy requires constant attention. A high-humidity room, tent, or croupette is mandatory to combat obstruction caused by tenacious tracheobronchial secretions. Catheter aspiration with 20 to 24 inches of negative pressure, using aseptic technique with sterile gloves on each occasion, reduces intercurrent infection. A thumb valve increases the efficiency of the aspiration procedure. Secretions are washed out with a half-normal saline solution instilled into the tracheal tube with a rubber-tipped medicine dropper or small syringe. The patency of the airway is judged by frequent auscultation of the chest. Obstruction should be suspected when the temperature, pulse, or respiratory rate begin to rise. Additional catheter suction or actual bronchoscopic aspiration is necessary under these circumstances. Aspiration procedures must be brief, effective, and atraumatic. It is actually possible to produce atelectasis by sucking the air out of an individual lobe. If the procedure is too prolonged or repetitious, without regard for the cardiac status of the debilitated infant, a cardiac arrest may be precipitated. The inner tube is changed and cleaned every half hour to two hours, depending on the amount of drying secretions present in each patient. The entire tube is changed on the sixth or seventh day and daily thereafter. As soon as the improvement of the normal airway and general condition is assured, extubation is attempted. This is begun by using gradually smaller tubes, permitting the resumption of laryngeal breathing as the obstruction caused by the tube itself is decreased. After a test period of 24 hours with a small tube that is completely closed off by having the inner tube taped, the tracheostomy may safely be discontinued. In tiny infants, when such taping of the tube is impossible because even the smallest tube occludes the trachea, it may be necessary to revisualize the larynx and trachea endoscopically to determine the functioning patency of the airway before final extubation. The wound is closed with adhesive and generally is airtight within a few hours. A cosmetic revision of the scar frequently is necessary, but it should be delayed a year or two to secure the best results.

PAUL H. HOLINGER

21

Malformations of the Neck

CYSTIC HYGROMA

The term cystic hygroma is apt, for "hygroma" is derived from a Greek word meaning "watery." The typical cystic hygroma being filled with fluid has a soft consistency and usually transilluminates light readily. This lesion was described more than 100 years ago, and the observation then was that the lesion occurred most commonly in the neck. While the association of this lesion with the lymphatic system had been mentioned earlier, Sabin was the first to study the origin of this lesion during her extensive investigations of the lymphatic system. Goetsch later published a clinical study (1938) and concluded that cystic hygroma was an infiltrating tumor and in this regard could be classed with the malignant growths. This conception of it is not shared by pathologists, who generally consider this lesion benign.

EMBRYOLOGY

An important part of the lymphatic system is in the neck, for in this region communication between the venous and lymphatic system is direct. Sabin (1904) found that there were five points of origin of the lymphatic system: the paired sacs in the neck in conjunction with the jugular vein, a single sac at the root of the mesentery, and paired sacs in relation to the sciatic veins. A majority of the cystic hygromas are found in the neck, the axilla, and the thoracic region. A few are in the lower portion of the trunk. Lymphangioma in the extremity is different from the cystic hygroma in gross appearance. However, there is increasing evidence that these various lymphatic malformations are related and perhaps are degrees of the same basic congenital malformation. Although there is some disagreement about the details of the embryological basis of cystic hygroma, it is generally agreed that it is related to the early formation of the lymphatic system and probably represents a true congenital malformation.

PATHOLOGY

Cystic hygromas are composed of thin walled cysts lined with flat epithelium and filled with yellowish fluid. Often the cysts have communications, for puncturing one cyst may drain the entire cystic hygroma. Interspersed in the cystic hygroma to a varying degree are areas of lymphatic infiltration. These may be quite extensive in some parts and may be the cause of the nodular components of the tumor. These lymphocytic infiltrations are more likely to be in the deeper portions of the lesion.

The relationship among the true cystic hygroma, the lymphangioma, and the lymphohemangioma has been debated. Landing and Farber (1956) believe that they are in essence the same basic lesion manifested in a variety of ways. Bill and Sumner (1965) have proposed that all these malformations represent blockages of the lymphatic system. Goetsch (1938) concluded from his studies that these were usually tumors that infiltrated tissue. It is true that within the stroma of the cystic hygroma may be nerves and muscle fibers as well as fibrous tissue. It is difficult to determine whether this indicates actual invasiveness or whether the lymphatics in the tissue that becomes cystic with dilation enmeshed normal structures. Many pathologists believe the latter is true. The cystic hygroma is a soft tumor and does not produce nerve damage despite the fact that the nerve may be encircled by the lesion. On the other hand, when the location is in the neck and thoracic inlet there may be compression of the trachea as well as involvement of the larynx sufficient to produce airway obstruction. There may on occasion be difficulty with swallowing.

DIAGNOSIS

Over 50 percent of cystic hygromas are present at birth, and practically all make their presence known during the first year of life. The massive swellings of the neck, axilla, upper trunk, and even of the face are quite disfiguring (Fig. 1). In those rare patients with bilateral involvement of the neck, the tongue and larynx are frequently involved (Fig. 2). The tongue may be very large and prevent the child from closing his mouth. Teeth may be lost because of the involvement of the peridental tissue or because of pressure by the large tongue to force them outward. Overgrowth of the lower jaw has been observed in such patients. The massive tongue plus extraneous pressure of the cystic hygroma on the airway or involvement of the larynx may produce airway obstruction. Untreated, the lesion is vulnerable to infection; this is not surprising, since it is related to the lymphatic system, which may transmit organisms, particularly during an upper respiratory or a pulmonary infection. Before antibiotics came into use, small babies with infections of extensive cystic hygromas were

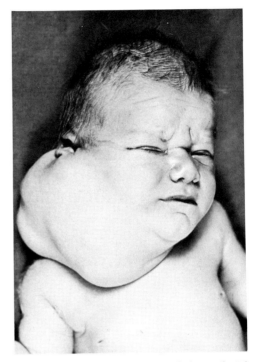

Fig. 1. Massive cystic hygroma of the neck. The major portion was on the right side.

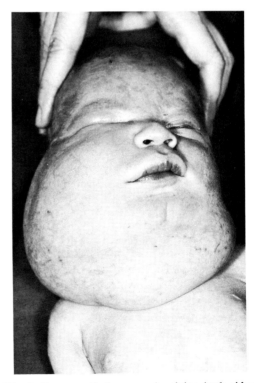

Fig. 2. Large cystic hygroma involving both sides of the neck.

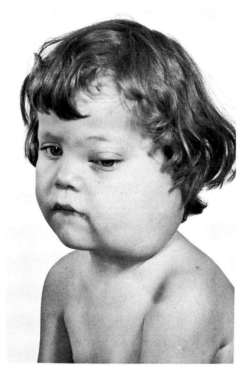

Fig. 3. Cystic hygroma which had decreased slightly in size.

Radiation therapy has had an extensive trial, and reports of success are rare. In view of the danger of inciting malignancy of the thyroid, it seems unwise to treat the cystic hygroma with radiation.

Injection of sclerosing fluid has been tried in the treatment of cystic hygroma, but with poor success. There is the danger of injected sclerosing fluid reaching the venous system, for there are communications with the venous system in some instances. Furthermore, the scarring produced yields an unacceptable cosmetic result.

About 75 percent of cystic hygromas appear in the neck, about 20 percent in the axilla, and 5 percent in the trunk (Figs. 4 and 5). Diagnosis usually presents no problem. The flabbiness of the tumor, its indefinite outline, and its ability to transmit light are so characteristic that the tumor can be identified in most instances. When the lesion is small and rather firm it may be confused with a branchiogenic cyst. However, the cysts are so constant in their location

faced with a high mortality rate. Undoubtedly many of these infants died, and this may account for the fact that these disfiguring lesions were rarely if ever observed in adults. Occasionally, in smaller lesions, repeated bouts of infection might destroy the lining of the lymphangioma and actually produce a reduction in the size of the lesion. Occasionally, spontaneous regression of a cystic hygroma has occurred (Fig. 3). This does not happen with sufficient frequency for it to be a factor in deciding whether therapy should be instituted or not. A number of the hygromas will increase in size, and procrastination may lead to a more difficult surgical endeavor when therapy is eventually undertaken.

One early form of treatment was aspiration. This may lead to the introduction of infection into the lesion. Instances have been reported of aspiration followed by serious hemorrhage into the cystic spaces, converting the soft mass into a larger, firm, blood-filled tumor.

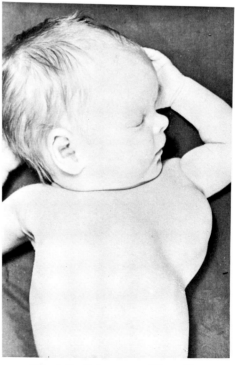

Fig. 4. Cystic hygroma of the axilla.

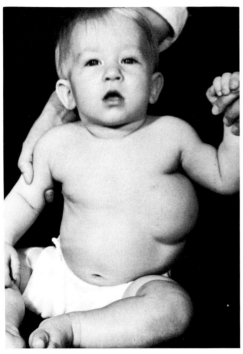

Fig. 5. Cystic hygroma of the trunk.

along the sternocleidomastoid muscle and
are so tense that a clear-cut differentiation
between the two lesions is usually possible.

Lipomas may be similar in texture and in
vague outline to cystic hygromas. The lipoma
is an unusual tumor in children and extremely
rare in the neonate. It becomes more of a
diagnostic problem when soft tumor masses
on the trunks or in the axillae of older children are being investigated, and in some
situations it may be impossible to determine
preoperatively which of the lesions is present. Occasionally, it is difficult to determine
whether a deep, soft, subcutaneous lesion is
a cystic hygroma or a hemangioma. Usually
where the lesion is predominently vascular,
there will be enlarged vessels in the skin and
a decidedly bluish cast of the overlying skin
that may enable the observer to identify the
lesion as being a hemangioma rather than a
lymphangioma.

TREATMENT

Surgical excision is the treatment of choice
and should be instituted as soon as the lesion

is detected. There is no value in delaying excision, for the lesions may increase in size
and make the surgical procedure more difficult. Since this lesion is nonmalignant, the
objective should be complete removal with
preservation of vital structures. The structures in the neck and face that are most vulnerable to damage during removal of cystic
hygroma are nerve elements. In the neck,
the spinal accessory nerve is one which
should be identified and preserved. Damaging this nerve produces far-reaching ill effects, for the patient develops a drooped
painful shoulder as he grows older. When
the lesion extends onto the face there is danger of injury to the facial nerve. Because of
the importance of preservation of these vital
nerves during excision, it is unwise to undertake such operations without having available a nerve stimulator so that every effort
can be made to identify and preserve these
nerves during the dissection.

A simple transverse incision is required
over the major part of the mass. We like to
protect the skin with a plastic drape so that
the face can be seen during the course of the
operative procedure. With such an arrangement, stimulation of portions of the facial
nerve will produce contractions of facial
muscles that can be observed through the
plastic drape. The alternative is to prepare
all of one side of the face and drape it as a
part of the operative field so that direct observation of the face is possible. The incision
through the skin should be made with care.
If it is made casually, not only the thin skin
but the superficial cysts will be opened. With
most benign tumors, one does not have to
worry about drainage of cyst fluid into the
wound. In this situation, however, it is rather
disastrous to have such drainage occur, for
the intercommunicating thin walled cysts
collapse, and it is impossible for the surgeon
to identify them, and a complete excision or
a satisfactory excision of the lesion is impossible under such circumstances. Skin hooks
are needed to hold the skin and to permit its
sharp dissection from the surface of the
cystic hygroma. Application of forceps or

other instruments to the cystic hygroma will cause perforation and tears and leakage of fluid. This can be avoided by using a dry sponge to hold and retract the tumor during the dissection. When the tumor overlies the facial nerve it is wise to proceed directly to identification of the trunk of the facial nerve. If this is not possible, it may be wise to identify the mandibular branch of the facial nerve and then to dissect proximally along this nerve until the main trunk is identified. Fibrous strands are numerous in cystic hygroma. It is impossible to visually identify small nerves, and therefore an electric stimulator is a requirement for this part of the dissection. Questionable structures are stimulated. If there is no response, the structure can be cut. Once the nerve trunks are identified, they can be dissected from the mass and in most instances preserved. It is wiser to leave small bits of the lesion behind than to risk dividing the facial nerve or its main branches. Undoubtedly in most operative removals of cystic hygroma there are minute bits of the tissue left in place. As long as this is kept to a minimum, good cosmetic results will follow. This should not give the surgeon license to be careless and to leave large amounts of the tumor in place, for then recurrence may take place, or the cosmetic result from the remaining tumor may be unacceptable. These are tedious dissections but are rewarding in that when the nerves are preserved, one can secure excellent cosmetic results. Often the cystic hygroma extends around the larynx into the base of the tongue. It is wise to remove as much of this extension as possible, taking care again to leave the vital nerve structures in the neck intact. Massive tongue enlargement must be treated surgically. Large V-shaped segments of the tongue can be removed to reduce the tongue size so that the mouth can be closed. Often more than one resection is required to reduce the tongue to a reasonable size. In massive cystic hygromas of the neck and face, the procedure may be too long for the patient to withstand at one time. One can do the operation in stages in such instances

and achieve good cosmetic results. Closure of the skin is best achieved with interrupted 5-0 silk sutures through the skin. Once the cystic hygroma has been completely removed, the problem postoperatively is that there will be in some instances accumulation of fluid in the wound, and this may be related to how much of the lesion has been left in place. We have found it helpful in those patients who tend to accumulate considerable fluid to insert a hemovac through a small stab wound. These plastic tubes with multiple perforations attached to gentle suction are effective in keeping the wounds from accumulating fluid and permitting the skin flaps to adhere to the deeper structures. We do not believe that they should be used routinely in the neck because of the rather poor cosmetic result which may be obtained, since the thin skin is plastered to all of the irregularities of the deep structures. Rather, we would delay inserting this apparatus for a day or two to determine whether this type of therapy will be necessary. In contrast, with the excision of cystic hygromas of the trunk, where accumulation of fluid is practically routine, the hemovac system should be inserted at the time of operation.

The cystic hygroma may extend into the thoracic cavity, and this should be suspected when the neck mass noticeably increases in size with increased intrathoracic pressure. A chest roentgenogram usually will detect such extension into the thoracic cavity.

Surgical removal may be accomplished when removal of the neck portion of the lesion is undertaken. When this is not possible thoracotomy must be done.

BRANCHIOGENIC SINUS AND CYST

The role of the branchial apparatus in the development of branchial sinuses and cysts is not clear. Information on this subject is based upon studies which were made years ago, for little investigative work has been done on these problems for many years. The branchial apparatus begins to develop on the fifteenth day of gestation and appears as five bars, or arches, of mesoderm separated by grooves or clefts. Externally the structure is covered by flat epithelium and lined by columnar epithelium. During the first half of the second month these disappear, except for the first, which forms the external auditory canal and the eustachian tube. Each arch contains a central cartilage, a blood vessel, and a nerve. The preauricular sinus and those sinuses extending downward and forward from the ear are considered to be related to the first arch, and the sinus and cysts lower in the neck are considered to be related to the second arch. The presence of cartilage in the cleft system offers an explanation for the cartilaginous remnants encountered in the neck.

Branchiogenic sinuses and cysts are lined with stratified squamous cells or columnar or ciliated epithelium and are surrounded by a muscular wall of varying thickness. The common form of the anomaly consists of a sinus tract which communicates with the skin anterior to the sternocleidomastoid muscle and above the clavicle in the middle and lower thirds of the neck; the other end of the sinus communicates with the pharynx at the base of the tonsil or posterior pillar. It is usually difficult to identify the opening in the pharynx. This communication is important clinically, for it is the portal of entry of material that may produce infection in the sinus.

The cysts usually do not communicate with either the skin or the pharynx—or the opening into the oropharynx is so small that it cannot be readily identified. It is possible to have a combination of both sinus and cysts in which the openings to the skin and pharynx are present but minute. The sinuses are noted early in life; cysts usually do not become clinically noticeable until the patient is in the late teens or early twenties.

DIAGNOSIS

The symptom commonly associated with a branchiogenic sinus is an intermittent discharge of mucoid material through a small opening of the skin of the neck, and there is a tendency for the material to dry about the orifice and form a white crust. Older patients may note a disagreeable taste in the mouth occasionally, caused by a discharge of material from the sinus to the mouth. Aside from these complaints the sinuses are asymptomatic except for infection, which takes place occasionally. During an episode of infection there is extensive redness and swelling of the neck; later, fluctuation and spontaneous rupture will occur unless incision and drainage are performed. Such episodes prior to surgical removal make complete excision of the sinus difficult and the probability of recurrence greater. The relationship of these sinuses to deep carcinoma of the neck is not proved, but the two conditions have been associated; this is an additional reason for surgical removal of the sinus.

In examining the patient with a branchiogenic sinus, the small pinpoint opening is observed in the lower portion of the neck anterior to the sternocleidomastoid muscle. Milking the tissue from above toward the cutaneous opening will usually produce a droplet of mucoid material (Fig. 6). By pull-

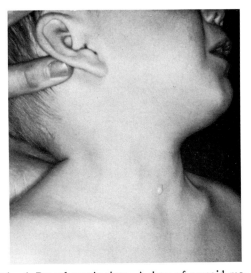

Fig. 6. Branchiogenic sinus. A drop of mucoid material has drained from the sinus, indicating its position on the surface of the neck.

ing the skin downward below the opening, it is possible to visualize the outline and palpate the firm sinus tract as it extends upward for a distance in the subcutaneous tissue. Branchiogenic sinuses are about as common on one side of the neck as on the other, and about 10 percent are bilateral. Patients with branchiogenic sinuses should be examined carefully for small sinuses in the lobe of the ear and anterior to the aural canal, for in some patients both anomalies are present. A branchiogenic sinus may be injected with radiopaque material, but this is of no practical value either diagnostically or therapeutically.

The diagnosis of branchiogenic cyst may be difficult. It appears as a painless swelling anterior to the sternocleidomastoid muscle. The cysts are usually thick walled and tense, and therefore on palpation the mass may seem solid rather than cystic.

Patients with uncomplicated branchiogenic cysts present no history of pain, tenderness, or redness of skin over the mass. Variation in size of the mass is unusual, although in some instances such changes may occur if the cyst communicates with the pharynx.

Frequently these cysts become infected, making impossible their differentiation from pyogenic adenitis; however, careful questioning of the parents may reveal a history of a preceding painless swelling of the neck. It is also difficult at times to distinguish the swelling from tuberculous adenitis. A negative intracutaneous tuberculin test is of value, for it is rare to have tuberculous adenitis without a positive skin test. It is also possible to confuse branchiogenic cyst with lymphoma, which may initially appear as a simple painless swelling in the neck. Generalized lymphadenopathy and splenomegaly support the diagnosis of lymphoma rather than branchiogenic cyst. A chest roentgenogram is of value to rule out mediastinal lymphoid enlargement, which would make the diagnosis of some form of lymphoma more likely than that of a branchiogenic cyst.

Treatment consists of surgical excision of the sinus or cyst. In the past there were some attempts made to eradicate the sinuses with sclerosing fluid. However, the cosmetic results were poor, for there was a tendency for a fibrous band to form that puckered and indented the skin at the site of the cutaneous opening. These lesions should be excised early in life to avoid episodes of infection which make the operative procedure more difficult, the likelihood of a complete excision less sure, and the cosmetic results less acceptable than is the case when the sinus is excised before infection has occurred. It is a simple technical procedure to excise these lesions in the first few months of life, for the sinus has considerable substance to it, and dissection can be done along an avascular plane adjacent to the tract.

OPERATION FOR BRANCHIOGENIC SINUS

A transverse incision is preferable to a diagonal incision along the anterior border of the sternocleidomastoid muscle, for the diagonal incision results in a tight cord that becomes prominent particularly when the head is turned. If the sinus opens low in the neck, it is advisable to make a short elliptical incision around the skin opening and then to dissect upward as far as possible. The second transverse incision is made in a normal fold of the skin of the neck. The sinus can be pushed up into this incision and the dissection continued. The usual course of the sinus through the neck is between the bifurcation of the carotid artery and above the hypoglossal nerve. Patients complaining of atrophy and deviation of the tongue postoperatively may have suffered hypoglossal nerve damage. The dissection must be made up to the pharyngeal wall to ensure complete excision of the sinus. It is helpful for the anesthesiologist to place his index finger in the patient's mouth with the tip of the finger in the tonsillar fossa, so that the operator can be informed when the dissection extends to this point (Fig. 7). The sinus is

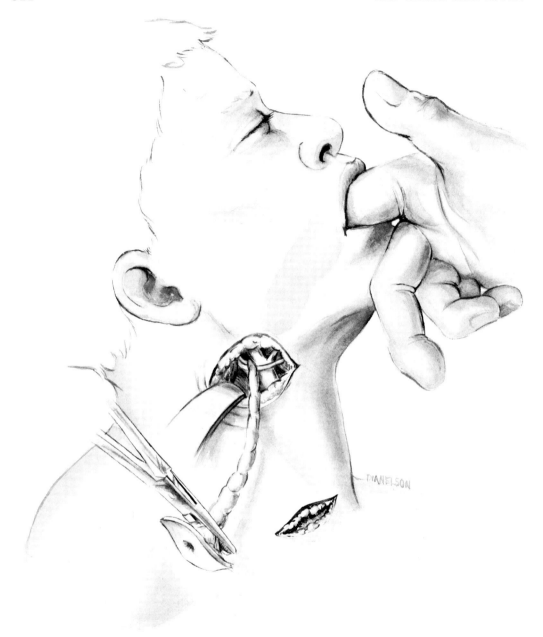

Fig. 7. Two incisions are usually required for good exposure after the tract is dissected beyond the bi-furcation of the carotid. The anesthesiologist can be of great help by inserting his finger into the patient's mouth and placing its tip in the tonsillar area; this aids the surgeon in making a complete removal of the tract.

ligated with a transfixing silk suture adjacent to the pharyngeal mucosa and divided beyond the ligature. The deep structures of the neck are approximated with a few interrupted fine chromic sutures. The platysma is approximated with interrupted 5-0 chromic sutures, the skin is brought together with continuous 5-0 plain catgut subcuticular sutures, and a collodion dressing is applied (Fig. 8). No drains are necessary. These patients are usually discharged on the third or fourth postoperative day.

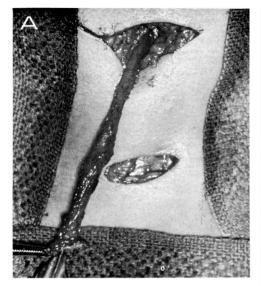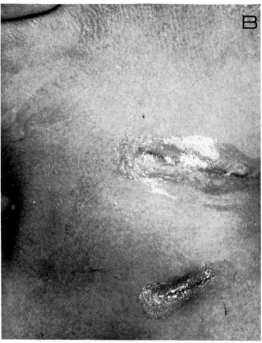

Fig. 8. A. Branchiogenic sinus dissected out, utilizing two short skin incisions. B. Flexible collodion has been painted on the skin incisions after subcuticular closure was accomplished.

OPERATION FOR
BRANCHIOGENIC CYSTS

Branchiogenic cysts are excised through a transverse skin incision. A superior cosmetic result can be obtained by placing the incision in a natural skin fold rather than over the most prominent portion of the mass. The dissection is made down to the cyst, which is deep to the sternocleidomastoid muscle and over the carotid sheath. In rare instances the mass may be so large that there has occurred a thinning out of the sternocleidomastoid muscle. The muscle is retracted laterally and the mass dissected out. Unless there have been bouts of infection, the plane of cleavage is avascular. Deep in the wound there will be a pedicle with a few vessels entering the cyst which require ligation. A search should be made for a sinus communicating with the pharynx, and if one is found it should be dissected down to the pharynx mucosa and dealt with in the same way as described for branchiogenic sinus, above. At times these cysts are so large that

it is advisable to deflate them partially by aspiration before removal is attempted.

The cysts contain a thin, yellowish-gray, opaque material which may be similar to that found in broken down tuberculous glands. However, smears will reveal no acid-fast bacilli, and there are no organisms present in a gram-stained smear.

A superior cosmetic result is secured by closing the wound with interrupted fine chromic sutures to the platysma and a running 5-0 plain catgut subcuticular suture. Collodion dressing on the incision immobilizes the skin edges and protects the incision for the first few days of healing.

BRANCHIAL ARRESTS

From time to time, patients are seen who have cartilaginous remnants under the skin of the neck. These remnants may be unilateral or bilateral, and they are objectionable from a cosmetic standpoint (Fig. 9). Surgical removal is simple. Fistulas are not connected with these lesions.

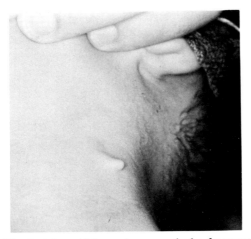

Fig. 9. A branchial arrest composed of a fragment of cartilage under the skin.

PREAURICULAR SINUSES

Preauricular sinuses are probably related to malformation of the first branchial cleft. They are common and at times are associated with branchiogenic sinuses (Fig. 10). Most of the preauricular sinuses are of little

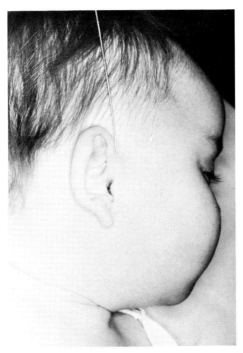

Fig. 10. Preauricular sinus. A probe has been inserted into the sinus to gauge its length, direction, and depth.

concern—they are small and are neither objectionable cosmetically nor likely to become infected. Occasionally, however, the sinus may be sufficiently deep for material to collect in it and infection to occur repeatedly, and in such instances the sinus should be excised. These sinuses are almost always more difficult to remove than is generally appreciated. Recurrence of infection is the rule unless a complete removal is accomplished. Preauricular sinuses should never be removed anywhere but in the operating room, with adequate instruments and assistance available. There are rare sinuses or cysts which open to the skin or are located just under the mandible. They may communicate with the aural canal.

Because they may be in close proximity to the facial nerves, care must be exercised during surgical removal to prevent nerve damage.

THYROGLOSSAL CYST

Thyroglossal cysts arise from remnants of the embryonic thyroglossal duct. During the fourth week of gestation the thyroid anlage forms as an evagination from the floor of the primitive pharynx between the first and second pharyngeal grooves and develops as a duct. Later the lumen is obliterated, and the structure remains as a solid cord extending from the foramen caecum of the tongue, usually through the hyoid bone (but occasionally anterior or posterior to it), to the pyramidal lobe of the thyroid gland. When the lining epithelium of the thyroglossal duct fails to degenerate, a cyst may form anywhere along the midline of the neck between the foramen caecum and the suprasternal notch. Most commonly, the rounded cyst is found in the midline, at or just below the hyoid bone. There may be slight lateral deviation of the mass, but this is not usually of such a degree as to cause confusion of thyroglossal cysts with branchial cysts, which are definitely in the lateral portion of the neck. Thyroglossal cysts may be lined by stratified squamous, columnar, or transitional epithelium. Following infection, heavy fibrous connective tissue may surround the tract.

There are few symptoms related to a thyroglossal cyst. Because of the cyst's usual position at the level of the hyoid bone or just below it, no pressure phenomena are produced, and because it develops slowly there is no pain. Cysts within the tongue substance above the hyoid bone may enlarge and produce symptoms of pharyngeal discomfort, including choking sensations and dysphagia. Such cysts can be seen when the back of the tongue is depressed with a throat stick. In rare instances, pressure on the cyst may produce a flow of fluid from the cyst through the foramen caecum into the mouth (Fig. 11).

Except for a small lump in the midline of the neck, the patient is often not aware that he has a thyroglossal cyst until a bout of infection occurs. The infection begins as cellulitis of the neck; later, unless incision

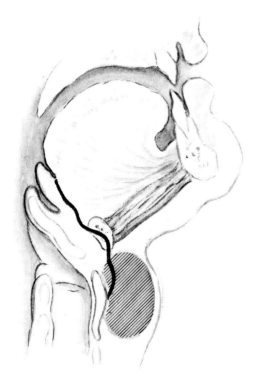

Fig. 11. Drawing indicating the relationship of a thyroglossal cyst and sinus to the hyoid bone and the tongue.

and drainage are performed, spontaneous rupture and formation of a fistula will occur. It is doubtful that a congenital fistula of this duct ever occurs, for in all instances the fistula is preceded either by incision and drainage or by spontaneous perforation from infection.

Thyroglossal cysts are in the midline of the neck below the hyoid bone. The cyst fluid is under pressure, so the mass usually cannot be distinguished from a solid tumor by palpation of the lesion. The cysts are nontender and move with deglutition. Movement of the cyst may be detected when the patient protrudes his tongue. There are only a few lesions which can be confused with thyroglossal cyst. Dermoids do not transilluminate light, and they are not attached to the hyoid bone and therefore do not move on deglutition. On physical examination it is impossible to differentiate an aberrant thyroid from a thyroglossal cyst—in the location and external appearance of the mass, the two conditions may be identical. Direct examination of the tumor should enable the surgeon to distinguish thyroid tissue from the smooth, avascular surface of the cyst. As a rule, patients with congenital malformation of the thyroid will have all the glandular tissue in a midline round mass. Removal of this mass under the mistaken impression that it is a thyroglossal cyst leaves the patient with hypothyroidism and even hypoparathyroidism. Therefore, if there is any doubt, the cyst should be aspirated to identify it, or a biopsy should be performed. Occasionally, the thyroglossal cyst is situated laterally to the midline, and in such a situation it is indistinguishable from a branchiogenic cyst until it is demonstrated at operation that the tract leads to the midportion of the hyoid bone. Once the diagnosis has been made, the thyroglossal cyst should be excised. Some surgeons believe that excision is not invariably indicated except in instances where the cosmetic situation requires correction. However, the incidence of infection is so high in this anomaly that it is wise to remove the lesion once the diagnosis has been established.

There have been a number of reports of carcinoma developing in the structure, and this is an additional reason for surgical removal.

If infection occurs, there may be extensive cellulitis of the neck, and the cyst cannot be detected on examination. The history of a nontender, small mass preceding the infection indicates the true nature of the lesion. Antibiotics are helpful in checking the cellulitis but will not completely control the infection. Incision and drainage are preferred to spontaneous rupture of the cyst because the duration of the illness is reduced and the patient is left with a more acceptable scar. In most instances, after either spontaneous rupture or incision and drainage, a cutaneous fistula is established. Repeated infection will occur until the tract, with its lining, is completely removed. Excision should not be attempted until at least six weeks after infection because of the edema which makes the operation difficult and which increases the likelihood of postoperative wound infection. Under no circumstances should a thyroglossal cyst be treated with the injection of sclerosing material. It is impossible for the necrotizing solution to reach all the crevices and minute projections along the tract and produce a cure. Furthermore, the resulting scarring may produce irregularities of the skin which are not cosmetically acceptable. Radiation therapy is also of no avail, for none of the histological components of the cyst is radiosensitive.

OPERATION

Surgical excision is a simple procedure; the cosmetic result is excellent, and recurrence is unusual. The patient is given anesthesia with an endotracheal tube in place. Sandbags are placed under the shoulders, and the head section of the table is lowered to hyperextend the neck. A transverse incision 3 to 4 cm in length is made over the mass, or, if a fistula to the skin exists, an elliptical incision is made around the opening. The subcutaneous tissue and platysma are reflected with the skin. The infrahyoid muscles are separated in the midline, and the cyst is exposed. The cyst is then dissected free. There is invariably a short stalk leading to the midportion of the hyoid bone. Even in those instances in which the tract does not clearly traverse the hyoid bone, it is advisable to remove the central portion of that bone (Fig. 12). Excision of the mid-

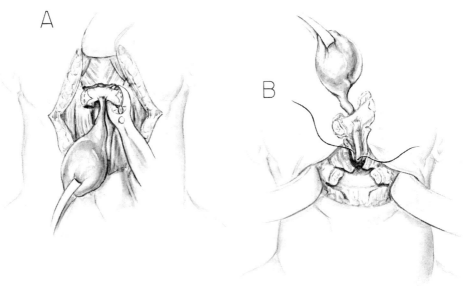

Fig. 12. A. Exposure of the thyroglossal cyst and the hyoid bone. Excision of the central portion of bone is necessary in this operation. B. The sinus has been dissected out of the tongue.

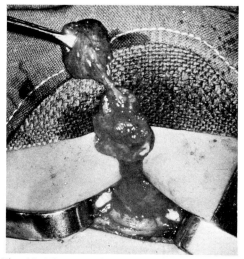

Fig. 13. The operative field after the hyoid bone has had a segment cut out of it as being part of the sinus tract.

portion of the bone will be facilitated by the partial detachment of the geniohyoideus and mylohyoideus from the superior surface of the hyoid bone and the sternohyoid from the inferior surface, thus exposing the thyrohyoid membrane below the bone. It is possible to remove a 1-cm portion of the bone in children under two years of age with a pair of heavy scissors. In older patients a bone cutter is required (Fig. 13). Amputation of this portion of hyoid does not interfere with any function after operation. Beyond the hyoid bone a friable tract is usually found, and it is necessary to remove some tongue sub-

stance with the tract to prevent tearing and to assure its complete removal. It is of great practical assistance to have the anesthesiologist place his index finger in the patient's mouth and press the foramen caecum downward and forward. This improves the exposure and permits the anesthesiologist to detect when the dissection approaches the mucosa of the tongue. This procedure assures a complete dissection of the tract and also prevents one from inadvertently making an opening into the mouth. It is not necessary to excise the foramen caecum. When the dissection is down to the mucosa of the tongue, the stalk is ligated with a transfixing silk suture and the lesion excised.

The hyoid bone is reapproximated with interrupted black silk sutures through the periosteum. The infrahyoid muscles are also brought together with interrupted black silk sutures and the skin closed with subcutaneous sutures of chromic and continuous 5-0 plain catgut subcuticular suture. The incision is painted with flexible collodion. A drain is unnecessary.

The recurrence rate is low, provided a complete excision of the tract including a generous portion of the tissue above and below the hyoid bone and at least 1 cm of the central portion of the bone is performed.

ORVAR SWENSON

REFERENCES

BAILEY, H. Clinical aspects of branchial fistulae. Brit. J. Surg., 21: 173, 1933.

BILL, A. H., Jr., and SUMNER, D. S. A unified concept of lymphangioma and cystic hygroma. Surg. Gynec. Obstet., 120: 79, 1965.

BOCHETTO, J. F., MONTOYA, A., and SUNDE, E. A. Papillary carcinoma of the thyroid in thyroglossal duct cysts. Amer. J. Surg., 104: 773, 1962.

BRIGGS, J. D., LEIX, F., SNYDER, W. H., and CHAFFIN, L. Cystic and cavernous lymphangioma. West. J. Surg. Obstet. Gynec., 61: 499, 1953.

CHILDRESS, M. E., BAKER, C. P., and SAMSON, P. C. Lymphangioma of the mediastinum; Report of a case with a review of the literature. J. Thorac. Surg., 31: 338, 1956.

CHISHOLM, T. C., SPENCER, B. J., and McFARLAND, F. A. Lymphangiomas. Pediat. Clin. N. Amer., 6: 529, 1959.

FLINT, C. Sinus of first branchial cleft. Amer. Surg., 48: 165, 1908.

FRAZER, J. E. Nomenclature of diseased states caused by certain vestigial structures of the neck. Brit. J. Surg., 11: 131, 1923.

GALOFRE, M., JUDD, E. S., PEREZ, P. E., and HARRISON, E. G., Jr. Results of surgical treatment of cystic hygroma. Surg. Gynec. Obstet., 115: 319, 1962.

GOETSCH, E. Hygroma colli cysticum and hygroma axillare; Pathologic and clinical study and report of 12 cases. Arch. Surg., 36: 394, 1938.

HARKINS, G. A., and SABISTON, D. C. Lymphangioma in infancy and childhood. Surgery, 47: 811, 1960.

HODGSON, E. H., et al. Hereditary hemorrhagic telangiectasia and pulmonary arteriovenous fistula. New Eng. J. Med., 261: 626, 1959.

KOTTMEIER, P. K., ROSENTHAL, S., and MINKOWITZ, S. Retropharyngeal abscess secondary to thyroglossal cyst. Amer. J. Dis. Child., 109, No. 2: 160, 1965.

LANDING, B. H., and FARBER, S. Tumors of the cardiovascular system. In Armed Forces Institute of Pathology, Section III, Fascicle 7, Washington, D.C., National Research Council, 1956.

LIERLE, D. M. Congenital lymphangiomatous macroglossia with cystic hygroma of the neck. Ann. Otol., 53: 574, 1944.

LYALL, D., and STAHL, W. Lateral cervical cysts, sinuses and fistulas of congenital origin. Int. Abstr. Surg., 102, No. 5: 417, 1956.

LYNN, H. B. Cystic hygroma. Surg. Clin. N. Amer., August: 1157, 1963.

PENICK, R. M. Preauricular sinuses; Diagnosis and treatment. Southern Med. J., 38: 2, 1945.

POTTER, E. L. Pathology of Fetus and Infant. Chicago, The Year Book Medical Publishers, Inc., 1961.

SABIN, F. R. On the development of the superficial lymphatics in the skin of a pig. Amer. J. Anat., 3: 183, 1904.

————. Development of the lymphatic system. In Keitel, F., and Mall, F. P., eds. Manual of Human Embryology. Philadelphia, J. B. Lippincott Company, 1912, Vol. 2, pp. 709–745.

————. Direct growth of veins by sprouting. In Contributions to Embryology, Washington, Carnegie Institution of Washington, 1922, Vol. 14, pp. 1–10.

SHAW, A., SANTULLI, T. V., and RANKOW, R. Cysts and sinuses of the first branchial cleft and pouch. Surg. Gynec. Obstet., 115: 671, 1962.

STARK, D. Congenital tract of neck and ear. Plast. Reconstr. Surg., 23: 621, 1959.

TANAKA, K., and CIVIN, W. H. Cancer arising in thyroglossal duct remnant. Arch. Surg., 86: 136, 1963.

WENGLOWSKI, R. Über die Halsfisteln und Cysten. Arch. Klin. Chir., 98: 151, 1912; 100: 789, 1913.

WILLIS, R. A. Pathology of Tumors, 2d ed. London, Butterworth & Co. (Publishers), Ltd., 1960.

22

Infections of the Head and Neck

ENLARGEMENT OF THE CERVICAL LYMPH NODES

Chronic enlargement of the cervical lymph nodes often poses a problem to the attending physician, for there is always the possibility of the change being caused by a malignant process. A child with an obvious nasopharyngeal infection or oral infection is expected to have some enlargement of the cervical lymph nodes, and when such infection is detected, enlarged lymph nodes are readily explained. It is in the situation where examination fails to reveal any cause for enlarged lymph nodes that the physician is understandably worried about the possibility of the nodes harboring some form of malignancy. A careful history should be taken from such patients. If there is a history of ingestion of raw milk or contact with a person with active tuberculosis, the possibility of cervical tuberculous adenitis is suggested. An intercutaneous tuberculin test will determine if the patient harbors tuberculosis. It is reasonable for the attending physician to observe a child with cervical lymph node enlargement without obvious etiology for a period of three to four weeks. If at the end of such a period of observation the lymph nodes have not decreased in size or if they have enlarged, and the Mantoux test is negative and careful examination of the oral and nasal cavities has revealed no tumor, biopsy is a wise course to follow. It is true that in most instances the removed lymph node will contain no evidence of malignancy but rather will show a hyperplasia which is perfectly innocent, nevertheless, it is impossible to be sure which category the lymph node will fall into without excision biopsy.

Chemotherapy is usually administered in the acute stage of cervical adenitis, and often this therapy is successful in eliminating the adenitis. At times the enlargement of the lymph nodes persists despite prolonged chemotherapy. In such situations the antibiotic has not eradicated the infection; rather, it has held it in check and there has been no resolution of infection. If the enlarged lymph nodes persist after three or four weeks of observation, excisional biopsy to rule out malignant disease is mandatory. This type of situation can be avoided by limiting the use of antibiotics for cervical adenitis to a relatively short course of therapy. If the antibiotic is not effective in a period of five to seven days, it is advisable to discontinue the medication and permit the lymph nodes to soften and eventually be incised and drained.

PYOGENIC CERVICAL ADENITIS

Infection of the cervical lymph nodes is frequently secondary to pharyngeal infection, particularly tonsillitis (Figs. 1 and 2). The causative organism is a streptococcus or a staphylococcus, and usually several lymph

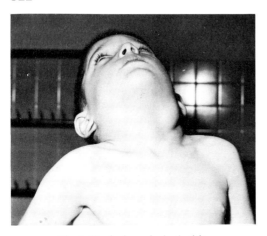

Fig. 1. Typical cervical adenitis.

nodes are involved on one or both sides of the neck. The pharyngeal infection which precedes the adenitis by several days may be mild and hardly recalled by the patient or observed by his parents. In small children a virulent form of the infection occurs with a sudden and high fever. Initially, only slight enlargement of the lymph nodes occurs, and a careful examination is necessary to detect the infected cervical nodes. As the disease progresses, the lymph nodes become enlarged, and there is considerable localized pain and tenderness, so that the patient limits his head movements. With further progress of the infection, cellulitis of the adjacent skin and subcutaneous tissue develops.

The diagnosis of pyogenic cervical adeni-

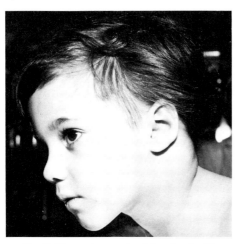

Fig. 2. Unusual posterior triangle adenitis.

tis is obvious from the short history, high fever, enlarged, painful, and exquisitely tender lymph nodes, and inflammation of the overlying skin. Later in the disease the hard enlarged lymph nodes become soft, and abscess formation takes place. It is usually simple to differentiate pyogenic from tubercular cervical adenitis because of the short history and the signs of acute inflammation. Cervical lymph nodes infected with tubercle bacilli enlarge gradually during a period of several weeks and are not painful or tender initially. Frequently there is a history of contact with tuberculosis or of ingestion of raw milk, and the intracutaneous tuberculin test is invariably positive.

Patients who have had repeated infection of the cervical nodes should have tonsillectomy and adenoidectomy performed as an aid in preventing recurrence, for the primary site of infection is thereby removed.

Moist heat can be used to hasten localization of the infection in the lymph nodes and to make the child comfortable. Incision and drainage are delayed until there is extensive softening within the lymph nodes and the skin is smooth, red, and shiny over the fluctuant area. A common mistake is to undertake drainage too early, before liquefaction within the lymph nodes has occurred, and consequently a prolonged period of drainage follows, with the inconvenience of repeated dressings.

OPERATION

A transverse incision is used to facilitate drainage. Particular care should be exercised to avoid dividing the mandibular branch of the facial nerve while draining fluctuant areas high in the neck. Such accidents can usually be prevented by making the incision through the skin with a scalpel and then by resorting to blunt dissection in the deeper tissue. This operation is preferably carried out under general anesthesia so that the compartments of the abscessed cavity can be broken down and the whole infected area converted into one cavity, which is then packed with a

¼-inch plain gauze strip. Two to three feet of packing is inserted into the abscess, depending on the size of the cavity. The advantage of this type of drain is that the pack will not come out until it is removed. Six to eight inches can be withdrawn each day, and with this program the drain will remain in place for four to five days. This is sufficient time for the abscessed cavity to contract considerably, so there is little or no drainage once the drain has been removed. If the drain is removed before drainage is completed, the skin may seal over, leaving a partially filled abscessed cavity that may require reincision and drainage.

Today, this disease process is not as frequently observed as it was formerly. This is probably related to the fact that antibiotics are administered to the patient with severe pharyngitis and other types of oropharyngeal infection, which undoubtedly plays a role in reducing the incidence of cervical adenitis.

TUBERCULOSIS OF CERVICAL LYMPH NODES

Tuberculous cervical adenitis, a rare condition in the United States today, was a prevalent disease 50 years ago. The control of bovine tuberculosis, the use of pasteurized milk, and the sanatorium care of tuberculous patients with open lesions have all contributed to this improvement. Pathological studies of tonsils and adenoids removed from children with tuberculous cervical adenitis often demonstrated the presence of acid-fast organisms, indicating that involvement of the lymph nodes is often secondary to pharyngeal infection. Today this may not be the invariable train of events, for indications are that the human strain is involved more frequently, whereas the bovine strain was common in the past. Involvement of lymph nodes in the anterior cervical triangle is secondary to both pharyngeal and tonsillar infection. The adenoids may also be a portal of entry, and in such instances the preauricular nodes and those of the posterior triangle are most commonly involved. This was the experience in the past when this lesion was common and often caused by the bovine strain.

Usually, the progression of infection is slow so that the glands gradually increase in size. Later, liquefaction occurs, and at this stage the nodes may rupture and the exudate may form an abscess in the neck which will necrose the superficial tissue. If this abscess is left unattended, spontaneous drainage through the skin will occur. The resulting sinus may discharge tuberculosis organisms. After prolonged drainage the sinus may eventually close spontaneously with unsightly scarring.

Initially, a child with cervical tuberculous adenitis usually has no complaints except the enlarged glands. There is often a history of ingestion of raw milk or contact with a person infected with tuberculosis. As the adenitis progresses there may be minimal generalized symptoms, such as malaise and low grade fever, and eventually abscess formation occurs, with localized pain and tenderness.

Early in the course of cervical tuberculous adenitis, diagnosis is problematic because the lymph node is discrete and shows no evidence of inflammation, and differentiation from glands enlarged with chronic pyogenic infection or some form of malignant disease is difficult. As the disease progresses, the diagnosis of tuberculous cervical adenitis is less difficult. This is the most likely diagnosis when a child has had unilateral, matted, nontender cervical lymph nodes for six weeks or more and has a positive intracutaneous tuberculin test. A history of contact with tuberculosis or ingestion of raw milk supports the diagnosis (Fig. 3). Cervical lymph nodes containing malignant disease are usually bilateral, discrete in outline, and unattached to the skin and deep structures, and the patient may have splenic enlargement. A negative intracutaneous test with a 1:100 dilution of old tuberculin used to be evidence that a tuberculin infection was not present. Today there are other strains of tuberculosis, and those, such as the Batty strain, should also be used as a skin test. If these are negative

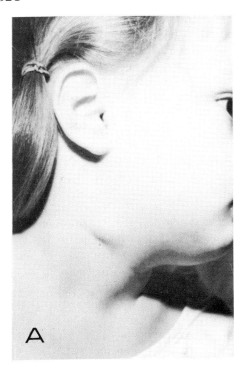

it is reasonable to assume that acid-fast infection is not present. A chest film is advisable before treatment is undertaken. In most instances, children with tuberculous cervical adenitis are not afflicted with pulmonary involvement. As a precaution, all siblings and the parents should have routine investigations for the detection of tuberculosis.

Tonsillectomy and adenoidectomy are indicated for patients with cervical tuberculous adenitis, for the primary lesions are often in the tonsils and adenoids, and, unless they are removed, recurrence is likely despite surgical removal of the cervical glands. If enlarged neck glands are present three weeks after tonsillectomy, the best treatment is surgical excision of the cervical glands. Only in instances in which the skin is thin over the lymph nodes and spontaneous drainage is imminent should tonsillectomy be deferred until after excision of the glands. For patients with cervical tuberculous adenitis whose tonsils and adenoids have been removed previ-

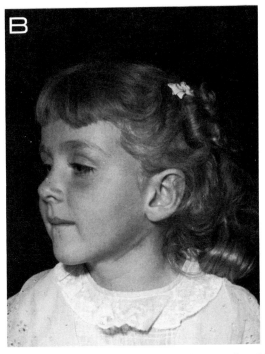

Fig. 3. A. Tuberculosis of cervical lymph nodes. Softening had occurred, and breakdown of the skin had begun. B. Patient after excision.

ously, surgical excision of the cervical nodes is the treatment of choice.

OPERATION

Tuberculous lymph nodes of the neck need not be removed by a block dissection such as that used for lymph nodes containing metastatic malignant implants. With tuberculous lymph nodes excellent results are obtained by excision of the involved glands, and no other structure need be sacrificed or damaged. A transverse incision in a skin fold provides adequate exposure and ensures an excellent cosmetic result. Incisions parallel to the sternocleidomastoid muscle are not satisfactory, for a prominent, diagonal, unsightly scar often results. If a sinus is present or the skin is thin and red, an elliptical incision is used so that the sinus or devitalized skin is removed with the lymph nodes. There is an intense periglandular inflammation about the superficial nodes so that they are matted together and adherent, requiring sharp dissection in their removal. Occasionally, caseous nodes are inadvertently opened, and the operative field is contaminated with exudate. Such contamination is tolerated by the tissue, and primary healing of the incision is the rule despite this complication.

In dissection of the superficial lymph nodes, particularly if they are high in the neck, damage to the mandibular branch of the facial nerve is possible. This branch traverses the neck considerably below the mandible, and since the nerve's smallness

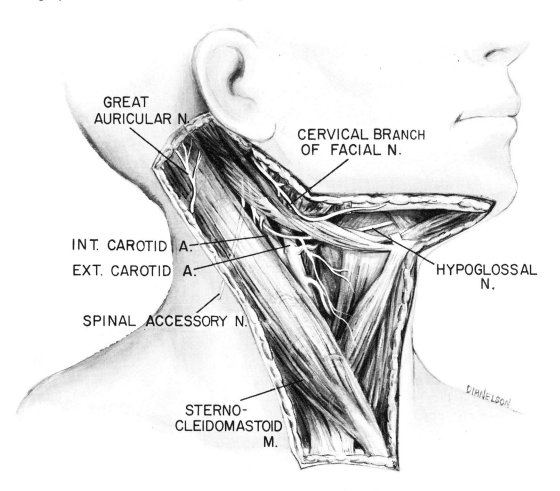

Fig. 4. Anatomical drawing of the neck.

precludes visual identification, the surgeon must depend on an electrical stimulator for its identification. Cutting of the nerve results in a cosmetically unacceptable dysfunction of the angle of the mouth (Fig. 4).

It is essential to isolate the spinal accessory nerve after the superficial nodes have been removed. It is a large nerve and is readily identified by dissection along the upper third of the anterior border of the sternocleidomastoid muscle. The nerve is usually superficial to the internal jugular vein and descends obliquely behind the digastric and stylohyoid muscles to enter the upper part of the sternocleidomastoid muscle. Division of this nerve in the child results in a painful depressed shoulder, a serious deformity which should be avoided.

As the carotid sheath is exposed, the lymph nodes are found to be smaller, less adherent, and more easily removed. The nodes deeper than the spinal accessory nerve and between the structure and the tip of the mastoid should be removed to prevent recurrence. The hypoglossal nerve should be identified as it emerges from between the internal carotid artery and the internal jugular vein, swings downward and forward, and becomes superficial below the digastric muscle. Damage to the hypoglossal nerve produces ipsilateral deviation and atrophy of the tongue. When all visible and palpable glands have been removed, complete hemostasis is secured by the use of fine catgut ligatures. The wound is closed with interrupted silk skin sutures. A drain is not left in the wound because it would promote the formation of a sinus. If fluid collects under the wound postoperatively, repeated aspiration is recommended until fluid no longer accumulates.

There are no objections to the use of isoniazid preoperatively, although our experience has indicated that such treatment is not of perceptible value. Streptomycin is not indicated because prolonged use of this antibiotic has been associated with hearing loss. The same is true postoperatively, although some complications, such as wounds that drain chronically, may be prevented if this drug is used. The excellent results of excision and the rare complications and recurrence make surgical treatment the best method of caring for children with tuberculosis of the cervical lymph nodes.

ACTINOMYCOSIS OF THE NECK

Actinomycosis is a growing problem in medicine. Although it is not as common in children as in adults, it does occur with sufficient frequency that physicians caring for children must be aware of this chronic infectious process. Actinomycetes are anaerobic to microaerophilic gram-positive organisms with branching filamentous mycelia and seem to be more related to bacteria than fungi. Bollinger (1877) was the first to recognize the organism as being related to a disease in cattle known as lumpy jaw. Israel (1878) was the first to recognize the organism in exudate from human material. An aerobic form of this same organism, nocardia, has been described and is now recognized as being the cause of disease in patients, which has been designated nocardiosis. In reported series of actinomycosis the cervicofacial area is most commonly involved; next is the abdominal form of the disease, and least common is chest involvement. This is a chronic disease which in some ways resembles tuberculosis. In the past the human disease has been closely associated with lumpy jaw in cattle. It is assumed that the bovine form of the disease is spread in straw and grasses. The organism which is invariably involved in human cases has never been found to grow outside the human body. Consequently the concept that this disease is related to the chewing of straws and grasses is not reasonable. Furthermore, the disease is just as prevalent in city areas as it is in the rural population. Chronic caries has been found to be related to the disease. Often, examination of the exudate about extracted teeth reveals the presence of the organism. It is now conjectured that this is the source of infection, and it would explain the prevalence of the cervicofacial type of the disease.

The disease makes itself known in the cervicofacial region by the swelling of lymph nodes. At first there may be a mass that gradually grows in size. There may be very little enlargement of the lymph nodes, the first indication of the disease being the development of a draining cutaneous fistula. In such patients careful examination of the exudate for sulfur granules is important, for this is a simple and positive way to establish the diagnosis.

In the abdominal form of the disease a draining fistula may develop in the right lower quadrant, for this is the area within the abdominal cavity most likely to be affected by actinomycosis. The fistula may be associated with a palpable mass. In the thoracic form of the disease there may be pulmonic infiltration and empyema, and frequently the disease process makes itself known in a chronically ill patient by spontaneous drainage of an empyema. In all situations where a chronic draining sinus presents, examination for sulfur granules is an essential diagnostic step.

TREATMENT

In the past, various forms of treatment were advocated. The administration of iodides was quite popular. It is now established that this does not have any direct curative action on the disease process. There were some patients who responded to sulfanilamides. It may well be that these were cases of nocardiosis rather than actinomycosis, for the latter does not regularly respond to the sulfa drugs.

In 1941 an Oxford group of investigators, including Sir Howard W. Florey (Abraham, et al., 1941), found that actinomycetes were killed by a concentration of 0.01 units of penicillin per ml of medium. In 1960, Peabody and Seabury stated that for the average case of actinomycosis penicillin remains the drug of choice. Two points in therapy with penicillin are important, the first being that the dosage must be quite high, 1 to 6 million units of penicillin being recommended daily for adults. In severe cases the dosage is increased to as high as 12 million units. The second point in the treatment is that penicillin must be given over a long period of time, at least six to eight weeks and frequently much longer.

There remains some place for surgical treatment. In the past, excision of the lesion has been possible in some situations where the mass is quite superficial and has not extended widely. Where abscess formation is detected, incision and drainage has proved beneficial. Curettage of chronic draining sinuses has been of some help. At the present time the role of surgery in the treatment of this disease is that of an adjunct to chemotherapy. In nocardiosis, the organism is not sensitive to penicillin. Patients afflicted with this organism should have sensitivity studies. Usually, one of the sulfa drugs is reasonably effective as a therapeutic agent.

SIALECTASIA

The most common cause of parotid swelling is sialectasia. The etiology is not clear, for infection does not invariably seem to be the causative agent. Few of the glands have been biopsied, and consequently there are few pathological data available. In the advanced stages of sialectasis, concretions form in large ducts. Allergy has been proved to be the etiology in rare instances.

With sialectasia, the patient has a relatively painless swelling of the gland. There may be some fever, but the temperature usually remains normal. The entire gland is swollen, and local tenderness is usually slight, although in some instances it is considerable. The opening of Stensen's duct may be a bit red, and pressure on the gland may produce a flow of cloudy fluid that on microscopic examination may be found to contain leukocytes. The swelling persists from several days to two or three weeks before subsiding, and it is usually followed by a recurrence of swelling in a few weeks to several months. The

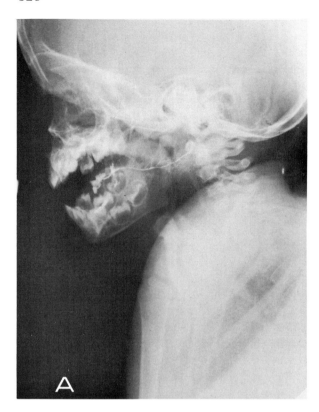

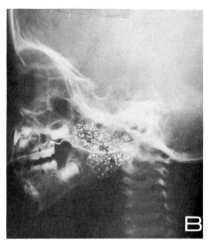

Fig. 5. A. A normal sialogram. B. This patient had a swelling of the parotid gland. The sialogram demonstrates dilatation of the duct system.

disease may progress with considerable enlargement of the ducts and the formation of concretions in the glands, and in this advanced form there may be considerable pain. The disease does not often progress to this stage, since in most patients it is mild and self-limited.

A sialogram will demonstrate enlargement of ducts similar to the enlargement of the bronchioles in bronchiectasis (Fig. 5). A blockage of Stensen's duct would also be detected in the sialogram.

The lack of sound etiologic data makes treatment unsatisfactory. Occasionally, a broad-spectrum antibiotic, such as Aureomycin, seems to alleviate attacks and diminish recurrences. In the advanced form of the disease, there may be considerable pain and chronic swelling which prove resistant to medical treatment. Stones are usually present in such glands. In such rare instances, when attacks become frequent and excessively painful, surgical excision of the gland may become necessary, and it can be accomplished without damage to the facial nerve.

OPERATION

Removal of the gland is performed through a vertical incision anterior to the ear. The incision curves behind and below the aural canal and then forward below the angle of the jaw. Preliminary ligation of the external carotid artery will reduce bleeding and is favored by some surgeons. The ligature can be conveniently placed between the superior thyroid and the lingual arteries. The trunk of the facial nerve should be identified as it passes between the two lobes of the gland so that the large superficial part of the gland can be separated and the isthmus divided without damage to this important structure. Identification of the facial nerve trunk is accomplished by careful dissection below the aural canal anterior to the

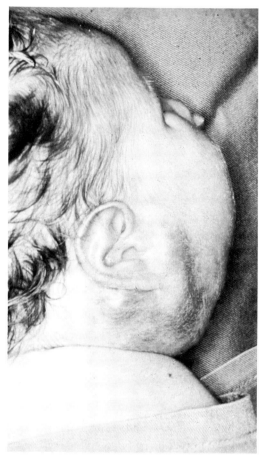

Fig. 6. An infant with a parotid abscess on the right side.

mastoid. The nerve is a large trunk that is usually deeper than anticipated. It is possible to identify one of the branches of the nerve, such as the mandibular branch as it passes over the caudal edge of the mandible and crosses the anterior facial vein. Identification is made simpler by the use of an electric stimulator. Once the branch has been identified the dissection is pursued proximally until all of the branch and the trunk is exposed. The dissection also removes the superficial part of the gland and permits ligation and division of Stensen's duct.

The smaller deep portion of the gland can then be removed, with care being taken to check frequently with the electrical stimulator to prevent damage to the facial nerve

branches. Stensen's duct and all bleeding points are ligated, and the wound is closed with interrupted silk sutures. A drain is unnecessary. A slight diminution of facial nerve function may be present in the first few postoperative days. Complete loss of function of all areas innervated by the facial nerve is evidence of division of the main trunk and is an indication for an exploration of the wound and a suturing of the divided nerve or for the insertion of a graft if a segment of a nerve has inadvertently been excised.

ABSCESS OF THE PAROTID GLAND

There seems to be a diminished incidence of parotid abscess at the present time. The disease is most frequently observed in infants (Fig. 6), and formerly it was associated with a high mortality rate. There may be extensive cellulitis and bacteremia, and intensive chemotherapy is usually effective for these aspects of the disease. However, localized collections of exudate will not be appreciably influenced by this therapy and will eventually require incision and drainage. It is advisable to perform a sialogram to demonstrate the patency of Stensen's duct, for if incision and drainage of an abscess is performed with the duct blocked, a salivary fistula will persist until patency of the duct is reestablished.

TRAUMATIC DIVISION OF STENSEN'S DUCT

Penetrating lacerations of the cheek may divide Stensen's duct, and unless this is recognized when the laceration is sutured, a salivary fistula to the face may result. If a laceration extends to or into the masseter muscle, it is advisable to identify Stensen's duct before suturing the laceration. Saliva in the wound may call attention to laceration of the duct. Usually there is division of one of the facial nerve branches, but repair of this is impossible and unnecessary, for functional return is the rule. The divided duct is sutured together with 5-0 plain catgut, and it is helpful to use a 4-0 ureteral catheter as a splint. This may be left in place a few days or re- moved immediately after the anastomosis has been accomplished.

ORVAR SWENSON

REFERENCES

ABRAHAM, E. P., CHAIN, E., FLETCHER, C. M., GARDNER, A. D., HEATLEY, N. G., JENNINGS, M. A., and FLOREY, H. W. Further observations on penicillin. Lancet, 2: 177, 1941.

BOLLINGER, O. Über eine neue Pilzkrankheit beim Rinde. Zentralb. Med. Wiss. (Berlin), 15: 481, 1877.

ISRAEL, J. Neue Beobachtungen auf dem Gebiete der Mykosen des Menschen. Arch. Path. Anat. (Berlin), 74: 15, 1878.

JURGENS, P. E. Cervico-facial actinomycosis, Report of a case. J. Oral Surg., 20: 345, 1962.

PEABODY, J. W., and SEABURY, J. H., Jr. Actinomycosis and nocardiosis. Amer. J. Med., 28: 99, 1960.

WEED, L. A., and BAGGENSTOSS, A. H. Actinomycosis: A pathologic and bacteriologic study of twenty-one fatal cases. Amer. J. Clin. Path. 19: 3, 1949.

WRIGHT, J. H. The Biology of the micro-organisms of actinomycosis. J. Med. Res., 13: 349, 1905.

23

Diseases of the Thyroid Gland

ECTOPIC THYROID

The thyroid gland develops from a midline pharyngeal diverticulum that extends caudally and becomes the thyroglossal cyst. Below the hyoid bone the end of the duct gives rise to the thyroid as a midline structure from which the lateral lobes develop. The pyramidal lobe and isthmus remain as parts of the original midline mass. On rare occasions the thyroid does not develop into the bilobed form but persists as a rounded midline structure in the neck. Despite this gross maldevelopment of gland configuration, the patients with this anomaly exhibit no symptoms or signs of thyroid dysfunction. Patients with this type of thyroid gland have an asymptomatic, rounded, midline mass below the hyoid bone in the neck. The mass is smooth in outline, firm in consistency, and unattached to the skin, and it moves on deglutition. The solid thyroid tissue transilluminates poorly, and this helps differentiate it from a thyroglossal cyst. In other respects these two conditions are indistinguishable on physical examination. A history of variation in size or development and of a gradual increase in the size of the mass after birth is important and indicates a thyroglossal duct cyst rather than ectopic thyroid.

A precise preoperative diagnosis between the two conditions is often impossible. However, it is of the utmost importance to differentiate the two conditions when the mass

is surgically exposed, or all of the patient's thyroid tissue might inadvertently be removed. Unfortunately, the midline mass usually comprises all of the thyroid tissue the patient possesses. If this is excised, daily administration of thyroid will correct the symptoms of hypothyroidism. The child will develop into a normal adult but with the handicap of necessary continuous medication. However, the situation becomes more serious in the rare situation in which all the parathyroids are intimately attached to the ectopic thyroid and are removed with the thyroid mass. This may result in an early postoperative demise, unless the situation is recognized by the presence of positive Chvostek's and Trousseau's signs. A fatality can be prevented, but the patient and his doctor are faced with the difficult problem of lifelong parathyroid substitution.

The surgeon who expects to find a thyroglossal duct should be suspicious when he uncovers a mass that has a fleshy consistency and vessels on the surface. The thyroglossal duct cyst has a perfectly smooth surface without vessels traversing its surface. If there is any question about the identity of the mass, aspiration may be resorted to. A thick, translucent fluid will identify the lesion as a thyroglossal duct cyst. If there is no fluid, a biopsy is advisable, and if this proves the tissue to be thyroid, the mass is left in place and a search made for additional thyroid tissue. If an adequate amount of thyroid tissue is found, the midline mass, which is objectionable cosmetically, may be removed. If no additional thyroid tissue is found (and this is usually the case), the midline thyroid mass is left in place. Some maneuver may be extemporized to dislodge the projecting mass to one side of the trachea and thus correct the cosmetically objectionable midline tumor. Another possibility is to split the gland in half and place one half in each side of the neck beside the trachea.

Lingual thyroid is another type of aberrantly positioned thyroid gland. It presents as a mass on the tongue in the region of the foramen caecum and is grossly indistinguishable from a thyroglossal duct cyst in this location. Needle aspiration will distinguish the two lesions. When a lingual thyroid is found, excision is not indicated unless the gland is producing symptoms. Scanning of the neck after the administration of a radioactive substance will establish whether there is thyroid tissue in the neck. When it is absent and when the lingual thyroid must be removed because of symptoms, substitution thyroid therapy must be instituted.

THYROTOXICOSIS

Hyperthyroidism in children is a rare systemic disorder of unknown etiology that involves principally the neuroendocrine systems. A reasonable but unproved theory is that the thyroid hyperfunction is secondary to excessive pituitary stimulation. The disease has been reported in infants and even in newborns. But the incidence increases with age, and a majority of cases are seen in the immediate prepuberal period. There is a greater incidence among females than among males, the percentage of females in some series being 80 percent. This disease is more common in the United States than in Europe, and it seems to be on the increase.

The disease in children is not greatly different from that observed in adults, except that children do not complain of the well-known symptoms of weakness, palpitation, and heat intolerance. In children there is usually a gradual onset, although in rare instances a crisis may be the initial symptom of the disease. The absence of complaints in the child makes the diagnosis more difficult than in adults. Restlessness, irritability, and constant movement are early symptoms of hyperthyroidism in children. Emotional upsets become commonplace in a formerly well integrated child, and if the patient is of school age, scholastic inadequacy becomes prominent. Unfortunately these neurogenic and psychic disturbances often precede the well-known eye signs, and at this early stage the diagnosis may be confused with chorea of a psychological disturbance. Such gastrointestinal symptoms as vomiting and diarrhea occur early, and in association with the neurogenic and psychic disturbances they should prompt a consideration of hyperthyroidism. There may be a loss of weight despite a large food intake. The child is usually tall and thin. In about one third of the cases a physical or psychic crisis precedes the onset of symptoms.

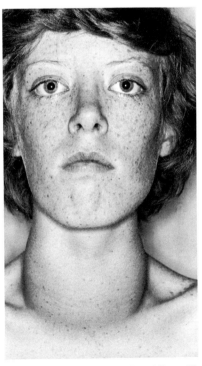

Fig. 1. A patient with hyperthyroidism. Note the profuse enlargement of the neck.

The physical signs develop gradually, and almost invariably there will be an increase in the size of the thyroid gland and the organ will be firmer than normal (Fig. 1). A thrill or bruit may be present. There is a fine tremor of the extremities, and the skin is flushed and moist. Gradually the classical eye signs, consisting of widening of the palpebral fissures, exophthalmos, lid lag, and failure of convergence, will develop (Fig. 2).

Because of the increased metabolic rate, the vascular system is overactive, with an increased pulse rate and cardiac output, which accounts for the high systolic pressure (140 or 150). The peripheral vascular dilation produces the warm, flushed skin and is an explanation of the low diastolic pressure (40 or 50).

The increase in the rate of basal metabolism, which has been of great value in confirming the diagnosis of hyperthyroidism, is difficult to test for and has largely been abandoned for the more reliable test for protein bound iodine. Normal values are 3.5 to 7.5 μg per 100 ml of blood; in most

series of reported cases the measured value in this disease ranges from 8 to 25 μg per 100 ml of blood. Any ingestion of inorganic iodine such as in some cough medicines results in spuriously high PBI levels. Blood levels of thyroxine have proved to be superior and are now coming into general use. There are other laboratory findings, such as a low blood cholesterol and an increased uptake of radioactive iodine by the thyroid, which support the diagnosis. The diagnosis can be made clinically in a child who has tachycardia that persists during sleep, a pulse pressure over 90, and enlarged thyroid, hyperkinesia, and a history of excessive nervousness and weight loss.

TREATMENT

Treatment should consist of bed rest and good general hygiene. Iodine can be used to produce a remission and at one time was an important part of medical therapy. Today propylthiouracil is more effective than iodine and should be given a trial in total amounts

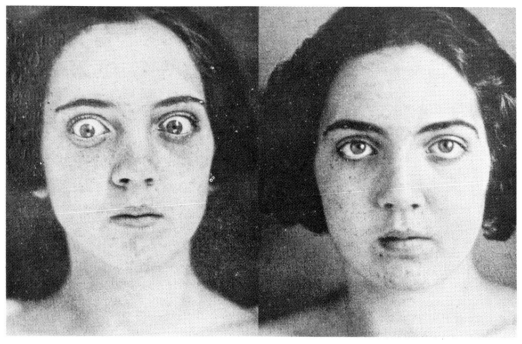

Fig. 2. Left. A girl with the typical signs of hyperthyroidism. Right. The same patient after treatment with propylthiouracil.

of 150 to 300 mg per day, divided into three doses. In most instances, remission can be produced, and after a year or more the drug can be diminished in amount and eventually discontinued. In some of these patients there may be permanent remission; in others a recurrence of hyperthyroidism may take place months after the drug is discontinued. When recurrence takes place, surgical therapy should be considered, particularly in cases where there is a recurrence following propylthiouracil therapy or where there has been a reaction to the drug. Instances of sensitivity to the drug are relatively infrequent and consist of skin manifestations or depression of blood-forming elements. Occasionally, propylthiouracil may produce a marked growth of the thyroid gland because of its goitrogenic effect. When this occurs it is advisable to discontinue the drug and institute surgical treatment. Surgical treatment of children with hyperthyroidism has lost favor in some quarters, probably because of the high rate of recurrence postoperatively.

Talbot and his group (1964) utilized surgical therapy in a majority of their patients (52 out of 70). Hypothyroidism was a common state after surgery, particularly when only 1 g of tissue was left in place. More distressing was a 10 percent instance of hypoparathyroidism that became permanent. There was one postoperative death, in a patient with rheumatic heart disease. Wilkins has used medical therapy for all his patients, persisting in the administration of propylthiouracil for many years in some patients. Most workers in the field report that about 40 to 50 percent of patients require surgical therapy. The indications for surgery are drug sensitivity, with a decrease in the white blood count and with skin lesions, a growth of the thyroid into a large goiter because of the goitrogenic effect of the drug, and a failure of the drug to produce a remission within a reasonable period of time. It is also agreed that in some irresponsible families who will not follow a medical program, surgical therapy may be the wisest initial course of action.

Crile (1964) has used radioactive iodine (I^{131}) as a treatment, and the clinical results have been good. The possibility of genetic injury has made many workers in this field advise against its use in patients under 40. This seems wise in view of the probability of increased radiation of the public in the modern world. A high percentage of such treated patients develop hypothyroidism.

SUBTOTAL THYROIDECTOMY

When surgical treatment is elected, the patient should be prepared for four weeks on propylthiouracil and for 10 to 14 days on iodine. The surgeon should be aware that recurrence is more likely to occur in children than in adults after surgery, and to prevent this a more radical thyroidectomy is indicated. If more than one tenth of the thyroid tissue is left in place, a recurrence is likely, and the patient has had the risk of a thyroidectomy without permanent benefit. Some authorities believe that unless hypothyroidism is a complication of thyroidectomy in children, the operation has been inadequate.

The technique of subtotal thyroidectomy in children is identical with that in adults; however, certain special points are pertinent because of the need for radical resection. A good exposure is essential, and this can be provided by division of the strap muscles. A careful search for the parathyroids should be made to guarantee that no trauma occurs to these vital structures. Thyroidectomy is performed by dissecting out the superior pole, placing three small curved clamps on the superior pole, and dividing the tissue between the second and third clamps. Two clamps thus remain on the divided superior thyroid artery. A tie is placed above these clamps, and one clamp is removed, leaving the second to control bleeding if the ligature breaks. By maintaining the dissection between the superior pole and trachea close to the superior pole, injury to the external branch of the superior laryngeal nerve is prevented. The trachea is identified below the isthmus, and the lower pole of the thyroid is dealt with by clamps being placed across the veins in this region. The gland is then pulled downward and outward and the recurrent laryngeal nerve identified as well as the inferior thyroid artery. The dissection is continued by clamps being placed into the capsule along the posterior lateral edge, with care being taken that parathyroid tissue is not damaged or removed. The dissection is then made directly across the gland, leaving about one tenth of each lobe behind. The isthmus and the pyramidal lobe are completely removed. Particular care is taken to ligate all bleeding points before the strap muscles are reapproximated with interrupted black silk sutures. The skin is brought together with a continuous 5-0 plain catgut subcuticular suture, and a collodion dressing is applied.

The dread complication of "storm" is not a problem in patients after thyroidectomy, provided that they have been prepared with propylthiouracil. Another complication to be watched for postoperatively is injury to a recurrent laryngeal nerve. A patient with this complication will have persistent stridor. If the patient can enunciate such vowel sounds as "i" and "e" clearly postoperatively, there need be no concern about recurrent nerve injury. The most serious postoperative complication is hypoparathyroidism. For diagnosis and treatment of this condition, see the discussion below of total thyroidectomy.

If the patient has increasing airway obstruction, hemorrhage into the wound with tracheal compression may be the cause and should be sought by careful inspection and palpation of the wound. Blood collecting in the wound will clot, and it can be removed only by reopening the incision and mechanically removing the clot.

PAPILLARY CARCINOMA OF THE THYROID

Papillary carcinoma of the thyroid is an epithelial neoplasm made up of cuboidal or columnar cells in papillary arrangement. The tumor occurs in children and young adults,

and for this reason a congenital origin is suspected. This nonencapsulated carcinoma is usually unilateral, or the major part of the involvement is in one lobe. Spread occurs first as lymphatic metastasis to the nodes of the neck. The behavior of this tumor sets it apart from most carcinomas. Growth is slow, and metastasis takes place late. Some patients have been observed for many years with little change in the main tumor mass or the involved lymph nodes. Such a benign course is not inevitable, for occasionally more rapid growth occurs locally, with tracheal compression and widespread hematogenous metastasis.

Patients have been observed with pulmonary metastasis that has made them dyspneic on excretion. After removal of the local tumor in the neck and treatment with high doses of thyroid extract, dyspnea has decreased, as has the pulmonary metastasis.

The relationship of this lesion to preceding radiation to the neck is now generally accepted. Usually relatively small doses of radiation under 500 rads have been administered for an enlarged thymus or for lymphoid tissue in the nasopharynx. It is unusual to have a history of more radiation than this, and usually the amounts are less. It has been noticed in some clinics that since this information became available and greater care has been taken in selecting patients to receive radiation to the neck the instance of papillary carcinoma of the thyroid has decreased.

There are no specific symptoms associated with early papillary carcinoma of the thyroid. The appearance and slow increase in size of a nodule in the neck usually prompts the parents to seek medical aid. On examination there will be a hard, nontender mass lateral to the trachea in the thyroid area that is attached to deep structures (Fig. 3). The hardness of the mass is its most characteristic feature. An absolute diagnosis cannot be made, but the presence of a hard mass of several months' duration on one side warrants biopsy. Unfortunately, there are no laboratory tests that are of aid in making the

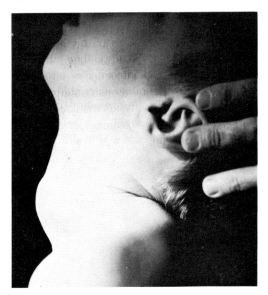

Fig. 3. Seven-year-old boy with papillary carcinoma of the thyroid.

diagnosis. However, provided the mass is small and not stone hard in consistency, it is permissible to treat the child with thyroid extract for four to six weeks. Failure of the

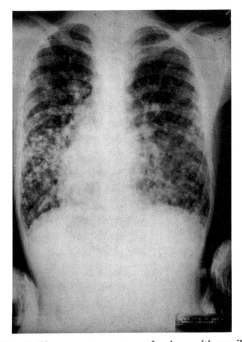

Fig. 4. Chest roentgenogram of a boy with papillary carcinoma of the thyroid and pulmonary metastasis.

nodule to regress on this therapy makes biopsy mandatory.

The lesion may cause widespread pulmonary metastasis late in the disease. It is remarkable how some children with many lesions in the lung will have minimal respiratory symptoms, consisting of slight shortness of breath (Fig. 4). Such lesions may regress with thyroid therapy.

TREATMENT

Papillary carcinomas are not affected by radiation. The best method of treatment consists of hemi- or sub-total thyroidectomy and removal of the enlarged lymph nodes. Incomplete excision of the tumor often accelerates its growth and makes subsequent excision of the recurrent mass difficult or impossible. A radical neck dissection is usually not warranted unless the patient is seen late in the disease with extensive lymph node involvement. When a hard nodule is discovered in the thyroid, surgical exploration is indicated. Excision of the lobe involved is to be preferred to biopsy. Crile (1964) has had great experience with this tumor and has objected to biopsy because of the spread of tumor which may take place. In some instances the tumor is completely unilateral, and hemithyroidectomy can be performed with satisfactory results. However, frequently there is extension into both lobes with deep projection of the tumor into the normal gland, and in these cases cure can be achieved only by sub-total thyroidectomy.

A careful search for enlarged lymph nodes is essential. These can be removed without the more extensive radical dissection of the neck.

SUB-TOTAL THYROIDECTOMY

The technique of sub-total thyroidectomy is available in texts on adult surgery. However, certain details are worthy of emphasis. An extensive exposure is essential and can be provided by dividing the strap muscles. The superior pole is isolated as in routine subtotal thyroidectomy, and then the inferior thyroid artery is identified as well as the recurrent laryngeal nerve. The artery should not be ligated, for it is the main blood supply to the parathyroid glands. The gland is freed by blunt dissection laterally and turned forward and medially, and a search is made for the parathyroid glands. Normally there are four parathyroid glands, brownish-yellow in color, ovoid in shape, and variable in location. Usually one pair is on the posterior aspect of the superior pole at the juncture of the middle and superior portions. The second pair is on the posterolateral aspect of the thyroid gland, at the junction of the middle and lower thirds of the gland, along the ramifications of the inferior thyroid artery. The lower set is far less constant in position than the superior set. Not until two, and preferably three, parathyroid glands have been positively identified is it advisable to begin excision of the thyroid gland. The removed thyroid tissue is carefully inspected by the surgeon, and it is our practice to have the pathologist, under sterile conditions, make a search of the tissue for parathyroid glands. Tissue suspected of being a parathyroid gland can be positively identified if a small slice is removed and subjected to frozen section study. If it proves to be parathyroid tissue, the gland is implanted in the sternocleidomastoid muscle.

At times the thyroid tissue is adherent to the trachea, and sharp dissection is required for removal. Histological study may demonstrate invasion of the trachea. However, invasion of the tracheal wall does not invariably indicate a poor prognosis, for such patients have been observed to live many years without evidence of local recurrence.

The dread complication of sub-total thyroidectomy is tetany; the symptoms usually appear during the first four days postoperatively but may come on more insidiously and not be recognized for two or three weeks. The first symptom is usually numbness, followed by cramps in the hands and feet. Early in the course of tetany, stimulation of the facial nerve by tapping over the main trunk pro-

duces a contraction of the facial muscles (Chvostek's sign), and a blood pressure cuff applied to the upper arm produces muscle spasm (Trousseau's sign). The serum calcium will be depressed and the phosphorus elevated. Treatment consists of intravenous calcium gluconate, which produces immediate relief. This should be followed by large oral doses of equal parts of calcium lactate and calcium carbonate, and of vitamin D. A fair number of patients with tetany recover, and in these instances it is postulated that operative injury to the parathyroids occurred and temporarily depressed their function. A. T. 10 is of some value, particularly in those patients who do not respond satisfactorily to oral calcium and vitamin D. The parathyroid hormones are of small help, since the patient soon develops resistance to them. These tumors appear to be extremely thyrotropin dependent. Therefore, postoperatively these patients should be given thyroid extract in doses of 2 to 3 grains per day to suppress secretion of TSH.

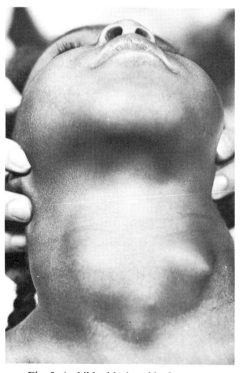

Fig. 5. A child with thyroid adenoma.

THYROID ADENOMA

Thyroid adenomas are uncommon in children; however, following puberty they occur and present a problem in diagnosis. Astwood (1956) treats such lesions with thyroid extract. Failure of regression with this therapy should prompt the physician to request a biopsy to rule out carcinoma. Most experts in this field advocate early biopsy rather than a course of treatment with thyroid such as is advocated by Astwood (Fig. 5).

ORVAR SWENSON

REFERENCES

ASTWOOD, E. B. The problem of nodules in the thyroid gland. Pediatrics, 18: 501, 1956.

BOYD, J. D. Development of the thyroid and parathyroid glands and the thymus. Ann. Roy. Coll. Surg. Eng., 7: 455, 1950.

CRILE, G., Jr. Late results of treatment for papillary cancer of the thyroid, Ann. Surg., 160, 2: 178, 1964.

———. Survival of patients with papillary carcinoma of the thyroid after conservative operations. Amer. J. Surg., 108, 6: 862, 1964.

———. Treatment of goiter in children. Cleveland Clin. Quart., 25: 210, 1958.

———. Treatment of hyperthyroidism with I^{131}. Amer. J. Surg., 107, 4: 545, 1964.

McRUER, E. E., and ROSS, M. D. Case of thyroid carcinoma in a newborn infant. Brit. Med. J., 2: 224, 1964.

PILEGGI, V. J., LEE, N. D., GOLUB, O. J., and HENRY, R. J. Determination of iodine compounds in serum. I serum thyroxine in the presence of some iodine contaminants. J. Clin. Endocr. 21: 1272, 1961.

SAXENA, K. M., CRAWFORD, J. D., and TALBOT, N. B. Childhood thyrotoxicosis: A long-term perspective. Brit. Med. J., 2: 1153, 1964.

WILKINS, L. The Diagnosis and Treatment of Endocrine Disorders in Childhood and Adolescence, 3rd ed. Springfield, Ill. Charles C Thomas, Publisher, 1966.

24

Tumors of the Head and Neck

Children are frequently brought to the physician for the evaluation of masses in the head and neck region. Most of these masses result from the enlargement of congenital cystic lesions or from chronically inflamed lymph nodes, but malignant neoplasms do occur, and, consequently, persistent growths in this region must be regarded with suspicion. Moussatos and Baffes (1963) reviewed the findings in 267 children with cervical masses seen at The Children's Memorial Hospital up to 1961. There were 190 with developmental cysts or chronic infection as a cause for the enlargement, and 77 with true neoplasms. Of the latter group, 44 had benign tumors, and 33 had malignant ones.

Rush, Chambers, and Ravitch (1963) have summarized the malignant head and neck lesions encountered in 103 children under the age of 15. The 62 primary tumors included neoplasms of the nasopharynx, the skin and subcutaneous tissues, the thyroid gland, and the deeper tissues of the neck. (Four cases of basal cell and two of squamous cell carcinoma were found in this group of patients.) At The Children's Memorial Hospital, 44 malignant tumors occurring primarily in the head and neck region have been seen during the past ten years (Table 1).

As a general rule, any type of tumor that occurs in adults may also be encountered in the pediatric age group; but certain neoplasms are much more likely to develop in children, and some of them are peculiar to this age group.

Metastatic lesions to the neck include neuroblastoma, lymphoepithelioma, and carcinoma of the thyroid. The lymphomas and also the reticuloendothelioses are relatively frequent. While these may occur primarily in the head or neck, more often they represent disseminated disease. About one half of

TABLE 1.   MALIGNANT TUMORS OF THE HEAD AND NECK, 1956–1965

SOFT TISSUE SARCOMAS (FIBROSARCOMA, RHABDOMYOSARCOMA, AND SO ON)		10
RETRO-OCULAR SARCOMA		3
NEUROBLASTOMA		6
Primary	4	
Secondary (neck mass first symptom)	2	
BONE SARCOMAS		5
Reticulum cell, maxilla	1	
Ewing's sarcoma, mandible	1	
Ewing's sarcoma, clavicle	1	
Neurofibrosarcoma, zygoma	1	
Fibrosarcoma, mandible	1	
CARCINOMAS		13
Of the thyroid	10	
Of the tongue	1	
Of the parotid	2	
MALIGNANT LYMPHOMAS		7
Lymphosarcoma	3	
Hodgkin's disease	4	
		—
TOTAL		44

339

the malignant lesions of the head and neck are secondary to some other focus of malignancy.

Tumors of the bones of the face or neck are not uncommon in children. Osteogenic sarcoma, fibrous dysplasia, dentigerous cysts, eosinophilic granulomas, adamantinomas, Ewing's sarcoma, and fibrosarcomas have all been seen in our clinics. These represent a special group of cases, for their treatment requires a broad understanding both of their neoplastic potential and of the changes in facial growth that may follow their surgical removal or their treatment by irradiation.

HISTORY AND PHYSICAL EXAMINATION

Children with tumors of the head and neck present with a visible mass, symptoms of nasal and oropharyngeal obstruction, or bleeding. Cervical lymphadenopathy is so common during childhood that its significance may be overlooked for considerable periods of time. Changes in the quality of the voice or nasal breathing are most often attributable to "adenoids." Enlarged tonsils are usually caused by chronic tonsillitis, but the enlargement may be caused by a tumor. When bleeding occurs from the nose or mouth the child is usually brought at once for evaluation. In most cases such bleeding is of no significance, but it may occasionally be caused by juvenile nasal angiofibroma in pubertal boys or by various types of sarcoma of the oral cavity or nasopharynx. Swelling of the tongue in infants and children is usually benign and caused by involvement by a hemangioma, lymphangioma, or cystic hygroma with extension into the floor of the mouth. The plexiform neurofibroma may involve the tongue as an isolated lesion, or it may be associated with the stigmata of von Recklinghausen's disease. Rhabdomyosarcomas often present as bulky lesions, and the leiomyosarcoma of the tongue frequently leads to ulceration.

The size and position of masses in the neck are of importance for diagnostic purposes. According to Moussatos and Baffes

(1963), most solitary masses anterior to the sternocleidomastoid muscle are benign. About half of the solitary masses lying posterior to the muscle are malignant, and tumors lying both anterior and posterior to it are nearly always malignant. Neuroblastomas of the neck are usually located in the posterior cervical triangle, and multiple firm, movable, rounded lymph nodes anywhere in the neck are most often due to metastatic papillary carcinoma of the thyroid. If there is enlargement or nodularity of the ipsilateral thyroid lobe in such cases, the diagnosis of thyroid carcinoma may be considered certain. About 50 percent of nodular masses found in the thyroid during childhood are malignant.

The methods of evaluation for tumors of the head and neck in children do not differ from those required for adults. The history of fever, pharyngitis, and local tenderness suggests an acute inflammatory process. Cervical lymphadenopathy is usually caused by chronic tonsillitis, but recently atypical myobacteria have been found to be a fairly frequent cause of cervical node enlargement. Weight loss, anorexia, and abdominal enlargement in conjunction with a cervical mass occur with metastatic neuroblastoma or other abdominal tumors. The complete physical examination should include careful palpation of the entire head and neck region and bimanual examination within the mouth. Mirror examination of the tonsils, larynx, and occasionally the nasopharynx can usually be carried out without anesthesia in children over the age of four. The nasopharyngoscope is useful for the evaluation of lesions of the nasal cavity. Laryngoscopy, when indicated for diagnosis, is best done with only light sedation, but general anesthesia is usually required for biopsy of any lesions which are found.

TUMORS OF THE SKIN AND SUBCUTANEOUS TISSUE

Perhaps surprisingly, the skin and subcutaneous tissue is the commonest location for tumors in the head and neck, as indicated by the figures of Rush, Chambers, and Ravitch (1963). The malignant epithelial tumors consist of basal cell and, more rarely, epidermoid carcinoma. These lesions when found are best treated by adequate surgical excision. An equally common lesion of the skin and subcutaneous tissues in this region is fibrosarcoma. This may present as a subcutaneous nodule, or there may be ulceration of the lesion so that it presents a chronic granulating surface. It is important in the treatment of these tumors, which are locally invasive, that wide local excision be performed to prevent recurrence. Irradiation therapy in this group is of no avail.

Many of the more common benign tumors of the skin and subcutaneous tissues are congenital and hamartomatous in nature. The hemangiomas that are present at birth or within the first few weeks of life commonly pass through a period of relatively rapid growth during the first six months. After this time central paling of the lesion reflects involutionary changes. Although slight extension at the periphery may still occur, the involution continues and in the majority of cases is complete by two to five years of age. With larger lesions about the face, the end result of spontaneous involution may be more acceptable than a long surgical scar. Lesions involving the scalp are probably best removed surgically before maximum growth has occurred because their involutional changes often result in atrophy of the dermal appendages and absence of hair. We do not advocate the use of carbon dioxide snow, since this often leads to deep scarring. X-radiation has only occasionally been used in our clinics in an attempt to retard growth during the normally active phase of the hemangiomas, but it may occasionally be indicated for rapidly invasive growth (Fig. 1). When ulceration of the tumor occurs, greater scarring usually results, and so the decision to excise the lesion should be made before large areas of the skin become necrotic and infected.

The lymphangiomas may be seen as diffuse involvements of the cheek with occasional infiltrations of the parotid gland. Cystic hygromas of the neck also frequently insinuate into the deep tissues of the neck and into the submandibular and sublingual areas, and they may occasionally involve the gingival tissues or tongue. The treatment of these conditions is discussed in Chapter 21.

Pigmented lesions about the head and neck are very common. McWhorter and Woolner (1954) reviewed a total of 172 pigmented lesions in children. There were 149 benign pigmented nevi, 7 blue nevi, 11 juvenile melanomas, and 5 malignant melanomas. In the past the juvenile melanoma has been considered to be histologically malignant but to have a benign course, but these authors place it distinctly apart from the malignant melanoma. It characteristically has a paucity of melanin and presents as a slightly elevated pink, red, pale brown, or colorless nodule about the neck and face. Of 11 such lesions in the series, 4 occurred on the cheek, 1 on the forehead, 1 on the nose, and 1 on the ear. The blue nevus is less common: of 7 lesions, 3 occurred on the cheek and 1 on the

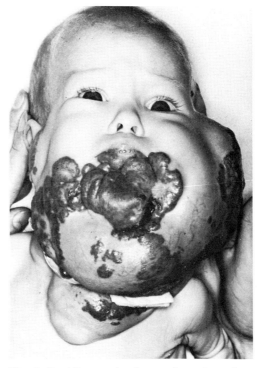

Fig. 1. Rapidly growing hemangioma in a three-month-old infant.

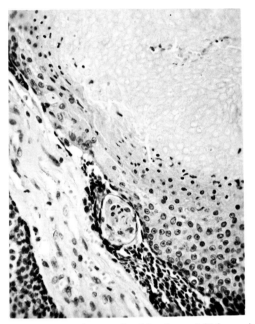

Fig. 2. Photomicrograph of benign calcifying epithelioma. This should not be mistaken for squamous carcinoma.

scalp. The 5 cases of malignant melanoma discussed by McWhorter and Woolner occurred mainly in the head region: 3 were present on the cheek and 1 on the ear. In reviewing 18 authenticated cases of malig-

nant melanomas during childhood listed in the literature, 10 were found to be in the region of the head and neck, and 5 were located on the cheek.

The benign calcifying epitheliomas are fairly common cutaneous tumors. These are often diagnosed preoperatively as sebaceous cysts. They are poorly encapsulated and present a dry, granular, cut surface. Proliferating epithelial cells of basal cell type are arranged in islands that have largely degenerated, giving rise to sheets of "shadow cells" (Fig. 2). Between the islands of epithelium a foreign body giant cell reaction is common, and calcification and even bone formation is noted to a variable degree. The tumor should not be confused with carcinoma.

As noted above, fibrosarcomas, rhabdomyosarcomas, hemangioendotheliomas, hemangiosarcomas (called "malignant hemangioendothelioma" by some authors), neurofibrosarcomas, and other malignant tumors of mesenchymal origin are occasionally seen during childhood. Aggressive surgical excision should be undertaken either at the time of biopsy or shortly after. While wide local excision of portions of the face may seem unnecessarily radical for these tumors,

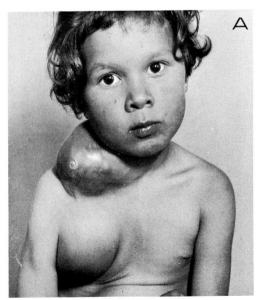
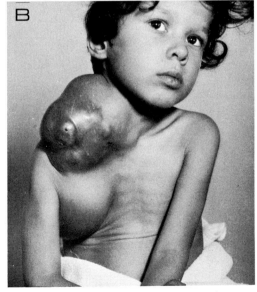

Fig. 3. Fibrosarcoma of neck. Photographs taken two weeks apart show the rapidity of growth that may occur.

the consequences of their local invasiveness may be considerably more difficult to deal with at subsequent operations. We have seen a child with a slow-growing malignant hemangioendothelioma arising in the upper cheek that after many local operations finally penetrated the skull to involve portions of the frontal lobe. The fibrosarcomas are usually curable by adequate wide excision, but some sarcomas may become wildly malignant after inadequate local excision (Fig. 3).

Often a child is seen with what appears to be an inoperable tumor of the head and neck. It is our policy in such cases to treat the patient vigorously with chemotherapeutic agents, either by general or local administration, in the hope that localization of the residual tumor will result, making possible an attempt at surgical cure. The agents that we have used, with their dosages, are discussed elsewhere. Admittedly it is rare to succeed with such aggressive therapy, but occasionally a child will be salvaged without excessive facial deformity.

NEUROFIBROMA

A neurofibroma may present as a part of von Recklinghausen's neurofibromatosis, or it may be a localized lesion in the head and neck region unassociated with the general disease. Although all neurofibromas fundamentally arise from proliferation of the nerve sheath cells of Schwann, they may present in a variety of forms. The more discrete solid masses are fusiform encapsulated tumors arising essentially from a portion of the nerve sheath. They grow by expansion, compressing the adjacent nerve. Histologically the discrete tumor may present a uniform interweaving fibrous pattern with clefts, or it may in addition show the features of palisading and focal degeneration so characteristic of the neurilemmomas (Fig. 4). This type is more amenable to surgical excision than are the other forms.

The *plexiform neurofibroma* is a frank longitudinal tumefaction of a nerve and its branches that may insinuate widely within

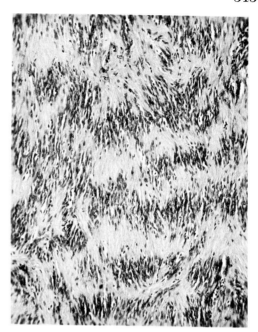

Fig. 4. Prominent nuclear palisading typical of the neurilemmomas. ×100.

the tissues. It contains residual nerve fibers but is largely composed of proliferating nerve sheath cells. These tumors may cause diffuse swelling of an eyelid, lip, cheek, or other portions of the face (Fig. 5). At times neurofibromas present as folds of thickened, slightly pigmented skin involving especially the scalp and eyelids. Treatment of this group of tumors is difficult and is often not effective. Surgical excision leaves a great deal to be desired. Occasionally such therapy has to be resorted to, despite the fact that recurrence is common and the cosmetic results are poor. Plexiform neurofibromas in the neck may penetrate into the extradural space through the intervertebral foramena (Fig. 6).

WENS

Dermoids, or wens, are common in children. A frequent location is the lateral quadrant of the eyebrow. The lesions consist of inclusion type cysts, skin-lined cavities that contain white putty-like or liquid material produced by the desquamation of epithelial

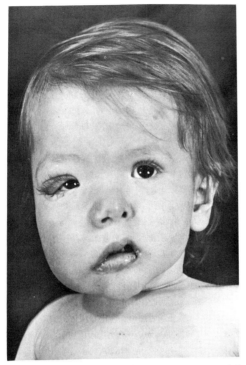

Fig. 5. Diffuse plexiform neurofibroma of right face. These are difficult to manage surgically.

cells and by secretion from the glandular structures. Another common location for these lesions is in various parts of the scalp. The swellings are painless, and infection is unusual until very late in their growth.

The dermoid of the eyebrow is usually oblong in shape, and many times it is fixed to the deep structures (Fig. 7). This is accounted for by the fact that it is usually attached to the periosteum of the orbital ridge and in some instances may actually occupy a depression in the bone. The scalp lesions may also be attached to the periosteum and may be partially submerged in the bone. They may even occupy the space between the inner and outer periosteum, and in such cases will appear in roentgenograms of the skull as smooth, punched-out areas in the skull. Some dermoids present in the midline of the neck and may be confused with the thyroglossal duct cyst, although they are usually lower in position. They can be differentiated from the thyroglossal duct cyst by their low location in the neck and by the

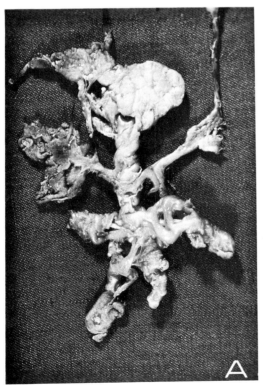

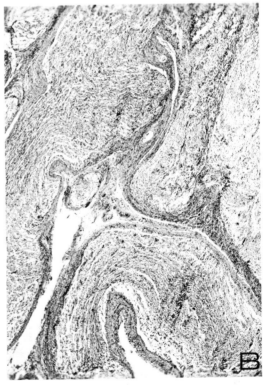

Fig. 6. A. Plexiform neurofibroma of neck that extended into cervical spinal canal. B. The micrograph demonstrates the characteristic interweaving of the neurofibromatous tissue bundles.

fact that they rarely move on deglutition or on protrusion of the tongue.

Surgical excision of dermoid cysts of the head and neck is indicated both for cosmetic reasons and because they may occasionally become infected. In excising the dermoids of the orbital ridge, it is advisable to make the incision within the hairline of the eyebrow so that the scar will be inconspicuous. It is inadvisable to shave the eyebrow because regrowth of the hair may be extremely slow. The lesions are usually thin walled and offer some difficulty in removal, since sharp dissection is necessary to detach them from the periosteum. All of the cyst must be removed, for persistence of even a small portion of its lining will lead to recurrence. After complete hemostasis is achieved, the wound is closed with 5-0 chromic catgut sutures to the subcutaneous tissue, and the skin is closed with a running 5-0 plain catgut suture. The incision is painted with flexible collodion, and pressure is applied to the

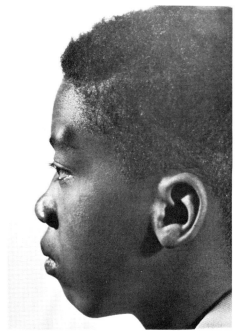

Fig. 7. Dermoid cysts are frequently located at the lateral superior side of the orbit.

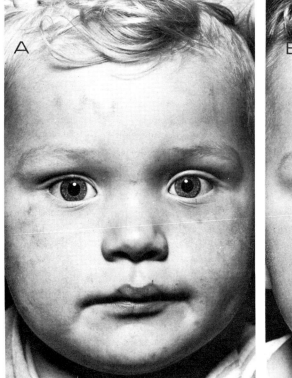
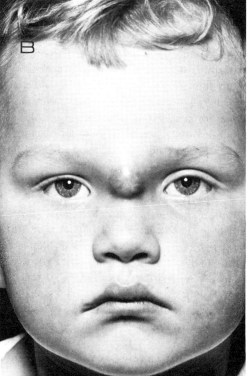

Fig. 8. A child in whom the small nasal dermoid sinus became infected prior to its removal. Note the initial small pit over the bridge of the nose.

wound with a gauze pack for three to four minutes. The patient may be discharged from the hospital on the day of operation. When the lesion is in the scalp, the same procedure is indicated. It is not necessary to remove the adjacent bone, since removal of the cyst lining is sufficient for cure. This is true even of those lesions that occupy the space between the dura and the external surface of the bone.

DERMOIDS OF THE NOSE

A dermoid of the nose, which has been called "external nasal glioma" by some authors, usually presents as a small opening on the bridge of the nose. Careful examination of the patient may reveal considerable widening of the nose, and this is usually an indication that there is a long deep projection of a sinus into the nasal structures. Infection of a deeper portion of the sinus tract may lead to abscess formation (Fig. 8). Very rarely the sinus may perforate the cribriform plate and extend into the intracranial cavity. When surgical excision of these lesions is considered, and particularly when there is radiographic evidence that the cribriform plate may be invaded, it is prudent to have a neurosurgeon available for assistance should there prove to be extension through the cribriform plate. In such cases the frontal lobes are retracted through a formal craniotomy exposure, and removal of the dermoid sinus is completed from above. Excision of these sinuses should always be undertaken with care, for their removal without extensive deformities to the nose presents certain technical problems. Short vertical incisions can be made about them, and by patient dissection the long sinus tracts can usually be removed. It is unwise in most instances to attempt removal of any of these lesions by the intranasal route.

TUMORS OF THE NASAL CAVITIES AND NASOPHARYNX

Nasal and nasopharyngeal growths are uncommon during childhood. The great ma-jority are benign and come to the attention of the physician because of nasal obstruction, external nasal deformity, or bleeding. Nasal polyps caused by allergy and granulomas secondary to foreign bodies or to trauma are the most likely causes of these symptoms. Other more serious conditions may occur, however, and these should be considered in the diagnostic evaluation (Table 2).

TABLE 2.   TUMORS OF THE NASAL CAVITIES AND NASOPHARYNX

CONGENITAL CYSTIC LESIONS
  Intranasal meningocele
  "External nasal glioma" (dermoid of the nose)
TUMORS ARISING FROM DEVELOPMENTAL ARRESTS
  Chordomas
  Teratomas
BENIGN FIBROMATOUS AND POLYPOID LESIONS
  Juvenile nasal angiofibroma
  Antral-choanal polyp
  Allergic polyp
  Nasal papilloma
TUMORS OF THE SOFT SOMATIC TISSUES
  Rhabdonyosarcoma
  Myxofibrosarcoma
  Lymphosarcoma
  Neuroblastoma
EPITHELIAL TUMORS
  Adenomas
  Tumors of the minor salivary glands
  Neuroepithelioma
  Carcinomas of the usual adult types
  Lymphoepithelioma

From the practical point of view, it is important first to determine whether a nasopharyngeal growth is likely to be benign or malignant and then to assess the risks of biopsy for diagnostic purposes. There are several pitfalls in the management of the nasopharyngeal tumors that are seen during childhood. Although the physician is often tempted to proceed at once to biopsy such lesions when the child is first seen in the office, it is generally better to evaluate the whole problem by means of a careful history-taking and physical examination. The biopsy should then be done in the operating room after pertinent laboratory studies and radiographs have been complete. A "polyp" arising high in the nasal cavity may in fact be one of the rare intranasal meningoceles, and its biopsy or attempted excision will result in cerebrospinal rhinorrhea or in an ascending meningitis. The juvenile angiofibromas of adolescent boys may appear innocent on first examination, but they are notorious for the severe hemorrhage that may occur after attempts at biopsy; and the "external nasal gliomas" at the base of the nose, which extend through the suture line of the nasal bones, will frequently recur after inadequate office surgery.

For all these reasons, caution should be the rule in one's approach to any growth within the nose or nasopharynx. An orderly history and physical examination will include indirect mirror examination, use of the nasopharyngoscope, and palpation of suspicious areas under topical anesthesia. Lederman has reviewed the diagnosis and treatment of tumors of the nose and nasopharynx in an excellent monograph (1961). The problems associated with the management of these tumors are no different in children than they are in adults. A few of the lesions that are peculiar to childhood will be considered briefly in the following paragraphs, and others will be discussed in other sections of the present volume.

JUVENILE NASAL ANGIOFIBROMA

The juvenile nasal angiofibroma is an uncommon lesion that is seen almost exclusively in adolescent and preadolescent males. Associated with increasing nasal obstruction and epistaxis, it is a smooth, red, highly vascular mass that usually protrudes downwards from the base of the skull at the spheno-occipital synchondrosis and extends either into the nasal cavity and sinuses or posteriorly into the nasopharynx. There is no clear agreement as to the site of origin of these tumors, for by the time they are diagnosed they have usually come to fill a great part of the cavity that contains them, and the severe bleeding that accompanies their surgical re-

moval tends to obscure the position of their base. Allen, who has managed several of these lesions, has expressed the belief that the majority arise from the base of the sphenoid, that there is nearly always a narrow pedicle from this site to the main body of the tumor, and that they may progress into the cranial cavity as well as outward into the nasopharynx. The pedicle contains two or three large arteries that can be tied off by ligature, with virtual elimination of the severe hemorrhage that usually attends the removal of the tumor. Carotid angiography reveals the extent of the lesion and some of the vessels (Fig. 9). The best approach is through the palate, achieved by the elevation of a palatal flap (Fig. 10). It is well, if possible, to stay away from the main body of the tumor until the ligation of its pedicle can be accomplished. Occasionally submucous resection of portions of the hard palate is required to enlarge the exposure, and it may also be necessary to perform the Caldwell-Luc procedure in some cases to push the

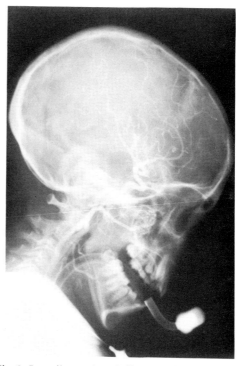

Fig. 9. Juvenile nasal angiofibroma of nasopharynx. The carotid angiogram reveals the extent of its vascular connections. (Courtesy of Doctors George Allen and John Bergan.)

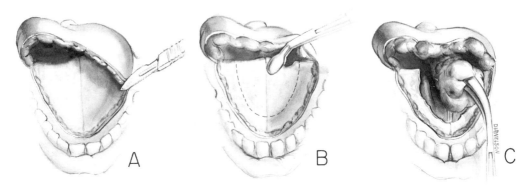

Fig. 10. Transpalatal approach to the juvenile nasal angiofibroma. A. The mucosa is elevated from the hard palate. B. It is often necessary to resect a portion of the hard palate. C. The tumor is exposed.

tumor out of a maxillary sinus into which it may have extended.

Earlier authors—for example, Figi and Davis (1950), who reported 114 cases of juvenile nasal angiofibroma from the Mayo Clinic in 1949—concluded that a combination of electrocautery and irradiation is the treatment of choice. These are not now recommended. In some cases testosterone therapy has appeared to cause regression of these tumors, and not infrequently they regress spontaneously with the attainment of maturity. In general, however, it is not safe to rely upon this possibility, and active treatment is indicated for repeated episodes of epistaxis or for increasing pressure deformity of the nasal and facial bones. If there is recurrence following the operation, testosterone is used in an effort to tide the child over in the hope that spontaneous regression may occur.

EPITHELIAL TUMORS OF THE NASOPHARYNX

Adenomas, tumors of the minor salivary glands, neuroepithelial tumors, and carcinomas may all manifest themselves by a combination of persistent nasal obstruction and varying degress of epistaxis. Whenever these symptoms appear to be progressive, a complete examination of the nose, paranasal

sinuses, and nasopharynx is essential. Sarcomas of various types and some metastatic tumors, particularly the neuroblastomas, may also give rise to these symptoms. Lymphoepitheliomas of the nasopharynx are often small and first manifest themselves by upper cervical adenopathy, particularly when the primary lesion lies in the region of the faucial pillars. When the site of origin of the tumor can be determined by careful examination, direct biopsy should be performed. If it cannot be located, it may be necessary to remove a cervical node to make the diagnosis. The lymphoepitheliomas are highly sensitive to irradiation and may occasionally be cured through its use. In the other types of tumors, appropriate combinations of surgical removal, irradiation, and chemotherapeutic agents may lead to arrest of the disease in a few of the children. The hideous deformity and the painful discomfort attending the progressive growth of these tumors, which kill usually by local extension and not by metastasis, demand that the most radical measures be employed to achieve a cure.

Chordomas of the base of the skull are slowly expanding tumors of notochordal origin that are rare during childhood. They arise from the spheno-occipital synchondrosis and protrude into the skull behind the optic chiasm or downwards into the nasopharynx in the midline. Their complete surgical removal is usually impossible, and irradiation therapy is of no value.

TUMORS OF THE ORAL CAVITY AND TONGUE

Although a squamous carcinoma of the lip or oral mucosa may arise during childhood, most of the neoplasms in this region are of mesenchymal origin. Fibromas and papillomas (Fig. 11) are common benign tumors, and, occasionally, large granulomas may form at the site of dental infection. An *epulis* is a fibromatous or peripheral giant cell reparative granuloma that arises at the sides of the teeth from the peridontal membrane. There is no bony destruction, but cure of these tumors usually requires the removal of the tooth contiguous to the lesion (Fig. 12). The rare condition of congenital epulis of the newborn, presenting as a pedunculated smooth mass arising from the maxillary or mandibular alveolar ridge, occurs almost exclusively in female infants. It is considered to be a variant of the granular cell myoblastoma, a benign tumor composed of large eosinophilic polyhedral cells that ordinarily arises in the skin and less frequently in the tongue. Benign hemangioendotheliomas, rhabdomyosarcomas, and other mesenchymal growths are found occasionally in the oral cavity or tongue. Neurofibromas occur not infrequently in this region in patients with von Recklinghausen's disease (neurofibromatosis), and they also occur in the tissues of the neck.

A small lymphosarcoma of the tonsil may remain localized within the deeper portions of the gland long after the appearance of large cervical metastases. For this reason, tonsillectomy is indicated whenever a lymphosarcoma of the cervical nodes is to be treated by either surgical excision or radiation therapy. Leukemia is sometimes first manifested by gingival swelling resulting from cellular infiltration. Other types of gin-

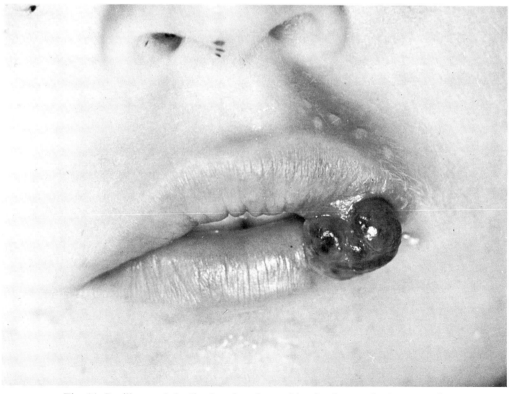

Fig. 11. Papilloma of the lip. Local wedge excision is adequate for its removal.

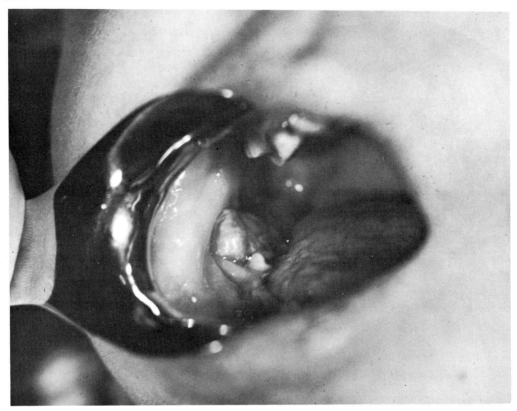

Fig. 12. Characteristic appearance of an epulis arising at the side of a lower tooth.

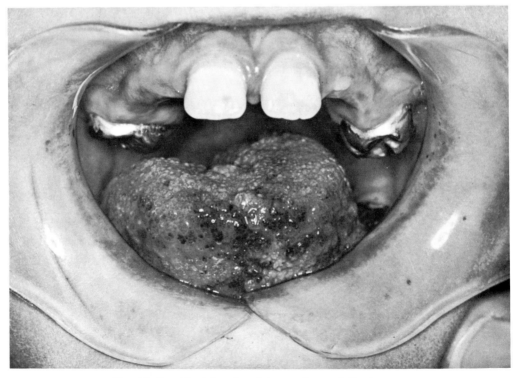

Fig. 13. Combined lymphangiohemangioma of the tongue.

gival thickening are those caused by diphenylhydantoin sodium (Dilantin) therapy or by vitamin C deficiency. In these conditions the biopsy reveals edema and perivascular round cell infiltration; in leukemia the massive small cell infiltration into the interstitial spaces is characteristic of this neoplastic disease.

The most common neoplastic enlargement of the tongue is that caused by involvement with lymphangioma or hemangioma. In many cases there is a mixture of the two, so that the small varicose and cystic lymph channels are partially filled with blood (Fig. 13). The condition usually involves the whole of the tongue, and its surgical treatment is therefore difficult and not entirely satisfactory. While some authors have advocated the use of radiation therapy, it is the consensus that the lesion is little affected by this mode of therapy and that its use may result in abnormalities of facial development and later cervicofacial malignancy. The operation is often bloody and tedious, but it is possible to bisect the tongue and remove considerable portions of the involved tissues in order to allow the child to close his mouth. The same surgical therapy is employed for those cystic hygromas of the upper midline of the neck that have invaded the tongue (Fig. 14). Resection of the cysts together with portions of the tongue can be combined with removal of the main mass through a transverse incision from below.

Rhabdomyosarcomas, leiomyosarcomas, and other malignant tumors involving the tongue or the buccal mucosa are diagnosed by biopsy, which is quite simply and safely done under local anesthesia. Their surgical treatment is feasible, for surprisingly large amounts of the tongue may be removed without impairing normal mastication and speech. Every effort must be made to resect these tumors with as large a margin of nor-

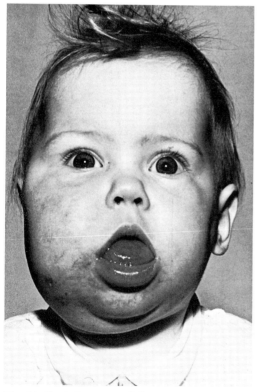

Fig. 14. Cystic hygroma of the upper neck invading the floor of the mouth. It had been unsuccessfully treated by radium implantation.

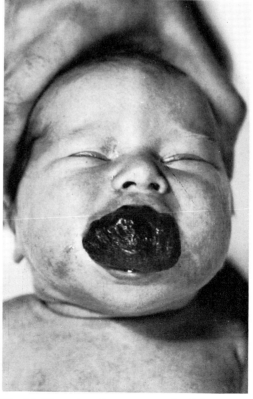

Fig. 15. Hamartomatous overgrowth of the tongue in a newborn infant.

mal tissue as possible. For those lesions occurring in the midline of the tongue, preservation of the lateral margins and the arterial and nerve supplies will generally result in a usable tongue and in satisfactory growth of the oral cavity. It is amazing how well small children adapt to the resection of 80 percent or even more of the tongue.

Enlargement of portions of the tongue may occasionally result from hamartomatous overgrowth. Usually the mass is just anterior to the circumvallate papillae, but it may involve the whole of the tongue (Fig. 15). Resection of the tumor mass can be accomplished safely, and recurrence is unlikely. It should be remembered that a mass at the base of the tongue may be a lingual thyroid and that its removal may lead in some cases to hypothyroidism (Ch. 23). In the anterior floor of the mouth, ranulas—cystic masses arising from the obstruction of one of the ducts in the sublingual glands—are frequently encountered. Their excision under local anesthesia is usually ineffective, but the use of a heavy chromic suture placed through them to form a new drainage tract may often be successful.

BONY TUMORS OF THE HEAD AND NECK

From the surgical point of view, tumors of the jaws and face may be classified into benign curable lesions, malignant lesions of poor prognosis, and lesions associated with generalized disease. Many tumors in this region—for example, the eosinophilic granulomas, the giant cell reparative granuloma of the jaw (epulis) arising in sites of chronic irritation, and several of the different types of dentigerous cysts are not considered to be neoplastic in nature, yet they may produce pain and swelling and bony abnormalities that are indistinguishable from the changes produced by neoplastic growths. It is important, therefore, that careful clinical and ra-

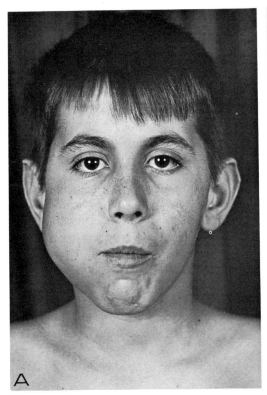
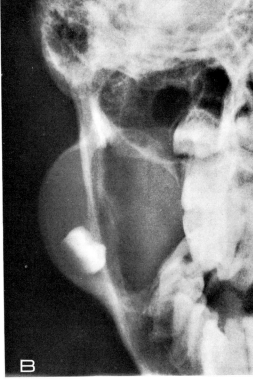

Fig. 16. A. Dentigerous cyst of the jaw. B. A tooth is seen at its inferior outer margin.

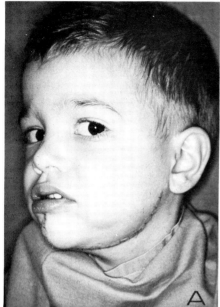

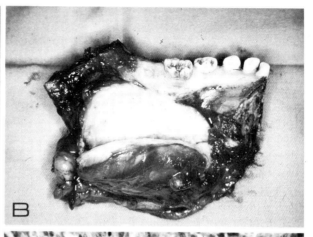

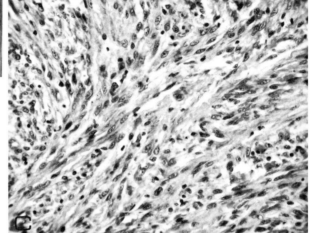

Fig. 17. Fibrosarcoma of the mandible. A. Appearance of patient after resection of the jaw. B. Section of mandible removed. C. Photomicrograph of the fibrosarcoma. (Courtesy of Dr. Clarence Monroe.)

diographic evaluation of all tumors of the jaw be followed by open biopsy and appropriate surgical or irradiation therapy.

Benign curable growths within the bones of the head and neck may be classified as cystic, fibrous, or granulomatous. Several types of odontogenic and nonodontogenic cysts occur in both the upper and lower jaws. These are generally single and are lined by nonkeratinizing squamous or columnar ciliated epithelium. The dentigerous cyst arises between the crown of a newly formed tooth and its enamel epithelium as a fluid-containing space lined by squamous epithelium. These cysts may attain a large size, with marked expansion of the bone of the jaw (Fig. 16), and may occasionally result in the formation of an ameloblastoma. The treatment of all non-neoplastic cysts of the jaws consists of their excision or of the unroofing of the bony wall of the cyst with removal of the epithelial lining.

FIBROSARCOMA

Fibrosarcoma of the jaw appears as a painless swelling of the mandible, causing deformity of that side of the face. When biopsy reveals a fibrosarcoma or neurofibrosarcoma the treatment is hemisection of the mandible. Anything less than this will result in recurrence. It is surprising how little deformity results from such operations providing the opposite side of the mandible is left to support the chin (Fig. 17). The insertion of bone grafts is not necessary, as the child does well without the adjunct during his growth. When full growth of the mandible is achieved, bone inlay grafts may be advisable for cosmetic reasons.

FIBROUS DYSPLASIA OF BONE

Certain benign non-neoplastic lesions of fibro-osseous character may affect the mandible, maxilla, or cranial bones. There has been a tendency to group these lesions under the all-inclusive term "fibrous (or fibro-osseous) dysplasia," but this concept is not universally accepted. True fibrous dysplasia of bone is considered to be hamartomatous and is characterized by fibroblastic proliferation and metaplastic bone formation. Most cases become clinically apparent during childhood or adolescence. When a single bone is involved (the monostotic variety) it is more

likely to affect the femur, a tibia, a rib, or a facial bone (particularly a jaw bone). With multiple bone involvement (polyostotic variety) there is a tendency to unilateral destruction within a limb, and when the upper limb is involved the skull is also frequently the site of lesions. The infrequent variant of polyostotic fibrous dysplasia that occurs in infancy together with cutaneous pigmentation, sexual precocity, and endocrine disturbances is referred to as Albright's syndrome. It has been seen almost exclusively in girls.

The lesions of fibrous dysplasia may be radiolucent or radiopaque. Those involving the facial bones and base of the skull are characteristically densely radiopaque and in these sites may be distressing to the patient and his family because of the severe deform-

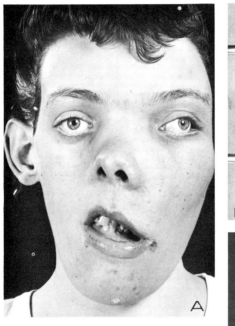

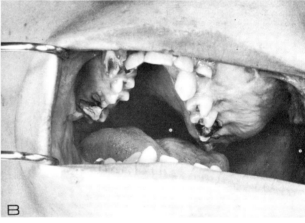

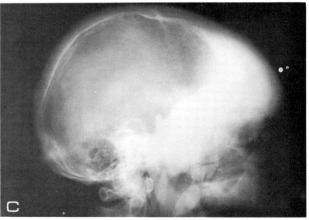

Fig. 18. *Leontiasis ossea* in a 16-year-old boy. The skull is extensively ossified (C) leading to deviation of the left eye (A) and massive enlargement of the left mandible (B). (Courtesy of Dr. F. Hoffmeister, Roswell Park Memorial Institute.)

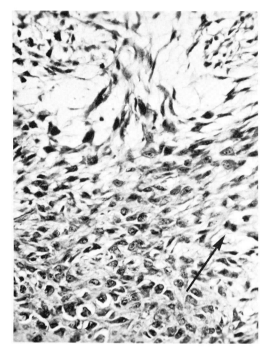

Fig. 19. Photomicrograph of highly cellular fibrous dysplasia. A mitosis is identified by the arrow.

ity, *leontiasis ossea,* that may be produced (Fig. 18). Since the growth of fibrous dysplasia often stops soon after puberty, some surgeons advocate simple contouring of the bone. The more rapidly growing lesions may demand a more aggressive approach. In the active or proliferative fibroblastic phase the tissue is highly cellular, and mitotic figures

may be found. In such cases a diagnosis of osteogenic sarcoma or fibrosarcoma is sometimes erroneously entertained (Fig. 19).

Although the fibrous osteoma, or ossifying fibroma, of the jaw is considered by many pathologists to be a variant of fibrous dysplasia, it has certain differentiating histological features that merit its being kept as an individual entity. These have been discussed by Jaffe (1958). The surgical treatment of these two lesions is similar. Since the margins are poorly delineated, complete surgical extirpation necessitates the removal of a larger margin of normal bone than one would anticipate. The lesion is recurrent unless total excision has been accomplished. In one case, such a lesion (Fig. 20) was cured only by subtotal mandibulectomy with subsequent insertion of a free bone graft, after its having recurred three times following lesser procedures.

The giant cell reparative granuloma of the jaw bones is a disease that is sometimes confused pathologically with the benign giant

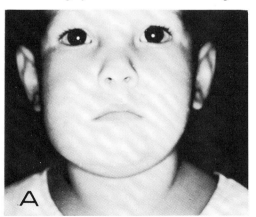

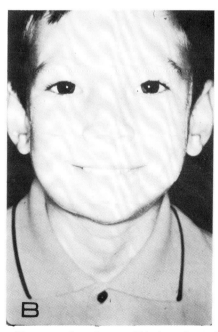

Fig. 20. Ossifying fibroma of the jaw. This type of growth will recur unless the mandible is excised with a wide margin. There is no true encapsulation. An excellent result was achieved by wide excision and subsequent bone graft.

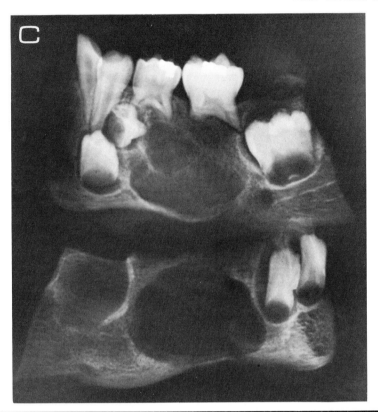

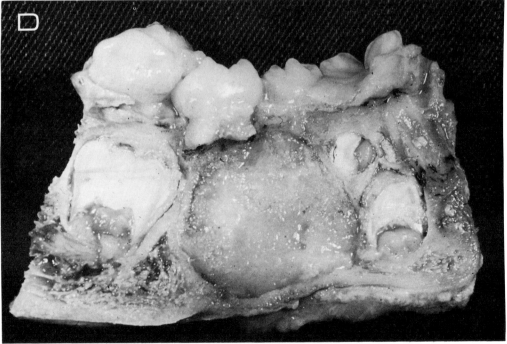

Fig. 20 (cont.). Ossifying fibroma of the jaw. This type of growth will recur unless the mandible is excised with a wide margin. There is no true encapsulation. An excellent result was achieved by wide excision and subsequent bone graft. (Courtesy of Dr. Harold Griffith.)

cell tumor of bone. Most authors believe that it results from trauma. It occurs more often in the mandible than in the maxilla, and the bicuspid and molar areas are the usual sites. The proliferating fibroblasts and osteoid are not as dense as they are in fibrous dysplasia, and the number and histology of the giant cells are different from those of true giant cell tumors. The presence of hemorrhages and hemosiderin pigment is common. According to Dahlin (1957), true giant cell tumors are extremely rare in the jaw bones. The distinction between these two lesions is of great importance, since the reparative granulomas almost never recur after complete excision, whereas true giant cell tumors are recurrent in 50 percent of the cases, and in 10 percent they become malignant.

Aneurysmal bone cyst is another entity that has been confused histologically with giant cell tumor. It usually has the characteristic radiological appearance of a well circumscribed and eccentric zone of rarefaction delineated peripherally by a thin shell of subperiosteal new bone formation. The metaphyseal regions of long bones and any of the vertebrae are sites of predilection, although infrequently the mandible may be involved. Two thirds of the affected patients in Dahlin's series were less than 20 years of age. The lesion is predominantly cystic, with numerous capillaries and large blood-filled spaces, but in the more solid areas vascular fibrous tissue, osteoid trabeculae, and multinucleated giant cells are prominent findings.

EOSINOPHILIC GRANULOMA OF BONE

The localized eosinophilic granuloma of bone is thought to be similar in nature to the disseminated visceral lesions that occur in Hand-Schüller-Christian disease and Letterer-Siwe disease. The bone lesion presents radiologically a rather sharply defined destructive process (Fig. 21). The tissue is grossly soft and friable, and it may be gray, pink, or yellow.

Microscopic examination reveals a basically histiocytic proliferation with associated fibroblasts and inflammatory cells, particularly the eosinophilic leukocytes. Focal areas of necrosis are common. The same picture may be seen in patients with overt visceral involvement, and therefore careful clinical followup is vital. One or several bones may be involved initially, following which a second or third lesion may appear while the

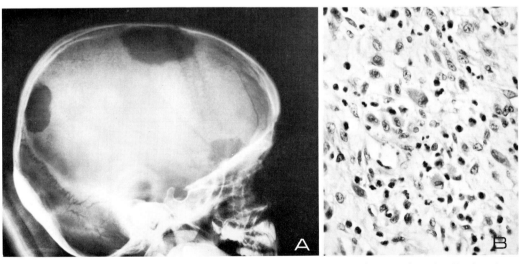

Fig. 21. Eosinophilic granuloma. A. Multiple eosinophilic granulomas that remained localized to bone over a considerable period of time. B. Photomicrograph of the eosinophilic granuloma showing the basic histiocyte pattern in which scattered eosinophils are seen.

disease continues to be localized to the skeleton. In the head and neck, the calvarium, the base of the skull, or the mandible are the usual sites of the lesion. When disseminated disease is present the patient often develops exophthalmos and diabetes insipidis. Unilateral or bilateral otorrhea is common with mastoid involvement, and when the mandible is affected the teeth often become loosened and the gums swollen and ulcerated.

The painful lesions of eosinophilic granuloma respond well to radiation therapy. Dosages in the range of 500 to 1,000 rads are usually curative. When the disease becomes disseminated such therapy may delay its course, but there is usually a fatal end after a period of one to several years. Chemotherapy and steroids have not markedly improved this gloomy outlook.

TRUE NEOPLASMS OF THE BONES OF THE FACE

True neoplasms of the bones of the jaws and face are about equally divided into benign and malignant varieties. Whether it is benign or malignant, any bone tumor in this area will recur after operations that do not accomplish complete removal of all of the neoplastic cells. The porosity of the bone marrow leads to much wider dissemination of the neoplasm than is anticipated from its gross appearance, and the excision of bone to a degree that may appear to be excessively mutilating is often essential for success.

Benign tumors of the bone in the region of the head and neck, such as the hemangiomas of bone, osteoid osteomas, chondromas, neurilemmomas, and hemangiopericytomas

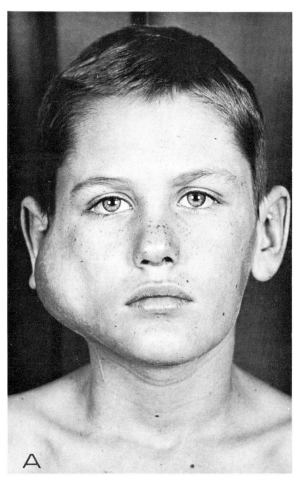

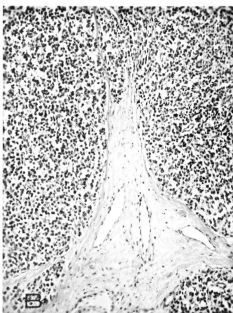

Fig. 22. A. Ewing's sarcoma of the mandible. Death occurred within five months. B. Photomicrograph of the sarcoma.

of bone, are infrequently seen. Benign osteoblastomas may arise in the calvarium or cervical vertebrae. True fibromas in this location are apparently rare. The adamantinomas of the bones of the jaw are of benign appearance but are usually classified with the malignant tumors because of their ability to invade locally. Following the excision of any of these tumors, appropriate reconstructive operations must be carried out in order to provide the best cosmetic and functional result. The writings of Converse and his associates (1964) are extremely valuable to the surgeon contemplating wide-scale ablative and reconstructive procedures about the head and neck.

Many of the relatively common bone tumors of adult life are rare in the head and neck region in children. Osteogenic sarcomas are not usually seen to involve the jaws during childhood, even though 75 percent of these tumors occur in the 10-to-20-year-old age group. Multiple myeloma is a disease of the third and later decades and is almost never found in children. As has been mentioned, giant cell tumors occur uncommonly in children and are in any case rare in the jaws at any age.

A primary lymphoma of bone in the head and neck region is usually a reticulum cell sarcoma and may involve the skull, mandible, or maxilla; but these are exceedingly rare tumors. They may be difficult to differentiate from Ewing's sarcoma.

Ewing's sarcoma involving the mandible or skull is fatal in almost every case within a period of 18 months. The tumor remains quiescent for a time, and sometimes it appears to be localized to a single area of bone, but soon more rapid growth occurs, and the patient succumbs either to the local disease or to generalized metastases (Fig. 22). There has been a recent revival of interest in radiation therapy for Ewing's sarcoma. It is also to be expected that more active chemotherapeutic agents will be developed during the next few years to manage this tumor, which histologically appears to be composed of a rather homogeneous and well-organized cellular pattern. Surgical therapy for this sarcoma has not been successful in our experience.

Neurofibromas may arise in bone or involve it secondarily. They are rapid in their growth, and, although moderately well encapsulated, they invade locally and may extend through the skull. Wide local excision sparing the facial nerve, with subsequent chemotherapy given intra-arterially, sometimes results in cure.

TUMORS OF THE MAJOR SALIVARY GLANDS

Of the major salivary glands, the parotid, the submandibular (submaxillary), and the sublingual, the parotid is more commonly associated with tumor formation than are the other two together. In addition to these major glands, which are of a compound racemose acinar type, and which have large duct systems, there are numbers of smaller glands of a similar nature lying within the submucosa of the mucous membranes of the

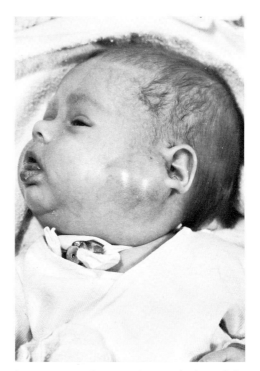

Fig. 23. Hemangioma of the parotid in an infant.

mouth, the interior of the lips, and the oropharynx. These minor salivary glands may occasionally be the site of any of the tumors that affect the major glands.

Neoplasms involving salivary glands in children are infrequently encountered. The various types and their relative incidence in children have been reviewed by Howard and his associates (1950) and by Byars, Ackerman, and Peacock (1957).

During infancy the most common tumor is the hemangioma. Many of these are present at birth or in the first few weeks of life. The majority become manifest by one year of age. The hemangioma frequently presents as a bulky, rapidly enlarging, unilateral swelling of the parotid that may be associated with overlying bluish discoloration or a superficial hemangioma of the skin (Fig. 23). It generally occupies the superficial lobe of the parotid and is grossly lobulated with no true capsule formation. Wide extension into the surrounding soft tissues may sometimes occur. Many of these tumors fall into the class of benign hemangioendotheliomas, characterized by solid masses of endothelial cells and anastomosing capillaries that re-

place the acinar structure of the parotid, leaving widely separated ducts. Mitotic figures may be numerous.

The rate of growth of hemangiomas should be carefully evaluated. In those tumors that are present in the neonatal period and that exhibit less aggressive growth, spontaneous involution can usually be expected to start by six months of age. For tumors that enlarge alarmingly or that exhibit extension beyond the gland, surgical excision is recommended. Radiation therapy has been used in an attempt to achieve growth restraint, but its effect is not predictable, and particular care must be taken to guard against damage to the underlying articular cartilages.

Beyond infancy a tumor of the parotid gland or other salivary glands is most likely to be a benign mixed tumor. These occur with increasing frequency after the age of nine years, but they may be seen at an early age. All other tumors of the parotid are more rare. Carcinoma may take the form of adenocarcinoma, epidermoid carcinoma, mucoepidermoid carcinoma, malignant mixed tumor, or cylindroma. Warthin's tumor (papillary cystadenoma lymphomatosum)

Fig. 24. A. Normal duct system in anteroposterior view. B. Sialectasia of the parotid with characteristic ectasis of the acini.

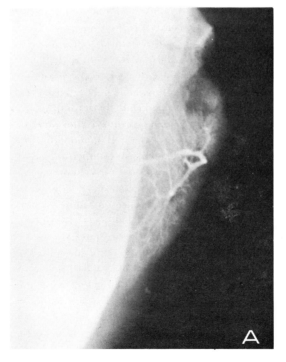

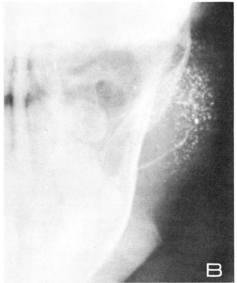

almost never occurs in children. Rarely, a lipoma or a parotid cyst may develop during childhood.

It is important to realize that not all chronic salivary gland swellings are caused by neoplasms. An important condition in this regard is chronic sialadenitis, the result of repeated bouts of inflammation, congenital stenosis of the ducts, or, occasionally, ductal obstruction caused by stone. The affected gland, usually the parotid, is firm, sometimes slightly tender, and may show progressive enlargement because of increasing edema and fibrosis. In some cases a localized swelling within the gland parenchyma is indistinguishable from tumor. We believe that sialography alone is sufficient for diagnosis in these cases, since the radiographic appearance is pathognomonic (Fig. 24). The acini are dilated, and the radiographic material collects and persists in them to form an unmistakable pattern.

TECHNIQUE OF SIALOGRAPHY

The process of inserting a blunt cannula or polyethylene catheter into the papilla of

Stensen's duct is nearly painless, and sialography can be carried out in children without great difficulty. The classic method is to introduce an olive-tipped cannula into the duct via the buccal papilla and then to inject directly 0.2 to 1.0 ml of *warmed* iodinated oil until discomfort is felt over the region of the parotid. (The other salivary glands are less easy to inject, and for practical purposes the procedure is restricted to the visualization of the parotid gland.) The armamentarium for such sialography is simple (Fig. 25).

Because the use of iodinated oil in sialography may result in an aggravation of chronic parotitis, attempts have been made to replace it by other radiopaque substances. Unfortunately, when water-soluble media are used, the material often runs out of the duct before satisfactory radiographs can be made. For this reason, Anderson and Byars (1965) have recommended the insertion of a polyethylene catheter into the duct after dilation of the papilla with fine silver probes. When this is done the duct will close firmly about the tube, and the radiographs can be made at leisure before the catheter is removed. Excellent sialograms can be made by this

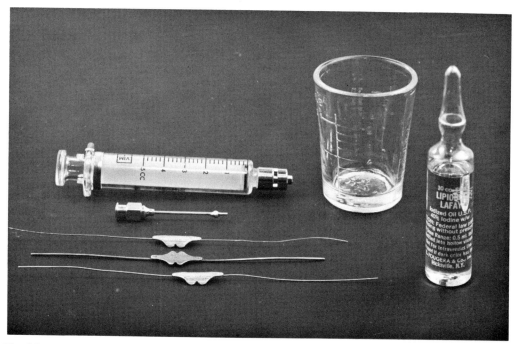

Fig. 25. Materials for sialography. The olive-tipped cannula occludes the opening of Stensen's duct during the injection.

method using 70 percent Diodrast without the dangers inherent in the use of oily contrast materials.

Aside from the acute parotitis caused by mumps, which is self-limiting, and the chronic parotitis diagnosable by sialography, all other parotid tumors should be diagnosed by biopsy. Particularly in children, little is to be gained by routine radiographs of the parotid or the submandibular region. Bimanual palpation of the face will show whether or not there is an intraoral protrusion of the tumor. In any tumor about the face, bone films are indicated to determine if there is erosion or direct involvement of the facial bones. The history and the physical examination are important in order to eliminate some diagnostic entities and also to enable the surgeon to familiarize himself completely with the patient and with the peculiar anatomy of his parotid or submandibular region, but the definitive diagnosis rests exclusively on the histological examination of the entire lesion.

Excisional biopsy of the affected salivary gland is carried out under general anesthesia in the operating room. It is distressing for the physician to attempt removal of a small parotid or submandibular swelling under local anesthesia in the office and then to find that it is more extensive than was anticipated or that one or more branches of the facial nerve have been inadvertently severed. Any swelling of the parotid region, unless it is clearly a sebaceous cyst and moves freely with the subcutaneous tissue, must be considered to require operating room conditions for its removal. This dictum is applicable not only to parotid swellings but also to cystic hygromas, the small preauricular sinuses that penetrate deeply and end around the cartilaginous portion of the ear canal, and to accessory auricles, whose cartilaginous component may have a similar deep origin.

PAROTID OPERATIONS

We prefer the S-shaped incision, carried anterior to the ear and curved posteriorly

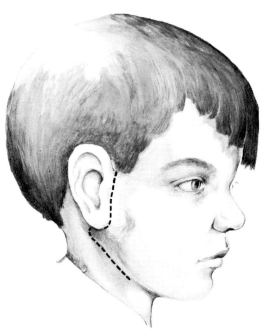

Fig. 26. Incision for parotid exploration. It can easily be extended superiorly into the temporal region.

behind the tragus, to the usual Y incision (Fig. 26). Its healing is better, and adequate exposure is obtained through its use. In children, the structures to be exposed are often extremely fine, and exceedingly careful dissection and the use of nerve stimulation are necessary for success. It is important for the surgeon to recognize the various tissues without stimulation, but where distortion of the anatomy has been caused by an expanding tumor it is comforting to be able to test each fine fibrous strand before it is sectioned. There are several nerve stimulators available that have proved valuable, provided they are calibrated for minimal effective voltage in each patient at the operating table by stimulation of a branch of the nerve that has been dissected free early in the course of the operation.

EXPOSURE OF THE FACIAL NERVE

There are two general methods for exposing the facial nerve. The main trunk can be picked up just anterior to the mastoid process as it emerges from the stylomastoid fora-men, or one of the minor branches can be exposed peripherally at two or three well defined points. Both of these methods must be mastered, since the surgeon will be faced with anatomic situations in which one or the other is unsafe or impossible to use. Tumors located posteriorly may impinge upon the mastoid to such an extent that the usual dis-section along its anterior border will neces-sarily injure the posteriorly compressed facial nerve. Conversely, generalized enlargement

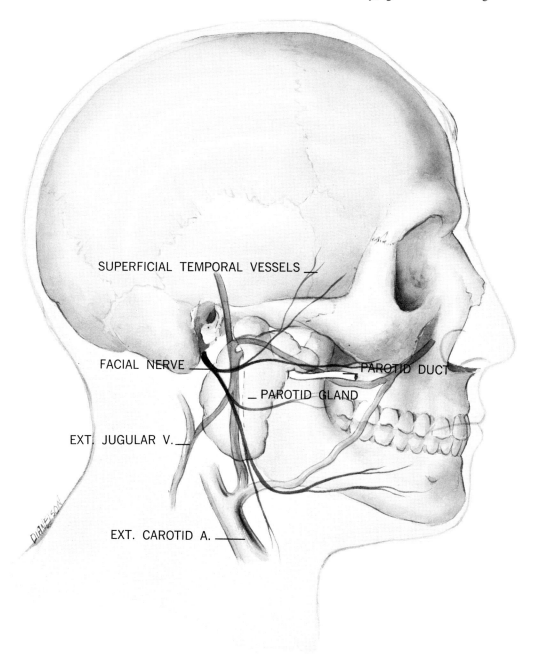

SUPERFICIAL TEMPORAL VESSELS

FACIAL NERVE

PAROTID DUCT

PAROTID GLAND

EXT. JUGULAR V.

EXT. CAROTID A.

Fig. 27. Possible sites to locate peripheral facial branches during parotidectomy. A. Preferred site at lower border of gland anterior to posterior facial vein. B. Localization of small branch above the parotid duct. C. Mandibular ramus is located by its proximity to facial artery and vein.

of the gland may obscure the usual land-marks of the anterior tertiary branches of the nerve and make the posterior approach more suitable.

Adson's method may be used to expose the main trunk of the facial nerve during parotid surgery. It is detailed in the paper of Beahrs and Adson (1958). Briefly, the nerve emerges from the stylomastoid fora-men between the mastoid process and the base of the styloid and passes forward and laterally superficial to the external carotid artery. Shortly after leaving the skull it en-ters the parotid substance and divides into two constant main branches, the *temporo-facial* and the *cervicofacial* divisions. These give rise to the tertiary branches within the parotid. It is necessary for the surgeon to have this pattern of division well in mind before approaching parotid surgery. When the anatomy has been worked out carefully on the skull and in the cadaver, dissection in this region is done much more confidently.

Peripherally, there are three sites in which the position of the facial nerve branches is sufficiently constant to provide for their safe exposure. The best method of exposing the entire facial nerve in a retrograde manner is to pick up the mandibular ramus or even the entire cervicofacial division at the lower pole of the parotid gland just anterior to the posterior facial vein, which makes its exit from the gland in this region (Fig. 27). The posterior facial vein is large, is easily identi-fiable, and has a constant relationship to the lower division of the facial nerve. Once one of the branches has been isolated and posi-tively identified by electrical or mechanical stimulation, it is possible to isolate the entire nerve by careful dissection along the course of the branches. A branch of the facial nerve commonly runs along the upper border of Stensen's duct at the anterior border of the parotid. This duct, which can be palpated in its subcutaneous position prior to elevation of the flaps, can be used to locate the small nerve branch that accompanies it. Both of these structures lie within a fascial sheath that surrounds the facial muscles, and they

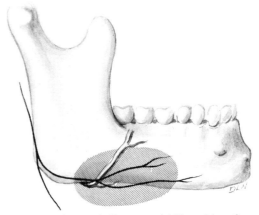

Fig. 28. Dark area indicates variability of location of mandibular ramus in vicinity of facial artery.

are usually not elevated with the skin flaps if care is taken in the initial dissection.

The third position in which it is possible to locate a branch of the facial nerve is said to be that point at which the mandibular ramus of the nerve crosses the anterior facial vein and artery. We have always found it somewhat difficult to locate the nerve by this approach, since it may lie within an area of 0.5 to 1.0 cm above the lower margin of the mandible and up to 1.0 cm below it (Fig. 28). Furthermore, the nerve may lie within or under a platysma muscle which is thick, or it may be immediately subcutaneous when the platysma is poorly developed. For these reasons, many surgeons consider it safer to seek the posterior facial vein as a landmark than to use the more anterior approach that is usually recommended. The excellent mono-graph of Anderson and Byars (1965) should be consulted for the details of these and other procedures related to the surgery of the parotid gland.

TREATMENT OF
SPECIFIC PAROTID TUMORS

Tumors of the parotid gland should be removed surgically. Radiation therapy is not indicated preoperatively in any child with a parotid tumor. It may be necessary postop-eratively under certain well defined condi-tions—for example, when a parotid malignancy has extended into the pterygoid fossa where its total en bloc removal is impossible. Surgical treatment combined with the use of such chemotherapeutic agents as actinomycin D, vincoblastine, and Cytoxan is occasionally successful. It is important for the physician to recall the effect of irradiation on the various growth centers about the face when considering radiation therapy, since the development of the face may be seriously impaired by damage to them. Certainly the use of radiation therapy is never indicated for benign lesions such as cystic hygromas or hemangiomas localized in the parotid parenchyma, nor for primary treatment of the benign mixed tumors of the mucoepidermoid group.

Wide local excision of the benign mixed tumor is the treatment of choice. In most cases this will require removal of at least the external lobe of the parotid. Since there may be irregular projections of the tumor outside its usual round, smooth exterior, these must be looked for carefully during the dissection. If the tumor lies anteriorly in the parotid, identification of the facial nerve branches in its vicinity is sufficient prior to its removal. When it is more posterior, it is easier to identify the main trunk and to proceed with the dissection with the major branches under direct vision. Some facial palsy will often follow exposure of the facial nerve or its branches, but if the various rami are known to have been left intact the surgeon need have no fear that normal function will return within a few days or weeks.

According to Anderson and Byars (1965), the usual cause of recurrence of the benign mixed tumor is inadequate excision of the tumor or the seeding of tumor cells through spillage at operation. These authors have recorded only one recurrence in a series of more than 350 benign mixed tumors treated primarily by them. We agree with them that careful local excision is equally as effective as total parotidectomy, provided that a wide margin is taken to ensure total removal of the tumor.

The recurrent mixed tumor presents sev-

eral difficult surgical problems. Not only is there considerable fibrosis underneath the scar and about the branches of the facial nerve, but the tumor itself may have penetrated near the nerve, raising the question of possible sacrifice of this important structure. While such cases should be evaluated on their merits, the surgeon who approaches the treatment of recurrent mixed tumor of the parotid should be well versed in immediate facial nerve grafting, so that he may deal with the problems resulting from the sacrifice of portions of the main branches of the nerve.

Mucoepidermoid tumors have an excellent prognosis in most cases when they are completely excised, even though many of them appear histologically to be of low grade malignancy. The lesions are usually small and are generally not well encapsulated. Often the zone of inflammation that surrounds them makes their removal more difficult than might be expected (Fig. 29). In the treatment of the rare tumors of high grade malignancy, which are usually associated with facial paralysis and fixation of tissues early in their course, sacrifice of the facial nerve is essential at the first operation.

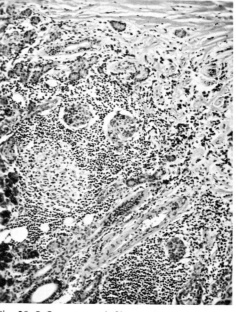

Fig. 29. Inflammatory infiltrate about extensions of mucoepidermoid tumor.

When the presence of a malignant tumor is suspected from the rate of growth and from physical signs, incisional biopsy is justified for definitive diagnosis. A vertical skin incision is made just anterior to the tragus, and after appropriate tissue has been obtained the wound is closed tightly. The entire biopsy tract excised with the specimen when the main portion of the tumor is removed together with the facial nerve.

presence of tuberculosis, other granulomas, or a tumor must be suspected. The necessary methods of investigation will include the tuberculin test, radiographs of the neck for vertebral involvement or calcification within the tumor mass, and finally the performance of an open biopsy.

Whereas in adults simple biopsy of masses in the neck is to be discouraged, in children the types of lesions that are encountered

TUMOR MASSES IN THE NECK

Masses in the neck occur so frequently in children that it is difficult at the outset for the physician to consider that serious disease may be present. On the one hand he wishes to avoid unnecessary or painful diagnostic test, but on the other hand he realizes that early diagnosis is the key to the successful treatment of many of the malignant lesions that may arise in this region.

Fortunately, in children the great majority of masses in the neck are benign. Most of them are either congenital cystic lesions or the result of infections within the lymph nodes. Moussatos and Baffes (1963) have reviewed 267 patients with cervical masses seen at The Children's Memorial Hospital between 1945 and 1961 (Table 3). The figures, modified from this series, reveal that 190 of the masses were non-neoplastic in nature and that of the 77 true neoplasms 44 were benign and 33 malignant. Malignant neoplasms, therefore, accounted for only 12.4 percent of all the cervical masses encountered in the study.

One's approach to cervical masses must be individualized. In most cases of acute infection of the lymph nodes, the rapidity of enlargement of the mass and the associated pain make the diagnosis obvious. Generally within two weeks there will be fluctuation or subsidence of the mass with adequate treatment by antibiotics (Ch. 22). If there is no change, or if the mass increases in size, an acute inflammation is less likely, and the

TABLE 3. CERVICAL MASSES OF THE NECK REGION, 1945–1961 *

DEVELOPMENTAL MASSES	
Thyroglossal cyst	70
Branchial cleft cyst	62
Inclusion cysts	8
Cyst of the parotid	1
Occipital meningocele	1
Ectopic cartilage	1
Number of cases	143
INFLAMMATORY MASSES	
Nonspecific lymphadenitis	26
Tuberculous lymphadenitis	18
Parotitis	3
Number of cases	47
BENIGN TUMORS	
Cystic hygroma	27
Hemangioma	4
Lipoma	1
Teratoma	1
Parathyroid tumor	1
Epithelial tumor	1
Thyroid adenoma	4
Neurogenic	5
Number of cases	44
MALIGNANT TUMORS	
Lymphosarcoma, Hodgkin's disease	20
Thyroid carcinoma	7
Neuroblastoma	5
Neurofibrosarcoma	1
Number of cases	33
Total	267

*Modified from Moussatos and Baffes. Pediatrics, 32: 25, 1963.

make this a safe and practical method of diagnosis. Most nodular masses in the adult are caused by metastasis from lesions of the oral or respiratory epithelium, and biopsy interferes seriously with the performance of a radical neck dissection in continuity with the tumor. In children, on the other hand, node enlargement from operable lesions in this region is rare. It is usual to do the operation under general anesthesia and to drape the entire region to be explored, so that a definitive procedure can be done if necessary. The availability of frozen section examination adds greatly to the usefulness of this type of exploratory biopsy. It is our practice to remove any cervical lesion entirely at the first procedure if this can be accomplished without damage to important structures. At this time the tissue planes and small structures can be followed much more easily than after a general fibrosis has developed in the area of the biopsy during the healing process.

BENIGN TUMORS OF THE NECK

Benign tumors involving the neck are legion. The most common are the lipomas, fibromas, neurilemmomas, hemangiomas, and cystic hygromas. Teratomas occasionally arise in this region, often from the thyroid gland (Ch. 23), and tumors of thymic origin are also encountered. The mass lying within the sternocleidomastoid muscle in cases of congenital torticollis (Ch. 79) is often indistinguishable from that of a primary tumor (indeed it may be a tumor of the desmoid group), and it may have to be removed for diagnosis or treatment. In all of these conditions, formal exploration through a transverse skin incision is the procedure to be followed. The surgeon undertaking the removal of benign tumors of the neck in children must be fully conversant with the normal anatomy and its variations in this important region, for the structures are often

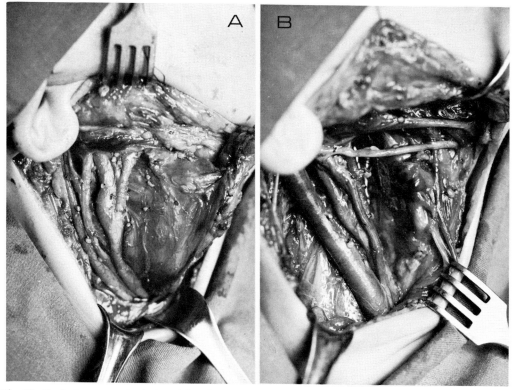

Fig. 30. Cystic hygroma. A. A deep-lying firm cystic hygroma. The carotid artery and jugular vein are stretched over the mass. B. The mass has been removed.

very small. Paralysis of the muscles served by the accessory nerve will lead to scoliosis and even asymmetrical growth of the head on the side of the deficit, and section of the phrenic nerve may also result in body asymmetry as the child grows. Figure 30 shows the degree of adherence of important structures in the neck to a deep-lying tumor, in this case a firm fibrous cystic hygroma.

The clinical differentiation between neoplasms and benign congenital cystic lesions of the neck, such as the thyroglossal and branchial cleft cysts, may sometimes be difficult. Maturing cystic hygromas may also present as firm masses that may be mistaken for tumors. Tuberculous lymph nodes can sometimes be confused with lymphomas localized to the neck, since in some cases the findings on physical examination are similar, and the tuberculin test may be negative. All of these non-neoplastic conditions are considered elsewhere in the book. The surgical problems associated with their removal are not different in principle from those presented by the benign tumors, which may also evidence inflammatory adhesion to surrounding structures, wide infiltration between tissue planes, and obliteration of important anatomic landmarks.

MALIGNANT TUMORS OF THE NECK

Malignant tumors of the neck in children (Table 4) usually show themselves by rapid and progressive growth. Aside from thyroid carcinoma and the rare mucosal epitheliomas, four main classes can be distinguished: primary mesenchymal growths, primary tumors of lymph node origin (the lymphomas), tumors metastatic to the nodes or soft tissues, and malignant lesions of the skin or subcutaneous tissues. In addition, the reticuloendothelioses, although of questionable neoplastic origin, are associated with the development of tumor masses and display a clinical course that justifies their inclusion with the malignant lesions of the head and neck.

Rush, Chambers, and Ravitch (1963) have presented important statistics in relation to head and neck cancer in children. It is evident from their review that metastatic tumors are at least as frequent as primary malignancies in this region. It is our impression, however, that malignant tumors of the neck are more likely to be primary than secondary, particularly if the cases of Hodgkin's disease and lymphosarcoma are considered with the primary group.

The most common malignancies of the cervical region are the lymphomas, thyroid carcinoma, and metastatic or primary neuroblastoma, in that order. Other occasional lesions are malignant neurilemmoma, fibrosarcoma, hemangiosarcoma (malignant hemangioendothelioma), malignant melanoma, and basal or squamous cell carcinoma. Lymphoepithelioma of the nasopharynx, tumors

TABLE 4.   MALIGNANT TUMORS
OF THE NECK

PRIMARY
 Skin
  Basal and squamous carcinoma
  Malignant melanoma
  Dermatofibrosarcoma protruberans
 Deeper soft tissue tumors
  Mesenchymal tumors
   Fibrosarcoma
   Rhabdomyosarcoma
   Hemangiosarcoma
  Neurogenic tumors
   Neurofibrosarcoma
   Neuroblastoma
   Ganglioneuroblastoma
 Malignant lymphomas
  Hodgkin's disease
  Lymphosarcoma
  Reticulum cell sarcoma
 Thyroid carcinoma
 Salivary gland carcinoma
 Laryngeal and hypopharyngeal tumors

SECONDARY
 Neuroblastoma
 Thyroid and salivary gland carcinoma metastases
 Lymphoepithelioma, and so on

that have metastasized from a lymphosarcoma of the tonsil, and squamous cell carcinoma of the larynx or hypopharynx may sometimes be found in a biopsied lymph node.

In dealing with a mass in the neck that is increasing in size, a routine pattern of investigation should be followed. We agree with Rush and his co-workers that "search for a primary head and neck lesion precedes biopsy of the cervical lymph node" and that "biopsy of the node usually precedes search for the primary elsewhere," although the experience of Moussatos and Baffes (1963) indicates that in children it is nearly always possible to identify the primary tumor with the usual diagnostic methods by the time cervical metastasis has occurred. There may occasionally be patients with small primary tumors elsewhere whose diagnosis can only be established by histological examination of the biopsied node.

TREATMENT OF MALIGNANT TUMORS OF THE NECK

The treatment of thyroid carcinoma, an important cause of enlarged cervical lymph nodes in children, is detailed in Chapter 23. Branchial cleft carcinoma is considered elsewhere. Of the remaining malignancies, most will require individualized treatment, depending upon the type of tumor and its tendency to disseminate. The reader is referred to survey articles listed in the bibliography for discussions of recent trends and the results of treatment. In the following paragraphs the management of the more common cervical malignancies will be described in some detail.

MALIGNANT LYMPHOMAS OF THE NECK

A cervical mass is frequently the presenting sign in patients with malignant lymphomas. This group includes Hodgkin's sarcoma, lymphosarcoma, and reticulum cell sarcoma. Obviously, the prognosis depends on whether the condition is localized to the neck at the time of diagnosis and on whether it disseminates from its primary site. There is some reason to believe that certain of the lymphomas may begin within the nodes of the neck and that early complete surgical excision of the diseased tissues will result in cure. This is particularly the case in Hodgkin's disease, which can serve as a model for the aggressive treatment of the lymphomas during childhood.

HODGKIN'S DISEASE. Since Hodgkin's disease is not common in children, there have been only sporadic reports of individual cases or of small series of cases. More recently, the literature has included clinical and pathological studies of large groups of cases, such as that published by Pitcock, Bauer, and McGavran (1959). Prior to these studies, there was a tendency to extreme pessimism regarding the treatment of Hodgkin's disease. This was a disservice to patients because it led to treatment that was palliative in its concept rather than more aggressive and possibly curative. In the modern literature five- and ten-year overall cure rates of up to 25 to 30 percent are being achieved by a combination of chemotherapy, irradiation, and surgery.

The peak instance of this disease in children seems to be between the ages of 5 and 10 years. Its slow progression is emphasized by the fact that some patients have a history of 6 years of cervical lymph node enlargement before coming for medical assistance. A predominant number of the cases occur in boys, the ratio usually being given as 3 males to 1 female. The disease is rare in children less than 4 years old, and the diagnosis is usually doubted when made in children below the age of 2 years, for no well documented account of a patient below this age has been published.

In the past, Hodgkin's disease was considered to be a generalized condition with initial manifestations in one area, but there are now some workers in this field who view the lesions as being localized at a very early stage to one set of nodes, which may successfully be removed or irradiated for cure.

This view has been important in prompting physicians and surgeons to be more aggressive in treatment. Both the clinical course of the disease and the histological characteristics of the involved lymph nodes separate this entity from the general lymphoma group. The lymph nodes contain reticulum cells, lymphocytes, eosinophils, and the scattered large mononuclear or multinucleated Reed-Sternberg cells (Fig. 31). The normal histological arrangement of the lymph node is replaced by the granulomatous lesions, and there is invasion of the capsule. In about one fourth of the patients in the pediatric age group, only enlargement of the cervical lymph nodes has been observed, without evidence of involvement of the other parts of the lymphoid and reticuloendothelial system. These patients present as normal children without symptomatology except for the persistent enlargement of the lymph nodes on one side of the neck. Where there is generalized involvement of the lymphoid system,

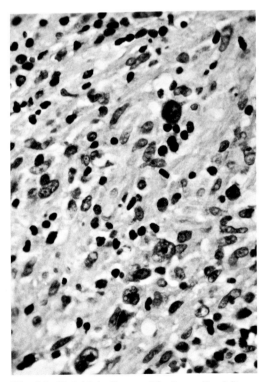

Fig. 31. Hodgkin's disease. The large Reed-Sternberg cells lie in a reticulum cell stroma.

there is usually low grade fever and general malaise. In such patients enlargement of the liver and spleen is common, and prominence of the mediastinal lymph nodes may be detected by chest roentgenogram (Fig. 32).

Peters and Middlemiss (1958) have analyzed Hodgkin's disease as occurring in three stages: when the disease is localized, when it involves more than one lymphoid area, and when it is generalized, with constitutional symptoms. This classification has value in prognosis. Where the disease is generalized, survivors are rare. Patients with clinical localization of the disease when the diagnosis is made have a somewhat better prognosis. There may be up to 60 percent 5-year survival in these cases. The duration of the disease before the diagnosis is made is another feature that may be used in prognosis. Generally, where there has been presence of the lymph nodes over a long period of time with slow growth, the prognosis is superior to the situation in which there is a short history and rapid growth.

Treatment. The best form of treatment for Hodgkin's disease is generally considered to be radiation therapy, though there has been a recent renewal of interest in surgical therapy for localized disease. In the past, rather small and inadequate dosages of radiation have been given. The work of Peters and Middlemiss (1958) and others indicates that larger doses of radiation have given better results. There is also a tendency now to irradiate contiguous areas of lymphoid tissue prophylactically, since this seems to increase the survival rate in large series of cases. While there may be late recurrences in the distant areas following the initial treatment, a vigorous attack upon these had led to further long periods of remission. The attitude toward the disease should now be to seek a cure and to abandon the past concept of palliation alone. This can only be achieved by tumor dosages of 3,500 to 4,000 rads of irradiation carried out over periods of three to four weeks.

There may be a place for surgical therapy

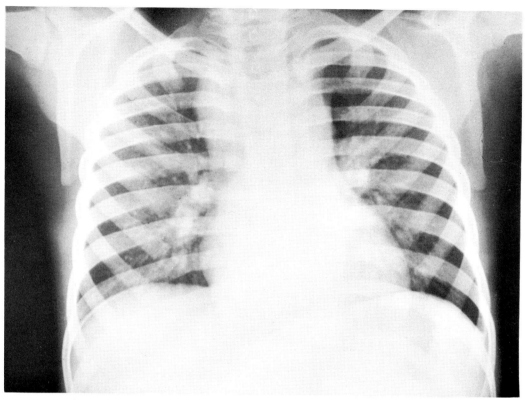

Fig. 32. Involvement of the mediastinum in Hodgkin's disease during childhood.

in the early localized stages of Hodgkin's disease. Sufficient follow up figures are not available to make a sound evaluation of this type of therapy, which was discarded in the past and has only recently been renewed by some authorities in this field. Slaughter (1958) has presented a five-year survival rate of 63.6 percent in patients treated primarily by surgery. Almost identical figures are provided by Lacher (1963) for irradiation therapy alone. It is our opinion that localized disease is best treated by surgical excision, so that further areas of recurrent disease can be subjected to adequate irradiation.

LYMPHOSARCOMA. Another primary malignancy of the lymph nodes is lymphosarcoma. The terminology and the division of the various types of this group of conditions into subdivisions are debated. In the pediatric age group, the disease appears first in the lymph nodes of the cervical region in 20 to 30 percent of the cases. In the more advanced forms of the disease, there is usually involvement of the lymph nodes of the mediastinum, and generally there is hepatosplenomegaly as well. Children with persistent enlargement of the lymph nodes of the cervical region and those with chronic progression of such enlargement should undergo biopsy to determine the true nature of the disease process. Bone marrow examination is important in all of the cases, for the lymph node enlargement may be associated with aleukemic leukemia, which can be diagnosed only by examination of the bone marrow.

A cure from surgical treatment of a lymphosarcoma is occasionally reported in the literature. Most such successes have been reported for lesions encountered in the gastrointestinal tract, and only very rarely has there been successful treatment by surgical excision of lymphosarcoma of the cervical lymph nodes. The authors have encountered one case where a single node was involved in the neck. This and the adjacent nodes were removed surgically followed by radiation therapy, and a five-year survival was achieved. Usually the surgeon's role in the management of cervical lymphosarcoma consists only of biopsy. There is generally widespread involvement of lymphoid tissue throughout the body, and therefore palliative radiation therapy or the concomitant use of chemotherapy provides the most sensible therapeutic approach. Frequently with lymphosarcoma a transition into a full-blown leukemia occurs, and in such cases the outlook is dismal. At The Children's Memorial Hospital rare instances have been observed where this leukemic phase has been reversed by antileukemic therapy, only to be followed by a second episode of lymph node enlargement. In no such case has a five-year survival resulted from this reversal to the localized form of the disease.

Surgical therapy of lymphosarcoma. While Smith and Klopp (1961) have recorded a 56 percent five-year cure rate for the surgical treatment of apparently localized lymphosarcoma, most authors have reported little success with surgery alone. Localized recurrence or dissemination of the process is the usual outcome of excisional therapy for this disease. This is not to say that wide excision or full-scale irradiation should not be tried in the individual case. Whenever the biopsy reveals lymphosarcoma in a cervical lymph node it is our practice to carry out tonsillectomy and a modified radical neck dissection on the involved side. In such cases, the sternocleidomastoid and accessory nerve are left intact, since extension of the malignancy into these structures is unusual except in very advanced disease. Local recurrences, disease on the other side of the neck, generalized metastases, and subsequent leukemia are treated by appropriate combinations of irradiation, chemotherapy, and surgical excision for their palliative effect.

RETICULUM CELL SARCOMA. Reticulum cell sarcoma has had the worst prognosis of all of the sarcomas. The tumor, which is composed of pleomorphic reticulum cells lying in an argyrophilic reticulum stroma (Fig. 33), is found in areas similar to those which become involved by lymphosarcoma and Hodgkin's disease. It tends to become generalized quite rapidly. The treatment is the same as that required for the lymphosarcoma. Leukemic transformation is less common in reticulum cell sarcoma than in lymphosarcoma, where it occurs in about 50 percent of the cases.

TUMORS OF NEUROGENIC ORIGIN. The *neurilemmomas,* or Schwann cell tumors, are malignant in about 10 percent of cases. They arise most frequently from the nerves of the cervical plexus and present usually as smooth, elongated, deep-lying masses beneath the sternocleidomastoid muscle. Occasionally a nodular mass may be seen. Nerve pain is uncommon unless malignant degeneration has occurred. Biopsy reveals sheets of fusiform cells within an eosinophilic mucoid stroma. The characteristic Verocay

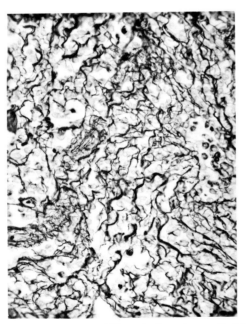

Fig. 33. The argyrophilic reticulum stroma that is characteristic of the reticulum cell sarcoma.

bodies are composed of cells of similar type arranged in parallel rows (Fig. 4) that form prominent palisades. The malignant tumors are composed of cells that are similarly oriented, but their pleomorphism, increased numbers of mitotic figures, and general irregularity indicate their malignant potential. These tumors are sometimes seen in association with von Recklinghausen's disease.

At operation the benign neurilemmomas are small fusiform structures attached to a peripheral or sympathetic nerve. It has been said that they can be removed with preservation of the nerve. In most cases it is probably wiser to resect the nerve in its entirety, provided that no serious muscular deficit will result, in order to ensure against recurrence. The malignant neurilemmomas have had a poor prognosis, and according to Michael (1964) the over-all five-year survival rate of 25 percent is considerably reduced in the pediatric age group.

Neuroblastomas in the cervical region may be primary or secondary. These tumors arise from primitive sympathetic neuroblasts (sympathogonia) that develop into ganglion cells or into cells of the chromaffin group. Although ganglion cells occur from the base of the skull to the sacral region, the overwhelming number of neuroblastomas and benign ganglioneuromas develop in the adrenal medulla.

The neuroblastomas developing primarily in the neck are similar in structure to the more common retroperitoneal variety. The key histological features are the eosinophilic neurofibrillary stroma and the characteristic pseudorosettes formed by 8 to 20 cells clustered together so that their elongated cytoplasm extends centrally while their darkly staining nuclei form the peripheral ring. The differentiation of this tumor from neuroblastoma, lymphosarcoma, Ewing's sarcoma, and the reticuloendothelioses may be difficult in some cases. In the usual type of tumor, surgical excision is followed by a significant number of cures, particularly when the patient is under the age of one year and when radiation therapy has been used postoperatively.

The treatment of choice for cervical neuroblastoma at The Children's Memorial Hospital has been total excision if possible, followed by irradiation to a tumor dosage of up to 3,000 rads in four weeks. A search is made by intravenous pyelography for a possible primary site in an adrenal. At present, three of four children with primary cervical neuroblastomas are alive and well at least five years after receiving this type of therapy.

The chemodectomas, or carotid body tumors, are uncommon during childhood but are now being reported more frequently in this age group. They have been discussed by Morris and his co-workers (1963) and by Wilson (1964). Resection of the mass along with adventitia of the carotid bifurcation is generally not followed by recurrence. These tumors are occasionally malignant even during childhood.

Fibrosarcoma, rhabdomyosarcoma, liposarcomas, hemangioendotheliomas, and other tumors of deep tissue origin may be discovered in surgical biopsy specimens. These are treated by wide excision if possible, followed by irradiation or chemotherapy. In general, these tumors respond poorly to irradiation. Two lipomyxosarcomas in the retroperitoneal area have apparently been cured in our clinics by partial excision followed by long term chemotherapy. If this type of tumor is found in the cervical region, therefore, this drug should be used during the postoperative period. The prognosis for most of the malignant tumors is poor, but it may perhaps be improved by a more aggressive surgical approach at the time of first treatment.

Thyroid carcinoma and other visceral malignancies are discussed elsewhere (Ch. 23).

WILLIAM L. DONNELLAN
JAMES M. KIDD
ORVAR SWENSON

REFERENCES

ANDERSON, R., and BYARS, L. T. Surgery of the Parotid Gland. St. Louis, The C. V. Mosby Company, 1965.

AVERY, M. E., McAFEE, J. G., and GUILD, H. G. The course and prognosis of reticuloendotheliosis (eosinophilic granuloma, Schüller-Christian disease and Letterer-Siwe disease). A study of 40 cases. Amer. J. Med., 22: 636, 1957.

BEAHRS, O. H., and ADSON, M. A. The surgical anatomy and technic of parotidectomy. Amer. J. Surg., 95: 885, 1958.

BHASKAR, S. N. Oral tumors of infancy and childhood. A survey of 293 cases. J. Pediat., 63: 195, 1963.

BRADLEY, J. L. Cysts of the jaw bones. J. Oral Surg., 9: 295, 1951.

BYARS, L. T., ACKERMAN, L. V., and PEACOCK, E. Tumors of salivary gland origin in children: A clinical pathological appraisal of 24 cases. Ann. Surg., 146: 40, 1957.

CONVERSE, J. M., ed. Reconstructive Plastic Surgery. Vol. 3, Head and Neck. Philadelphia, W. B. Saunders Company, 1964.

DAHLIN, D. C. Bone Tumors. General Aspects and an Analysis of 2,276 Cases. Springfield, Ill., Charles C Thomas, Publisher, 1957.

DARGEON, H. W. Tumors of Childhood; A Clinical Treatise. New York, Paul B. Hoeber, Inc., 1960.

FIGI, F. A., and DAVIS, R. E. The management of nasopharyngeal fibromas. Laryngoscope, 60: 794, 1950.

FOOTE, F. W., Jr., and FRAZELL, E. L. Tumors of the major salivary glands. Atlas of Tumor Pathology, Section IV, Fascicle II. Washington, D.C., Armed Forces Institute of Pathology, 1954.

HÄRMÄ, R. A. Nasopharyngeal angiofibroma. A clinical and histopathological study. Acta Otolaryng. (Stockholm), Supplement 146, 1958.

HARRISON, D. F. N., and TUCKER, W. N. The role of chemotherapy in advanced cancer of the head and neck. A Review of Eighty Cases. Brit. J. Cancer, 18: 74, 1964.

HOWARD, J. M., RAWSON, A. J., KOOP, C. E., HORNE, R. C., and ROYSTER, H. P. Parotid tumors in children. Surg. Gynec. Obstet., 90: 307, 1950.

JAFFE, H. L. Fibrous dysplasia. In Tumors and Tumorous Conditions of the Bones and Joints. Philadelphia, Lea & Febiger, 1958, Ch. 9.

LACHER, M. J. Role of surgery in Hodgkin's disease. New Eng. J. Med., 268: 289, 1963.

—— and DURANT, J. R. Combined vinblastine and chlorambucil therapy of Hodgkin's disease. Ann. Intern. Med., 62: 468, 1965.

LEDERMAN, M. Cancer of the Nasopharynx. Its Natural History and Treatment. Springfield, Charles C Thomas, Publisher, 1961.

LICHTENSTEIN, L. Histiocytosis X. Integration of eosinophilic granuloma of bone, "Letterer-Siwe disease" and "Schüller-Christian disease'" as related manifestations of a single nosologic entity. A.M.A. Archives Path., 56: 84, 1953.

MacCOMB, W. S. Juvenile nasopharyngeal fibroma. Amer. J. Surg., 106: 754, 1963.

McCONNELL, E. M. Nasopharyngeal carcinoma in children and young adults. Brit. J. Cancer, 12: 195, 1958.

McGAVRAN, M. H., and SPADY, H. A. Eosinophilic granuloma of bone. A study of twenty-eight cases. J. Bone Joint Surg. (Amer.), 42-A: 979, 1960.

McWHORTER, H. E., and WOOLNER, L. B. Pigmented nevi, juvenile melanomas and malignant melanomas in children. Cancer, 7: 564, 1954.

MICHAEL, P. Tumors of Infancy and Childhood. Philadelphia, J. B. Lippincott Company, 1964.

MORRIS, G. C., Jr., PANAYOTIS, E. B., COOLEY, D. A., CRAWFORD, E. S., and DeBAKEY, M. E. Surgical treatment of benign and malignant carotid body tumors: Clinical experience with sixteen tumors in twelve patients. Amer. Surg., 29: 429, 1963.

MOUSSATOS, G. H., and BAFFES, T. G. Cervical masses in infants and children. Pediatrics, 32: 251, 1963.

PETERS, M. V., and MIDDLEMISS, K. C. H. A study of Hodgkin's disease treated by irradiation. Amer. J. Roentgen., 79: 114, 1958.

PETTET, J. R., WOOLNER, L. B., and JUDD, E. S., Jr. Carotid body tumors (chemodectomas). Ann. Surg., 137: 465, 1953.

PICKRELL, K. L., MASTERS, F. W., GEORGIADE, N. G., and HORTON, C. E. Tumors of the head and neck in infancy, childhood and adolescence. Plast. Reconstr. Surg., 12: 10, 1953.

PIMPINELLA, R. J. The nasopharyngeal angiofibroma in the adolescent male. J. Pediat., 64: 260, 1964.

PITCOCK, J. A., BAUER, W. C., and McGAVRAN, M. H. Hodgkin's disease in children: A clinicopathological study of 46 cases. Cancer, 12: 1043, 1959.

RICHARDSON, R. J., ROBINSON, D. W., and MASTERS, F. W. Tumors of the mandible in children. Plast. Reconstr. Surg., 23: 576, 1959.

RUBIN, P., ed. Current concepts in cancer. 2. Hodgkin's disease. Curability of localized Hodgkin's disease by surgery, radiotherapy and chemotherapy. 3. Advanced Hodgkin's disease. Chemotherapy, radiotherapy and special considerations in pregnancy and childhood. J.A.M.A., 191: 25, 314, 1965.

RUSH, B. F., Jr., CHAMBERS, R. G., and RAVITCH, M. M. Cancer of the head and neck in children. Surgery, 53: 270, 1963.

SLAUGHTER, D. P., ECONOMOU, S. G., and SOUTHWICK, H. W. Surgical management of Hodgkin's disease. Ann. Surg., 148: 705, 1958.

SMITH, D. F., and KLOPP, C. T. Value of surgical removal of localized lymphomas. Surgery, 49: 469, 1961.

SMITH, J. F. Fibrous dysplasia of the jaws. Arch. Otolaryng. (Chicago), 81: 592, 1965.

STOBBE, G. D., and DARGEON, H. W. Embryonal rhabdomyosarcoma of the head and neck in children and adolescents. Cancer, 3: 826, 1950.

WILSON, H. Carotid body tumors: Surgical management. Ann. Surg., 159: 959, 1964.

25

Respiratory Emergencies in the Newborn

Respiratory insufficiency is the major cause of death in the neonatal period. It may be produced by defective functioning of the central nervous system or by peripheral abnormalities of the respiratory passages and pulmonary parenchyma. Ineffective or absent respiratory efforts suggest central nervous system damage. Labored breathing, in contrast, is frequently an indication of peripheral defects of the respiratory mechanism.

CLASSIFICATION

From the surgical point of view it is convenient to list the causes of neonatal respiratory distress topographically, in the manner outlined by Schaffer (1965) (Table 1).

Surgical conditions leading to neonatal respiratory distress do not usually produce symptoms until after the first hour of life. The exceptions are those congenital abnormalities which lead to complete obstruction of the airway and total compression of the pulmonary parenchyma. Of the correctable lesions only laryngeal atresia, diaphragmatic herniation of the entire abdominal viscera, and occasionally severe tension pneumothorax produce immediate and nearly total obstruction to alveolar air entry. These must be diagnosed and treated within the first few minutes of life. The remaining conditions permit some oxygenation of the baby and are usually associated with increasing dysp-

nea for periods of several hours or days before the correct diagnosis is made.

SIGNS AND SYMPTOMS

The signs of neonatal respiratory distress are an abnormal cry, grunting breathing or stridor, an increasing respiratory rate, flaring of the nostrils, violent respiratory efforts accompanied by retraction of the chest, excessive mucus, tachycardia, irritability, and cyanosis. Bradycardia, irregular breathing, and lethargy are late signs which indicate serious metabolic decompensation. It is essential to prevent the occurrence of these late signs by appropriate initial treatment, since the mortality rate and the development of late neurological sequelae are directly related to the length of time during which they are present. For this reason prompt reoxygenation is the key to proper management. Such reoxygenation is possible only when the level of the obstruction to pulmonary gas exchange has been determined without doubt.

DIFFERENTIAL DIAGNOSIS

The following remarks apply to the development of respiratory difficulties either in the delivery room or, later, in the newborn nursery. It is important first of all to gain control of the pulmonary aeration by proving potency of the upper airways, and then to

TABLE 1. CAUSES OF LABORED RESPIRATION IN THE NEWBORN *

OBSTRUCTION TO THE AIRWAY

In the mouth, nose, and pharynx
  Macroglossia
  Micrognathia
  Congenital atresia of posterior choanae
  Cysts and tumors, including aberrant thyroid

In the neck
  Congenital goiter
  Cysts and tumors

In the larynx and trachea
  Congenital laryngeal stridor
  Congenital anomalies of the larynx or trachea
    Laryngeal webs
    Laryngeal stenosis
    Tracheal stenosis
      Congenital stenosis
      Compression by neighboring structures
  Cysts and neoplasms of the larynx
  Vocal cord paralysis
  Neurogenic stridor
  Acquired laryngeal lesions

In the chest
  Massive aspiration of amniotic, vaginal, or
    oropharyngeal contents
  Atelectasis
  The emphysema group
    Interstitial
    Mediastinal
    Blebs and bullae
    Pneumothorax
    Unilobar emphysema
  The hyaline membrane syndrome
  The Wilson-Mikity syndrome
  Pneumonia of the newborn
    Intrauterine
    Intranatally or postnatally acquired
  Pulmonary agenesis and hypoplasia
  Disorders of the diaphragm
    Hernia
    Paralysis
    Eventration
    Accessory diaphragm
  Tracheoesophageal fistula
  Pulmonary cysts
  Intrathoracic tumors and fluid-filled cysts
  Accessory and sequestered lobes
  Chylothorax and pleural effusion
  Pulmonary hemorrhage

TABLE 1. (CONT.) CAUSES OF LABORED RESPIRATION IN THE NEWBORN *

CONDITIONS PRODUCING DYSPNEA WITHOUT OBSTRUCTING THE AIRWAY

  Intracranial hemorrhage
  Cardiac failure

* From Schaffer. Diseases of the Newborn. 2nd Ed. Courtesy of W. B. Saunders Co.

demonstrate the degree of pulmonary expansion by roentgenological examination. If after the usual methods of resuscitation of the newborn infant the respiratory function remains abnormal, patency of the airway is proved by a catheter being passed through the nostril to eliminate the possibility of choanal atresia or an obstructing tumor, and then by examination of the oropharynx, larynx, and trachea with the laryngoscope. As noted previously (see "Technique of Laryngoscopy"), the tip of the blade should be placed in the right vallecula between the epiglottis and the tongue rather than directly beneath the epiglottis, since this structure is small, curved, and narrow in newborn infants, and it easily slips off the blade when it is lifted up directly. After the inspection of the larynx has been completed a soft plastic catheter is placed into the trachea through the glottis, and 100 percent oxygen is introduced into the system.

While the laryngoscopy is being performed, provisions are made for portable radiographic examination of the chest. Considerable information about the aeration of the chest can be obtained by physical examination alone, but it is not sufficient for an accurate diagnosis. Chest films, by contrast, reveal not only the degree of pulmonary aeration but also the presence or absence of localized intrathoracic lesions, the position and size of the heart and mediastinum, and the position of the diaphragms. These details permit a provisional diagnosis to be made.

A complete examination of the baby may reveal persistent tachypnea and cyanosis despite intubation. Other signs of hypoxia are flaring of the nostrils and tachycardia. The neck is palpated for the presence of tumors or cysts. Percussion of the chest may reveal dullness on one side when a space-occupying mass is present. When a tension pneumothorax or increasing expansion of a lung cyst is present, hyperresonance on one side is combined with displacement of the cardiac impulse to the outer margin of the opposite thorax. In the massive aspiration syndrome apparent overexpansion of the chest is combined with paradoxical dullness to percussion.

Examination of the abdomen provides useful information. If extreme distension of the stomach is found, its deflation may cure the respiratory distress. The size of the liver must be determined. A large liver usually signifies cardiac failure, but it may also be a sign of sepsis, of a hemolytic disorder, or of congenital leukemia. Abdominal masses should also be excluded. In one of our patients a huge hydronephrosis so compressed the diaphragm that extreme respiratory embarrassment developed.

Palpation of the pulses is essential. In congenital coarctation of the aorta, which may be associated with rapidly developing congestive heart failure, the femoral pulses are absent or markedly diminished. They are less prominent than usual in the presence of pulmonic stenosis without a sepal defect. If a significant arterio-venous shunt is present, the pulses are collapsing in nature. When these findings are combined with examination of the heart and liver, the diagnosis of cardiac failure as a cause for the dyspnea may be confirmed or ruled out.

RADIOLOGICAL FINDINGS

In general the chest radiograph reveals displacement of normal structures, pulmonary consolidation, atelectasis or emphysema, the presence of space-occupying masses and abnormalities of the cardiac shadow. The position of the trachea, the mediastinal shadow, and the diaphragm must be evaluated first, the cardiac shadow next, and finally the lung fields in the anteroposterior and lateral views. Herniation of the lung across the upper mediastinum is a sign of pulmonary overdistension. It may be produced by obstructive emphysema on the affected side (Fig. 1) or by overdistension of a lung resulting from contralateral atelectasis. This distinction is an important one to make, since the diagnosis and treatment are entirely different in the two conditions.

It should be remembered that the pulmonary parenchyma is not entirely expanded for two to four days after birth. Weymuller and his associates determined as early as 1928 that patchy mottling of the lung fields, a large globular heart, and a broad mediastinum are usual on the day of birth (Weymuller et al., 1928). The normal appearance is only gradually assumed as adequate breathing continues. The diagnosis of congenital pneumonia with cardiac failure may be erroneously entertained in normal babies unless these peculiarities of the newborn chest radiograph are appreciated.

Thoracic lesions of direct surgical significance can usually be demonstrated unequivocally in chest radiographs. Tension pneumothorax, an enlarging lung cyst or congenital emphysema, opacity owing to chylothorax, and diaphragmatic herniation are the usual surgically treatable causes of serious respira-

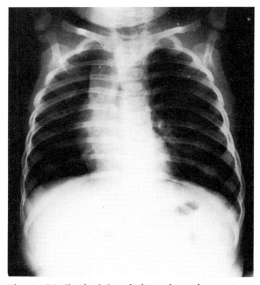

Fig. 1. Mediastinal herniation of emphysematous left lung to right chest.

tory distress in newborn babies. Less severe dyspnea may be the result of localized atelectasis or of pneumonia associated with the presence of a tracheoesophageal fistula with or without esophageal atresia.

INITIAL MANAGEMENT OF NEONATAL RESPIRATORY DISTRESS

PHYSIOLOGICAL CONSIDERATIONS

Regardless of the cause of insufficient pulmonary function in newborn infants, the resulting physiological events are predictable and progressive. Inadequate gas exchange leads to hypoxemia and to retention of carbon dioxide. This initial respiratory acidosis is rapidly increased by the metabolic acidosis resulting from anaerobic glycolysis in anoxic tissues. Acidosis diminishes both the efficiency of the respiratory center and the effective cardiac output, and thus the tissue oxygen deficit is intensified. This vicious circle of events may lead to the death of the infant or to permanent cerebral damage unless it can be rapidly reversed.

hypoxia-------acidosis

respiratory center depression

acidosis-------tissue hypoxia

Studies of normal newborn infants have revealed that all babies undergo extreme hypoxia during the delivery period. James and his co-workers (1964) and other authors find that the pH of the blood frequently falls to 7.0, the oxygen content is often less than 10 percent, the carbon dioxide partial pressure rises to 100 mm Hg, and the available buffer base is reduced to 30 mEq/l from a normal of 42 M/l. When organic causes are present which limit pulmonary gas exchange, these values may not be corrected in the normal way.

Anoxia has its primary effect on the individual cell. If adequate oxygen is not available to the cell, the capture of electrons to produce the high-energy molecule adenosine triphosphate (ATP) is an inefficient process. This molecule, which appears to be absolutely essential for the transfer of energy and the cellular synthetic functions, is produced aerobically from adenosine diphosphate (ADP) by the following reaction:

$$glucose + O_2 \text{ --------- } 6\ CO_2 + 38\ ATP$$

Under the conditions of anoxia, energy transfer can still occur anaerobically, but it is very inefficient:

$$glucose \text{ ------ } 2\ lactic\ acid + 2\ ATP$$

Although energy is derived in other ways from carbohydrate metabolism, the general decrease in normal energy transfer is apparent. Not only is the production of the high-energy mediator ATP only about 1/16 of that which occurs under aerobic conditions but also lactic acid, which cannot be excreted by the lungs, is produced instead of CO_2. The buffer systems of the body are soon saturated with excess hydrogen ions, and metabolic acidosis ensues, leading to defective cardiac function, alterations in the pulmonary hemodynamics, and further tissue

diminished cardiac output
(plus increased right-to-left shunting)

anoxia. Quite obviously the treatment of anoxia requires reoxygenation of the blood. If improvement of oxygenation is not immediately possible, elevation of the lowered pH of the body fluids by the administration of base in the form of sodium bicarbonate may serve to improve the baby's condition temporarily, as demonstrated by Usher (1963).

One should remember that fetal hemoglobin is a more efficient carrier of oxygen than adult hemoglobin. According to Klaus and Meyer (1966) it binds more oxygen than the adult type at any oxygen partial pressure (PO_2) below 100 mm Hg. The fetal arterial PO_2 is always somewhat lower than it is in the adult by the time cyanosis is observed, since hemoglobin saturations of 75 to 85 percent are equivalent to oxygen tensions of only 32 to 42 mm Hg on the fetal oxyhemoglobin dissociation curve. This PO_2 is about the level at which defective tissue oxygenation occurs. It is the *oxygen tension* in tissue fluids rather than the *total oxygen content* that conditions the movement of oxygen across cellular membranes.

An important response of the newborn baby to anoxia is an exaggerated constrictive response of the pulmonary vasculature. At birth the pulmonary and systemic circuits are quite similar in pressure, but the pulmonary resistance then decreases and shunting across the foramen ovale ceases, although left-to-right shunting may still occur through the ductus arteriosus and perhaps also within the lungs. Such shunting may amount to as much as 20 percent of the cardiac output during the first few days of life. Hypoxemia and lowering of the pH of the blood both combine to increase the pulmonary vascular resistance and pulmonary artery pressure. This may lead to increased right-to-left shunting, which further aggravates the hypoxemic state. Oxygen therapy may improve the baby's condition not only by increasing the oxygenation of the hemoglobin but also by decreasing this shunting of unoxygenated blood into the systemic circulation, since significant reduction of the pulmonary vascular pressure usually occurs when oxygen is given to anoxic infants.

These general considerations indicate the need for oxygen therapy whenever any degree of respiratory insufficiency is present in newborn infants. In most of the cases the need for oxygen is short-lived. Failure to provide it may lead to serious acute metabolic abnormalities, chronic brain damage, and poor postoperative responses in the babies requiring surgical procedures. The problem of excessive oxygen administration is discussed elsewhere in this book. It is now possible to monitor the blood pH and PO_2

and to keep them within reasonably normal ranges by oxygen therapy and in this way to avoid the dangers of hyperoxygenation. (See "Inhalation Therapy.")

FIRST STEPS IN RESUSCITATION

The necessity for the immediate and effective administration of oxygen is apparent whenever respiratory distress or cyanosis develops in a newborn infant. If this measure does not improve the general condition dramatically, endotracheal intubation is essential to provide for positive pressure respiratory assistance. A tube should also be passed into the stomach to decompress the upper abdomen. A venous catheter in the saphenous vein at the ankle provides a route for the administration of fluids and electrolytes, epinephrine or other stimulants, blood and plasma, and buffer bases designed to reduce the acidosis. Base-line serum electrolyte values and measurements of the blood pH, PO_2, and PCO_2 serve to determine the need for specific fluid administration and to define the adequacy of the therapeutic program.

When the blood pH is below 7.2, cellular enzyme functions are impaired. The cardiac function and the activity of the central nervous system decreases. The use of buffers such as sodium bicarbonate* and trishydroxymethylaminomethane (Tris or THAM) may sometimes allow the infant to survive until the primary lung defect can be corrected. This is the basis for the treatment of the hyaline membrane syndrome with intravenous sodium bicarbonate in addition to the use of a high-oxygen environment. It applies equally well to surgical problems. During the period of diagnosis and preoperative preparation the acidosis can be partially corrected by the following formula:

0.58 g $NaHCO_3$ per kilogram

elevates serum CO_2 1 mEq per liter

---

* Commercial sodium bicarbonate ampules contain 3.75 g (44.6 mEq) $NaHCO_3$ in 50 ml of solution, or 0.075 g $NaHCO_3$ per ml.

The amount of bicarbonate calculated to correct the acidosis about 25 percent is diluted in an equal amount of 10 percent glucose solution and infused within five minutes. Bicarbonate rather than lactate is used because infants metabolize lactate rather slowly. Subsequent amounts of buffer are based on pH and carbon dioxide content measurements. Since neonatal acidosis is a mixed one, including both respiratory and metabolic components, the carbon dioxide content is not actually a good guide to management. It is of some value in initiating therapy, however, particularly if the pH is measured concomitantly. It is this latter value which must be watched carefully, since the creation of an alkalosis by excessive bicarbonate administration will almost certainly lead to tetanic convulsions from low serum calcium ion concentration.

When Tris is used for the buffer, it is given as a 0.5 M solution with 3.5 percent glucose in the dosage of 12 ml per kg over a period of two to four minutes. This buffer has proved dangerous under certain conditions, and we continue to prefer sodium bicarbonate for the acute correction of acidosis.

Positive pressure respirators are discussed in Chapter 8. These machines are of increasing value in the management of respiratory paralysis and for temporary airway or pulmonary parenchymal dysfunction. Their safe use requires constant observation of both the machine and the patient and considerable knowledge of respiratory physiology on the part of the attendants.

Laryngoscopy and bronchoscopy are valuable adjuncts to the pre- and postoperative management of respiratory problems in infants. Repeated direct endotracheal aspiration can be performed either through an indwelling endotracheal tube or by exposing the larynx with the laryngoscope. Formal bronchoscopic aspiration at intervals permits observation and cleansing of the major bronchi. No anesthesia is required. It is essential that soft rubber catheter tips be employed in order to avoid serious tracheal and bronchial mucosal abrasion. Another problem which arises after successful surgical correction of many intrathoracic obstructions is prolonged and excessive bronchial secretion and often pulmonary infection, both of which may be greatly relieved by bronchoscopic cleansing of the airway.

The infant must be kept warm. It is now clearly established that the need for oxygen increases considerably when a baby's temperature is lowered below the normal range. This increased need for oxygen may aggravate the metabolic acidosis of a normal newborn premature infant, and may prove disastrous when the infant is unable to compensate for it by increased pulmonary gas exchange.

SURGICALLY CORRECTABLE LESIONS

Most infants with respiratory difficulty at or shortly after birth do not have surgically correctable problems. The hyaline membrane syndrome, massive atelectasis, aspiration obstruction, and neonatal pneumonia have been mentioned as the major causes of respiratory difficulty in this age group. Most of the other responsible conditions are discussed in other parts of this book. Among these are the congenital diaphragmatic hernias, esophageal atresia with tracheoesophageal fistula, obstructive congenital anomalies of the larynx and tracheobronchial tree, constricting vascular rings, the Pierre Robin syndrome, and masses in the neck and mediastinum such as cystic hygromas, hemangiomas, teratomas of the thyroid, and congenital cysts of various types. There remain a heterogeneous group of conditions which, while not of frequent occurrence, are important to the general discussion of respiratory distress in the newborn infant.

LUNG CYSTS AND CONGENITAL LOBAR EMPHYSEMA

Lung cysts occur infrequently. Aside from the bronchogenic cysts, which do not communicate with the air passages, and the pneumatoceles which follow staphylococcal pneumonia, there are two forms of true congenital lung cysts. One or more dysplastic lobes may be made up of numbers of small cysts filled with mucus and air (Fig. 2), or there may be only one large cavity that communicates with the bronchial tree. Both these lesions may so compress the normal pulmonary parenchyma that serious respiratory difficulty occurs. The treatment is surgical excision. A delay in operation may lead to serious infection within the cyst and subsequent pneu-

monia in the postoperative period due to seeding of the normal lung during the thoracotomy.

CONGENITAL LOBAR EMPHYSEMA

Congenital lobar emphysema is an interesting and not infrequently lethal condition that results from obstruction to the expiration of air from the affected pulmonary lobe. Inspiration is normal, and so an increasing

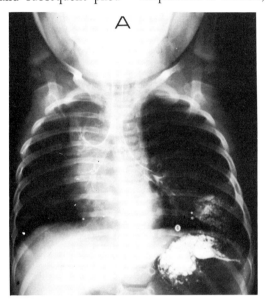

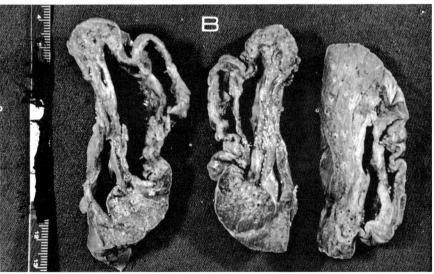

Fig. 2. Large multilocular lung cyst. A. The cyst caused deviation of the heart to the right. B. Internal structure of the cyst.

distension of the lobe ensues that may ultimately lead to compression of the unaffected lung. The upper lobes are most frequently involved. Although a temporary bronchial obstruction by mucus may produce the condition, it is usually caused by a congenital deformity of the proximal bronchial cartilages. The affected bronchus opens normally on inspiration but is closed by the raised intrathoracic pressure of expiration.

Whenever increasing respiratory distress in a newborn infant is found to be associated with hyperresonance on one side and deviation of the heart contralaterally, congenital lobar emphysema or a tension pneumothorax is the usual cause. Chest radiography is essential to differentiate the two conditions (Fig. 3).

The treatment of congenital lobar emphysema is surgical excision under general endotracheal anesthesia. It is obvious that excessive endotracheal pressure to "improve" the baby's air intake can only result in further overinflation of the lobe. For this reason rapid thoracotomy through the fifth intercos-

tal space should follow the anesthesiologist's intubation.

Some authors recommend deflation of the emphysematous lobe by an intercostal needle. Although this may give temporary relief and may occasionally be necessary in desperate circumstances, it is our opinion that surgical removal of the lobe is a safer and more definitive procedure. Bronchoscopy just prior to the thoracotomy may make it possible to avoid operation in those few infants in whom a mucous plug rather than defective bronchial cartilages is the cause of the ball-valve obstruction.

POSTPNEUMONIC PNEUMATOCELE

The pneumatoceles that follow staphylococcal and occasionally other pneumonias do not usually enter into the diagnosis of neonatal respiratory distress. They develop during the healing process and are not seen for several days after the initial pneumonia. The infection, however, may be contracted in the

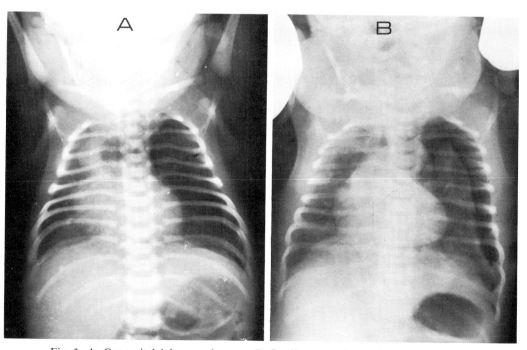

Fig. 3. A. Congenital lobar emphysema. B. Small pneumothorax in newborn infant.

newborn nursery and develop at home, the child being admitted later with the radiographic evidence of a lung cyst. The differentiation of pneumatoceles and congenital cysts of the lung may be difficult, but, in general, the older infant with a symptomatic congenital lung cyst is getting worse because of the associated infection, while the infant with a pneumatocele is getting better (Fig. 4).

When a pneumothorax is present in addition to the cyst, the diagnosis of poststaphylococcal pneumatocele is the more likely one.

The treatment of pneumatoceles is expectant. Oxacillin is the antibiotic of choice to clear up the infection. If serious tension de-

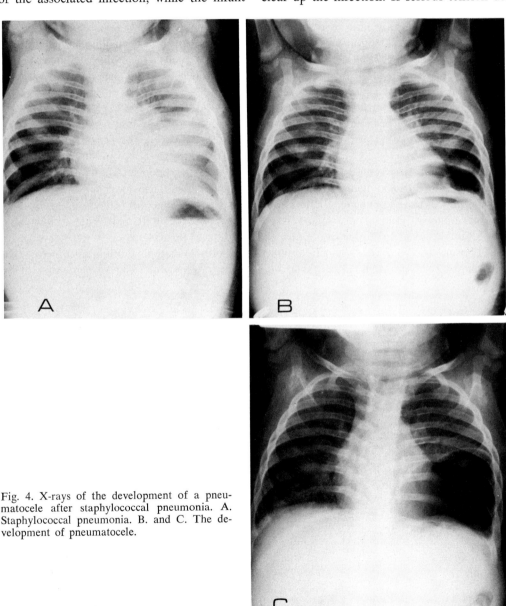

Fig. 4. X-rays of the development of a pneumatocele after staphylococcal pneumonia. A. Staphylococcal pneumonia. B. and C. The development of pneumatocele.

velops in the cyst or a pneumothorax super-venes, intercostal catheter drainage and continuation of the antibiotic are indicated. Oxygen therapy with high humidity is often necessary during the first few days of treatment. Pneumatoceles almost invariably recede and do not require excision. On rare occasions chronic infection may develop in a cyst and excision may be required.

TENSION PNEUMOTHORAX

During its passage through the birth canal the emerging infant sometimes experiences sharp compression of the thorax. If the lungs have been partially filled with air, a pneumothorax may occur. Other causes of pneumothorax are excessive respiratory efforts associated with amniotic fluid aspiration (the initial breath may develop as much as 70 cm H_2O negative pressure) and overinflation of the lungs by enthusiastic attempts at resuscitation. When a single episode of air leakage

is followed by sealing of the pleural or peri-bronchial opening, there is no significant impediment to breathing. Occasionally, however, the rent acts as a one-way valve, and a tension pneumothorax with peribronchial, mediastinal, and subcutaneous emphysema may develop (Fig. 5).

In infants a tension pneumothorax or great emphysema leads to complete compression of the contralateral lung and heart against the opposite thoracic wall because of the lack of stability of the mediastinum (Fig. 6). Rapid deterioration of these infants occurs. When the mediastinum is filled with air, compression of the great veins is a complication that produces a serious decrease in the venous return to the heart.

A small pneumothorax does not require surgical treatment. If the baby's condition is stable, collapse of one lung of up to 50 percent is well tolerated, and the air can be expected to resorb within a few days. An increase in the environmental oxygen to 35 or 40 percent will hasten its disappearance. When the pulse rate rises and tachypnea

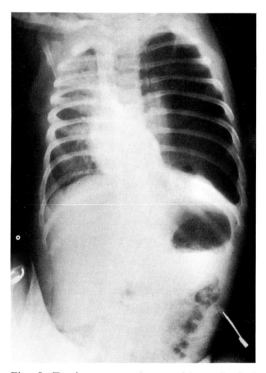

Fig. 5. Tension pneumothorax with mediastinal herniation of the lung.

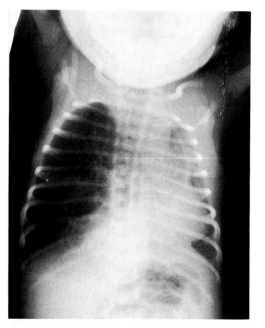

Fig. 6. Compression of the heart and right lung by a huge emphysematous left lung.

with cyanosis develops, chest radiography will reveal an increase in the pneumothorax. Under these conditions it is safe to introduce a small # 10 French catheter through the second intercostal space anteriorly. This catheter is connected to underwater-seal drainage. If the dyspneic condition is not relieved, low-pressure, high-volume suction by means of an Emerson aspirator should be utilized. The important consideration is to expand the lung as quickly as possible so that the two pleural surfaces can come together to seal the leak. Very occasionally the bronchopleural opening persists, and thoracotomy is required to close the defect.

CONGENITAL CHYLOTHORAX

Collections of lymph within the thoracic cavity occasionally cause dyspnea in newborn infants. Most of the cases appear to be due to rupture of the thoracic duct during delivery, because of either direct trauma to the duct or temporary intense venous hypertension associated with passage through the birth canal. The condition is almost always unilateral, and symptoms appear after the first few hours of life rather than immediately following the delivery.

Dyspnea in association with dullness to percussion and with deviation of the cardiac impulse to the opposite side is probably due to chylothorax. On roentgenological examination the costophrenic sulcus is obliterated, and the affected chest is opaque. Fluid is easily obtained. It is slightly yellowish in color before feedings are begun, but later it assumes the characteristic milky color of chyle.

In the treatment of congenital chylothorax it is recommended that repeated daily aspirations of the fluid be performed. In most of the cases no more than 3 to 8 aspirations are required. If the condition does not clear up within ten days, however, a serious loss of nutrients results from further removal of the chyle. In a recent study of chylothorax in all age groups, it was found that immediate intercostal suction drainage of the fluid led to sealing of the leak more rapidly, with less total loss of fluid than did repeated thoracentesis. For this reason we believe that aspiration should be done only for four consecutive days. If the opening remains and fluid collects rapidly again, a # 10 French catheter should be placed into the chest laterally at the sixth intercostal space and connected to suction. The fluid obtained in this manner may be discarded for a further three days. If there is no diminution of flow during this period, the chyle is collected under sterile conditions into plastic blood transfusion bags and reinfused into the baby intravenously.

Although it is stated that the leaks close spontaneously in all cases of chylothorax if sufficient time is allowed, there have been several reports of fatalities in newborn babies after several weeks of aspiration. Some authors therefore recommend earlier exploration and surgical closure of the defect. While this method is a definitive one if the opening can be found, either it imposes the burden of thoracotomy on an already depleted infant or it results in an unnecessary operation when it is done too soon. The middle course of reinfusion of the nutrient materials may make it possible to avoid early operation and to preserve the nutritional state of those babies ultimately requiring operation.

PHRENIC NERVE PALSY AND EVENTRATION OF THE DIAPHRAGM

Newborn infants breathe mainly by diaphragmatic activity. With paralysis of one or both phrenic nerves this mechanism is impaired, and serious respiratory distress may occur. Phrenic nerve palsy is a result of trauma in the great majority of cases. It may occur alone or in association with damage to the brachial plexus, the so-called Erb's palsy. The symptoms are those of insufficient entry of air into the lungs: poor cry, tachypnea, cyanosis, and subsequently periods of apnea. The chest roentgenogram often reveals a normal or only slightly raised diaphragm, and frequently there are areas of atelectasis or pneumonia. At fluoroscopy paradoxical motion of the paralyzed diaphragm can be observed: it *rises* on inspiration as the result of the increasing negative intrathoracic pressure (Fig. 7). Unless fluoroscopic examination or inspiration-expiration films are made in addition to the routine chest radiographs, the diagnosis is likely to be missed.

Although usually later in occurrence, the symptoms and signs of eventration of the diaphragm are similar to those of phrenic palsy, and indeed many authors consider the two conditions to be the same. In eventration the muscular portions of the diaphragm are absent or diminished, and the diaphragm is formed only by the cohesion of the pleura and peritoneum into a thin fibrous diaphragmatic septum. Some of the cases are associated with persistent brachial plexus palsy, but most are apparently due to the failure of development of muscular elements within the embryonic pleuroperitoneal membranes and septum transversum, and no brachial palsy is present. Paradoxical motion does not usually occur in eventration, since the defective diaphragm is elevated to its fullest extent by the normal negative intrathoracic pressure.

The treatment of phrenic nerve palsy and eventration is expectant. In the former condition nerve activity usually resumes in from two weeks to several months, and the babies can be tided over by oxygen therapy, humidification of the environment, and frequent aspiration of the tracheobronchial tree. Aspiration is required because of impaired drainage from the lung on the affected side. Pulmonary infection should be treated only when it appears, for prolonged prophylactic antibiotic therapy may lead to serious complications in small babies.

Hashida and Sherman (1961) described an accessory diaphragm in a newborn infant who died of respiratory difficulty at five hours of age. Roentgenological changes were

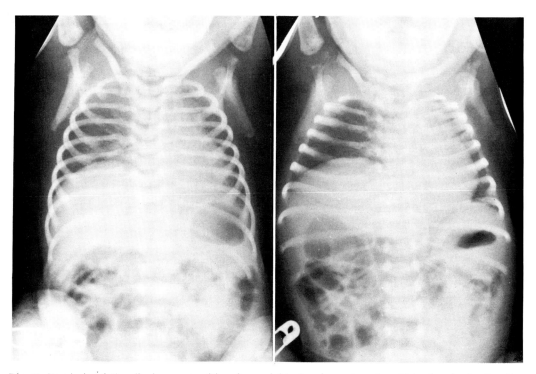

Fig. 7. Paralysis of the diaphragm resulting from right phrenic nerve palsy. Note the rise in the diaphragm on inspiration shown at right.

those of pneumothorax, but the condition did not respond to aspiration. At postmortem examination a septum was found midway in the left chest through which the lower lobe bronchi and pulmonary vessels extended to the lower lobe.

PULMONARY ARTERIOVENOUS FISTULA

The occurrence of congenital arteriovenous fistulas in various parts of the body is not uncommon. These may produce acute heart failure with dyspnea and cyanosis in the newborn period. Such lesions in the lungs may be single but are more usually multiple, involving one lung or even both lungs. The chest radiograph reveals one or more lobulated densities connected to the hilum by a cordlike opacity. The heart is usually enlarged. A continuous murmur may be heard over the mass. Resection of the larger aneurysms is not difficult, but the presence of multiple lesions may make a cure impossible to achieve. About one sixth of the reported cases have been associated with the Osler-Weber-Rendu form of hereditary telangiectasis.

WILLIAM L. DONNELLAN

REFERENCES

AHVENAINEN, E. K. Clinical symptoms of respiratory disorders in the newborn: VI Symptoms suggestive of anoxic damage. Ann. Paediat. Fenn., 5: 98, 1959.

APGAR, V., and JAMES, L. S. Further observations on newborn scoring system. Amer. J. Dis. Child., 104: 419, 1962.

BOYDEN, E. A. Bronchogenic cysts and the theory of intralobar sequestration; New embryonic data. J. Thorac. Cardiov. Surg., 35: 604, 1958.

BRODIE, H. R., CROSS, K. W., and LOMER, T. R. Heat production in newborn infants under normal and hypoxic conditions. J. Physiol. 138: 156, 1957.

BROWN, R. J. K. Respiratory difficulties at birth. Brit. Med. J., 1: 404, 1959.

BURNARD, E. D. The pulmonary syndrome of Wilson and Mikity, and respiratory function in very small premature infants. Ped. Clin. N. Amer., 13: 999, 1966.

CRAIG, J. M., KIRKPATRICK, J., and NEUHAUSER, E. B. D. Congenital cystic adenomatoid malformation of the lung in infants. Amer. J. Roentgenol., 76: 516, 1956.

DITCHBURN, R. K., HULL, D., and SEGALL, M. M. Oxygen uptake during and after positive-pressure ventilation for the resuscitation of asphyxiated newborn infants. Lancet, 2: 1096, 1966.

EMERY, J. L. Interstitial emphysema, pneumothorax, and "air-block" in the newborn. Lancet, 1: 405, 1956.

GANS, S. L., and HACKWORTH, L. E. Respiratory obstructions of surgical import. Pediat. Clin. N. Amer., 6: 1023, 1959.

HASHIDA, Y., and SHERMAN, F. E. Accessory diaphragm associated with neonatal respiratory distress. J. Pediat., 59: 529, 1961.

HUTCHISON, J. H., KERR, M. M., DOUGLAS, T. A., et al. A therapeutic approach in 100 cases of the respiratory distress syndrome of the newborn infant. Pediatrics, 33: 956, 1964.

JAMES, L. S. Onset of breathing and resuscitation. Pediat. Clin. N. Amer., 13: 621, 1966.

——— and ADAMSONS, K., Jr. Respiratory physiology of the fetus and newborn infant. New Eng. J. Med., 271: 1352, 1403, 1964.

KAPLAN, S., FOX, R. P., and CLARK, L. C., Jr. Amine buffers in the management of acidosis; Study of respiratory and mixed acidosis. Amer. J. Dis. Child., 103: 4, 1962.

KLAUS, M., and MEYER, B. P. Oxygen therapy for the newborn. Pediat. Clin. N. Amer., 13: 731, 1966.

MALAN, A. F. Respiratory rates and patterns in normal newborn infants. Their relationship to prematurity, sex, difficult labor and some maternal conditions. Clin. Pediat., 5: 593, 1966.

NELSON, N. M. Neonatal pulmonary function. Ped. Clin. N. Amer., 13: 769, 1966.

OYAMADA, A., GASUL, B. M., and HOLINGER, P. H. Agenesis of the lung. Amer. J. Dis. Child., 85: 182, 1953.

REID, D. H. S., and TUNSTALL, M. E. Treatment of respiratory distress syndrome of newborn with nasotracheal intubation and intermittent positive-pressure respiration. Lancet, 1: 1196, 1965.

RICHARDSON, W. R. Thoracic emergencies in the newborn infant. Amer. J. Surg., 105: 524, 1963.

——— Surgical complications of staphylococci pneumonia in infants and children. Amer. Surg., 27: 354, 1961.

ROOPENIAN, A., and STEMMER, A. L. Congenital posterior choanal atresia. Amer. J. Surg., 96: 802, 1958.

ROWE, R. D., and JAMES. L. S. Normal pulmonary artery pressure during the first year of life. J. Pediat., 51: 1, 1957.

RUDOLPH, A. J., DESMOND, M. M., and PINEDA, R. G. Clinical diagnosis of respiratory difficulty in the newborn. Pediat. Clin. N. Amer., 13: 669, 1966.

SCHAFFER, A. J. Diseases of the Newborn, 2nd ed. Philadelphia, W. B. Saunders Co., 1965.

SCHIFRIN, N. Unilateral paralysis of the diaphragm in the newborn infant with and without associated brachial palsy. Pediatrics, 9: 69, 1952.

STRANG, L. B. The pulmonary circulation in the respiratory distress syndrome. Pediat. Clin. N. Amer., 13: 693, 1966.

THOMSON, J., and FORFAR, J. O. Regional obstructive emphysema in infancy. Arch. Dis. Child., 33: 97, 1958.

USHER, R. Reduction of mortality from respiratory distress syndrome of prematurity with early administration of intravenous glucose and sodium bicarbonate. Pediatrics, 32: 966, 1963.

WEISBROT, I. M., JAMES, L. S., PRINCE, C. E., HOLADAY, D. A., and APGAR, V. Acid-base homeostasis of the newborn infant during the first 24 hours of life. J. Pediat., 52: 395, 1958.

WEYMULLER, C. A., BELL, A. L. L., and KRAHULIK, L. Roentgenographic changes in the thorax of normal newborn infants. Amer. J. Dis. Child., 35: 837, 1928.

26

The Chest Wall

LESIONS OF THE BREAST

The breast is identical in male and female at birth, being composed of ducts lined with epithelial cells interposed in a fibrous stroma. This connecting duct system communicates with the surface at the nipple, and in the deeper portions there are solid epithelial buds that will form the ancini in the female at puberty. There are no significant changes in the breast until puberty; the minor changes are predominantly in the female but may occur in males. In the male at puberty a mild form of change takes place and rapidly regresses. This occurs later than the breast growth that takes place in the female at puberty. Neonatal enlargement of the breast in both sexes within a few days after birth, associated with secretion of a cloudy fluid that has been referred to as "witch's milk," is common. This change is attributed to estrogen and prolactin from the maternal circulation. The swelling is usually soft and diffuse and nontender but may progress to a state of some hyperemia and local tenderness in some infants. It may precede pyogenic infection, but a definite relationship cannot be established.

BENIGN TUMORS OF THE BREAST

Tumors of the breast in children are rare, and the majority of those encountered are benign.

ADENOFIBROMA

Adenofibromas are composed predominantly of fibrous elements, and the rate of growth may be surprisingly rapid and appear to be malignant from this characteristic alone. Supporting this impression is the common presence of enlarged axillary glands. This tumor is encountered in girls prior to puberty but usually beyond ten years of age. The tumor is firm and the rate of growth is variable, but often the increase in size is rapid. There may be tenderness and some tenseness and shininess of the skin overlying the mass. Treatment consists of surgical excision. In most instances the tumor mass will shell out, and the essential portions of the breast tissue are left undisturbed (Fig. 1). Whenever possible, the areola and the duct system of the gland should not be disturbed. However, at times the tumor may be massive, and its removal is essentially a simple mastectomy.

CYSTS

One of the commoner lesions in the breast is a small cyst. It may be about 0.5 to 1 cm in its greatest diameter. Usually it is oblong, and it may be tender. The lesion is under the nipple, freely movable and without attachments to the skin or chest wall. These cysts are quite characteristic and will usually disappear over a long period of time. Cysts may be larger than this, but such lesions are

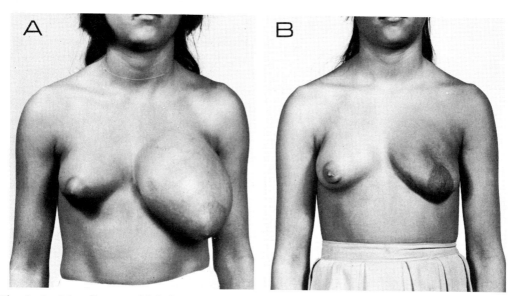

Fig. 1. A. Adenofibroma of left breast. B. Same patient at discharge from hospital following surgical removal.

extremely rare. Treatment is unnecessary in all situations, except with the rare large cyst, because they disappear spontaneously. Biopsy is unwarranted, for it may result in considerable destruction of breast tissue. The larger cysts can be aspirated, and this may result in their permanent elimination. Cases of lipoma, hemangioma, and lymphangioma have been reported in the breasts of children, both male and female. Usually they are found soon after birth. Lipomas and lymphangiomas should be removed surgically, care being taken to preserve the normal breast tissue. This can usually be accomplished by a circular incision below the breast or in the quadrant where the tumor exists. The treatment of hemangioma should be expectant. It is now widely recognized that hemangiomas in children usually grow in size until the child is about six or seven months of age, following which there is gradual regression. Not all hemangiomas follow this pattern. When there is rapid growth or growth beyond the anticipated period of activity, surgical excision has to be undertaken.

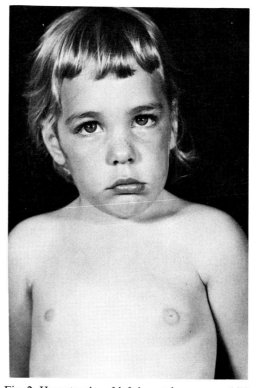

Fig. 2. Hypertrophy of left breast in a young child.

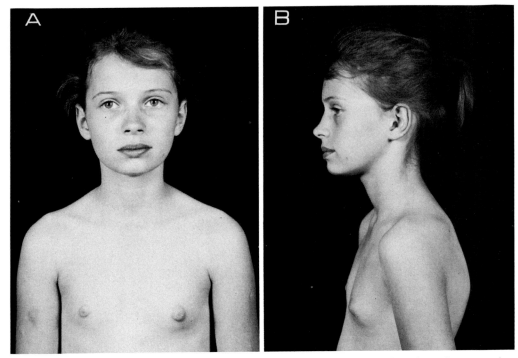

Fig. 3. A. Front view of older child with hypertrophy of left breast. B. Side view of same patient.

ENLARGEMENT OF THE BREAST IN CHILDHOOD

Enlargement of the breast may occur in children, particularly in females, without an abnormality of any other associated secondary sex characteristics. Initially there may be a tender nodule under the areola, and gradually the enlargement takes place. This may proceed for a time and then spontaneously subside. This can occasionally be seen in male children but is more common in females (Fig. 2). In other female children there may be an enlargement of the breasts without the painful tender nodule as a prerequisite; rather, a general enlargement, unilateral or bilateral, takes place. It is most disturbing to a girl when it is unilateral (Fig. 3). Usually, as the patient develops during puberty, the other breast will enlarge and symmetry will be established. Microscopically, this lesion is a fibrous tissue hyperplasia. It has been referred to by some as a form of mastitis. This is not primarily an inflammatory lesion.

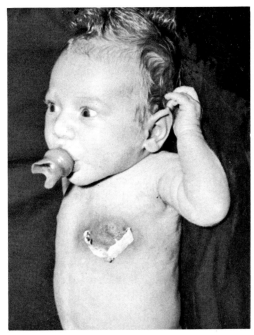

Fig. 4. An extensive breast abscess. Note two incisions placed some distance from center of breast. To maintain the drain in place, the ends are fastened together.

Treatment of this condition should be to reassure the parents that it has no significance and to persuade them that a biopsy is unnecessary. Doing a biopsy on the breast, particularly of a small child, may result in considerable damage to the duct system and in deformity of the breast after puberty.

ABSCESS OF THE BREAST

Abscess of the breast is most frequently seen in small infants and may be related to the hyperplasia that is seen in 50 percent or more of the affected infants. Usually there is a history of enlargement of the breast in the first few days after birth. When the lesion is small a broad-spectrum antibiotic is of value. Despite such treatment an abscess may develop and incision and drainage be required. It is important when draining these lesions that every effort be made to preserve the breast tissue. To accomplish this, small incisions are made some distance from the areola and the abscessed cavity entered in this

way. Usually a single drain through two small openings with the two ends attached together is preferable in order to maintain the drain in place (Fig. 4). The advantage of leaving a drain in place is that evacuation can be accomplished through relatively small incisions and the drain kept in place for several days so that the abscess cavity is completely evacuated and premature sealing of the wound will not occur with reaccumulation of exudate in the abscess cavity. The alternative is a large incision, which will be cosmetically objectionable.

GYNECOMASTIA IN THE YOUNG MALE BREAST

It is recognized that during puberty in the male there is some enlargement of the breast that normally regresses. In some boys, this growth may be quite excessive and persist for a considerable length of time (Fig. 5). It is usually seen after puberty. However, it may be observed in boys five and six years of age

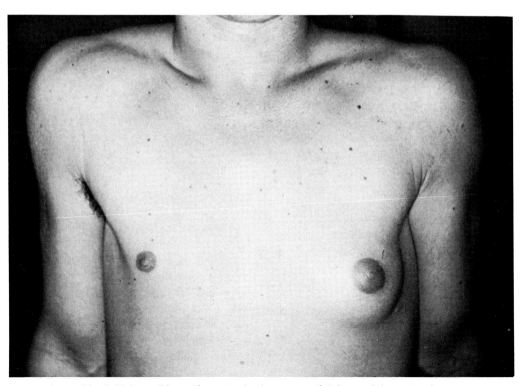

Fig. 5. Unilateral breast hypertrophy (gynecomastia) in an adolescent male.

In these younger children it may be transient or persist for a considerable length of time. In the boy beyond puberty the growth of the breast may be most marked in muscular boys where virilization is strong. Usually the persistence of the enlarged breast is unilateral. On occasions it may be bilateral. It is well to observe these for a period of time in order to take advantage of the normal regressions that usually occur. When this is not the course of events, the treatment is surgical removal. This should be accomplished through a small circular incision below the areola so that the normal configuration of the male breast will not be disturbed. On histological section of the removed breast, some increase in ductal elements and hyperplasia of the ductal epithelium are seen. The primary change is hypertrophy of the fibrous tissue stroma. The etiology of this gynecomastia, which is literally "woman's breast," is obscure.

MALIGNANT LESIONS OF THE BREAST

There has been considerable debate about the presence of true mammary cancer in children before puberty. It is now well documented that this lesion does occur and may be seen quite early in life. The distribution of the tumor is equal between males and females. This is in contradistinction to the lesion in adults, where perhaps 1 percent of the lesions appear in males. The appearance of the tumor is that of a nodule, with lymph node enlargement in some cases. It soon develops the characteristics of adult carcinoma becoming attached to the skin and producing a local depression. Lymph node enlargement is common. Treatment has consisted of radical mastectomy. The number of cases have been small in number, fewer than 30 being reported in the literature. Survival seems to be better than with the same lesion in adults.

SARCOMA OF THE BREAST

Sarcoma of the breast is less frequent than carcinoma of the breast in children. The mass is hard, and the skin tends to have enlarged vessels. Location of this tumor tends to be away from the nipple. Axillary lymphangography is the rule. Radical mastecomy is the treatment.

SUPERNUMERARY BREASTS

In some children there may be accessory nipples and breast tissue. These are found along the level of the normal nipple from the axilla to the abdomen. When these are definitely identified removal is advisable.

CONGENITAL DEFORMITIES OF THE CHEST WALL

Obvious lesions on the surface of the body have been known from antiquity. The correction of such defects was begun some fifty years ago, and now such procedures are common. The defects of the chest wall can be classified into the sternal defects and the rib defects. In the sternal group there is the most common depression deformity, known by a variety of terms and most usually by the term "pectus excavatum." There is the protrusion deformity known as "pectus carinatum," or "pigeon breast." There is a third group of deformities related to the sternum that consist of complete absence of the sternum or of a full or partial cleft of the sternum. In the rib defects there are absences of ribs and deformities of ribs.

EMBRYOLOGY OF THE STERNUM

According to Hansen, the sternum arises independently of the ribs as laterally situated sternal bands. At the cephalic end, a median anterior rudiment develops that is intimately associated with the shoulder girdle. By the end of the ninth week of embryonic life the sternal bands are united in the midline, forming the sternum. At a later date transverse division of the cartilaginous sternum results in segmental division. The usefulness of this description of the formation of the sternum is not great. It does give a possible explanation for cleft sternum, complete or partial.

DEPRESSION DEFORMITIES

Depression deformities are generally referred to as pectus excavatum. The deformity is primarily of the sternum. The cartilaginous ends of the ribs partake in the deformity in that they are bent inwards to meet the depressed central portion of the sternum. The deformity is observed in all degrees from a gentle depression to a deep cavity. Usually the deformity is deepest superior to the junction of the xiphoid (Fig. 6). During infancy there is an inward movement of the sternum during inspiration, accentuating the degree of deformity. Where a precise history can be obtained, the deformity dates from birth, and in most instances the depression becomes less

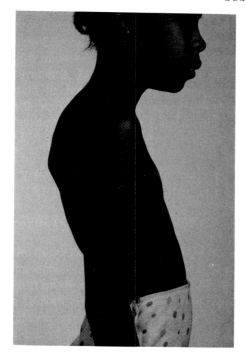

Fig. 7. Typical poor posture in a patient with pectus excavatum.

severe with age. There may be displacement of the heart associated with the deep lesions. An integral part of this deformity is poor posture. There is excessive abdominal protuberance and lordosis, with the head being held forward (Fig. 7).

ETIOLOGY

The causes of the deformity are debated. By some it is claimed that there is a deep sternal band that deforms and holds the sternum in its curved position. Among persons who have corrected a number of these deformities there is no unanimity of opinion regarding the presence of such a band. It is interesting that a number of careful observers of laryngeal anomalies believe that in pectus excavatum there is an inadequacy of airway that accounts for the lesion. Certainly in the small baby it is well to have the upper airway carefully studied to eliminate this as a cause for the deformity. The most plausible explanation for the lesion is an overgrowth of the ribs and a subsequent backward deformity.

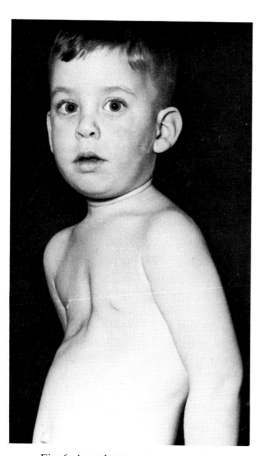

Fig. 6. A moderate pectus excavatum.

The patient with the depression type of deformity of the sternum often has a poor posture, with lordosis, protrusion of the abdomen, and the shoulders and head held forward.

SYMPTOMATOLOGY

There is a considerable difference of opinion about what symptoms may be related to this lesion. Some surgeons with a lot of experience in the operative treatment of the disease, such as Ravitch, are adamant in their statement that relief of such symptoms as cardiac irregularities, even heart failure, and pulmonary insufficiency are complete with surgical correction of the lesion. However, objective measurements of defects of cardiac function or of pulmonary function are striking by their absence. It is the opinion of some workers in this field that at no time is the pectus excavatum the cause of either pulmonary or cardiac symptoms. It would appear that there are patients with cardiac symptoms, and it is well to have such individuals carefully appraised by careful cardiac studies to ascertain the precise cause for the cardiac disability, for the association of a congenital heart lesion with pectus excavatum is known. In the past there have been no well-documented published cases of studies including catheterization with selective angiocardiography and pressure studies to substantiate the claim that there are cardiac irregularities and insufficiencies caused by the external compression of the sternal bone. Equally important would be postoperative studies documenting a return to normal of these objective measurements after correction of the pectus excavatum. There has been a study by Polgar (1963) in which ten children had pulmonary function studies with varying degrees of severity of pectus excavatum. It could not be demonstrated by well-accepted, standard pulmonary function tests that there was any real deficiency in these patients. Furthermore, postoperative studies failed to reveal a decided improvement in function. It is well to caution the reader that these studies, while important, do not exclude the possibility that as the patient grows older defects in pulmonary or cardiac function may develop. While many opinions have been expressed, the solution of the problem must await further careful preoperative and postoperative studies in various age groups. Most important would be such careful studies of cardiac and pulmonary function in adults who seem subjectively to have symptoms related to the pectus and who experience relief of their symptoms after operation.

There is no doubt that the psychological problem associated with a pectus excavatum, particularly in a boy, can be a major disturbance. In the well-adjusted, outgoing boy with a pectus excavatum there need be little fear of psychological disturbances. However, the insecure child may have a considerable problem with the deformity as far as his psychological attitudes are concerned. Some patients, particularly those with severe lesions, are extremely sensitive about their deformity and resist disrobing to be examined.

INDICATIONS FOR OPERATION

There is a wide variety of opinion regarding the advisability of repairing pectus excavatum. In most large series there are postoperative deaths reported. Ravitch (1949) had one death in 130 patients. Welch (1958) reports one death in about 100 patients. Probably the mortality is about 1 percent. Another factor in considering surgical correction of this lesion is recurrences. Some workers such as Ravitch report large series with few recurrences. Welch is less confident of uniformly good postoperative results. Other surgeons with perhaps less experience have given their recurrence rate as high as 50 percent. With these facts at hand, it becomes difficult to urge all patients with pectus excavatum to have correction of the deformity. Data on the number that will have serious pulmonary and cardiac difficulties in adult life would be helpful. A word of caution should be raised regarding the correction of this defect in patients with Marfan's syndrome. Cardiac anomalies in this group tend to be frequent, and a mortality in correction of the deformity with this basic disease has occurred with greater frequency than in the normal patient with pectus excavatum.

Our present state of knowledge indicates a more conservative approach than surgical correction of all these deformities. It is interesting that some Australian workers have added physiotherapy to the postoperative regime, and this may be a factor in their good results. The role of physiotherapy in the patient with a mild lesion certainly should be given serious consideration and can do no harm in all patients. Certainly, strengthening the abdominal musculature by sitting-up exercises and leg-raising exercises, along with deep-breathing exercises have theoretical merit. Probably the severe lesions should be considered for operation on the basis that the deformity may produce some symptomatology in later life. However, it is well to have the patient's parents well informed on all aspects of the problem so that they are acquainted with the facts, particularly with the fact that recurrence is not too uncommon after operation. Correction of the lesion in girls is not required in most instances, since it is not an important cosmetic problem with them (Fig. 8).

SURGICAL TREATMENT

The basic procedure for the correction of depression deformities is now pretty well evolved and consists of subchondral removal of the cartilaginous portions of the ribs that are deformed (Fig. 9). It is important that the segments be removed laterally a sufficient distance to remove all of the deformity. Usually the fourth through the seventh ribs must be dealt with, and occasionally ribs as high as the third must be handled. The xiphoid can then be removed, and by blunt dissection the sternum is freed from the mediastinal structures. This should be performed gently and carefully to prevent production of a pneumothorax, which may occur despite

caution, particularly on the right side. An osteotomy is then performed on the sternum. Most authors advise that this be done on the anterior surface of the sternum by removing a transverse wedge of bone. The sternum can then be hinged forward and the deformity obliterated. The periosteum on each side of the wedge is then sutured together with interrupted silk to firmly hold the sternum in its new alignment. It is a wise practice to take the soft tissue, particularly the endochondral portions of the rib beds, and to suture them together posterior to the sternum so that the retraction of the sternum into its former depressed position is discouraged. This is superior to using a foreign body such as a steel pin or Kirschner wire to maintain the sternum in position. The use of a resected rib as a strut is troublesome and probably not more effective than the suturing of the soft tissues behind the sternum.

There has been considerable discussion of the use of the vertical versus the transverse incision. The lesion is far more readily ex-

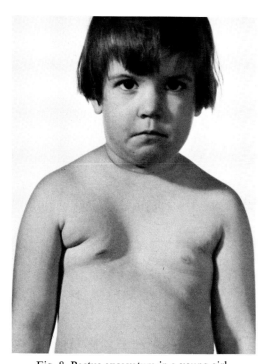

Fig. 8. Pectus excavatum in a young girl.

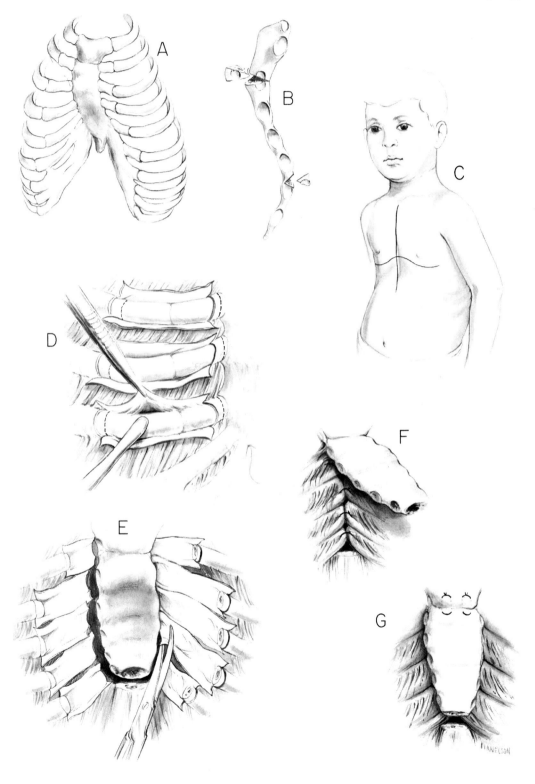

posed by the vertical incision. However, keloid formation is more troublesome, and therefore some surgeons have used a transverse submammary incision. Certainly in girls this incision has much in its favor. This is an operation of some magnitude. There may be considerable loss of blood, and provision should be made for replacement in all cases.

Chest films postoperatively are helpful in determining whether a pneumothorax is present or not. This should be a routine part of the postoperative care of the patient within a few hours after the end of the operation. Another important adjunct in the treatment of these patients, as outlined by Russell Howard of Australia, is that if there is any indication of a recurrence, vigorous physiotherapy is instituted. This may be an important factor in accounting for his good cosmetic results and the low instance of recurrences.

PROTRUSION DEFORMITIES

The so-called pigeon breast is not as common as the depression deformity (Fig. 10). The physician appraising the patient with pigeon breast should be aware that there is a considerable instance of cardiac anomalies associated with this, and hence a careful survey for defects in the cardiac system should be a routine part of the preliminary preoperative evaluation of these patients. In this group of patients there seems to be an overgrowth of the ribs adjacent to the sternum and a protrusion forward. It may be that in some of these patients, because of cardiac lesions, enlargement of the heart has played some role in forming the protrusion. The symptomatology associated with the pigeon breast is again debatable and is less documented than in the group of pa-

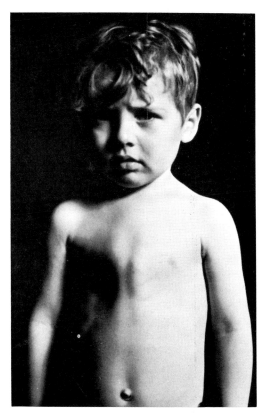

Fig. 10. Pigeon breast. (Courtesy of Dr. K. Welch.)

tients with depression defects. Here again the cosmetic problem is a real one, and in severe situations correction is indicated. Resection of the cartilaginous and bony portions of the ribs, subperiosteal for the entire length of the deformity, is the wise surgical maneuver. Osteotomies must then be performed on the sternum to bring it into a normal position. To prevent recurrence, suture of the chest wall structures made up of the beds of the resected ribs should be sutured together in the midline anterior to the sternum to help hold it in a depressed but normal position. Generally, the cosmetic results are more satisfactory in this group than in those with a depression deformity.

Fig. 9 (opposite page). Correction of depression deformities. A. A drawing indicating the rib and sternal deformity in pectus excavatum. B. The position of the osteotomies. C. The operation can be performed either through a transverse or vertical incision. D. A subchondral excision of the deformed portions of the ribs is accomplished. E. The sternum is freed. F. An attempt is made to suture the soft tissue behind the sternum as an added safeguard against recurrence. G. The osteotomy is sutured together to hold the sternum in a normal position.

DEFORMITIES OF THE RIBS OR ABSENCE OF THE RIBS

Absence of the ribs may not be associated with any abnormality, such as with paradoxical movement of the chest wall in the defective area. These movements are usually observed when there are defects in the upper ribs. There may be muscular defects associated with the bone lesion. The patient with absence of the ribs may have considerable separation of the bony thoracic cage in the region of the defect, and there may be excessive protrusion and inversion with respiratory movements. Usually this is not excessive and does not call for surgical correction. However, there are situations where the separation is great and where movement of the chest wall is considerable. Some improvement can be achieved by bringing the rib edges present into closer approximation, or bone grafts can be resorted to. Deformed ribs, either protruding or inverting, can be resected subperiosteally and the new rib formed in a more normal position. There may be unusual lesions associated with the rib anomaly, such as hemivertebra, which may lead to severe and intractable scoliosis.

CONGENITAL ABSENCE OF RIBS

Rickham has defined congenital absence of the ribs as lung hernia, which is a descriptive term. Actually the pathology consists of the absence of several ribs. This may extend to the sternum anteriorly and involve the absence of the cartilaginous portions of the ribs as well. These patients have excessive paradoxical motion of the soft tissues overlaying the defect with respirations. It is technically easier to repair these in the neonatal age group than to wait until the child is older. Attempts to cover the defect with fascialata have not proven successful. Ravitch (1961) suggests that a normal rib from the opposite side be resected, split, and used as struts across the defect.

In patients with hemivertebra, there actually may be a lung herniation without any defect in the number of the patient's ribs. The positions of the ribs are such that they deviate, leaving a wide gap through which lung herniates. In these situations, osteotomies of the ribs can be performed so that they can be brought into more normal positions and the defect closed.

STERNAL CLEFTS

According to Hansen, the sternum forms independently of the ribs as two lateral buds. The anterior thoracic is completed when the lateral centers join to form the sternum, and the growing cartilaginous ribs attach to the newly formed sternum. At a later date, transverse divisions of the cartilaginous sternum form the sternal segments. Gradually this cartilaginous structure becomes ossified, and at three years of age it contains some bone marrow. The ossification is not completed until after puberty. This formation process gives an explanation for incomplete and even complete lack of fusion of the two bands.

COMPLETE FAILURE OF STERNAL FUSION

In the past, complete failure of sternal fusion has been reported as ectopia cordis because of forward displacement of the heart, which is made possible by the sternal split that is an unusual clinical finding. Severe intracardiac malformations often incompatible with extrauterine life have prevented survival after surgical closure of the split sternum. Maier (1949) has reported a case of complete lack of sternal fusion where he was able to achieve a repair. The apparent anterior protrusion of the heart proved to be a large outpouching of the pericardium. Experience indicates that these should be treated promptly, since delay of several weeks makes it virtually impossible to bring the separated sternal segments together.

CEPHALAD STERNAL CLEFTS

Cephalad sternal clefts are the most common ones involving the sternum (Fig. 11)

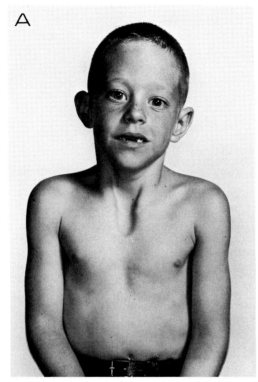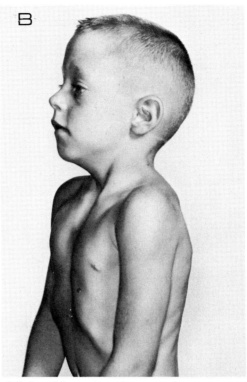

Fig. 11. A. Patient with cephalad sternal cleft. B. Oblique view of same patient.

and have been reported in the past as cervicothoracic ectopia cordis. Absence of a bony cover for the mediastinum permits pulsation of the cardiac impulse to be such that to the examiner the heart seems displaced cephalad. Anatomic dissection has proven that the heart is anatomically in a normal position. Successful closure of these defects can be accomplished with greater ease in the first few days of life than when the infant is older. The structures become more rigid as the child grows older, and Sabiston (1958) found in a three-year-old child that there was considerable difficulty in bringing the sternal separation together. However, when the procedure has been performed in the neonatal period the closure has been simple. This is verified by Longino and Jewett (1955), who operated on a patient at six days of age with virtually a complete separation of the sternum and successfully united the sternal segments. However, Rehbein (1957), in correcting a similar

lesion in a nine-year-old child, resorted to inserting stainless-steel mesh to close the defect. The outcome was satisfactory cosmetically; however, a direct repair using the patient's tissue is preferable.

CAUDAL STERNAL CLEFTS

Caudal sternal clefts have been reported in the past as thoracoabdominal ectopia cordis. Here again, the failure of a bony covering for the heart gives the examiner the impression that the heart has moved cephalad from its normal position. In these patients there is a defect in the diaphragm and upper abdominal wall in addition to the cleft in the lower sternum. The rectus muscle, while normally attached to the pubis, will extend upward and is separated, attaching to the thoracic cage at about the level of the anterior axillary line. In these patients there is a high instance of intracardiac malformations, which cannot be definitely related to

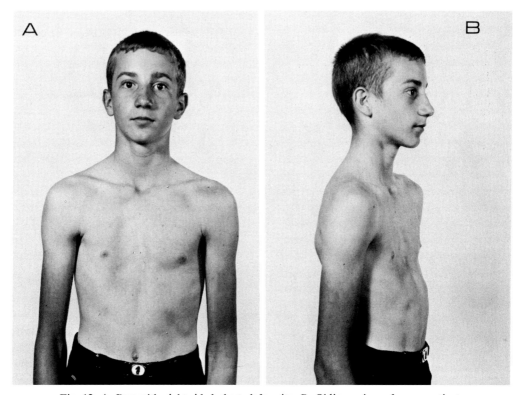

Fig. 12. A. Boy with right-sided chest deformity. B. Oblique view of same patient.

the structural defects in the sternum, diaphragm, and anterior abdominal musculature. An intraventricular septal defect has been present in 70 percent of these patients; 50 percent according to Ravitch (1952) have an atrial septal defect, and valvular or infundibular pulmonary stenosis occurs in 33 percent. Tetralogy of Fallot was observed in 20 percent of the patients. As these figures indicate, multiple intracardiac lesions are common. Early correction is advisable. Whether the intracardiac lesion should be repaired when the abdominal wall and sternal defects are approximated is debated. Ravitch has practiced correcting the defect of the sternum, the diaphragm, and anterior abdominal wall, leaving the intracardiac lesions for repair at a later date. Mulder (1960) has reported a 15-month-old child in whom he closed the defect, excised a diverticulum of the left ventricle, and closed a ventricular septal defect. When the abdominal defect is small, the rectus muscles are readily brought together. However, when the defect is large, relaxing incisions may be required as an assist in bridging the defect. It may be necessary to turn the anterior rectus sheaths from both sides medially to cover the defect.

LATERAL CHEST DEFORMITIES

There may be deformities of the thoracic cage limited to one side (Fig. 12). These can be corrected surgically by subpericostal resection of the ribs.

ORVAR SWENSON

REFERENCES

HANSEN, J. L., and JACOBY, O. The respiratory function before and following surgery in cases of funnel chest. Acta Chir. Scand., 3: 226, 1956.

———— Pulmonary function in pectus excavatum deformity. Acta Chir. Scand., 111: 25, 1956.

HOWARD, R. Pigeon breast (protrusion deformity of the sternum). Med. J. Aust., 2: 664, 1958.

LONGINO, L. A., and JEWETT, T. C. Congenital bifid sternum. Surgery, 38: 610, 1955.

MAIER, H. C., and BORTONE, F. Complete failure of sternal fusion with herniation of pericardium. J. Thor. Surg., 18: 851, 1949.

MULDER, D. G., CRITTENDEN, I. H., and ADAMS, F. H. Complete repair of a syndrome of congenital defects involving the abdominal wall, sternum, diaphragm, pericardium and heart; excision of left ventricular diverticulum. Ann. Surg., 151: 113, 1960.

POLGAR, G., and KOOP, E. E. Pulmonary function in pectus excavatum. Pediatrics, 32: 209, 1963.

RAVITCH, M. M. The operative correction of pectus carinatum (pigeon breast). Ann. Surg., 151: 705, No. 5, May, 1960.

———— Pectus excavatum and heart failure. Surgery, 30: 178, 1951.

———— The operative treatment of congenital deformities of the chest. Amer. J. Surg. 101: 588, 1961.

———— Operative treatment of pectus excavatum. Ann. Surg., 129: 429, 1949.

———— Unusual sternal deformity with cardiac symptoms; operative correction. J. Thor. Surg., 23: 138, 1952.

REHBEIN, F., and WERNICKE, H. H. The operative treatment of the funnel chest. Arch. Dis. Child., 32: 5, 1957.

RICKHAM, P. P. Lung hernia secondary to congenital absence of ribs. Arch. Dis. Child., 34: 14, 1959.

SABISTON, D. C. The surgical management of congenital bifid sternum with partial ectopia cordis. J. Thor. Surg., 35: 118, 1958.

WELCH, K. J. Satisfactory surgical correction of pectus excavatum deformity in childhood. J. Thor. Surg., 36: 697, 1958.

27

Infections of the Chest

BRONCHIECTASIS

Bronchiectasis was originally described by Laenned in 1829, on the basis of postmortem studies. It was not until Sicard and Forestier, in 1922, introduced contrast material to outline the bronchial tree that the clinical diagnosis could be made with accuracy. Publication of the report of the first successful pneumonectomy by Graham (1935) and of the first successful lobectomy by Churchill (1937) in the 1930's offered new hope in the treatment of a disease that had a poor prognosis with nonsurgical treatment. Lanman was the first to perform a large number of lobectomies on children for bronchiectasis. There has been a decided decrease in the incidence of this disease during the past decade and a half. This coincides with introduction of antibiotics for the treatment of upper respiratory and pulmonary infections, which suggests that such treatment may be the chief factor in the decreased incidence.

PROGNOSIS

Several long-term studies have appeared in the last few years that have traced the course of this disease from early childhood to the middle twenties. In most instances the disease has its onset in children under five. Following the onset there is a gradual intensification of the disease. At puberty there is a distinct alteration for the better in the course of the disease. This amelioration of the symptoms and arrest of progression of the disease may be hormonal in its cause or related to the stronger cough reflex present in the older child. Following this period of remission, there may be increased difficulty in the twenties. What happens to these patients in adult life has as yet not been documented.

Prior to surgical treatment and antibiotics, the disease commonly resulted in the patient's death from overwhelming pulmonary sepsis or from spread of infection, particularly to the central nervous system. The present outlook for these patients is vastly improved. With careful medical treatment and judicious selection of patients for surgical lung resections the mortality should be less than 5 percent.

ETIOLOGY

The etiology of this disease is not related to only a single factor; rather, a number of situations may produce this chronic disease of the bronchi. Over 30 percent of the patients with bronchiectasis have had definite bouts of pulmonary consolidation. In an equal number there is a history of atelectasis. In about half this number measles with its exudative pulmonary lesion seems to be a causative factor. In an equal number there is a history of pertussis. In about 3 percent, postoperative atelectasis seems to be the causative factor. In a small number of patients a foreign body is the cause of the bronchiectasis. A variety of objects have caused bronchiectasis, the chief reported one being the tasseled end of timothy grass, the multiple projections of which serve to anchor it in the bronchus. Each forceful inspiration propels the foreign body still deeper into the lung, and the projecting barbs prevent its expulsion on expiration.

There may be a congenital factor in a small number of patients in whom the disease begins shortly after birth and for whom there is no clear-cut history of pulmonary infection. In addition, in such situations it is postulated that there may be a defect in the composition of the bronchial wall that predisposes it to dilation and chronic infection.

Atelectasis or collapse is a definite cause of bronchiectasis. If bronchograms are made, even in relatively short periods of atelectasis, there is some bronchial dilation observed which returns to normal in most instances, provided that the preceding collapse has not been excessive in duration.

Mucoviscidosis is one of the common causes of the disease today. It is assumed

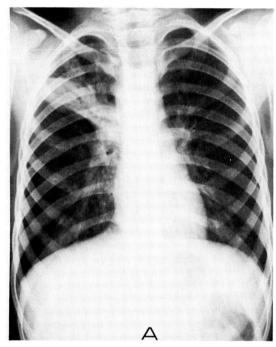

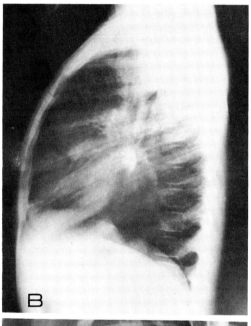

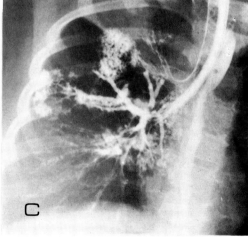

Fig. 1. A. Chest film of a patient with atelectasis of the right upper lobe. B. Lateral film of the same patient. C. Bronchogram of the same patient. Poor filling of right upper lobe with some bronchial dilation.

that the abnormally thick secretion blocks the airway and prepares the way for infection (Fig. 1). With an increasing survival rate among children with pancreatic fibrosis there are more children that develop bronchiectasis as a result of their pulmonary pathology. In them the disease is widespread, with some predilection for the upper lobes. This may be explained by the fact that in infants upper lobe atelectasis is common, in contrast to older children, in whom the middle and lower lobes are the common sites.

Tuberculosis may be associated with bronchiectasis. Enlarged lymph nodes producing external pressure on the bronchial branches is held to be the cause of the bronchial dilation. Endobronchial tuberculosis may also play a role by scarring and narrowing a major bronchus.

Agammaglobulinemia is understandably associated with this chronic pulmonary disease. A considerable number of patients with this congenital inability to cope with infection develop recurrent bronchitis and eventually bronchiectasis.

PATHOLOGY

The actual mechanics of production of bronchiectasis is debated. However, the common findings of some bronchial dilation following atelectasis, particularly that of some duration, indicates that where the parenchyma has collapsed, increased space is provided for the bronchioles to dilate as atmospheric pressure is asserted. This is now accepted as one of the mechanical factors producing the lesion. Once dilation has occurred, stasis and poor emptying sets the stage for chronic infection. The normal ciliated bronchial lining is destroyed and replaced by granulation tissue. Healing occurs with cuboidal cells forming a new lining. The infection spreads, and lung parenchyma is destroyed, a process which becomes irreversible. Vascular changes are not uncommon in the affected areas. The destruction of tissue may be of sufficient depth to destroy the cartilage rings.

Infection, bronchial obstruction, and stasis accentuate destruction of tissue and weakening of the bronchial wall, all of which contribute to bronchiectasis. The time factor in such situations is probably important. One cannot definitely rule out the possibility that in some patients there may be a congenital defect in the bronchial structures of a minor nature which permits the infection to be more destructive and to produce bronchial dilation more rapidly.

Bronchiectasis is a generalized disease in some patients, and the causative agents are not completely understood. In the generalized form there may be constant progression regardless of therapy. Although the intensity of the process may be more pronounced in some parts of the pulmonary system than in others, there is a steady progression of disease with the eventual involvement of all parts of the lungs.

The disease is most prevalent in the left lower lobe and next most common in the right lower lobe. In some reports the right middle has been involved more frequently than the right lower lobe. The explanation given for the predilection for the left lower lobe is that the bronchus that enters the left lung forms a greater angle with the trachea than does the bronchus to the right lobe, and consequently the left lung does not clear well with coughing, predisposing it to retain secretions; the right lower lobe clears secretions more effectively and thus protects itself from chronic disease more successfully than the left lower lobe does. On the other hand, foreign bodies tend to lodge in the right lower lobe. Again, this is probably related to the direct anatomical route from the trachea to the right lower lobe.

The chronic infection produces destruction of the bronchial wall lining, and the inevitable granulation tissue may be the cause of hemoptysis, a symptom in 10 to 15 percent of the patients.

CLINICAL COURSE

The onset of this disease in children primarily occurs below the age of five years,

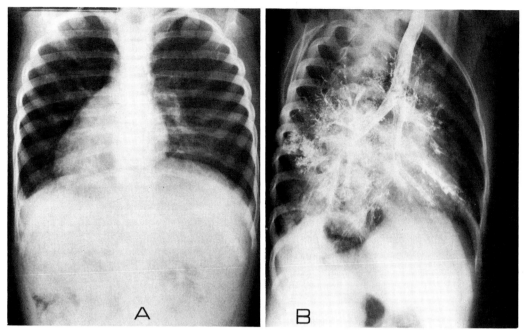

Fig. 2. Kartagener's syndrome. A. Chest film of a patient with Kartagener's syndrome; note the dextrocardia. B. Bronchogram of the same patient outlining bronchiectasis.

and in most instances below the age of three years. The onset in about 90 percent of the patients is preceded by pulmonary infection, atelectasis, pertussis, or measles. Cough is the universal symptom. Productive cough is unusual in small children, but after the age of five or six this symptom becomes prevalent. The sputum may be yellowish and not particularly foul, but in advanced cases it may be greenish and foul smelling. The children are pale and either lose weight or fail to gain. In a number of the patients there is clubbing of the fingers, a finding not related to the extent of the disease. A number of children have dyspnea that is out of proportion to the observed lung involvement. Wheezing is seen in 10 to 20 percent of the patients and has a bad prognosis.

Slightly blood-tinged sputum is common, and true hemoptysis occurs in 10 to 15 percent of the patients.

Sinusitis is not unusual and may be a part of the generalized form of the disease. On examination, there are breath sound changes and moist, coarse, sticky rales, most prevalent in the areas of greatest involvement.

There is an interesting syndrome, described by Kartagener, which consists of bronchiectasis, dextrocardia, and sinusitis (Fig. 2). In a series of 187 cases at Boston Children's Hospital 6 patients exhibited this syndrome. In this same group there were 4 patients that had agammaglobulinemia as a part of the disease. It is interesting that in the older age group 8 out of 13 children had bronchiectasis following oral surgery. One child was said to have had a vascular anomaly with pressure on the bronchi producing the bronchiectasis.

There have been a number of reports of this disease in patients with pancreatic fibrosis. Here, as noted above, the bronchiectasis is probably related to the thick, tenacious mucus that is abnormal and that probably causes partial obstruction and sets the stage for chronic infection in these patients with generalized mucoviscidosis. The bacteriology has been extensively studied. Because many of the reports are retrospective the bacteriology cannot be interpreted with certainty or translated into present terminology. Suffice it to say that a number of organisms are involved, among them streptococcus, staphylococcus, and some gram-negative organisms.

DIAGNOSIS

The patient who has had recurrent pulmonary infection or atelectasis in the same area of the lung field is likely to have localized bronchiectasis. While it is perfectly possible and probably true in most instances that such lesions regress and do not lead to chronic infection, persons who suffer from them are possible candidates for bronchiectasis and should be considered for definitive diagnostic studies should other symptoms, such as chronic productive cough or hemoptysis, develop. Plain chest roentgenograms usually contain no definite indication of bronchiectasis. There may be increased streaking and greater hilar density. A series of films is valuable in detecting persistent atelectasis. When bronchiectasis is suspected, the definitive diagnosis is established by bronchography. Lipiodol or the water-soluble opaque material Dionisil or the newer product iodinized oil may be used to outline the bronchial tree. The disadvantage of Lipiodol is that it distorts the roentgenograms of the chest for a period of three to six weeks, which is the time it takes for the body to eliminate it. It is well, in patients having suggestive generalized disease, to outline all parts of the bronchial system before a course of therapy is begun. With care this can usually be accomplished at one sitting. In making the bronchograms care should be taken not to overfill the bronchus and saturate the small bronchi and alveolar spaces, thus blurring the outline of the larger bronchi, which are the sites of the disease (Fig. 3). The finding of dilated sacculated bronchi in the bronchogram is diagnostic of bronchiectasis (Fig. 4). The former division of bronchiectasis into various types has largely been discarded, for it has no clinical value. The examination must include bronchoscopy to exclude the presence of a foreign body, to identify any endobronchial anomalies, and to secure adequate specimens for culture.

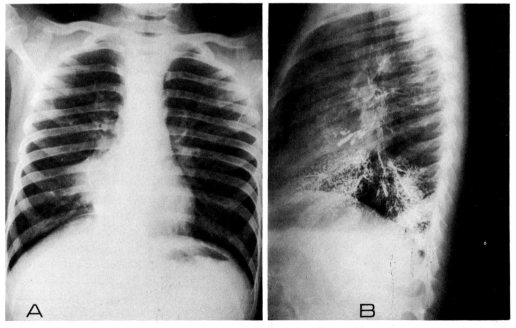

Fig. 3. A. Chest film of a patient with atelectasis of the right middle lobe. B. Bronchogram of the same patient outlining bronchiectasis in the right middle lobe.

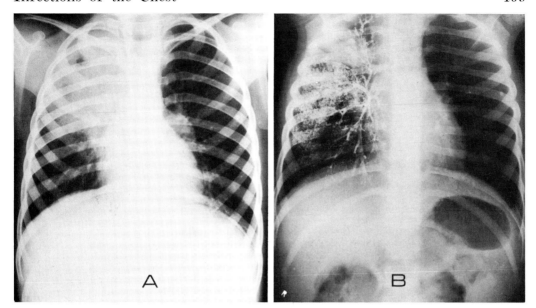

Fig. 4. A. Atelectasis of the right middle lobe. B. Bronchogram outlining bronchiectasis in the same area.

TREATMENT

In the 1930's and the early 1940's there was enthusiasm for lobectomy and even pneumonectomy in the treatment of bronchiectasis, and consequently virtually all patients were subjected to surgery. Followup of the children revealed that surgery failed to produce permanent improvement in a number of instances. This may have been due to one of several causes. In the early days of surgical treatment of this disease, a limited area—that is, the area suspected of having the heaviest involvement—was outlined by bronchography; it was not a common practice to survey the whole bronchial tree. Consequently, one cannot say with certainty whether there was widespread mild disease preoperatively in the patients that failed to gain relief from surgical therapy. The other possibility is that some of the patients had generalized disease that was progressive, and, although the initial site or the most severe disease process in one lobe was removed, the inevitable progression of the disease was not halted. Williams and O'Reilly (1959) have proposed that therapy be based on the historical origin of the disease and its degree of localization. They believe that the best candidates for surgical therapy are those patients having collapse or atelectasis and chronic involvement of a limited area and in whom bronchography demonstrates normal bronchi in the rest of the pulmonary tree. This group includes the patients who have aspirated foreign bodies, of course. They believe that the patients with generalized disease should not be subjected to surgery. Other students have failed to find this distinction useful in their management of patients with bronchiectasis. In particular, Clark (1963), who has treated a large number of patients in England, has taken this position.

MEDICAL TREATMENT

It is generally agreed that the mild cases and the early cases should be given vigorous medical therapy before considering surgical therapy. The medical treatment consists of postural drainage and the use of antibiotics and expectorants, as well as general care of the patients. Postural drainage is difficult to perform, particularly in younger children. A definite program should be outlined for the patient, and equipment should be provided so that he can be in the extreme Trendelenburg position for a period of time with reasonable comfort. A period of 15 minutes, three times a day, should be devoted to this aspect of treatment. Such therapy should be started in the hospital, and the parents should be taught to supervise it; the same type of equipment used in the hospital should be sent home with the patient. Along with the postural drainage, expectorants can be used to thin the pulmonary secretions and thus promote drainage of the diseased lung segment.

Antibiotics have been used to control the recurrent pulmonary infection that is such a prominent part of the disease entity. The wide-spectrum antibiotics have found greatest use. As yet no large group of patients has been tested on a long-term, continuous program of antibiotic administration to prevent recurrent attacks of infection. The fear of giving such agents over a long period of time because of the possible development of more resistant strains or bacteria in the diseased area has prevented most workers in the field from using the antibiotic agents for any but acute episodes of infection. The general hygiene of the patient should be supervised. Attention should be given to any sinusitis that may be present. Even with the best of medical care there is no guarantee that all patients will improve. A certain number will deteriorate; for instance, in a series of 79 patients studied by Clark (1963) with medical therapy, 46 revealed no change, 27 deteriorated, and 7 improved. In one five-year period of this study, 3 patients died of pulmonary infection.

SURGICAL TREATMENT

It is generally agreed that in those in whom the disease is localized and has failed to respond to medical therapy, surgical excision has much to offer. This is also true of the patients with aspirated foreign bodies and in whom the disease is progressing, and of those who failed to recover from the disease despite removal of the foreign body. In some reports, a majority of patients who had the foreign bodies removed still had persistent disease and required lobectomy or segmental resection. In patients with recurrent hemoptysis surgical therapy is advisable. Resection should be delayed until the patient

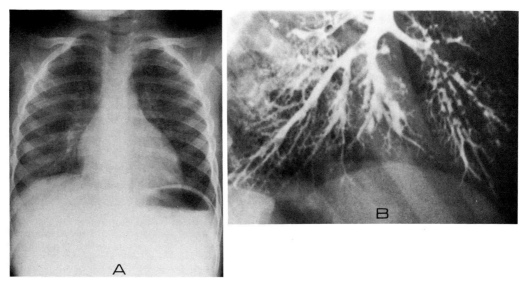

Fig. 5. A. Chest film of a patient with bronchiectasis limited to the medial basal segment of the right lower lobe. B. Bronchogram of the same patient.

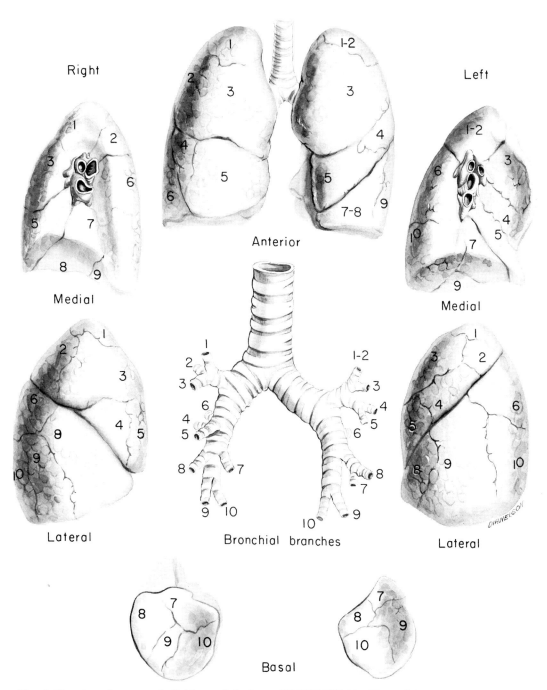

Fig. 6. Drawing of segmental divisions of the lung. RIGHT LUNG: Upper lobe segments: 1. apical, 2. posterior, and 3. anterior. Middle lobe segments: 4. lateral, and 5. medial. Lower lobe segments: 6. superior, 7. medial basal, 8. anterior basal, 9. lateral basal, and 10. posterior basal. LEFT LUNG: Upper division of the upper lobe: 1 and 2. apical posterior, and 3. anterior. Lower division of the upper lobe: 4. superior, and 5. inferior. Lower lobe: 6. superior, 7 and 8. anterior medial basal, 9. lateral basal, and 10. posterior basal.

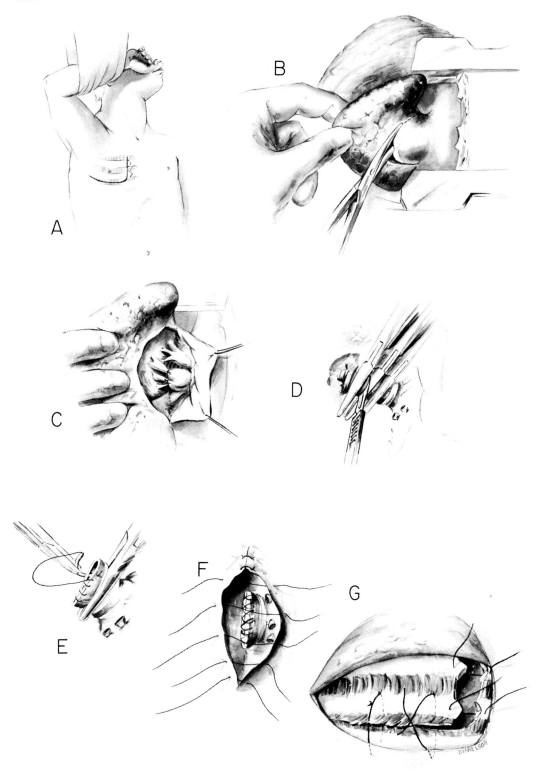

A

B

C

D

E

F

G

is in optimum condition. Culture should be obtained prior to operation and sensitivity studies performed. It is well to place the patient on chemotherapy 24 hours before operation.

OPERATIVE TECHNIQUE

In operating on patients with extensive bronchiectasis, there is considerable difficulty for the anesthetist in managing the secretions present in these patients. Consequently, careful postural drainage before operation is necessary. It may be necessary actually to perform bronchoscopy on the patient and to achieve bronchial toilet with this technique. It is wise either to position the patient so that the opposite lung will not be flooded during the operative procedure or to intubate the opposite main bronchus and thus have the patient respire with one lung during the procedure. Occasionally this is feasible in children, but at other times it provides insufficient pulmonary function for the patient to be maintained safely during lobectomy. Where such unilateral intubation is unsuccessful, it is well either to have the patient in the face-down position on the special table described by Overholt (1947) or to operate on the patient flat on his back, using an anterolateral approach.

SEGMENTAL RESECTION

The commonest operative procedure is lobectomy. However, in the type of patient seen at the present time, the disease may be more localized, and surgical therapy may be limited to a segmental resection (Figs. 5 and 6). Pneumonectomy is occasionally performed for widespread disease. The operation can be performed through a lateral approach or through an anterolateral approach, the type of incision popularized by Gross for ligation of the patent ductus (Fig. 7). In this type of incision the appropriate intercostal space is entered, and the cartilaginous portions of the anterior rib above and below the incision can be divided. This approach has the advantage of having the patient flat on his back so that spillage into the opposite lung is not promoted by gravity. Upon completion of the exposure, the lung should be carefully examined. If the bronchogram indicates that a segmental resection can be performed, the possibility should be explored. In such instances there is usually atelectasis of the segment involved, which gives the surgeon a clear outline of the lesion and important help in performing segmental resection (Fig. 8). It is well to ligate the vessels and bronchus at the apex of the segment and then to dissect out the segment. This can readily be accomplished because the firmness and dark blue color of the atelectatic segment make its outline clearcut in relation to the adjacent normal pink distended lung. If care is taken, air leaks should be minimal and small and should close readily without requiring suturing. Care should be taken to clamp all small vessels and to ligate them with fine 6-0 silk sutures, in order to reduce blood loss in the postoperative period. Segmental resection has the advantage of conserving lung tissue and a slight disadvantage in that complications occur somewhat more frequently than with lobectomy. The bronchus should be closed with interrupted fine silk sutures. It is well to cover the bronchial stump with pleura and adjacent tissue to reinforce the bronchial closure, an important step in preventing bronchopleural fistulas.

LOBECTOMY

In performing lobectomy the hilum is exposed. A small amount of lung parenchyma

Fig. 7 (opposite page). Operative technique for segmental resection of the lung. A. Outline drawing indicating the position of the incision. B. Pleura at the base of the lobe is mobilized to provide a cover for the closed bronchial stump. C. The vessels are individually ligated and divided. D. Three small clamps are placed on the bronchus, and the incision is made between the first and second clamp, removing the lobe. E. One clamp is removed, and the stump is closed with an interrupted or a continuous 5-0 silk suture. F. The pleura is closed over the bronchial stump. G. The chest incision is closed.

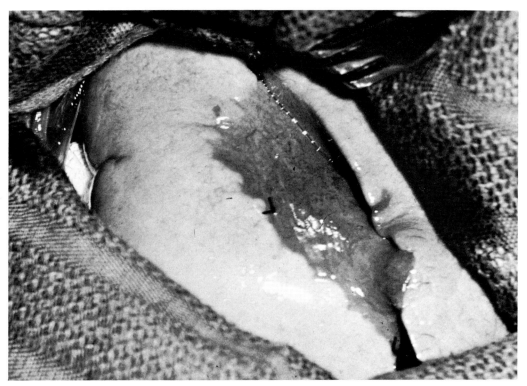

Fig. 8. Atelectasis of the medial basal segment of the right lower lobe.

and pleura is dissected toward the hilum to serve as a flap to cover the closed bronchus at the end of the procedure (Fig. 8). The vessels are then individually exposed and ligated. The bronchus can be clamped with either hemostats or Potts' clamps and the end closed with interrupted fine silk sutures. It is important to place the pleural flap over the closed bronchus to reinforce the closure and to prevent the formation of a fistula. The same procedure is followed in performing a pneumonectomy.

A drainage catheter must be left in the chest. It should be led out in a relatively dependent position and preferably through a stab wound rather than through the incision itself. Postoperatively a negative pressure of 10 to 15 cm of water is maintained on the chest catheter. The chest is closed in layers. The ribs are brought together with sutures placed around the adjacent ribs. It is well to use 3-0 chromic catgut for these large peri-rib sutures. The intercostal muscle may be closed with a running chromic catgut suture. The muscular layers should be closed with interrupted 4-0 or 5-0 silk, depending on the size of the patient, and the skin approximated with interrupted 5-0 silk sutures.

POSTOPERATIVE CARE

These patients may have considerable respiratory difficulty and should be watched carefully to be sure a patent airway is maintained. To dilute the patient's pulmonary secretions, mist is administered in a tent. Oxygen is usually not required. If there is any question of spillage during the operation into the opposite, normal lung, aspiration with the use of a bronchoscope may prevent serious postoperative complications. In Clark's series of 80 resections (1963), which included segmental resections, lobectomy, and pneumonectomy in children, there were 2 postoperative deaths. Forty-two had some atelectasis postoperatively, 6 had pneumonia,

3 had a noninfected effusion in the pleural space, 1 had frank empyema, and 1 had a bronchopleural fistula.

The treatment of these complications should be prompt and vigorous. It is well to have the chest tube in place a little longer in patients with segmental resections to prevent pneumothorax and collection of blood or fluid in the chest. Should there be recurrence of fluid or evidence of empyema, these should be dealt with promptly with the use of intercostal drainage tubes.

Bronchopleural fistula is a serious complication that was common in the days of mass ligation of the bronchial vessels and trachea. With individual ligation of the vessels and direct closure of the trachea with silk sutures and careful reinforcement with a pleural flap, bronchial fistula has practically been eliminated. It is impossible to outline any rules of management once this complication occurs. Usually, the best approach is to attack the lesion directly and to close the fistula soon after it is detected. Delay carries considerable risk and makes eventual closure of the fistula more difficult. It is true that some of the fistulas will close without assistance; however, this is a prolonged process, and direct attack has some advantages.

RESULTS OF SURGICAL THERAPY

It is generally agreed that over 50 percent of the patients treated surgically are returned to completely normal health and that about 75 percent are improved. With careful selection of patients these figures can be improved upon, particularly if lobectomy and segmental resection are reserved for those patients with definite, sharply localized disease processes and for those with aspirated foreign bodies and hemoptysis.

LUNG ABSCESS

Lung abscess is an entity that has diminished in incidence during the past few decades. With earlier detection of the lesion and thorough antibiotic therapy, the need for surgical treatment has also decreased.

ETIOLOGY

In a large majority of children the etiology is pneumonia. In a small number of cases the lesion follows an operation, particularly one involving the upper airway. A foreign body is also an occasional etiological agent in producing a localized abscess in the lung. This disease had a 75 percent mortality rate at the Massachusetts General Hospital prior to 1923. In a small series reported in children by Moore and Battersby (1960), the nonsurgically treated patients all died before the era of antibiotics. Today, the treatment of this disease in medical centers results in a mortality of about 5 percent.

PATHOLOGY

In the majority of instances the abscess follows pneumonia and consequently is most likely to be found in the lower lobe. Those following operative procedures and those due to foreign bodies have a predilection for the right side of the chest. It is interesting that in the past decade there has been a tendency for a predominance of lesions in the upper lobes rather than in the lower lobes, which previously were the sites of predilection. This may be an indication that the abscess occasionally seen today is related to a hematogenic spread of organisms rather than to local disease. In the formation of the abscess in the lung there is at first an intense area of inflammation, then breakdown of tissue in the center of the inflammatory area, and then formation of an abscess cavity. There may be a communication with the bronchial system, and in such an instance the patient may cough up considerable sputum. The presence of air fluid levels in roentgenograms is evidence that a bronchial fistula communicates with the abscess cavity.

CLINICAL COURSE

The patient usually has an antecedent history of pneumonia or is in the postoperative period. There is onset of septic fever, with elevation of temperature in the afternoon.

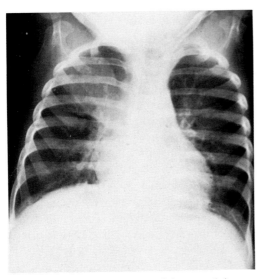

Fig. 9. Lung abscess in the right upper lobe.

peripheral portion of the lung and contain fluid (Fig. 9). Breath sounds are diminished in the area. Diagnosis depends upon radiological examination of the patient. In the early stages there will be consolidation, with an irregular outline. As the disease becomes more pronounced, localization occurs, and a more sharply demarcated outline of the abscess cavity is visible on the roentgen films. There may be a fluid level, which is evidence of communication with a bronchial system. After clearing of a lung abscess, there may be bronchiectasis (Fig. 10).

NONOPERATIVE TREATMENT

As soon as the diagnosis is made, an attempt should be made to secure bacteriological studies. This is particularly important if there is evidence of a communication with the tracheobronchial tree. Streptococcus has been a common offender, as has *Staphylococcus aureus*. In others, fusiform bacillus may be found. Early treatment with broad-spectrum antibiotics is indicated. These can

The patient develops a cough and loses weight, and in about 20 percent of the patients, hemoptysis occurs. There may or may not be clubbing of the fingers, depending on the impairment of the pulmonary function. By careful percussion, one may outline abscess cavities, particularly if they are in the

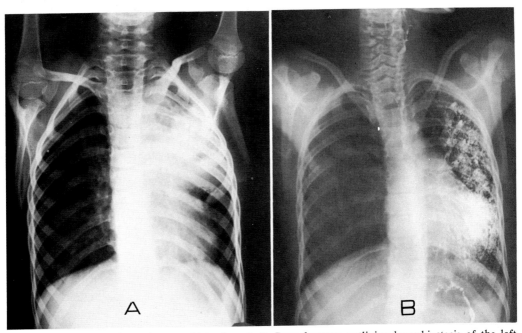

Fig. 10. A. A chronic lung abscess which cleared. B. Bronchogram outlining bronchiectasis of the left upper lobe. This was the residual of a lung abscess.

be altered once the bacteriology is definitely established and sensitivity studies have been made. In the days before antibiotic therapy, the mortality was extremely high with non-operative therapy. Today, with early detection of the lesion, administration of antibiotics is an effective form of therapy in the majority of patients. When the lesion becomes chronic, the possibility of influencing the situation with antibiotics becomes progressively less.

SURGICAL TREATMENT

On the basis of a review of a series of patients treated with drainage procedures, these procedures, although better than non-surgical therapy in the preantibiotic era, are not to be advocated today. The removal of the diseased lobe or segment of lobe containing the abscess has yielded far better results (Fig. 11). It should be possible to re-duce the mortality rate to about 5 percent in patients with lung abscess.

Complications from lobectomy and segmental resection are those commonly encountered in pulmonary surgery: pneumothorax, empyema, and bronchial fistula. With preoperative therapy with antibiotics and careful surgical techniques, these complications should be reduced to a minimum. However, it is good practice to insert one or two tubes through the thoracic wall to ensure drainage. Some surgeons put these tubes under mild negative pressure to ensure that there is no pneumothorax and consequently that the space available for infection to occur is minimized. The complications of the disease itself are brain abscess and meningitis. Hemorrhage was a really serious problem in the days before antibiotics and surgical therapy. Rupture of an abscess into a bronchus may be quite dramatic and may produce an acute clinical situation.

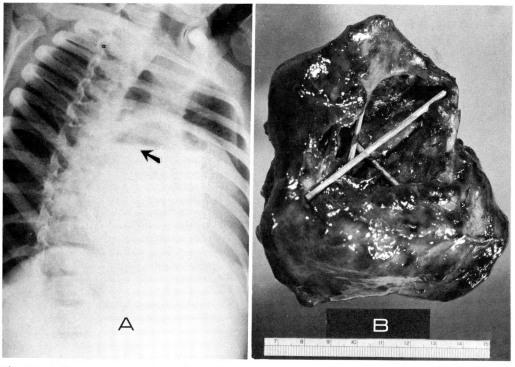

Fig. 11. A. Roentgenogram of a patient with a chronic lung abscess. Note the fluid level (arrow). B. Specimen removed at operation. Patient's recovery was uneventful after lobectomy.

PULMONARY TUBERCULOSIS

SURGICAL INDICATIONS IN THE TREATMENT OF TUBERCULOSIS

Pulmonary tuberculosis is an uncommon disease in children. Cameron, Hay, and Temple (1957) reviewed the records of 409 children under 16 years of age with pulmonary tuberculosis and attempted to outline the indications for surgical treatment. Only 36 cases of segmental lesions deserved consideration for surgical treatment. Only 5 patients had resection for severe irreversible lung damage, 4 for the removal of right middle and right lower lobes that were bronchiectatic, and 1 for the removal of the left upper lobe, the site of bronchial occlusion.

CLINICAL INDICATIONS FOR SURGICAL TREATMENT

Today, the treatment of pulmonary tuberculosis is extremely effective, particularly since the advent of Isoniazid. Streptomycin used over long periods of time led to com-

plications with hearing and vestibular problems. PAS (para-aminosalicylic acid) can be used, but it has some unpleasant side effects, chiefly gastrointestinal upsets, and the additional disadvantage of development of sensitivity to the drug. Isoniazid is the best drug; it is effective and has few complications.

There are limited indications for surgical treatment of tuberculosis in children. Primarily, the diagnosis of tuberculosis must be firmly established. In pulmonary tuberculosis localized disease that has been proved by a series of chest films to be chronic or that contains considerable calcium should be considered for resection (Fig. 12). In chronic disease with localized bronchiectasis surgical resection can be expected to provide considerable benefit. In chronic lung disease with cavitation the indications for surgical resection are similar to those in adult medicine (Fig. 13). Persistent narrowing of a bronchus with localized disease is another indication for surgical resection. It is rare today in the pediatric age group to see complications of tuberculosis leading to surgical therapy.

SURGICAL TREATMENT

Two types of surgical therapy should be given consideration. The first of these is bronchoscopy. In certain forms of tuberculosis, there may be granulation tissue and caseous material that perforate and occupy the bronchial lumen. In such patients collapse occurs, accompanied by all the problems that follow an atelectasis of any duration. It has been suggested that it is possible to remove endobronchial granulation tissue and caseous material by the use of bronchoscopy (Fig. 14). This method is held in high favor by some experts in this field but felt to be of little use by other workers. Since there does not seem to be any serious complications to its use, it would appear reasonable, in carefully selected cases, to consider this form of treatment when there is endobronchial involvement.

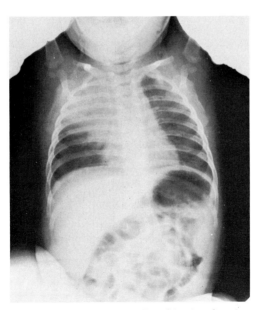

Fig. 12. Chest film of a child with chronic tuberculosis of the right upper lobe. Resection of the right upper lobe resulted in cure.

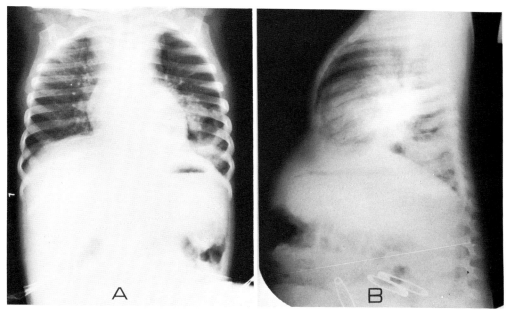

Fig. 13. A. Chest film of patient with tuberculosis of the left lower lobe with abscess formation. Cavity is air-filled. B. Lateral view of the same patient.

SURGICAL RESECTION

The indications for surgical resection vary considerably. Some workers caution that frequently there is such a severe inflammatory and fibrotic process in the hilar area of the lung that it is not unusual for the surgeon to begin with a segmental resection and end with pneumonectomy. It is generally agreed that where there is chronic disease and bronchiectasis develops, either segmental resection or lobectomy is indicated.

The causes of the middle lobe syndrome have been extensively discussed; it is probably related to the smallness of the bronchus to this lobe plus the angular configuration of the larger bronchi as they enter the main bronchus. At any rate, the middle lobe collapse is a well-known syndrome and occurs in children. Generally, resection is indicated where there is a narrowing or stenosis of the bronchus that is presumed, on the basis of its having been present for a reasonable length of time, to be caused by scar. A large amount of calcium within an obstructed area is a clear indication of surgical intervention,

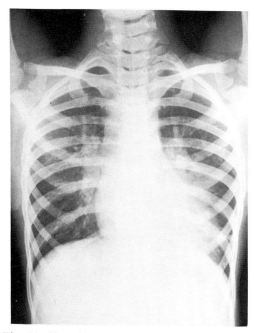

Fig. 14. Chest film of patient with tuberculosis of the left lower lobe. The left mainstem bronchus is partially occluded by granulation tissue. This tissue was removed bronchoscopically and proved to contain acid-fast organisms.

for this is evidence of chronicity. The resection of fibrotic disease with cavitation is rare in children. When a clear-cut example of this condition is encountered, the indications for surgery in children are essentially the same as those in adult patients. In such situations it is important, if possible, to cause conversion to a negative sputum. If this is impossible, surgical resection should be performed when the patient has been prepared with a course of chemotherapy. It is also wise to be sure there is a normal bronchus at the point of resection so that closure can be accomplished without the severe complications of bronchopleural fistula.

Occasionally, pressure on the major bronchi by enlarged glands produces severe stridor, and in such rare instances thoracotomy and adenectomy may be indicated. Rupture of large caseated glands with asphyxia has been reported in children. Adenectomy is difficult to perform because there are adhesions to the blood vessels, and hemorrhage has been a problem in some reported cases. Decortication of the lung after empyema with thickened pleura is rarely needed in children, and extensive operations to remove the constrictive pleuritis have rarely been performed. This is probably related to the fact that children in general progress much more favorably with

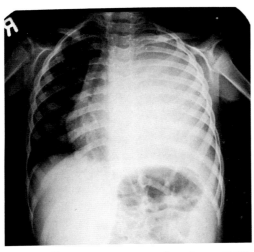

Fig. 15. Chest roentgenogram of postpneumococcal pneumonic empyema.

thickened pleura than adults do. The operation of choice is lobectomy rather than segmental resection in most cases. Lobectomy is tolerated well by children with very little if any diminution in pulmonary function. The reason for choosing lobectomy rather than segmental resection is that there are fewer complications following lobectomy than following segmental resection. Resection should not carry a mortality over 1 percent, a figure arrived at by considering that the known mortality in adults is 2 percent; although there are no reliable statistics in children, they are known to tolerate lobectomy better than adults. The chief difference between lobectomy in children and in adults is that the hilar node involvement is much greater in children, which constitutes a complicated technical problem during resection.

EMPYEMA

Empyema is a collection of exudate in the pleural space. Formerly, this disease was one of the commonest surgical conditions encountered in children and in a vast majority of cases was secondary to pneumococcal pneumonia. The use of antibiotics and chemotherapy in the treatment of pneumonia has proved so effective that postpneumococcal pneumonic empyema (Fig. 15) has been virtually eliminated. The rare pediatric patient with empyema today is far more likely to be infected with staphylococci or other bacteria than with pneumococci.

STAPHYLOCOCCUS EMPYEMA

As just noted, the common form of empyema today is caused by staphylococci. In most instances, the initial symptoms of staphylococcic pneumonia are mild. However, as the respiratory rate increases and the fever becomes elevated, the infant usually receives a potent antibiotic, and the classic signs and symptoms of pneumonia fail to develop because of the drug's effectiveness. While the diffuse part of the infectious process in the lung tissue is controlled, small abscesses probably remain in the lung parenchyma, as is frequently the case in any tissue invaded by staphylococci. These abscesses are relatively isolated from the bloodstream, and the inability of the antibiotic to permeate the abscess is the probable explanation for their subsequent enlargement and rupture into the alveolar spaces and bronchioles. Rupture of abscesses adjacent to the pleura accounts for empyema and bronchopleural fistula. The constant appearance of strains of staphylococci resistant to all antibiotics may be an additional cause of the increase in number of such patients.

The formation of an empyema makes the infant seriously ill, with increased respirations and a septic fever. Frequently, the situation is suddenly complicated by the formation of a bronchopleural fistula and the development of a pyopneumothorax. A tension pneumothorax quickly occurs with mediastinal shift, and unless this added complication is promptly recognized and treated, the infant may die of respiratory failure.

Examination of the small infant with pyopneumothorax will reveal tympany to percussion and diminished breath sounds. The

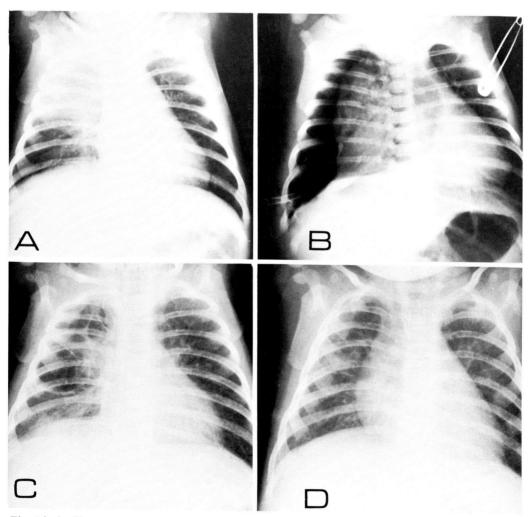

Fig. 16. A. Chest roentgenogram of a patient with staphylococcus pneumonia. B. The same patient after the development of pyopneumothorax. An intercostal catheter has been inserted. C. Reexpansion of the lung has occurred. Note the development of multiple cysts. D. The same patient two months later. The cystic structures have disappeared spontaneously.

difficulties of precise elucidation of such complicated pulmonary pathology in infants on the basis of physical examination alone make chest roentgenograms mandatory (Fig. 16). Prompt treatment is instituted not only to relieve the acute respiratory derangement caused by the tension pneumothorax but also to evacuate the empyema, for the exudate becomes thick and organization occurs early, and these developments complicate treatment.

TREATMENT

Treatment of staphylococcus empyema with or without pneumothorax consists of drainage by means of an intercostal catheter with a water seal. The technique of inserting an intercostal catheter is not difficult and can usually be managed in the treatment room with local anesthesia (Fig. 17). The patient is maintained upright, the skin is prepared, and local anesthesia is injected. A # 19-gauge needle is then inserted in the anterior axillary line in the fifth or sixth interspace, and 5 ml of exudate is removed for culture and sensitivity studies. The common cause for a dry tap when there is good evidence of an empyema, particularly in an infant, is that the chest has been needled at too low a level. Once the empyema is lo-

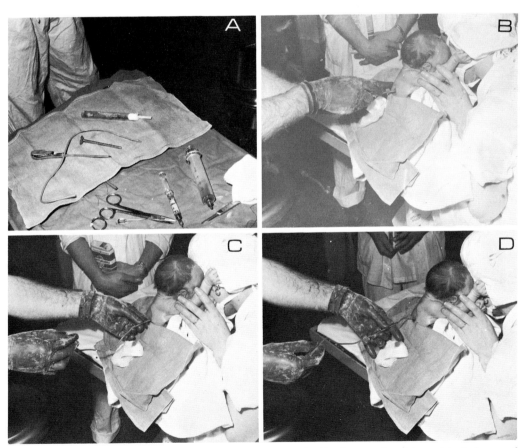

Fig. 17. Intercostal drainage of staphylococcus empyema. A. Equipment for intercostal drainage of staphylococcus empyema. A catheter is selected that can be passed through the sheath of the trocar. B. The skin is infiltrated with 1 percent procaine at an area in which a thoracentesis has recovered exudate. A 0.5-cm incision is made through the skin, and the trocar is inserted a sufficient distance to recover exudate. C. The catheter is inserted through the sheath of the trocar for a predetermined distance. D. The trocar sheath is removed, leaving the catheter in place.

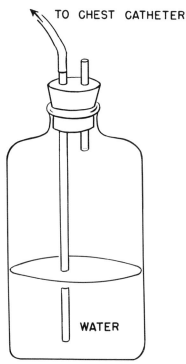

TO CHEST CATHETER

WATER

Fig. 18. A bottle arranged for an underwater seal. Air or liquid can drain from the pleural space, but the water seal prevents air from reentering the chest.

cated, the needle is withdrawn and a trocar is selected through which a catheter can be inserted through the shield when the central stylet is removed. Usually a # 12 or # 14 French rubber catheter is used, and three additional openings are made in the distal 2 inches of the catheter. The flaring end of the catheter is sacrificed to permit the trocar shield to be withdrawn over the catheter. A mark on the catheter at a point where it enters the trocar, with 3 inches of the catheter protruding from the trocar, is of help in estimating when the catheter has been inserted a sufficient distance through the chest wall to permit free drainage through the multiple openings in the end of the catheter. The assembled trocar is then inserted through a 0.5-cm skin incision (made with a scalpel) and pushed into the pleural cavity. The stylet is removed and the catheter inserted the predetermined distance. The trocar shield is then removed, leaving the catheter in place. The catheter is attached to the skin with a silk suture and connected to an underwater seal system (Fig. 18).

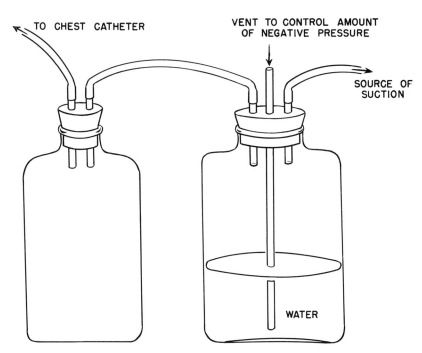

TO CHEST CATHETER

VENT TO CONTROL AMOUNT OF NEGATIVE PRESSURE

SOURCE OF SUCTION

WATER

Fig. 19. Diagram of an arrangement for chest suction. The bottle at the left is a reservoir for exudate that may drain from the empyema. Suction is attached to the bottle at the right, and the suction can be controlled by varying the water level.

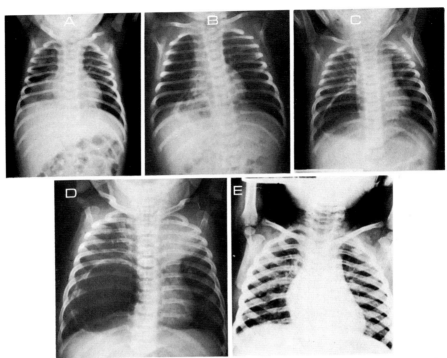

Fig. 20. Pneumatoceles. A. Chest roentgenogram of an infant with staphylococcus pneumonia. B. Beginning of cyst formation in the right lower lobe. C. Further development of the cyst. D. The cyst has progressed in size, and atelectasis of the left upper lobe has developed. Because of the steady progression in the size of the cyst and recurrence of pulmonary trouble, the cyst was removed with a segment of the right lower lobe. E. A roentgenogram taken several weeks after operation. By this time the baby had begun to gain weight.

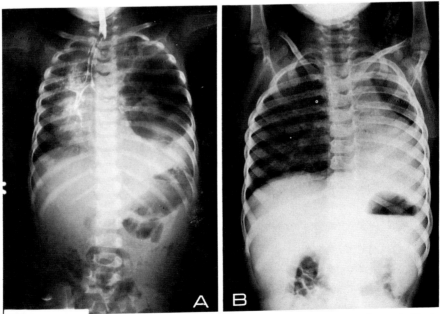

Fig. 21. A. Roentgenogram of a child with staphylococcus pneumonia and a massive cyst. During a six-month period of observation the child remained chronically ill and failed to gain weight. B. Roentgenogram two years after left pneumonectomy. Note that curvature of the spine is minimal.

USE OF PROTEOLYTIC ENZYMES

Thick exudate and fibrin occasionally form in the empyema, and evacuation of the cavity is consequently incomplete. Provided that the bronchopleural fistula has been closed for 36 to 48 hours, it is possible to inject an enzyme through the catheter and to clamp

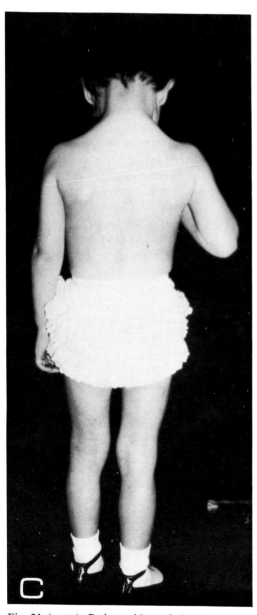

Fig. 21 (cont.). Patient with staphylococcus pneumonia and a massive cyst. C. The patient two years after pneumonectomy. The child's growth and development were normal.

the tube for 2 to 4 hours to permit digestion of the thickened exudate in the pleural space and then to reapply suction. Once organization of the exudate has occurred (this takes place in 5 to 7 days), the enzyme treatment is of no avail. Furthermore, the fistula may reopen, or there may be a severe febrile reaction. If this technique fails to prevent the formation of a thickened pleura and a residual cavity, an open operation is indicated, with removal of the thick exudate and pleura. This operative procedure is easier to accomplish 10 days to two weeks after onset of the empyema than later. Frequently, in small children a thickened pleura remains; however, as long as no cavity is associated with it, decortication is unnecessary because this will gradually disappear and be no hindrance to the patient. Simple intercostal drainage is usually sufficient, and evacuation of the empyema is accomplished in a few days to a week. When no further fluid is demonstrable by chest roentgenogram and there is no air or exudate draining, the tubes can safely be removed. Throughout this period, the antibiotic which has been proved by sensitivity tests to be effective is administered.

MANAGEMENT OF BRONCHOPLEURAL FISTULA

The treatment of bronchopleural fistula has three immediate objectives: (1) to decompress the pleural space and relieve the tension pneumothorax, (2) to permit lung reexpansion, and (3) to encourage the bronchopleural fistula to close. By checking the drainage apparatus and determining when air is no longer exhausted from the intercostal tube, one can surmise when the bronchopleural fistula closes. When the fistula has remained closed for 12 hours, gentle suction may be applied to the intercostal tube so that complete lung reexpansion will occur promptly (Fig. 19). If 4 to 6 inches of negative pressure causes air to be withdrawn constantly from the pleural space, it is advisable to discontinue the suction and to permit the fistula to close more firmly by returning to the simple underwater seal type of drainage.

At times this rule must be discarded because accumulation of air takes place with simple drainage, and mild suction may be

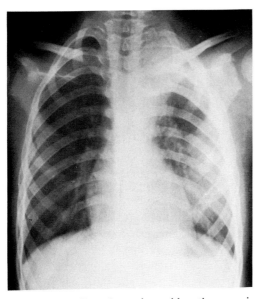

Fig. 22. Chest film of a patient with actinomycosis of the left upper lobe.

required to reduce the pneumothorax. In our experience such drainage measures are sufficient to treat the bronchopleural fistula. When the fistula persists, surgical closure must be accomplished.

DEVELOPMENT OF PNEUMATOCELES

In a large number of infants with staphylococcus pneumonia, multiple cysts develop in the lung. These may occasionally be single and quite large, and the possibility of a true congenital cyst is to be considered in the differential diagnosis. Clinically, congenital cysts are present in the first few days of life, and there is no history or clinical evidence of pulmonary infection. As a general rule, cysts following staphylococcus infection gradually subside after the infection is eradicated. This process may be slow; a year or more may be required for the air-filled cyst to disappear completely. No active treatment is required as long as the patient is asymptomatic.

On rare occasions, spontaneous regression of the cyst may not occur (Fig. 20), or the cyst may be the cause of the patient's failure to recover good health (Fig. 21). Under such circumstances, excision of the cyst must be undertaken. At operation, the cyst usually can be removed with a segmental resection. Occasionally, a more radical removal of pulmonary tissue, such as a lobectomy or a pneumonectomy, may be required.

Actinomycosis of the chest is rare today. It may be related to the prevalence of penicillin therapy, which is specific in most instances (Fig. 22).

REFERENCES

AVERY, M. E., RILEY, M. C., and WEISS, A. The causes of bronchiectasis in childhood. Bull. Hopkins Hosp., 109: 20, 1961.
Bronchiectasis in childhood. Lancet, 2: 498, 1959.
CAMERON, J. K., HAY, J. D., and TEMPLE, L. S. A critical examination of the role of surgery in the treatment of primary pulmonary tuberculosis in children. Thorax, 12: 329, 1957.
CARTER, M. G., and WELCH, K. J. Bronchiectasis following aspiration of timothy grass. New Eng. J. Med., 238: 832, 1948.
CLARK, N. S. Bronchiectasis in childhood. Brit. Med. J., I: 80, 1963.

CHURCHILL, E. D. Lobectomy and pneumonectomy in bronchiectasis and cystic disease. J. Thoracic Surg., 6: 286, 1937.
ERIKSEN, K. R., JENSEN, H. E., and AMDRUP, E. Nonspecific abscess of the lung: 129 Cases. II. Bacteriology. Acta Chir. Scand., 127: 495, 1964.
FIELD, C. E. Bronchiectasis: A long-term follow-up of medical and surgical cases from childhood. Arch. Dis. Child., 36: 587, 1961.
FILLER, J. Effects upon pulmonary function of lobectomy performed during childhood. Amer. Rev. Resp. Dis., 89: 801, 1964.

GLAUSER, E. M., et al. Bronchiectasis: A review of 187 cases in children with follow-up pulmonary function studies in 58. Acta Paediat. Scand. Suppl. 165: 1, 1966.

GORGENYI-GOTTCHE, O. G., and KASSAY, D. Importance of bronchial rupture in tuberculosis of endothoracic lymph nodes. Amer. J. Dis. Child., 74: 166, 1947.

GRAHAM, E. A., SINGER, J. J., and BALLON, H. C. Surgical Diseases of the Chest. Philadelphia, Lea & Febiger, 1935.

JOFFE, N. Cavitating primary pulmonary tuberculosis in infancy. Brit. J. Radiol., 33: 430, 1960.

LAFF, H. I., HURST, A., and ROBINSON, A. Importance of bronchial involvement in primary tuberculosis of childhood. J.A.M.A., 146: 778, 1951.

LANMAN, T. By personal communication.

LINDSKOG, G. E., and SPEAR, H. C. Middle lobe syndrome. New Eng. J. Med., 253: 489, 1955.

LINCOLN, E. M., HARRIS, L. C., BOVORN-KITTI, S., and CARRETERO, R. Endobronchial tuberculosis in children. Amer. Rev. Tuberc. 77: 39, 1958.

MOORE, T. C., and BATTERSBY, J. S. Pulmonary abscess in infancy and childhood: Report of 18 cases. Ann. Surg., 151: 496, 1960.

OVERHOLT, R. H., and LANGER, L. A new technique for pulmonary segmental resection. Its application in the treatment of bronchiectasis. Surg. Gynec. Obstet., 84: 257, 1947.

POTTS, W. E. Tuberculosis in childhood. Postgrad. Med. J., 39: 316, 1966.

ROTHMAN, P. E., JONES, J. C., and PETERSON, H. G., Jr. Endoscopic and surgical treatment of pulmonary tuberculosis in children. Amer. J. Dis. Child., 99: 315, 1960.

RUBIN, M. The role of resection for pulmonary tuberculosis in children and adolescents. Amer. J. Surg., 89: 649, 1955.

SCHWEPPE, H. I., KNOWLES, J. H., and KANE, L. Lung abscess. An analysis of the Massachusetts General Hospital cases from 1943 through 1956. New Eng. J. Med., 265: 1039, 1961.

SICARD, J. A., and FORESTIER, J. Méthode générale d'exploration radiologique par l'huile iodée (Lipiodol). Bull. Soc. Med. Hop. Paris, 46: 463, 1922.

STEINER, N., and COSIO, A. Primary tuberculosis in children. I. Incidence of primary drug-resistant disease in 332 children observed between the years 1961 and 1964 at the Kings County Medical Center of Brooklyn. New Eng. J. Med., 274: 755, 1966.

TABER, R. E., and EHRENHAFT, J. L. Chronic lung abscess. Arch. Surg., 67: 259, 1953.

WILLIAMS, H., and O'REILLY, R. N. Bronchiectasis in children: Its multiple clinical and pathological aspects. Arch. Dis. Child., 34: 192, 1959.

WILSON, R. Tuberculous atelectatic bronchiectasis. J. Pediat., 14: 368, 1939.

28

Tumors of the Chest

Space-occupying lesions in the thoracic cavity are not uncommon in infants and children, and a good proportion of them are malignant tumors. In infants and children, unlike in adults, pain is not a predominant symptom of malignancy within the thoracic cavity. In the pediatric age group the presence of the lesion usually comes to the attention of the physician because of cough or some other respiratory problem. Equally frequent as a signal of the presence of such a tumor are repeated bouts of pulmonary infection, which prompt the physician to have roentgenograms of the chest made, and the unsuspected tumor is thus detected. In a small percentage of the patients there may be Horner's syndrome, particularly if the lesion is posterior mediastinal in location and high in the chest. At times the growth of the tumor within the chest cavity may be of such a magnitude that protrusion through the thoracic inlet occurs and a palpable mass presents in the lower portion of the neck.

In evaluating these lesions the possibility of chronic infection must be given attention. This is particularly true of cystic lesions of the lung where the pathology is the result of staphylococcus pneumonia. There are other obscure and rare granulomatous lesions of the chest that may simulate tumors, and the diagnosis may be impossible unless a direct biopsy is made.

NEUROBLASTOMA

Neuroblastoma is one of the most unpredictable tumors in the pediatric age group.

R. E. Gross (1959) found that out of 217 cases, 11 percent presented as a primary chest lesion. This tumor has great latitude in its behavior and may be extremely malignant with widespread metastasis occurring early in the course of the disease. On the other hand, there are more instances of spontaneous regression of this tumor than of any other. Cole (1966) has studied the spontaneous regression of malignant tumors, and in his carefully selected cases neuroblastoma is the most common to undergo this type of change. There is pathological evidence to support this, for the tumor at times is mixed with a mature histological arrangement of ganglion cells and at times is entirely this benign form, known as ganglioneuroma. It is postulated that sometimes the malignant portions of these tumors undergo changes that cannot be explained at the present time but whose result is benign ganglioneuroma. The prognosis in this disease is related to the patient's age; in the very young, particularly those under one year of age and to a lesser extent those under two, the prognosis is considerably better than in older children.

PATHOLOGY

Neuroblastoma presents some characteristics on gross appearance that make possible the identification of the tumor upon examination. The mass is often smooth in outline and reddish gray. It is usually quite soft, and as the lesion grows the smooth outline disappears and the surface becomes multilobulated. In the early stages of the disease, the capsule is quite substantial. Later there is a thinning out of the capsule, and during surgical manipulation the tumor may readily be broken into, causing spread of the soft tumor tissue. The tumor arises from the sympathetic nervous system in any part of the body, and this accounts for its wide distribution. In the thoracic cavity the majority arise from the sympathetic chain in the posterior mediastinum, actually in the thoracic gutter (Fig. 1). There is no good explanation of the fact that most of these tumors arise in the superior portion of the thoracic cavity, most often just below the thoracic inlet. There have been a number of classifications of neuroblastoma. It is probable that pheochromocytoma, ganglioneuroma, neuroblastoma, and sympathogonioma are all variants of the same tumor. The first of these, pheochromocytoma, releases epinephrine and norepinephrine, which are the hormones detectable in the bloodstream and urine. To a lesser extent, abnormal secretion of these hormones occurs in the other forms of the tumor. It has now been established that in some patients with neuroblastomas there is a detectable substance in the urine that is the end metabolic product of epinephrine and norepinephrine. The difference between

a neuroblastoma and a sympathogonioma is of no practical importance as far as clinical diagnosis and management are concerned.

The histological appearance of this tumor includes great cellularity, evidence of rapid growth, and infiltration of adjacent structures. Invasion of blood vessels is not uncommon. Mitotic figures are frequent. In some zones, cells are arranged in so-called rosettes, and a number of cells become elongated or fusiform and contain neurofibrin. The identification of rosettes and neurofibrils attached to the cells is considered evidence for establishment of the diagnosis of neuroblastoma.

Spread of this tumor is primarily by way of the bloodstream; however, lymphatic spread takes place as well. The tumor has a predilection for bone metastasis, liver metastasis, and orbital metastasis. Pulmonary metastasis is less common.

SYMPTOMS AND DIAGNOSIS

In the reported series there is no outstanding symptom that calls attention to neuroblastoma of the thoracic cavity. Usually the patient is not doing well and has anemia. More frequently, the patient has bouts of pul-

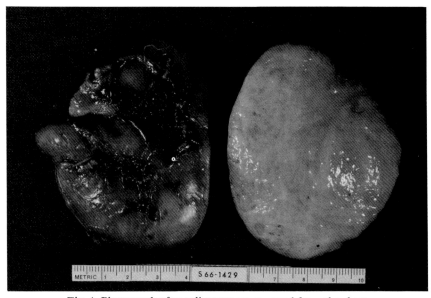

Fig. 1. Photograph of ganglioneuroma removed from the chest.

monary infection that may lead to roentgenograms of the chest being taken and thus to the detection of the tumor. Occasionally the trachea may be compressed to such an extent that there are respiratory difficulties, but this is unusual because the tumor arises in the gutter, not in the thoracic inlet itself. There may be cough, general malaise, and a failure to gain weight. In rare instances there may be a Horner's syndrome. Some reports state that the better survival rate in patients with intrathoracic neuroblastoma is due to the fact that intrathoracic neuroblastoma is detected earlier than intra-abdominal tumors. It may be that there is a real difference in growth characteristics of the tumor in the chest that accounts for the apparently better survival rate in this group of patients. Diagnosis depends upon roentgenograms of the chest. Usually the mass occupies the upper portion of a hemithorax rather than being a mass in the mediastinum (Fig. 2). On lateral projections of roentgenograms, the mass is posterior (Fig. 3).

Compression of the spinal cord may call attention to the thoracic neuroblastoma. The tumor can extend between the ribs and invade the spinal canal (Fig. 4). Chest films may show separation of the ribs, and a myelogram, invasion of the spinal canal. Such tumors may be referred to as dumbbell tumors.

Before therapy is undertaken, bone survey and chest films are mandatory. When there are definite bone lesions the prognosis is extremely grave. Bone marrow aspiration and examination for tumor cells is now widely practiced, and undoubtedly the tumor can be detected by this technique in the bone marrow at an earlier stage than by roentgen examination. As yet there is no unanimity of opinion among pathologists about the reliability of the diagnosis by bone marrow aspiration. Consequently, it is advisable to have biopsy material taken from the tumor before initiating therapy. Greenberg (1959) and Voorhees (1961) found that some ganglioneuromas and neuroblastomas produced sufficient norepinephrine and epinephrine to make their end product 3-methoxy-4-hydroxymandelic acid (VMA) detectable in abnormal amounts in the urine. A 24-hour urine collection analyzed for VMA is of value, for in many patients it will be elevated. Successful therapy will be accompanied by a fall to normal, and recurrence will again cause a rise in VMA.

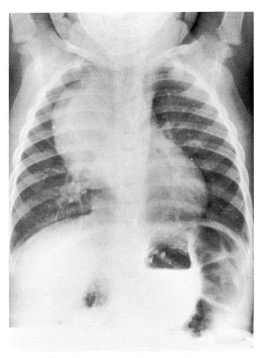

Fig. 2. Large neuroblastoma of chest.

TREATMENT

Surgical excision is the most successful method of treating these tumors. Recently, in a large study from the Children's Medical Center in Boston, it was found that with clean surgical excision followed by radiation therapy, the survival was 88 percent. In the patients in whom the tumor was massive but in whom there was no evidence of bone metastasis, partial resection of the neoplasm followed by radiation therapy resulted in a 64 percent survival rate. In those patients in whom biopsy was performed without extirpation of any portion of the tumor, therapy being limited to radiation, the cure rate was 38 percent. It would therefore seem that the

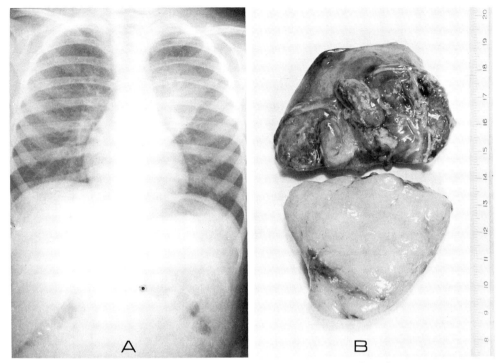

Fig. 3. A. Ganglioneuroma of chest. B. Photograph of specimen.

surgeon should make a determined effort to remove the tumor completely. On the other hand, there is considerable evidence that radiation therapy is almost as effective as surgical extirpation in the treatment of this disease. Consequently, the surgeon is unwise to make heroic efforts which endanger the patient's life in order to achieve a total resection of the tumor. It would seem appropriate in such situations to excise the major portion of the tumor and then to rely upon radiation therapy. Although the figures quoted above seem to indicate that partial removal of the tumor is beneficial, it is questionable whether this is the explanation of the observed therapeutic result. The age of the patients in the

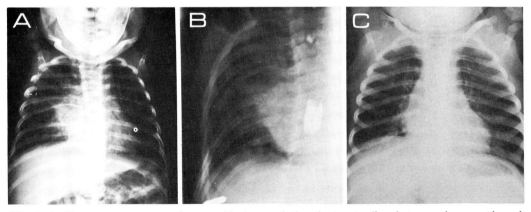

Fig. 4. A. Chest roentgenogram of a neuroblastoma of the chest extending between the seventh and eighth ribs posteriorly. B. Extension of the tumor into the spinal canal outlined by a myelogram. C. Chest roentgenogram of the same patient one year after removal.

group under therapy would have a significant influence on the results, for the tumor is more benign in children under two years of age. In patients in whom the tumor has grown and invaded the great vessels of the mediastinum and the trachea and major bronchi, a surgical extirpation is impossible. In such patients removal of the major portion of the tumor followed by radiation therapy is the wise course to follow.

When a dumbbell tumor is encountered, laminectomy should be performed as the initial step. Usually a complete removal is not possible. The chest tumor is then removed. When the excision has been incomplete, which is usual in this situation, radiation therapy is required.

SURGICAL APPROACH

In these patients we have found the anterior thoracic approach quite satisfactory. This is an incision popularized by Gross for ligation of the patent ductus. A curved anterior incision beginning close to the midline and curving under the nipple and extending into the axilla is useful. The cartilaginous portions of the third and fourth ribs or second and third ribs are divided as dictated by the position and size of the tumor, and an incision is made below these divisions in the intercostal space. The anterior thoracic muscles are spared to a large extent, and good exposure of the tumor mass is achieved. Care should be taken in dissection not to disturb the sympathetic system in the apex of the chest, for this may result in Horner's syndrome. On the other hand, in order to achieve a clean surgical excision, this complication should not prevent the surgeon from accomplishing a complete removal. It is surprising how few troublesome blood vessels enter the tumor when it is small. Later, when the tumor is large, there may be large, thin-walled vessels entering the mass which are quite troublesome for the surgeon to deal with. The chest should be closed without drainage, provided that the operative field is dry. In patients in whom there has been par-

tial removal of the tumor and hemostasis has not been ideal, a chest tube can be left in the thoracic cavity for drainage. It is our practice to close the skin with a subcuticular plain 5-0 catgut suture and a collodion dressing. This permits radiation therapy to be given promptly after operation. The amount of radiation varies, but often the total dose is in the vicinity of 3,000 to 3,500 rads.

The use of chemotherapy in the treatment of this disease has been extensive, yet no specific drug has demonstrated a consistent ability to destroy the tumor. On the other hand, with some nitrogen mustard derivatives such as Cytoxan, patients with widespread metastasis have been palliated for long periods of time. There is in our series at The Children's Memorial Hospital one patient with bone metastasis who has survived for more than five years. Generally, with this tumor, which is relatively rapid in growth, a two-year survival is considered to be adequate for cure. Again, one may apply Collins' law, which holds that the patient's age plus nine months equals the period of high risk after therapy is begun. This rule has proved reliable in determining the high-risk period, for very few patients have developed metastasis and died after this time interval.

The measurement of the breakdown products in the urine has been advocated by some workers in this field. It has been hoped that this would be a method not only of supporting the diagnosis but also of determining when recurrence takes place. As yet there has not been a large series of patients studied by this technique. Undoubtedly there is considerable variation in the ability of these tumors to produce the substance which is detected in the urine. It is interesting to note that in those patients in whom a preoperative 24-hour-urine test demonstrates the presence of these substances, after complete extirpation of the tumor or successful radiation therapy these substances disappear from the urine and reappear when metastasis takes place. In selected cases this can be a significant help in following the patient and an aid in guiding therapy.

THYMIC TUMORS

The infrequent occurrence of thymic tumors makes it difficult to outline clearly the pathology and clinical picture of these lesions. Many questions remain unanswered, even such basic ones as whether a truly malignant thymic tumor exists. In addition to the new growths there are granulomatous tumors, and the relationship of these to Hodgkin's disease is still unsettled. The relationship of these tumors to myasthenia gravis is not constant, since less than half the tumors so far described have been associated with it. More recently, in adults, a relationship between aplastic anemia and thymoma has been reported.

Enlargement of the thymus is not unusual in infants. In the past the enlarged thymus was considered to be a common cause of tracheal compression and sudden demise. This led to the practice of radiation therapy of the enlarged thymus, and it became a routine procedure before any surgical operation was undertaken. Today it is held that sudden deaths ascribed in the past to thymic tumors probably resulted from overwhelming infections and were not related to the enlarged thymus. It may be that in such patients there was a generalized enlargement of lymphoid tissue that included the thymus. Treatment of enlarged thymic shadows by radiation is today considered to be unwarranted. It is interesting that 60 percent of children with papillary adenocarcinoma of the thyroid seen at The Children's Memorial Hospital had some form of radiation therapy to the neck. In most instances this was low in dosage, such as is given for thymic enlargement.

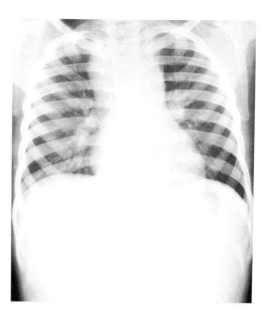

Fig. 5. Hodgkin's disease of the mediastinum.

size and pattern of arrangement. Occasionally these arrangements may suggest abortive Hassall's corpuscles. Lattes' classification divides the tumors into predominantly lymphoid, predominantly spindle cell, predominantly epithelial, and predominantly rosette-forming. In the last group there is confusion with the neurogenic tumors, such as the neuroblastoma. There are two unusual and rare groups, the granulomatous-like tumor and the seminoma-like tumor. The granulomatous-like thymoma, which has some characteristics of Hodgkin's disease histologically, differs from it in clinical behavior in that it remains local for long periods of time and is a tumor of great chronicity (Fig. 5). This should be appreciated, for the therapy should aim at excision or curative radiation therapy.

PATHOLOGY

Thymic tumors are classified by Lattes on the basis of histological configuration. Thymomas are fairly easily recognized on microscopic examination, having a dual composition of lymphoid elements and epithelial elements. The epithelial cells vary greatly in

SYMPTOMATOLOGY

About half the tumors so far recorded have presented because of respiratory complaints, consisting of cough or dyspnea. In some there has been mild compression of the venous return from the head and neck. The remaining tumors either have been found at autopsy or have been detected on routine chest roentgenograms. In the pediatric age group there has been no clear-cut, established case of myasthenia gravis associated with a tumor. If one takes the criteria of malignancy to be lymph node metastasis and blood-stream metastasis, it may be difficult to prove that any of the thymomas are malignant. On the other hand, if one considers the growth of the tumor and its local invasiveness as evidences of malignancy, then one has to classify some of the thymomas as malignant, for there have been reported cases of spread into the pleural cavity in the form of metastasis.

In x-rays these tumors tend to have a smooth outline, and they are seen in the anterior mediastinum (Fig. 6). They may be so large that they project into the thoracic cavity. There may be calcification, and this makes difficult their distinction from teratoma and dermoid cysts, which also tend to occur in the superior-anterior mediastinum and to contain calcification.

TREATMENT

A review of the literature indicates that surgical extirpation is the treatment of choice. The approach should be suited to the particular tumor. If the tumor is limited to the mediastinum, medial sternotomy can be used. Such an incision with a lateral extension is useful in patients in whom the tumor extends into a thoracic cavity. In the benign form of the tumor, surgical extirpation may be quite simple. In the malignant or invasive form of the disease, there may be such involvement of the great vessels and trachea and esophagus that extirpation becomes extremely difficult or impossible. In such situations, radiation therapy should be used, the doses being in the vicinity of 3,000 to 6,000 rads. The evidence so far suggests that x-ray therapy is a real adjunct to surgical therapy where extirpation is incomplete.

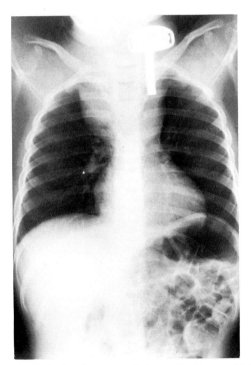

Fig. 6. A thymic tumor of the mediastinum which produced airway obstruction.

SUPERIOR MEDIASTINAL SYNDROME IN CHILDREN WITH MALIGNANCY

In the last few decades a syndrome consisting of venous engorgement of the veins of the head and neck, cyanosis of the head and neck, stridor, dyspnea, and edema has been designated as superior mediastinal syndrome. This set of symptoms is rare in adults and less often encountered in children. Recently, there has been a report by D'Angio of nine children, all boys, who presented with the superior mediastinal syndrome. These cases were among 607 patients with malignant diseases. The tumor which caused the symptoms was lymphosarcoma in all instances. Patients with this condition initially begin to cough, with or without expectoration and shortness of breath. The tumor may grow quite rapidly, and the edema of the face and venous engorgement develop with considerable speed. In such patients there may be hepatosplenomegaly or enlargement of nodes in other areas. Generally the diagnosis is suspected when a chest roentgenogram is made because of the pulmonary complaints.

TREATMENT

The treatment of this group of patients has posed quite a problem. The airway obstruction is such that to proceed with biopsy of the tumor directly with the use of general anesthesia may be disastrous. Where there are lymph nodes in other areas which are enlarged, biopsy of such lesions can be accomplished without general anesthesia and a tissue diagnosis made. When this is not possible, it has proven practical to give radiation therapy and to depend on the response to radiation for a diagnosis. It is recommended by some that small doses be started with and that as these are tolerated the dosage be rapidly increased. In the past, small doses have been given over a long period of time, and this has failed to be effective in relieving the symptoms. The rationale of this program was that radiation therapy would produce swelling and aggravate the obstructive symptoms. Actually this has not proved to be the case, and once radiation therapy is started, the dose is increased rapidly and beneficial results are observed in 48 hours or less. Although this gives symptomatic relief it has failed to produce any significant long-term cures. Often these patients will have recurrence or may reappear with acute leukemia. In patients with mediastinal tumors where there is no compression of the tracheal structures, biopsy should be performed before therapy is instituted. D'Angio has also given steroids during the radiation therapy. It is his belief that this potentiates the effect of radiation and also reduces edema. One of the results of radiation may be hyperuricemia and uric acid nephropathy. During treatment it is essential to ensure adequate hydration and to alkalize the urine.

DERMOID CYSTS AND TERATOMAS OF THE MEDIASTINUM

Dermoid cysts and teratomas of the mediastinum are rare in children. Rusby (1944), in a review of 174 collected cases from the literature for whom the age was recorded, found that 17 were between the ages of birth and 9 years. Most of these tumors become clinically apparent in the decade between 20 and 30. Of the 174 patients, 68 fell into this age group. Nevertheless, there are recorded cases in which the lesion grew to such size during intrauterine life that at birth it produced respiratory obstruction and prevented the establishment of normal respirations. A rare case has been recorded in which the newborn survived for a few hours, and in some other situations surgical excision has successfully been performed.

PATHOLOGY

The lesion is usually divided into two types, the dermoid cyst and the teratoma. The dermoid cyst is a single cavity containing sebaceous material, but it may be bilocular or multilocular. It is interesting that often there are daughter cysts adjacent to and completely isolated from the major lesion. These lesions increase slowly in size and may not become apparent until middle life. The cystic structures may become infected and undergo a spectacular increase in size during such a process. The dermoid cysts are usually benign and relatively simple tumors, the lining being stratified squamous or transitional in character—that is, cuboidal and high columnar, with or without cilia. These tumors are located in the anterior-superior mediastinum. Often growth predominates on one side, and on roentgenographic examination the lesion appears to be completely within one thoracic cavity. In such situations it has been demonstrated, at autopsy or at operation, that the lesion originates in the mediastinum and has a pedicle projecting into the thoracic cavity to which is attached the major portion of the tumor. These simple cysts are at times a little more complicated, as shown by the fact that ectodermal structures, such as salivary glands, pancreas, thymus, thyroid, and intestine, may be represented. Actually there is probably a transition from the simple cyst to the solid form of the teratoma, in which all three elements of the germinal layers are represented. A significant difference between the two groups is that the dermoids are rarely malignant, whereas the teratomas tends to have a high rate of malignancy—in some series as high as 70 percent in the solid teratoma but substantially less than half of this in the dermoid type.

ETIOLOGY

There is a great deal of debate about the origin of these structures. The fact that they are in the midline and anterior make them similar to the dermoid cysts, which are accounted for by the inclusion phenomenon. The fact that they are deep to the sternum does not falsify this explanation, for in some cases dumbbell structures have been described in which there is a portion in the subcutaneous tissue with a stalk through the sternum and an enlargement in the mediastinum. In other situations there is a defect in the sternum at the site of the mediastinal lesion. These findings support inclusion as a mechanism in the formation of these lesions.

CLINICAL BEHAVIOR

An analysis of the symptomatology places cough, with or without expectoration, as the commonest individual symptom. Dyspnea with cough is also a common complaint. In the older patient pain is next most common, and it resembles the pain of pleurisy. In some the pain has been described in the shoulder

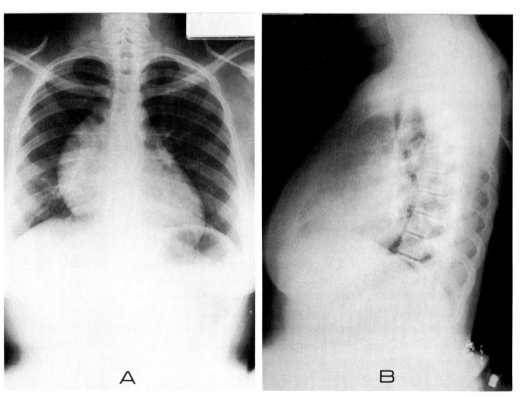

Fig. 7. Dermoid cyst of the chest. A. Chest film of patient with a large dermoid cyst of the chest. B. Lateral view of the same patient.

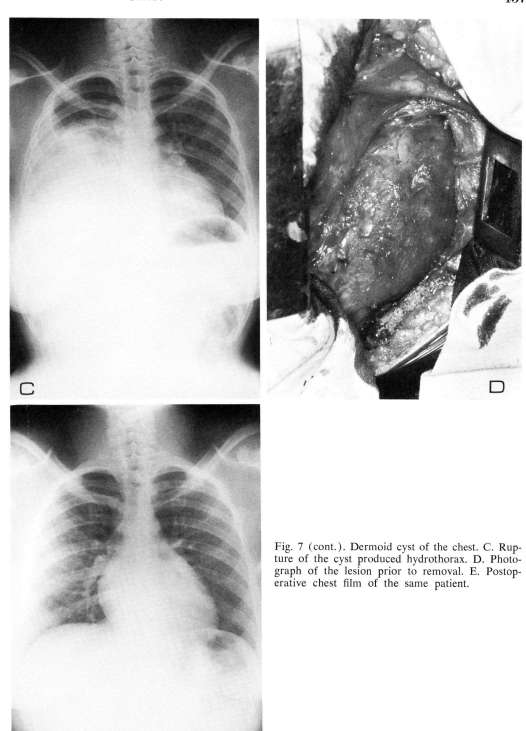

Fig. 7 (cont.). Dermoid cyst of the chest. C. Rupture of the cyst produced hydrothorax. D. Photograph of the lesion prior to removal. E. Postoperative chest film of the same patient.

girdle with radiation down the ulnar side of the arm. In the very large midline tumors there may be some elements of the superior mediastinal syndrome with engorgement of the vein of the neck. Horner's syndrome, because of compression of the stellate ganglion, has also been described. There may be alterations in voice related to compression of the recurrent laryngeal nerve.

Usual symptomatology occurs when the cysts become infected. Such a process may lead to rapid enlargement of the cyst or actual perforation of the cyst with formation of an empyema or rupture into the bronchus. When this occurs there may be bleeding in the initial episode. It has been observed in some patients that a leak of cyst fluid may take place into the thoracic cavity without infection. Other factors such as tissue necrosis with increasing pressure within the cyst or the presence of enzymes in the fluid from pancreatic tissue may play a role. When this occurs there is a rapid accumulation of fluid in the pleural space which is identical to the cystic fluid. In situations where the process is more gradual the perforation may take place into a bronchus and be associated with the development of a cough and sputum containing hair. Originally, before this had been described in the literature, physicians were perplexed by the history of the patient's coughing up hair. In the early recorded cases physicians were able to explain this phenomenon upon postmortem examination, when the dermoid cyst of the superior mediastinum was found to have perforated into a bronchus and thus to have been the source of hair in the sputum.

The diagnosis is established by roentgen examination, which reveals a large shadow in the mediastinum that is anterior and that often contains calcified material (Fig. 7). This material may resemble recognizable portions of bone or may be only specks of calcification. When this is found the possibility of definitely establishing the diagnosis of dermoid cyst or teratoma is enhanced. Often the radiologist is misled in that the major portion of the tumor mass projects into one thoracic cavity. This is not unusual, for large dermoids or teratomas may actually grow into one of the thoracic cavities; actually, the lesion originates in the mediastinum and projects into one of the thoracic cavities.

TREATMENT

Surgical excision is the treatment of choice and should be performed as soon as the diagnosis is made and preferably before the complication of infection and perforation takes place. Today the wide use of chest roentgenograms has led to the early diagnosis of this lesion, and perforation is rarely observed today. Surgical excision may be quite difficult, since the lesion may be extensive and adherent to the great vessels and the pericardium of the heart. In other situations the lesion may readily be separated from the mediastinal structures and present very little of a technical problem. The surgical approach when the lesion is primarily in one thoracic cavity should be through that side. The anterolateral approach is found to be effective in these situations. It also permits one to cross the sternum and gain a good exposure when this is required. When the lesion is primarily midline, a sternal splitting incision can be used quite effectively and has the advantage of providing excellent exposure of the mediastinal structures. Careful examination of the specimen, particularly of the teratoma, should be done to ascertain whether malignant cells are present. If they are, radiation therapy should be considered in the postoperative care of the patient.

RARE TUMORS OF THE LUNG

Primary tumors of the lung in infants and children are extremely rare. Medical literature reveals that practically all the lesions known to occur in adults will on rare occasions be encountered in children. The vast majority of malignant lesions of the lung in children represent pulmonary metastasis. In this group, those originating from Wilms'

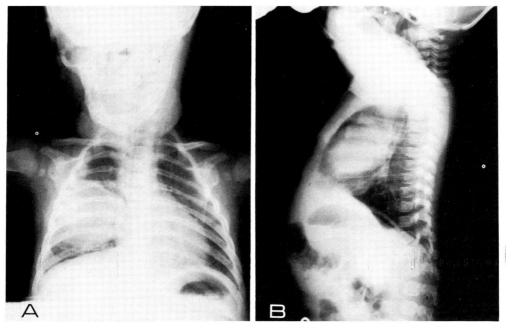

Fig. 8. A. Chest film of a patient with a hamartoma of the right chest. B. Lateral view of the same patient.

tumor are in the majority. Other tumors, such as rhabdomyosarcoma, osteogenic sarcoma, and, to a lesser extent, neuroblastoma, may give rise to pulmonary metastasis.

On rare occasions, hamartomas occur in the lung (Fig. 8). These are malformations consisting of normal tissue which is compounded into tumorlike malformations. These tumors are extremely rare, and no successful resections have been reported. They have been found in newborn children who have died of respiratory distress. There may be smooth muscle and connective tissue tumors such as have been described by Holinger (1960), who found two leiomyosarcomas that undoubtedly arose from the anterior wall of the trachea. He was able to resect them through the bronchoscope successfully, and there was no recurrence. Of the eight cases of fibrosarcoma of the bronchus described by Holinger, four were in patients under 15 years of age, and two of these patients survived operative treatment. These patients had obstructive symptoms with cough and repeated infection. There

has been one case reported in which the entire tumor was coughed up and the patient survived.

Bronchial adenomas are extremely rare; Ward (1954) found eight reported cases in

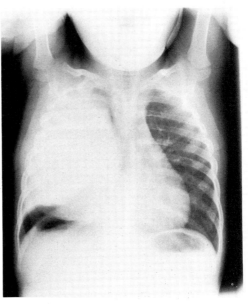

Fig. 9. Carcinoma of the lung in a child.

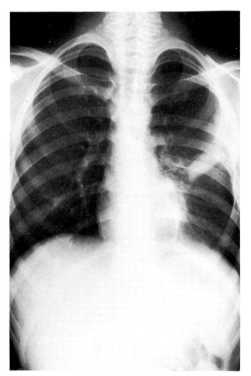

Fig. 10. Chest film of a child who proved to have Ewing's tumor of the rib.

dobronchial tumors are the common ones. The paucity of experience with this lesion in children makes it difficult to state whether there is eventual metastasis from these lesions. However, the experience with adults indicates the definite possibility of metastasis from such lesions, and consequently it is advised that treatment be vigorous.

Carcinoma of the lung is extremely rare in children, but it has been reported (Fig. 9). Cayley (1951) collected a series of 16 such lesions in the lungs of children with an age range of 15 months to 14 years. The histological diagnosis was adenocarcinoma, squamous cell carcinoma, epithelioid carcinoma, and oat cell carcinoma. Only one patient was reported alive. Ewing's tumor has been reported in the rib. There may be a considerable amount of soft tissue tumor projecting into the thoracic cavity, and the bone changes may be attributed to the adjacent soft tissue tumor. Furthermore, the bone changes are not characteristic of those usually observed in Ewing's tumor of long bones.

The tumor is usually of rapid growth, and survival is rare.

children and added one that he had observed. The predicted symptoms of atelectasis from obstruction with bleeding from ulcerated en-

Ewing's tumor of the rib is an unusual lesion of the chest wall. The patients have

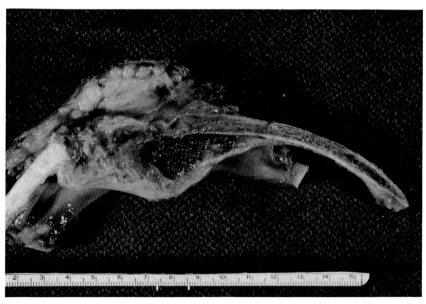

Fig. 11. Cross section of resected rib.

discomfort, and this may call attention to this new growth. Chest films may reveal a considerable soft tissue mass, which overshadows the rib involvement. Careful examination of the chest film or of a special film for bone detail usually suggests the correct diagnosis (Fig. 10). Resection was performed on our two patients, followed by radiation therapy (Fig. 11). Neither patient survived beyond 18 months.

CHYLOTHORAX

Spontaneous accumulation of chyle in the chest is an extremely rare clinical occurrence. It is almost invariably found in the neonatal age group and may be caused by birth trauma. In these patients there is a rapid onset of dyspnea, displacement of the mediastinal structures to one side, and a chest that is flat to percussion. Large amounts of fluid are seen on the chest film. Of the few cases that have been reported in the literature, the majority have occurred on the right side. Gross (Randolph and Gross, 1957) has explored two patients and thought that the defect was closed in one. Both patients recovered. Most reported cases have been treated by repeated aspiration. In a majority of the instances only a few paracenteses have been required to free the chest of fluid. In some, particularly that reported by Boles and Izant (1960), a prolonged period of therapy was required. In such instances the nutrition of the infant becomes a problem because of the considerable loss of fat and protein in the aspirated fluid.

IATROGENIC CHYLOTHORAX

In the course of various thoracic operations, injury to the thoracic duct may occur. In some instances the operator becomes aware of the injury and may be successful in ligating the thoracic duct below the opening. In most instances the patient accumulates fluid postoperatively that on aspiration proves to be chyle. In the patients with spontaneous chylothorax, repeated aspiration usually clears the chest, and operative intervention is not required. In resistant cases operative therapy is indicated. It is important that the patients be given a fat meal prior to operation so that the thoracic duct will become more prominent. Ligation of the defect is all that is required.

Maloney and Spencer (1956) reported 13 cases, 11 of which cleared with repeated aspiration and 2 of which required ligation of the duct.

ORVAR SWENSON

REFERENCES

BOLES, E. T., and IZANT, R. J., Jr. Spontaneous chylothorax in the neonatal period. Amer. J. Surg., 99: 870, 1960.

CAYLEY, C. K., KSCAEZ, H. J., and MERSHEIMER, W. Primary bronchogenic carcinoma of the lung in children. Amer. J. Dis. Child. 82: 49, 1951.

DANIEL, R. A., Jr., DIVELY, W. L., EDWARDS, W. H., and CHAMBERLAIN, N. Mediastinal tumors. Ann. Surg., 151: 783, 1960.

EVERSON, T. C., and COLE, W. H. Spontaneous Regression of Cancer. Philadelphia, W. B. Saunders Company, 1966.

FRIEDMAN, N. B. Tumors of the thymus. J. Thorac. Cardiov. Surg., 53: 163, 1967.

GREENBERG, R. E., and GARDNER, L. I. New diagnostic test for neural tumors of infancy: increased urine excretion of 3-methoxy-4-hydroxy-mandelic acid and norepinephrine in ganglioneuroma with chronic diarrhea. Pediatrics, 24: 683, 1959.

GROSS, R. E., FARBER, S., and MARTIN, L. W. Neuroblastoma sympatheticum. A study and report of 217 cases. Pediatrics, 23: 1179, 1959.

HOLINGER, P. H., JOHNSTON, K. C., GOSSWEILER, N., and HIRSCH, E. C. Dis. Chest, 37: 1, 1960.

MALONEY, J. V., Jr., and SPENCER, F. C. The nonoperative treatment of traumatic chylothorax. Surgery, 40: 121, 1956.

RANDOLPH, J. G., and GROSS, R. E. Congenital chylothorax. Arch. Surg., 74: 405, 1957.

RUSBY, N. L. Dermoid cysts and teratomas of the mediastinum. J. Thoracic Surg., 13: 169, 1944.

VOORHEES, M. L., and GARDNER, L. I. Urine excretion of norepinephrine, epinephrine and 3-methoxy-4-hydroxymandelic acid by children with neuroblastoma. J. Clin. Endocr., 21: 321, 1961.

WARD, D. E., Jr., BRADSHAW, H. H., and PRINCE, T. C., Jr. Bronchial adenoma in children. J. Thoracic Surg., 27: 295, 1954.

29

Congenital Malformations of the Esophagus

TRACHEOESOPHAGEAL FISTULA AND ATRESIA

Considerable interest was aroused in tracheoesophageal fistula and atresia three decades ago when Ladd (1944) and Levin (1941), working separately, had patients who survived the correction of this malformation. The lesion has been known for generations. Mackenzie (1884) gives Durston (1670) the credit for the first description of this malformation. Martin (1821) published the first clinical case. The lesion was not given clinical attention until the development of roentgen techniques and the use of contrast material. Earlier, a number of surgeons were interested in the lesion but did not succeed in having a survival despite the fact that a number of operations were performed. This is notably true of Lanman (1940), who published a series of unsuccessful cases that he had treated by performing closure of the fistula and end-to-end anastomosis of the esophagus. This experience led his colleague Ladd to initiate a staged method of treating the lesion, and it was with this technique that the first survivals were achieved. At the first operation the fistula was divided. A few days later a gastrostomy was performed, and the upper esophagus was exteriorized in the neck. At a later date, an esophagus was made. Similar work by Levin produced survivals. Haight (1944) was the first to report a survival following closure of the fistula and end-to-end anastomosis of the esophagus.

The occurrence rate of this lesion is debated. It is considered by some to occur once in 1,000 births, however most reviews place the incidence at about one in 3,000 births.

ETIOLOGY

The mishaps in embryological development that result in this lesion are as yet not clearly established. E. Ide Smith (1957) published a thorough review of the early development of the trachea and esophagus in relation to atresia of the esophagus and tracheoesophageal fistula. This study was based on five early embryos that contained the anomaly. It was possible for Smith to have three of the early embryos for detailed study, and it is this material that is described and that led to the conclusion that overgrowth of epithelium was important in the formation of this anomaly. A number of different explanations have been proposed to account for this overgrowth. It has been suggested that occlusion of the lumen of the esophagus is present in the 19- to 20-mm-stage embryo and that subsequently vacuolization reformed the lumen. Such a process could account for the formation of tracheoesophageal fistula and particularly for atresia of the esophagus. Subsequent work has cast doubt upon this as a possible etiology for the lesion. Although the vacuolization does occur, it is questionable whether complete occlusion is inevitably a part of the normal embryological development of the esophagus. Furthermore, even if it were always present it would not lead to a clear-cut explanation of tracheoesophageal fistula.

There have been a number of publications that have suggested that intraembryonic pressure may lead to the development of this anomaly. Schmitz in 1923 postulated that the pressure of the heart may produce this lesion, and anatomically this relationship seems reasonable. Pressure from abnormal vessels has been given as the possible explanation. While it is true that abnormal vessels are occasionally found in association with tracheoesophageal fistula and atresia of the esophagus, the association is by no means constant. Yemaski in 1933 felt that the lesion may be related to dysfunction of active cellular proliferation. Gruenwall in 1940 suggested that a delay in the separation of the esophagus and trachea might be accompanied by a rapid elongation of the trachea, which may carry the developing digestive tube with it, and therefore the common tube loses its ability to differentiate into a separate normal esophagus. This may be the explanation for the tracheoesophageal fistula. Rosenthal in 1931 expressed the judgment that the defect was caused by faulty union of the epithelial ridges which divide the foregut. The present state of knowledge indicates that the defect may result from either genetic or environmental causes or from a combination of both.

PATHOLOGY

The anatomical arrangement of this anomaly is quite constant. Over 90 percent of the patients have a tracheoesophageal fistula situated on the posterior tracheal wall above the carina and communicating with the lower esophageal segment. The upper esophagus ends in a dilated, obstructed pouch (Figs. 1, 2A, and 2B). In rare instances there may be atresia of the esophagus without a tracheoesophageal fistula. In these cases there is variable length to the upper esophagus, and the same may be true of the lower esophagus, although a number have very short lower esophageal segments, often no more than a

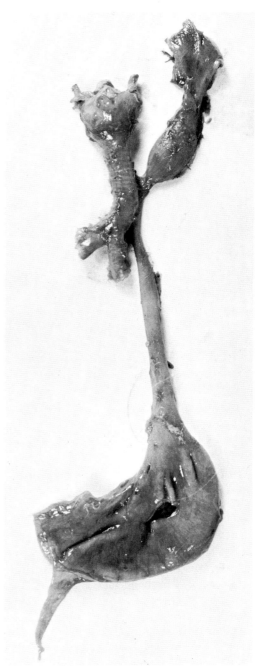

Fig. 1. Pathological specimen that includes the upper esophagus, which ends blindly but is attached by muscular bands to the trachea. The lower esophagus communicates with the trachea.

centimeter or so in length (Figs. 3A and 3B). Occasionally there is considerable length to the lower esophageal segment, and this may be associated with a quite long upper esophageal pouch, making end-to-end anastomosis possible.

In another group of patients the lesion is a tracheoesophageal fistula without atresia of the esophagus. In this group of patients there is communication from the esophagus to the trachea (Fig. 4A). Usually the fistula is slanted in a diagonal manner so that the esophageal opening is inferior to or below the level of the tracheal opening (Fig. 4B). This probably accounts for the fact that this lesion has been observed in adults and has not given a great deal of trouble to the patients until middle age is attained, when the structures become more lax and the fistula more functional. The position of the fistula is often quite high and may be above the second dorsal vertebra, so that is can be more con-

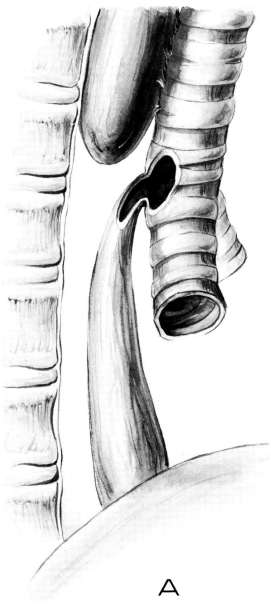

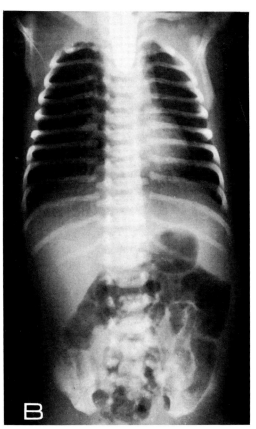

A

Fig. 2. A. Diagrammatic sketch of the common form of esophageal atresia and tracheoesophageal fistula. The lower esophageal segment enters the posterior tracheal wall just cephalad to the tracheal bifurcation. B. Roentgenogram of a patient with this type of lesion. The Lipiodol outlines the blind esophageal pouch in the upper chest. Air in the intestinal tract is evidence that a tracheoesophageal fistula is present. This form is found in 93 percent of the patients.

veniently approached through a neck incision than through a thoracic incision. In a fourth group of patients the lower esophageal segment does not communicate with the trachea, and the situation is reversed from the common form in that the upper esophageal segment communicates with the trachea (Figs. 5A and 5B). In a rare form that probably comprises about 1 percent of the patients there is a double fistula, one communicating with each segment of the esophagus (Figs. 6A and 6B).

The other associated pathological abnormalties are stricture associated with the tracheoesophageal fistula and, on rare occasions, small duplications.

Prematurity is commonly associated with the lesion, being reported in the vicinity of 20 to 25 percent of the patients (Fig. 7). In the whole group of patients there is a relatively high instance of associated congenital malformations, the figure given usually being in the vicinity of 40 percent. As is the case with many anomalies, the smaller the baby

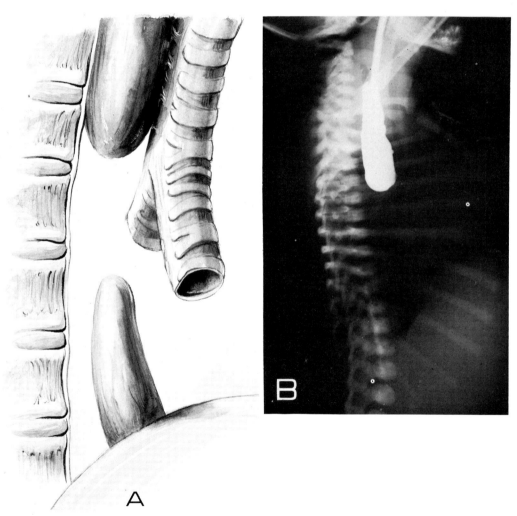

Fig. 3. A. Diagram of esophageal atresia without tracheoesophageal fistula. B. Chest roentgenogram of a patient with this type of lesion. The Lipiodol fills the upper blind esophageal segment. There is no air in the upper intestinal tract. Three percent of the patients have this form of anomaly.

and the shorter the period of gestation, the greater the chances of associated serious anomalies. These are hemivertebra, congenital heart lesions, atresias of the intestine, and anomalies of the perineum, the most common one being imperforate anus.

CLINICAL PRESENTATION

Attention may be called to these babies by the presence of large amounts of amniotic fluid. The absence of this in the mother does not exclude the diagnosis; however, when it is present, and it is in about half the affected infants, a search should be made for an obstructing gastrointestinal lesion. The cause of this associated hydramnios is a blockage in the infant's gastrointestinal system that prevents amniotic fluid from being freely ingested and reabsorbed through the infant's intestinal tract and returned to the placental circulation.

The presence of other congenital malformations in the family is another indication for attending physicians to be on the alert for anomalies in siblings. Although it is rare

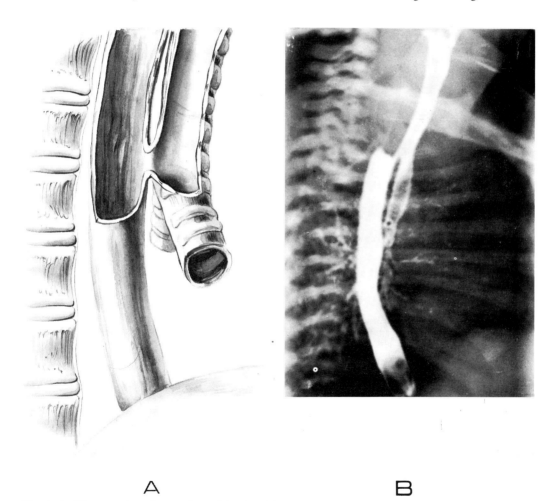

A   B

Fig. 4. A. Diagram of tracheoesophageal fistula with an otherwise intact esophagus. B. Roentgenogram of such a patient. There is a small fistula between the trachea and the esophagus. The course of the fistula is oblique, with the tracheal side being more cephalad. Two percent of the patients have this form of anomaly.

for this specific lesion to occur in the same family, the presence of serious malformations in previous siblings should nevertheless be a warning that a thorough examination for obstructive lesions in the newborn should be made. This lesion has been reported in twins. In some instances the lesion has been present in one twin, despite the fact that the infants appeared quite identical with similar blood types. However, there have been reports on identical twins where the lesion was present in both neonates.

At birth these infants are essentially normal in appearance. Some of them seem to have excessive amounts of saliva; this is not actually the case, rather it is inability to swallow their saliva, which is normal in amount. Nevertheless, what appears to be excessive amounts of saliva should be a warning to the attending physicians and nurses that an atresia is present, and it should prompt them to pass a catheter down the esophagus to determine if an obstruction is present.

The symptom that is pathognomonic of

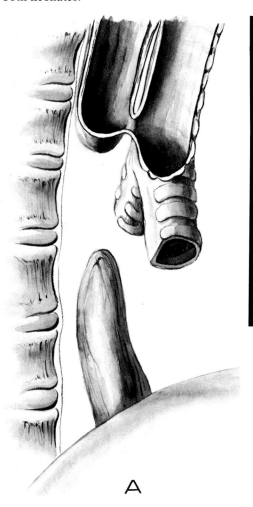

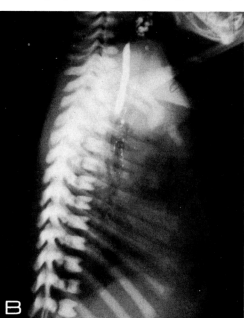

Fig. 5. A. Diagram of a rare form of tracheoesophageal fistula with esophageal atresia. The fistula in this situation communicates with the upper esophageal segment. B. Roentgenogram of such a patient. The Lipiodol in the upper segment and the communication with the trachea and absence of air in the intestine proves there is no fistula from the trachea to the lower segment. This type of fistula is seen in 1 percent of the patients.

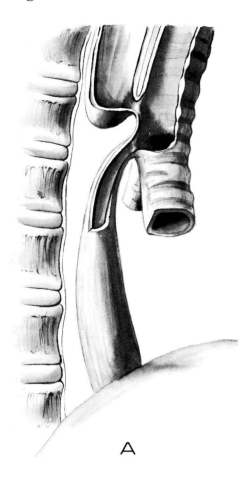

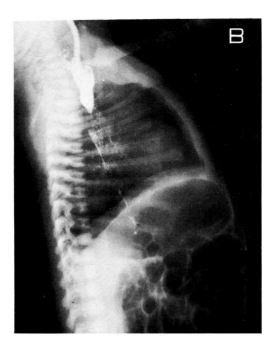

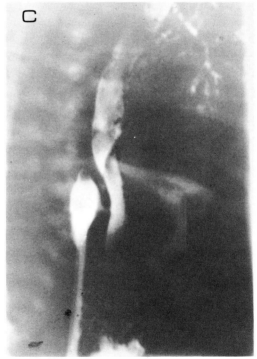

Fig. 6. A. Diagram of another rare form of tracheoesophageal fistula with atresia of the esophagus. There is a double fistula with communications between the trachea and the upper and lower segments. B. Roentgenogram of such a patient. The Lipiodol from the upper segment has entered the trachea and escaped into the lower esophageal segment. Air in the intestinal tract is proof of a fistula between the lower esophageal segment and the trachea. This type of fistula was encountered once in 100 patients. C. An unusual double fistula. The fistula from the upper segment arises from the side rather than from the bottom of the upper blind segment. Such lesions will be missed unless contrast material is used to outline the upper segment.

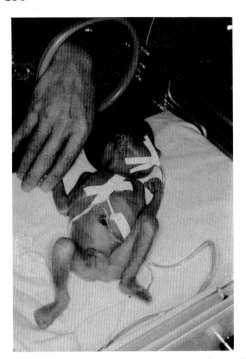

Fig. 7. A premature baby weighing less than 2 lb with atresia of esophagus and tracheoesophageal fistula.

tracheoesophageal fistula with atresia of the esophagus is a bout of severe cyanosis following attempted feedings. Typically, these infants will be offered their first feeding and take several milliliters quite normally and then cough and become cyanotic. If left alone they usually will recover from the bout of severe bronchial spasm, and a normal color will return to the skin. Often, suctioning and the start of various resuscitative measures may hasten the return from cyanosis to a normal skin color. Such an episode is so characteristic of atresia of the esophagus that the attending nurses and physicians should immediately pass a catheter down the esophagus, and, if there is any suggestion of an obstruction, a roentgenogram with contrast material or at least a plain roentgenogram of the chest should be made with a catheter in place, and it will often be found to be curled backward from the atretic esophagus. There is nothing on the external examination of these infants that is characteristic. There may be abdominal distension caused by a large

tracheoesophageal fistula through which excessive amounts of air enter the gastrointestinal tract. On examination of the chest there may be atelectasis, particularly of the right upper lobe.

DIAGNOSIS

The diagnosis rests on the passage of a catheter down the esophagus. One can be misled at times in using a soft small catheter that curls in the dilated upper segment and gives the impression to the examiner that it is passed into the stomach. Consequently it is well to use a fairly stiff rubber catheter of size 8 to 10. Initially, in the study of these infants barium was given to them by mouth, filling the upper esophageal segment and demonstrating the lesion quite dramatically. Objection to this technique was based on the observation that ingestion of the barium was often associated with overflow of the contrast material into the bronchial system. There has been considerable debate on the effect of barium in the tracheoesophageal tree, some believing that it is innocuous, others that it might produce harm. Nevertheless, the use of barium has been discouraged, and radiopaque oils have been substituted. More recently, water-soluble opaque solutions have had preference. Some workers do not believe that any contrast material should be used but rather a catheter should be passed down the esophagus, and, if obstruction is met, radiopaque examination should be made of the chest to determine the level of the obstruction. The disadvantage of this technique is that the occasional fistula from the upper esophageal segment to the trachea is not outlined. It would seem more profitable to have a small catheter in place in the upper esophageal segment, and with fluoroscopic control a small amount of water-soluble radiopaque material can be injected through the catheter and an examination of the baby made, particularly with cinefluorography, to determine if there is a fistula from the upper segment to the trachea. The contrast material can immediately be retrieved by suction on the tube, and aspiration of the contrast material by the patient is prevented.

An essential part of the examination is the chest film, which gives an idea of the extent of pulmonary involvement. Some degree of infection or atelectasis is present in a large majority of these patients, and the favorite site of these processes is in the right upper lobe.

The roentgenographic examination should include a plain film of the abdomen to determine whether air is present in the gastrointestinal tract. Absence of gastric and intestinal air proves that the infant has esophageal atresia and no tracheoesophageal fistula.

The added advantage of a roentgenogram of the abdomen is that associated obstructive lesions of the intestine can be detected. While it is not common for there to be atresias or other obstructive lesions, they have been reported and should be searched for in routine abdominal films of these infants before surgical therapy is undertaken.

PREOPERATIVE TREATMENT

Infants with tracheoesophageal fistula and atresia are usually detected in the first few days of life. The extent of preoperative therapy largely depends on the age at which the lesion is detected, on the presence and extent of pulmonary infection, on associated malformations, and on the degree of prematurity. It is quite well recognized that not a great deal is gained, and probably there is some disadvantage, in declaring these infants surgical emergencies and operating on them shortly after admission to the hospital. There is some evidence from studies in England that the lowest mortality is achieved in those patients operated on at three days of age. Whether or not this can be substantiated remains to be seen. However, there is a strong suggestion in the study from Great Ormond Street Hospital for Sick Children that there is some advantage in delaying operation until the third day of life. Other studies have indicated that survival is greater on the second or third day and falls

after that period. The evaluation of these studies is extremely difficult because of the fact that associated lesions, prematurity, and the presence of infection are all factors that would influence recovery and that are hard to evaluate in relation to the time of operation. Nevertheless, many of these infants are transported for some distance, and it appears to be the general consensus that surgery should be performed promptly but not on an emergency basis. The tendency is to treat these babies for a period of 12 to 24 hours giving them fluids, administering antibiotics, and performing tracheal toilet to diminish pulmonary atelectasis so that the baby becomes a better surgical risk. The administration of fluid during this period may be advantageous, particularly in the infant two or three days of age. It would appear that the best program is to place these babies in an isolette with a reasonable amount of oxygen and humidity and with the head elevated in order to discourage by gravity the flow of material from the stomach to the tracheal system. To prevent aspiration a tube can be placed in the upper esophageal segment on suction so that the saliva is removed in this way and aspiration is discouraged. Parenteral fluids, antibiotics, and, in some instances, blood can be administered during this period of preparation. Such a program usually permits the infant to be taken to the operating room during the day, when the most experienced personnel are available, particularly in the field of anesthesia. Some clinics perform a gastrostomy in the hope of lessening gastric reflux into the trachea, thus permitting a more prolonged period of preparation. This may have some merit, particularly in babies with severe pulmonary infection.

SURGICAL TREATMENT

Intubation of these patients was not practiced 20 years ago; rather, the anesthesia was administered with a tight-fitting mask. Today the operation is safer with intubation of all these patients. There has been considerable controversy about the method of repairing this congenital malformation. Initially a retropleural approach was used. Then many surgeons began to use the transpleural approach, and undoubtedly in a number of institutions recovery rates improved with this change of technique. However, that this represented an advantage of the transpleural approach over an extrapleural route is questionable because many other factors, such as experience with the lesion and improvement in anesthesia and in postoperative care, undoubtedly played a larger role in the improvement in the recovery rates. Some surgeons have tenaciously held to the extrapleural approach, tenacity vindicated by the large study conducted by the surgical section of the American Academy of Pediatrics (Holder, 1964). This study demonstrated that two thirds of the patients survived with a transpleural approach, whereas with the extrapleural approach three fourths of the patients survived. Our experience, which goes back 20 years and includes all of the affected infants regardless of weight, amount of infection, or associated anomalies, indicates that a 78 percent survival rate can be achieved with the extrapleural approach. The reason for the greater survival rate with the extrapleural approach is that when a leak occurs the complication is not fatal. An esophagocutaneous fistula is established, which hurts the pride of the surgeon considerably but does little harm to the infant. However, when this complication occurs with the transpleural approach there is the likelihood of an esophagopleural fistula, which can be fatal. The performance of these babies is uniform once a fistula of this type has been established. Feedings placed in the infants' stomachs regurgitate up through the esophagus into the chest and out the thoracic catheter. The cause of this constant performance may be related to the negative pressure in the pleural cavity, which promotes the flow of fluid in this direction. A number of restorative measures have been attempted once this complication has occurred, but none has proven entirely effective. Consequently, these infants die of inanition after a period of four to six weeks.

Several workers have now attempted to combine the two approaches, approaching the lesion transpleurally and at the completion of the operation closing the pleura and placing an extrapleural drain down to this area so that any leak might be converted into an esophagocutaneous rather than an esophagopleural fistula. It would seem that the tried and tested procedure of extrapleural approach has the distinct advantage, since it does deliver a higher rate of survivals. While it may be harder technically for the surgeon to perform the operation extrapleurally, the objective of surgical therapy is to have the highest possible rate of survival.

OPERATIVE TECHNIQUE

There are two distinct techniques used in the extrapleural approach. The original technique was to resect short segments of two or three ribs posteriorly and to push the pleura away in order to achieve an exposure of the pathology (Fig. 8A). More recently, resection of one rib over a long segment and then extensive freeing of pleura to achieve an exposure has been advocated. Which of these are used depends upon the surgeon's experience. Certainly resection of two ribs posteriorly places the incision much closer to the pathology than does the other technique (Fig. 8B). With care, the pleura can be pushed from the chest wall (Fig. 8C). The important point is to resect the rib segments posteriorly and then with a scalpel to divide the periosteum of the rib bed posteriorly and thus begin the dissection of the pleura from the chest wall. The muscular bundles can then be divided and the rib resected down to the articulation. It is not advised to disarticulate the ribs, for a pleural tear is often made. The pleural dissection proceeds readily until the region of the sympathetic ganglia and nerves is approached. The pleura is more adherent in this region, and particular care must be exercised not to tear it. The azygos vein is then exposed, and in order to improve the exposure it is ligated with 6-0 silk and divided. The mediastinum can be readily exposed, and the large vagus nerve is identified. Imme-

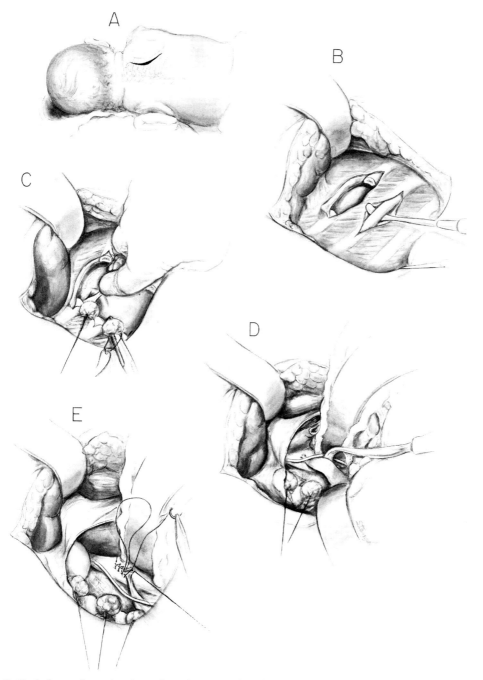

Fig. 8. Technique of repair of esophageal atresia. A. The baby is positioned on his side with the left side down. B. Short segments of two ribs are resected. C. The pleura is pushed from the thoracic wall. D. The lower esophageal segment is dissected free. It is adjacent to the vagus nerve. E. The tracheal portion of the fistula is oversewn as the fistula is divided.

diately deep to this nerve in the operative field will be found the lower esophageal segment (Fig. 8D). It can readily be dissected out, and a web tape or rubber drain can be placed around it for traction. The esophagus is then freed up to the fistula, and a 6-0 silk suture is placed adjacent to the trachea and tied. It is then advisable to cut the fistula par-

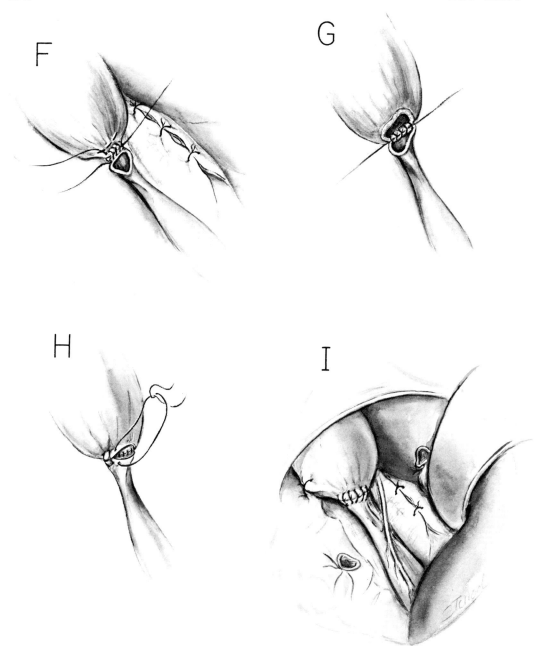

Fig. 8 (cont.). Technique of repair of esophageal atresia. F. The tracheal side of the fistula has been covered with adjacent tissue and the two segments brought together with interrupted 6-0 silk through the muscular coats. G. The upper segment has been opened and the mucosa approximated with 6-0 silk. H. The anastomosis is completed anteriorly with a completion of the silk sutures to the muscular coats. I. The completed anastomosis. One traction suture has been placed between the paravertebral fascia and the upper segment. This takes some tension from the anastomosis.

tially across and to close the opening as the dissection progresses with a continuous 6-0 silk suture (Fig. 8E). By placing the suture before any cut is made, there is assurance that the fistula will be completely closed. Care in dividing the fistula at the proper level is important. If it is cut at the level of the tracheal surface, closure of the defect may result in stenosis of the trachea and recurrent pulmonary infection. However, leaving too much of the fistula permits a pocket to develop that can be a source of infection and of disturbing noisy respirations. It is well to divide the fistula about one eighth of an inch beyond the tracheal surface, to oversew this with 6-0 silk, and to turn the tissue in with a second continuous 6-0 silk suture.

The distal segment tends to retract away from the field when it is cut across, and, therefore, it is well to place a 6-0 silk suture through an edge so that it can be readily retrieved when it is needed for the reconstruction. It is also well to take a culture from the open end of the trachea to serve as a guide in chemotherapy postoperatively. By dividing the fistula during an initial part of the operation, one improves the infant's respiratory function.

Attention is now directed to the upper pouch. Usually it is readily identifiable. If there is any problem, a catheter can be passed down by the anesthesiologist, which identifies the upper segment. In order to prevent trauma to it, a dependent portion is selected and a 6-0 silk traction suture is placed through the hypertrophied upper segment. This serves as a method of maneuvering the upper segment during its freeing and obviates the necessity of frequently traumatizing it through the use of forceps. The upper esophageal segment should be freed high into the neck. This can be accomplished quite readily in all quadrants except that adjacent to the trachea. Here it is usually quite adherent and requires careful sharp dissection so that neither tracheal nor esophageal lumen is opened. The adherence of the two segments is most dense at the lower end of the pouch. Once the two structures have begun to be separated, the dissection is easier the higher it progresses into the neck. Every effort should be made to achieve as much length from the upper segment as possible.

Management of the lower segment is debated. Some surgeons believe that considerable freeing of the lower segment is advisable to gain length. However, it has been found that extensive mobilization of the lower segment potentiates a hiatus hernia and dysfunction of the esophagus of a degree that can be troublesome postoperatively. For this reason, extensive freeing of the lower segment has been abandoned by most surgeons. Some surgeons free the lower segment very little. If it is to be freed moderately, there is usually loss of a short segment from ischemia. However, this has some advantage because a larger, somewhat thicker structure is thus made available for the anastomosis.

While it is quite convenient to place clamps across the lower esophageal segment to hold it in place during the anastomosis, this undoubtedly has some detrimental effect on this delicate structure. Therefore it is our practice to perform the anastomosis without any crushing clamps on the esophagus. The upper segment is dealt with by cutting out a circular bit of the hypertrophied muscular wall. Care must be taken to grasp the mucosa and not to permit it to slip away so that it cannot be used for the anastomosis. Often, before the mucosa is opened a 6-0 silk suture is placed through it so that once it is opened the edge can be retrieved for the anastomosis. The first muscular layer of sutures is through the muscular coat of the two segments, and it is preferable to place five or six sutures and then to draw these together gently so that the strain is distributed over a considerable portion of the lower esophageal segment (Fig. 8F). This is particularly true when a gap of 2 to 3 cm must be overcome. Once the five or six sutures posteriorly are tied, the two end sutures are left for identification. The mucosa of the two segments is then brought together with a row of interrupted 6-0 silk sutures and the anastomosis completed with a row of interrupted 6-0 silk sutures to the muscular segments of the two parts of the esophagus (Figs. 8G and 8H).

Various maneuvers have been suggested to prevent the recurrence of tracheoesophageal fistula, a complication reported as high as 5 percent in some series. In our own experience, it has not occurred. We have practiced stabilizing the upper thickened esophageal segment by placing one or two sutures through the muscular coat and attaching it to

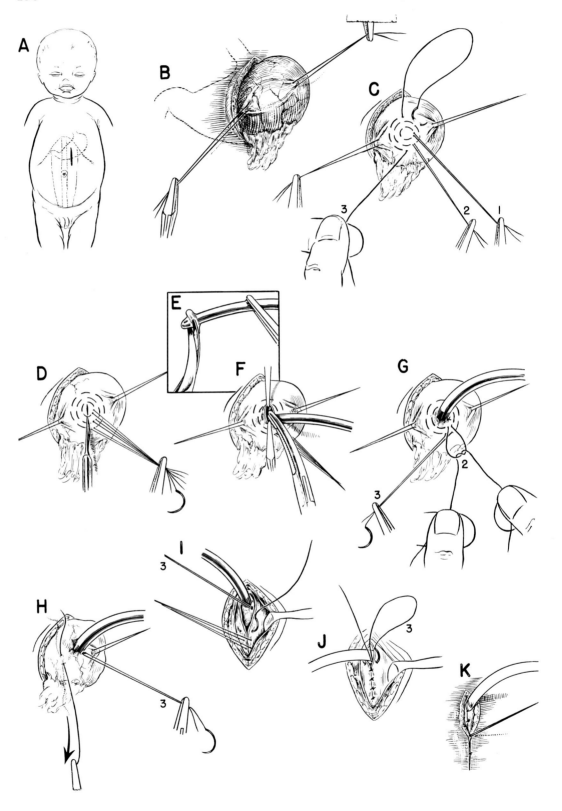

the paravertebral fascia, drawing it away from the tracheal closure. This stabilizes the anastomosis and also places the anastomosis 1 cm or more away from the tracheal closure, thus minimizing the possibility of a recurrence (Fig. 8I).

It is our practice to place a thin rubber dam drain down to the anastomosis. While the exposure using the extrapleural technique is somewhat more time-consuming than a transpleural approach, the closure is simple, and considerable time can be gained in this stage of the operation. Closure is accomplished by bringing the muscular layers back together with a row of 5-0 silk sutures. The skin is brought together with interrupted silk sutures. Should a small opening have been made in the pleura, it is best to enlarge it away from the site of the anastomosis. The baby's crying as soon as he recovers from anesthesia will push the air out through the drain. The tortuous drain route prevents re-entry of air into the retropleural space.

POSTOPERATIVE CARE

The first step in the postoperative care is to clean the mouth and pharynx carefully after removal of the endotracheal tube. There may be particles and congealed mucus that can either be inhaled or enter and obstruct the new anastomosis.

During the course of the operation, all sponges used should be weighed, and blood should be administered in an amount equal to this weighed volume plus 25 percent. Postoperatively, the baby should be placed in an oxygen tent with cold vapor and given fluids sparingly. A total of 100 to 125 ml of fluids parenterally per day is usually sufficient. A gastrostomy should be performed under local anesthesia 24 hours after the chest operation. A short, vertical, left rectus-splitting incision beginning 1 cm below the costal margin is preferred (Fig. 9). A simple Stamm gastrostomy is serviceable and easily made in these infants, whose stomachs are small. Three concentric pursestring sutures of 5-0 silk are used, and an opening into the stomach is made in the center of these. A small mushroom catheter is preferable for the gastrostomy. Cutting half the mushroom away decreases the likelihood of the tube becoming blocked by a curd clot in the distal end of the tube. Gastrostomy feedings are started six hours after completion of the gastrostomy; at first glucose water is used, then full formula. This permits discontinuation of parenteral fluid and supplies the infant with his caloric needs. On the tenth postoperative day, oral feedings are begun, and the infant will take a full formula by mouth within 48 to 72 hours. When oral feedings are well established the gastrostomy tube is removed, and leakage from the fistula rarely persists for more than 12 to 24 hours. In some instances where there is no tension on the anastomosis, gastrostomy can be dispensed with and oral feedings begun 24 hours after operation.

The patient is then placed in an isolette with high humidity. The object of the humidity is to thin bronchial secretions so that they can be dealt with effectively by the infant. Oxygen is given as needed. When there is no cyanosis and when respirations are not labored or increased in rate, little is accomplished by administering oxygen. Obtaining blood from a heel prick for the determination of pH and PCO_2 values is important. The presence of respiratory acidosis indicates that

---

Fig. 9 (opposite page). Technique of gastrostomy. A. The position of the incision is indicated. B. The fundus of the stomach has been delivered, and two traction sutures of 4-0 silk have been placed. C. Three concentric purse-string sutures of 5-0 black silk are placed. D. An opening is made through the stomach inside the silk sutures. E. The distal half of the mushroom catheter is excised. This is to prevent milk curds from forming and plugging the catheter. F. The mushroom catheter is inserted into the stomach. G. The first purse-string suture has been tied. H. All of the purse-string sutures have been tied. The last one is not cut. I. The peritoneum is closed with interrupted 5-0 black silk sutures. J. The last purse-string suture is used to attach the gastrostomy site to the anterior abdominal wall. The fascia is then closed with interrupted black silk sutures. K. The skin is closed with interrupted black silk subcuticular sutures. The wound is painted with collodion.

respiratory assistance must be provided. Initially, this can be accomplished by means of an endotracheal tube. It is only after this has been used for a considerable period of time that tracheotomy is resorted to. Should the patient be placed on assisted respirations repeated determinations of PCO_2 must be performed to test the adequacy of the assisted respirations. Preventing cyanotic episodes in the postoperative period is very important. Once these occur and are repeated, there seems to be an inevitable course of events with respiratory apnea causing an eventual demise. Paying more attention to the PCO_2 should reduce the frequency of this complication. Constant nursing attention is imperative. A small bit of mucus can produce a cyanotic episode, and unless a nurse is readily available it may result in a fatality. It is our practice to monitor these babies with various devices so that the heart rate is constantly known. This is important, for a slowing of the heart rate often warns the attending nurse that respiratory function is inadequate and gives her an opportunity to call for help before a disaster occurs.

The fluid requirements of these babies postoperatively is not great. Certainly it is better to keep them rather dehydrated than to provide excess amounts of fluid. We have found that our computed value of 1,200 ml per square meter is certainly adequate and can be reduced somewhat without detrimental effects on the patient and with some advantages.

It is our practice to perform a gastrostomy 24 to 48 hours after the initial repair. This is usually performed with local anesthesia. Some surgeons perfer to use a nasogastric polyethylene tube that traverses the anastomosis. We believe that such a tube may be an embarrassment to the child's pulmonary function, and since this is his most vulnerable area, we prefer to omit its use in these critical situations. When there has been an ample anastomosis with no tension, feedings can be started on the seventh or eighth day. In all patients we start feedings on the tenth postoperative day. If a leak occurs, feedings

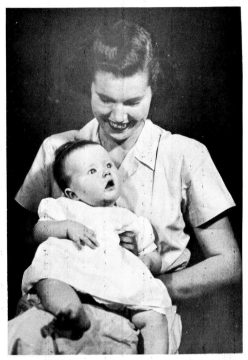

Fig. 10. Photograph of a baby who had a tracheo-esophageal fistula repaired.

are delayed until the leak has closed and radiographic examination reveals that there is no pocket at the area of the anastomosis (Fig. 10).

COMPLICATIONS

These infants are subject to the most bizarre postoperative complications. Extensive mediastinitis has not been a complication, probably because drains have been used. The drain has been removed on the fifth or sixth day after operation, and there have been esophagocutaneous fistulas in several patients, but all closed spontaneously. Recurrence of the tracheoesophageal fistula (Fig. 11) was not observed in a group of 78 patients. In this series of 78 patients, 18 postoperative deaths occurred, and 12 of these were caused by the development of infection in patients on whom the diagnosis of fistula was made later than the fourth day of life. In the other six, prematurity, malformations of the heart, and other serious deformities of

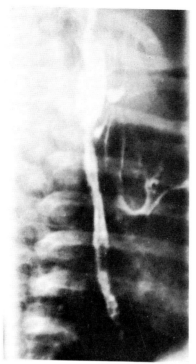

Fig. 11. Roentgenogram demonstrating a post-operative recurrent tracheoesophageal fistula.

the gastrointestinal tract were factors contributing to the fatal outcome. Prematurity was frequently a complicating cause of death. Infants who develop repeated bouts of cyanosis postoperatively rarely recover. These bouts of cyanosis are not directly associated with pulmonary pathology but seem rather to be related to defects in the central nervous system. Chemotherapy should be carefully administered postoperatively, penicillin and streptomycin being most satisfactory.

About one third of the patients required one or two dilations postoperatively. In determining which patients need dilation, one must rely entirely upon the patient's clinical behavior, not upon esophagograms (Fig. 12). If the roentgen criterion were used exclusively, one would dilate practically all these patients. Dilation is accomplished under general anesthesia. Utilizing a small bronchoscope, the esophageal stricture is visualized and a urethral filiform is passed through it. A small dilator is attached to the filiform

and, as the filiform tip is through the stricture, the dilation is readily and safely accomplished, provided that the procedure is terminated when more than gentle force is required to push the dilator through the stricture or when bleeding occurs.

ARTIFICIAL ESOPHAGUS

There are rare anomalies of the esophagus, such as the absence of a long distal segment in patients who have no tracheoesophageal fistula, that require that substitution for the esophagus be made if the child is to eat normally. Rarely is the gap between the two segments in a patient with atresia and tracheoesophageal fistula of a length to preclude end-to-end anastomosis. In the author's experience, only one such situation was encountered in 78 patients. A surgeon operating on these patients should make every

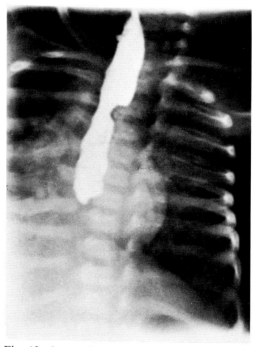

Fig. 12. An esophagogram on a patient who has had a tracheoesophageal fistula repaired. Note the narrowing at the suture line. This is not sufficient indication for dilation. It is far better to evaluate the patient's symptoms and to perform dilations on such grounds rather than on the appearance of esophagograms.

effort to achieve end-to-end anastomosis, for, if he is unsuccessful and the infant survives, there will eventually be the problem of how to make it possible for the child to eat normally. There is no easy solution to this situation despite the attention this problem has received from surgeons for several decades.

ANTERIOR THORACIC ESOPHAGUS

Any artificial esophagus, regardless of whether it is a skin tube or intestine, does not function well if attached directly to the stomach. The reflux of acid secretions into the artificial esophagus produces stricture, ulceration, and even perforation. To prevent such disastrous complications, the artificial esophagus can be attached to the proximal jejunum, thus bypassing the stomach. However, this anatomical arrangement, too, has unexpected disadvantages. The first is a tendency for the children to be thin and below average in weight and height. Some have also developed a pernicious anemia-like blood picture despite the fact that the stomach is in place. Presumably, this is related to the fact that the stomach is bypassed. The anemia is fairly resistant to treatment, although some help is derived from vitamin B_{12}.

Sweet (1964) suggested moving the stomach into the chest and anastomosing it to the esophageal segment in the neck (Fig. 13). This is an extensive but feasible procedure. Postoperatively, these infants have difficulty taking normal amounts of formula, but as they grow older they become able to eat fairly normal-sized meals. There is also a tendency for stricture formation at the esophagogastric anastomosis.

A subcutaneous esophagus made of skin or small intestine is successful, provided that it is connected to the proximal jejunum rather than to the stomach. Full-thickness skin is required if a dermal esophagus is contemplated. The defect in skin is conveniently covered with a Thiersch graft. A simpler method involves using proximal jejunum, and in all but exceptional situations a length can be developed long enough to be anas-

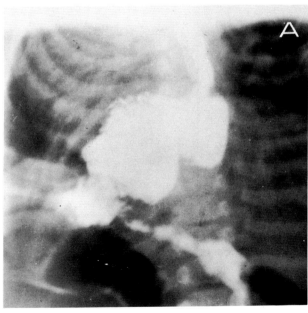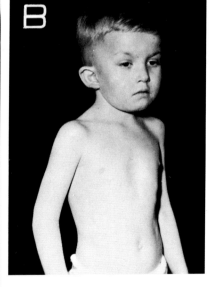

Fig. 13. A. Roentgenogram of patient with atresia of the esophagus without tracheoesophageal fistula. Repair was accomplished at five days of age. The entire stomach was brought into the chest and anastomosed to the upper esophageal segment. B. The patient at five years of age. He is somewhat below normal in size and weight.

tomosed to the esophagus in the neck (Fig. 14). This length is developed by dividing three or four mesenteric vessels, leaving an arcade to supply the freed jejunum.

Theoretically, the best procedure would be to use a segment of small or large intestine to bridge the gap between the two esophageal segments, utilizing the lower esophageal segment as well as the proximal one. This would preserve a normal esophagogastric junction and would prevent the complications of direct anastomosis to the stomach. It would also avoid the long-term problems associated with bypassing the stomach.

The great disadvantage is the immediate danger of the operation, which stems from the fact that the vitality of the intestine is dependent on a long single vascular pedicle that extends from the abdominal cavity through the diaphragm into the chest. In a series of patients in whom I used small intestine subcutaneously in the anterior chest wall, the blood supply failed in one. Resection of the subcutaneous necrotic intestine was accomplished, and the child lived. If the blood supply failed with intestine implanted to the mediastinum, a fatality would be almost inevitable.

Balancing all of these factors, it seems that the use of transverse colon to bridge the gap in the esophagus is the most desirable procedure, with the lower esophagus preserving the normal esophagogastric junction. In a personal communication to the author, Waterston notes success with this method in a large series of patients. The greater immediate risk of this procedure compared with that of the subcutaneous esophagus is accepted in the hope of more normal deglutition and fewer delayed complications (Fig. 15).

The most popular operation for esophageal reconstruction consists of using the transverse colon retrosternally as a segment uniting the upper esophagus and the stomach. The transverse colon is divided a few centimeters from the cecum and again in the distal transverse colon. Some surgeons use the ileocecal valve dividing the intestine a few centimeters above the cecal junction.

This has the advantage of limiting gastric reflux into the upper esophagus.

The distal part of the colon is anastomosed away from the pylorus in order to minimize reflux during gastric peristalsis. This is a two-layer anastomosis using 6-0 or 5-0 silk interrupted sutures, the first layer to the mucosa and the second layer to the seromuscular coats.

An incision is then made below the sternum and the mediastinal tissue pushed from the under sternal surface by blunt dissection. A similar incision is then made to accomplish a similar dissection from above. Ample room must be provided for the colon, yet openings into the pleural spaces must be guarded against. Pulling the colon through the retrosternal space must be done with gentle traction to prevent damage to the segment's precarious blood supply.

When the colon is in place an anastomosis is made to the upper esophagus, provided that the blood supply is adequate in the colon. When it is questionable, the anastomosis is delayed for two or three weeks. The anastomosis is made with two layers of interrupted 6-0 silk, one to the mucosa and the second to the seromuscular layers. This operation is associated with many complications, the commonest ones being leaks at the esophagocolonic junction, stricture at the anastomosis, and gastric reflux. Originally the colon mucosa was considered immune to gastric secretions. With longer postoperative follow-ups, this assumption has been proved incorrect, for troublesome erosions of the colon above the gastric junction have been reported.

H-TYPE FISTULA

There are three groups of patients who require special attention. First is the group of patients with the H-type fistula. This lesion is often overlooked for several days or weeks. There is invariably a history of coughing with feedings. Any neonate who consistently coughs immediately following or during feedings should be carefully exam-

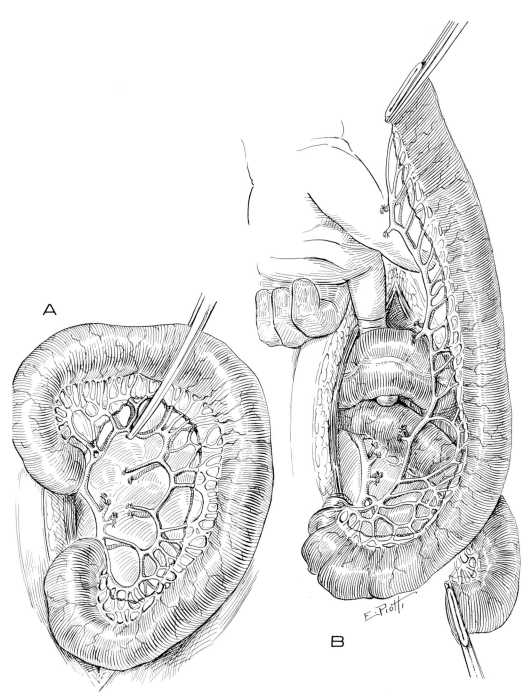

A

B

Fig. 14. Anterior thoracic esophagoplasty. A. The beginning step in the preparation of a loop of proximal jejunum. Note that the intestinal vessels have been ligated close to their points of origin so that
an arcade is maintained intact to supply the freed segment of jejunum. B. The vessels have been ligated,
and the bowel has been divided between clamps. The bowel passes posterior to the colon through the
mesocolon.

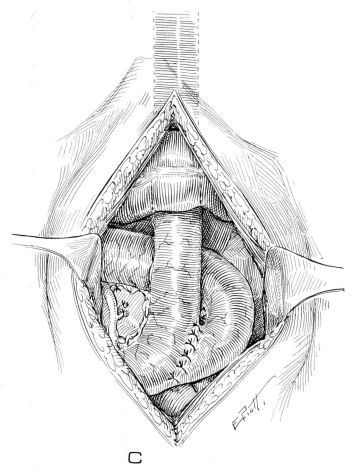

C

Fig. 14 (cont.). Anterior thoracic esophagoplasty. C. The end-to-side anastomosis has been made to restore continuity of the intestinal tract. The freed end of jejunum is brought up through the abdominal wall into the subcuticular tissue. If the end of jejunum is long enough and has an adequate blood supply, it can be anastomosed to the esophageal stoma in the neck. If the end of jejunum is not long enough, the gap between the esophageal fistula and the end of the jejunum may be bridged with a skin tube.

ined. The most effective method of locating this lesion is to have the patient ingest contrast material during an examination with cinefluorography. Often the lesion is not detected at the fluoroscopic screen. Rather it is identified when the cine films are reviewed. This is the type of lesion that can be overlooked and that has been undetected until adult life. The level of the lesion is important to determine, for this establishes the method of repair. When it is in the chest below the second or third dorsal vertebra it can be most conveniently approached through the chest. Here again a retropleural

approach is used in our clinic. Other centers use the transpleural approach. The important thing is to expose the lesion and to dissect above and below the fistula before it is divided. This gives control of the situation and assures that complete closure of both sides of the fistula is accomplished. This cannot invariably be done when the fistula is approached from one side only and cut without the other edge being exposed. It is our practice to use a continuous 6-0 silk suture on the tracheal side and to reinforce this with slight turn-in of the first row with a second continuous silk

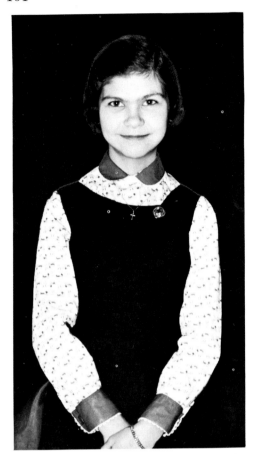

Fig. 15. Dr. Ladd's first successful repair of tracheo-esophageal fistula. This patient has an anterior thoracic esophagus that functions satisfactorily.

suture. The esophageal side is closed with two layers of interrupted silk sutures, one to the mucosal layer and the second to the muscular layer.

When the lesion is above the second dorsal vertebra, it can be conveniently approached from a cervical incision. It is preferable to approach it from the right side. A short transverse incision is made and the esophagus and trachea are exposed. Again the fistula is delineated by dissections above and below it, and then division and closure is done in a similar manner to that described for the chest approach. A drain is left in place so that development of a leak at the closure will result in an avenue of escape rather than in the development of a pocket and mediastinitis. These patients can oc-

casionally be managed without gastrostomy, particularly if a good closure has been achieved. In such situations feedings can be started on the first or second postoperative day.

ATRESIA OF THE ESOPHAGUS WITHOUT TRACHEOESOPHAGEAL FISTULA

Atresia of the esophagus without tracheo-esophageal fistula can be diagnosed by failure to pass a catheter into the stomach and by obtaining a roentgenogram of the abdomen. The absence of any air in the gastrointestinal tract establishes this diagnosis. The management of patients with this condition is different in some details from that of the average patient. It is known that in a considerable number of these patients the length of the lower esophageal segment varies a great deal. It may be of considerable length, but usually is not more than 1 or 2 cm in length. The length of the lower esophageal segment is important, and some surgeons advised that a thoracic exploration be performed to determine the extent of the lower segment. This does not seem to be a reasonable procedure, since the length of the lower esophageal segment can be determined in a simpler manner. These infants require gastrostomy, and at the time the gastrostomy is made a small cannula can be passed into the esophagus and the length of the esophagus determined by a roentgenogram with the probe in place. If necessary, it is possible to put a catheter up into the lower esophageal segment and to inject contrast material to delineate it completely. This is a far more simple procedure than subjecting the infant to a thoracic exploration. When the lower esophageal segment is only 1 cm or so in length and there is not an excessively long upper esophageal segment, it is best to exteriorize the upper esophageal segment. To assume that it is necessary to mobilize the upper esophageal segment through a chest incision in order eventually to exteriorize the esophagus to the surface of the neck is incorrect. We have exteriorized a considerable number of upper esophageal segments by a dissection limited to the neck. We prefer the right-sided approach. It is important to make a V-shaped incision in the skin so that there will be an adequate skin margin. Considerable contraction takes place, and unless this precaution is taken there will be a stricture of the esophagus at the cutaneous opening, which is disadvantageous to the patient. These patients are candidates for some type of procedure to provide an esophagus.

Howard (1965) published his experience with a patient of this type where the blind segments of the esophagus, particularly the upper segment, were elongated by dilation. Each day a weighted mercury bougie was passed into the upper segment, and by gentle pressure considerable elongation of the pouch took place (Fig. 16). We practiced

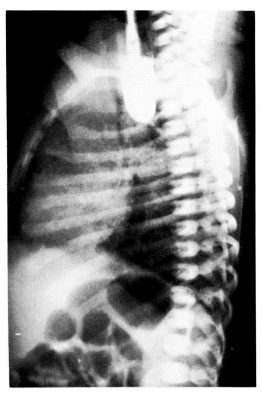

Fig. 16. Roentgenogram of a child with atresia of the esophagus. The upper segment contains some radiopaque material. A dilator is used to stretch and elongate the upper segment.

this and also gentle dilation of the lower segment, and in a selected case this has made it possible to perform an end-to-end anastomosis in a situation where we would previously have used elaborate procedures to construct a new esophagus. Certainly this is an adjunct to the care of these patients and should be tried when the lower esophageal segment is 3 or 4 cm long.

SPECIAL MANAGEMENT OF THE PREMATURE INFANT

It is generally known that the premature infant with this lesion suffers a higher mortality than does the full-term infant. Consequently it has been suggested by Holder (1962) that a staged repair would have some advantages, particularly in the very premature infant. It is proposed that the patient have a division of the tracheoesophageal fistula and then gastrostomy; then the patient is placed on suction to the upper esophageal segment. A word of caution is necessary. Repeatedly there have been reports of attempts to ligate the fistula. The instance of recurrence of the tracheoesophageal fistula is so high that this technique should be abandoned. Rather the tracheoesophageal fistula should be divided and the fistula on the tracheal side closed as well as the esophageal end. It is a practice when this technique is utilized to wait until the child weighs 6 or 7 pounds before attempting a repair by direct anastomosis between the two segments. At the present time there is not a sufficiently large number of patients reported to determine whether this is superior to direct anastomosis. It would appear from the information available at this time that a somewhat better salvage rate can be achieved.

GENERAL CONSIDERATIONS

Attention recently has been called to the problems that these infants face after discharge from the hospital. Holinger (1965) has pointed out that anomalies of the larynx and trachea are not unknown in this group of patients and may be the cause of repeated bouts of pulmonary infection. All that one can do with this group of patients is to treat them as effectively as possible during these bouts. It has been his experience that if the infants survive for a year or more, the tracheal and laryngeal structures become adequate and the instance of pulmonary infection subsides.

A more serious delayed complication is stricture formation, and this occurs in a considerable number of the patients. It is reported by the combined study of the American Academy of Pediatrics that this occurs more frequently when the extrapleural route is used (Holder, 1964). This is probably related to the fact that survival occurs with that technique in a group of patients with a long gap between the two segments. Such patients are more susceptible to stricture formation. When the transpleural approach is used, such patients may not survive. It is wise to follow these patients carefully and to initiate early dilation when a stricture develops. Clatworthy (1955) pointed out the importance of this and of even returning and excising a stricture that will not yield to repeated dilation. This has considerable advantage. When the stricture is excised, it is found that there is adequate length to the esophagus, so that a new anastomosis can be made without tension and without recurrence of the stricture.

WINDOW COMMUNICATION BETWEEN THE TRACHEA AND ESOPHAGUS

A few cases of window communication between the trachea and the esophagus have been reported in the literature, and we have observed one patient. The defect consisted of the larynx and upper trachea and adjacent esophagus forming a common lumen. On radiographic examination our patient was diagnosed as having a simple H-type fistula. At operation performed through the neck the full extent of the lesion was exposed. The two structures were separated, and the larynx and trachea were made into normal tubular structures. These structures functioned satisfactorily. The esophagus was also reconstructed; however, the child could not swallow, and the inevitable aspiration resulted in recurrence and finally a fatal pneumonia.

CONGENITAL ESOPHAGEAL STRICTURES

The embryology of the esophagus offers no simple explanation for the occurrence of congenital esophageal strictures. A congenital stricture of the esophagus is usually a diaphragm-like structure with a small opening at one point, and this structural detail may be the explanation of why this obstruction is so readily corrected by one or two dilations.

Infants with esophageal strictures have few symptoms during the first 24 hours of life. If the stricture is very narrow, there may be excessive mucus because the normal oral secretions are prevented from passing through the esophagus into the stomach, but this phase of the symptomatology is rarely sufficiently dramatic to attract attention. Most infants with strictures will vomit after feeding begins, but since the amount may be small, both the parents and the physician may disregard it. It is important to question the mother about the type of vomitus, for if the regurgitation is caused by esophageal stricture the material will not be soured or curdled, since it has not entered the stomach and been subjected to the acid digestive juices. During a small feeding, there may be no vomiting, for these babies are able to retain a considerable amount of formula in the dilated esophagus. As the esophagus becomes filled, the feeding may regurgitate into the oropharynx, and the baby will gag and empty the dilated esophagus. The infants gain poorly or fail to gain at all, and aspiration pneumonia is a common complication. If the stricture is moderate, clinical manifestations may not appear until solid foods are eaten.

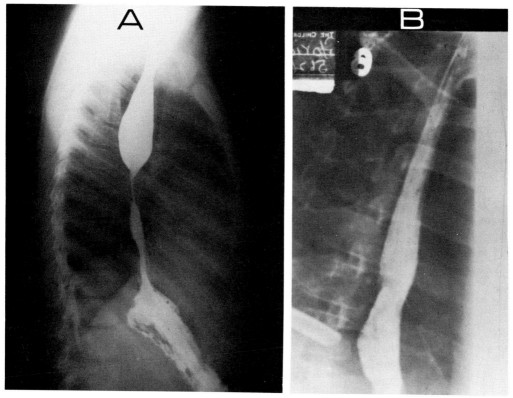

Fig. 17. A. Roentgenogram of a patient with stricture of the esophagus. Repeated dilations failed to correct the situation. B. Esophagram of same patient ten days after resection and end-to-end anastomosis of the esophagus.

DIAGNOSIS

The diagnosis depends upon a gastrointestinal roentgenogram, and the physician should specify that the esophagus be examined. Frequently, a gastrointestinal study is ordered for an infant with this type of vomiting. The routine in some hospitals is to give the barium solution on the ward, and the fluoroscopic examination is limited to the stomach and duodenum; consequently, defects of the esophagus may be overlooked. The diagnosis is obvious when the esophagus is examined fluoroscopically or when roentgenograms are made (Fig. 17). There is a widening of the esophagus above the stricture, and it is usually difficult to secure a clear outline of the stricture's length because the slow dribble of opaque material passing through the narrow point inadequately fills the esophagus beyond the obstruction.

The differential diagnosis should include pyloric stenosis and chalasia, both of which can be eliminated by a gastrointestinal radiographic examination. Another cause of esophageal obstruction is anomalies of the great vessels and aortic arch. The obstruction caused by a vascular ring is in the upper part of the esophagus, an infrequent site for a congenital esophageal stricture. Stridor and repeated bouts of pulmonary infection are associated with a vascular ring. Traumatic strictures of the esophagus frequently result from the ingestion of caustic material and tend to be multiple. These lesions are more often seen in the older age group, particularly in $2\frac{1}{2}$- to $3\frac{1}{2}$-year-old children who can move about and gain access to harmful solutions. Hiatus hernia may be associated with a stricture of the lower end of the esophagus that is caused by chronic esophagitis, but it is rarely encountered in the first week of life.

In this condition it is common for the vomitus to contain streaks of blood. Chalasia or reflux through a patent cardia will cause vomiting in young babies. Fluoroscopic examination of the esophagus with barium will demonstrate reflux of gastric contents into the esophagus when intra-abdominal pressure is increased or when the patient is placed in the Trendelenburg position.

The progress of patients with esophageal stricture depends on the degree of the obstruction. Some do quite well as long as the diet is entirely liquid. Others with a more severe degree of narrowing have difficulty even with liquids. Often, a single dilation will effectively eliminate the obstruction in those whose stricture is composed of a diaphragm with a small opening. If the obstruction consists of a thickening of the esophageal wall for a distance of 1 cm or more, several dilations may be required. The esophagus should be dilated at four-week intervals. A few patients with long strictures derive no permanent benefit from dilation. After a series of six to eight dilations without relief of symptoms, the surgeon should consider resection of the stricture with end-to-end anastomosis. Since the strictures are seldom excessive in length, they can be satisfactorily treated in this manner. The operation does not disturb the esophagogastric junction, and consequently it is not complicated by gastric reflux into the esophagus. Esophagogastrostomy is technically a sound operation for excision of strictures of the lower esophagus, but it may be complicated by free gastric reflux into the esophagus. Esophagogastros- and stricture formation. A surprisingly long segment of the esophagus can be removed and a successful end-to-end anastomosis accomplished. In a 1-year-old infant, 1 to 1½ in. of esophagus can be removed and the segments above and below mobilized sufficiently to permit end-to-end anastomosis. Segmental esophageal resection should be preceded by gastrostomy and the patient's general condition brought as near normal as possible before definitive treatment is instituted. By inserting a catheter through the gastrostomy into the esophagus and injecting barium into it, one can secure a roentgenographic outline of the lower part of the esophagus. When this is compared with roentgenograms made after a barium swallow, the length of the stricture can be determined.

OPERATION

The operation can be performed transpleurally. However, the extrapleural route has this advantage: If a leak develops at the suture line, an esophagocutaneous fistula forms, which is no hazard to the patient. However, if a fistula occurs when a transpleural approach has been used, a fatality may result. Intratracheal anesthesia should be used, and a vein cannula for administration of blood is mandatory. If the lesion is in the middle third of the esophagus, it can be approached most conveniently from the right side; if it is in the lower third, the left-side approach is preferable. Segments of two ribs as close to the vertebral bodies as possible are resected at the appropriate level. The muscle bundles between the ribs are ligated and divided, permitting the operator to separate the parietal pleura from the thoracic wall with a blunt dissector. Once this cleavage plane is established, the pleura is readily dissected from the thoracic wall, and the esophagus is exposed. Frequently, the external appearance of the esophagus does not indicate the site of the stricture. The anesthesiologist can readily pass a large rubber catheter down the esophagus; when the catheter arrives at the stricture, the surgeon, by palpation, determines the level of the lesion. After the position of the stricture has been determined, the esophagus is mobilized sufficiently to permit the ends to be sutured together with a minimum of tension (Fig. 18). If a 2-inch segment is to be resected, it is necessary for the thoracic esophagus to be freed by blunt dissection up to its cervical portion and down to the diaphragm. The esophagus in children has an excellent blood supply, as is demonstrated by the free bleed-

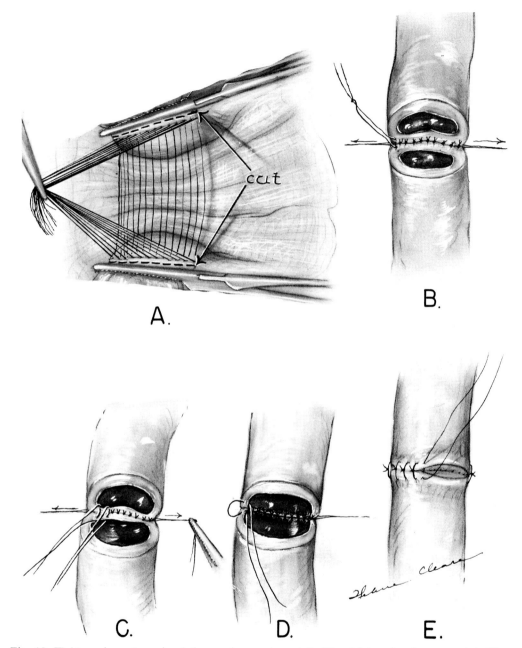

Fig. 18. End-to-end anastomosis of the esophagus. A. and B. The stricture has been resected. Clamps remain on the cut ends of the esophagus while the first row of interrupted silk sutures is placed. Before these sutures are tied, the esophagus is cut adjacent to the clamp so that there is a fresh cut edge of tissue for the anastomosis, the crushed tissue already having been resected with the clamps. The sutures are then brought together and tied as shown in B. C. The mucosa is sutured together with interrupted 5-0 silk sutures. D. The sutures through the mucosa on the posterior aspect have been placed and tied. E. After the mucosa has been brought together with interrupted silk sutures, the anastomosis is completed with interrupted silk sutures to the muscular coats. No cuff of tissue is turned in to obstruct the lumen of the diaphragm.

ing of the cut ends after the thoracic esophagus has been mobilized. It is convenient to place a pair of clamps across the esophagus on each side of the stricture and to excise the stricture by cutting between each pair of clamps. The pathologist should examine the resected segment immediately to determine that all the stricture has been excised. If an inadequate resection is made, the lumen at the site of the anastomosis will be narrower than the full size of the esophagus, and the postoperative result will be poor. It is convenient to leave the clamps on each end of the esophagus while the first row of interrupted silk sutures is placed through the muscular coats of the two segments. Thus, contamination is minimized. When the sutures have been placed on the posterior side, the esophagus again is cut across along the clamp, releasing the clamps and providing untraumatized tissue for the anastomosis. The row of sutures previously placed through the muscular coats posteriorly is now tied. The mucosal layers of the two segments are approximated with interrupted 6-0 silk sutures, with the knots placed inside the lumen to reduce the amount of foreign material in the tissue at the suture line. The anastomosis is completed by approximating the muscular coat with interrupted black silk sutures. This type of anastomosis does not turn in a diaphragm; consequently, a large functional stoma is provided. Animal experiments and clinical experience have demonstrated that the esophagus can be sutured under considerable tension with primary healing, provided that a meticulous water-tight anastomosis is made. A soft rubber drain is left in the wound, with the end adjacent to the anastomosis. The intercostal muscle, the muscular layer superficial to the ribs, and the skin are reapproximated with interrupted black silk sutures. Removal of the drain is advisable on the fifth postoperative day. After the patient is fed by gastrostomy for ten days, oral feedings are begun, and, if they are well tolerated, a full diet including solids is permitted. The patient is urged to take solids, since this provides a bolus that helps maintain adequate size of the lumen at the anastomosis. When oral feedings are fully established, the gastrostomy tube is removed. When the esophagus has been freed extensively and separated from the vagus nerves, there may be some difficulty in swallowing because of defective peristaltic activity. This will subside in three to four weeks.

DUPLICATIONS OF THE ESOPHAGUS

The development of duplications of the esophagus can readily be explained on an embryological basis. Although the esophagus has a lumen initially, it becomes partially solid during its subsequent development. The final lumen is established by the formation of vacuoles that coalesce. One of several vacuoles may fail to become connected with the esophageal lumen and remain as an isolated cyst adjacent to the esophagus. The duplication has a common muscular wall with the esophagus, and the lining membrane of the cyst frequently is partially composed of gastric mucosa, which accounts for the acid fluid in the cyst. Consequently, an intrathoracic cyst can often be identified by the aspiration of fluid and the determination of its pH. The acid fluid also accounts for such complications as ulceration, hemorrhage, and perforation of the duplication. Perforation is usually a slow process preceded by an inflammatory reaction, so that the duplication adheres to the lung, and the perforation takes place into the pulmonary tissue, eventually forming a communication between the duplication and one of the minor bronchi. Dysphagia is an unusual symptom, for the duplication rarely obstructs the esophageal lumen. The mass is more likely to exert pressure on the bronchial system and indirectly be the cause of repeated pulmonary infection. Occasionally, following several bouts of pneumonitis, chest films are taken and a smooth rounded tumor mass is revealed projecting into the lung field from the mediastinum (Fig. 19). Frequently, the lesion is discovered on a routine chest roent-

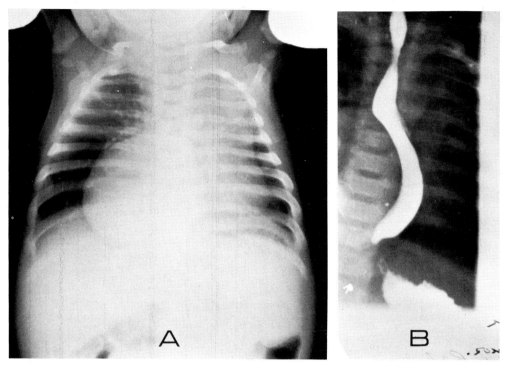

Fig. 19. A. Roentgenogram of chest outlining a duplication extending into the right chest. B. Esophagram of same patient.

genogram. In rare instances when perforation of the duplication occurs and a communication with the tracheobronchial tree is established. the patient may not only have symptoms of chronic pneumonia in one lobe but may also produce a copious amount of blood-tinged sputum. Unfortunately, when this complication has occurred, the pulmonary consolidation blurs the outline of the duplication, and for this reason the underlying cause of the pulmonary infection may remain obscure. The presence of a large, smooth mass projecting from the midline into the thoracic cavity is most likely an uncomplicated esophageal duplication. If an esophagogram is taken, the esophagus may be deviated from the midline because of pressure from the duplication. In the differential diagnosis, branchiogenic cysts should be considered. These tend to be in the midline in the area of the trachea bifurcation, projecting little if at all into the lung field. Dermoids the size of duplications rarely are encountered in children and are usually in the anterior mediastinum. Ganglioneuromas and neuroblastomas, which are often accompanied by erosion of either vertebral bodies or ribs, tend to be in the posterior mediastinum. They are irregular rather than smooth in outline. Likewise, lymphomas are irregular in outline because the tumor is composed of a mass of enlarged lymph nodes. Patients with lymphomas frequently have enlargement of the liver and spleen as well as generalized lymphadenopathy. Because duplications of the esophagus may increase in size and because those with gastric mucosa may ulcerate, causing perforation, it is advisable to remove them once the diagnosis is established.

OPERATION

Formerly, there was a tendency to marsupialize duplications to the skin of the chest wall and then to hope to destroy the mucosa with repeated curettage and application of a necrosing solution, such as tincture

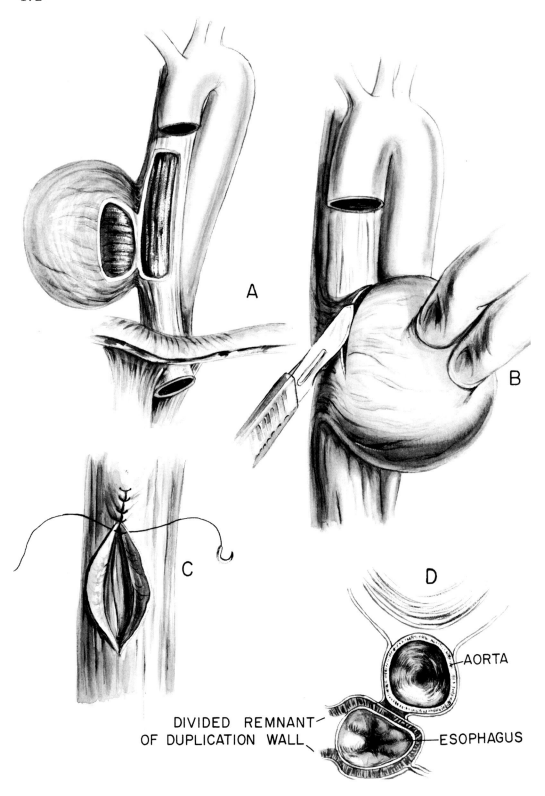

DIVIDED REMNANT
OF DUPLICATION WALL

AORTA

ESOPHAGUS

of iodine. This method of treatment was tedious and was often accompanied by excessive bleeding. Repeated treatments were necessary, and even then the duplication was not always eradicated completely. Consequently, excision is preferable when possible.

The operation is performed through an intercostal incision placed over the center of the duplication (Fig. 20). Usually, the lung is not attached to the duplication except when perforation has taken place, and, when this complication has occurred, lobectomy may be necessary. When dealing with large cysts, the exposure can be improved by aspirating a quantity of fluid, thus reducing the duplication in size. The pleura is incised over the duplication and the cyst mobilized except where it is attached to the esophagus. Since the esophagus and the duplication have a common muscular coat, there is no normal cleavage plane between the two structures, and this complicates the procedure of separating them. An incision should be made 1 or 2 cm from the esophagus on the cyst wall through the muscular coat to the mucosa of the duplication. The mucosa of the duplication is not opened but is separated from the muscular coat along this line of cleavage. Thus, the duplication can be removed without disturbing the esophageal wall. Occasionally, a line of cleavage can more readily be followed between the muscular wall and the esophageal mucosa. When the excision is performed in this manner, the muscle is sutured to cover the esophageal mucosa in order to restore the esophageal wall to normal thickness. If the esophageal mucosa is inadvertently opened, little harm results, provided that the perforation is carefully closed with interrupted silk sutures. After the duplication has been removed, the pleura is closed with interrupted silk sutures, the chest incision is closed, and

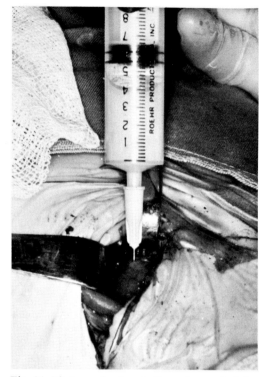

Fig. 21. Photograph of aspiration of a cervical duplication of esophagus.

a catheter is left in the pleural space for postoperative suction. This is particularly advisable when an opening has been made into the lumen of the esophagus. Oral feedings are offered 24 to 48 hours after operation.

On rare occasions a duplication of the esophagus will be found in the neck. These can be removed via a transverse neck incision. Identification of the cyst as a duplication is accomplished by aspiration of fluid and by determination of the fluid pH. An acid fluid identifies a duplication. This maneuver also decreases the size of the mass so that its removal by the same technique as described for intrathoracic duplication can be accomplished (Fig. 21).

Fig. 20 (opposite page). Operation for excision of esophageal duplication. A. A duplication of the esophagus. Note that there is a common muscular wall between the duplication and the esophageal lumen. B. An incision is made through the muscular wall of the duplication adjacent to its base. C. The duplication is removed as shown. The esophageal mucosa is left intact. D. The muscular layer is closed over the exposed esophageal mucosa with interrupted black silk sutures. Should the esophageal mucosa be inadvertently opened, it is likewise closed with interrupted 5-0 black silk sutures.

PERFORATION
OF ESOPHAGUS

If a foreign body is not removed, perforation of the esophagus occurs. If the perforation takes place where the pleura is adjacent to the esophagus, an esophagopleural fistula may develop with pyopneumothorax in addition to mediastinitis. Such complications are rare today; but when they do occur, the mortality is high. Treatment consists of inserting an intercostal catheter into the pleural space. The catheter is attached to an underwater seal system to which negative pressure can be applied if necessary to evacuate the pyopneumothorax.

Because of the chronic infection that is inevitably present with slow esophageal perforations, it is usually futile to attempt to close them surgically. Frequently, the fistula recurs as a large opening, and the child has only been made worse by an extensive operative procedure.

In those instances in which esophageal perforation occurs into the mediastinum, severe and spreading infection will occur. Such patients will have a septic type of fever and an elevated white blood count without detectable evidence of local infection. Chest roentgenograms will often reveal a widening of the mediastinal shadow. These patients should be treated by intensive administration of a wide-spectrum antibiotic. If these measures fail to control the infection and particularly if a mediastinal abscess develops, drainage should be undertaken. A paravertebral extrapleural approach is used, with resection of one or two ribs posteriorly at the level indicated by the widening of the mediastinum on a chest roentgenogram. Great care must be exercised to preserve the parietal pleura, and a Penrose drain filled with gauze should be left in place.

Traumatic perforation of the esophagus is usually caused by a complication of instrumentation. The patient will develop fever, or, if the tear communicates with the pleura, a tension pneumothorax will develop, which can prove fatal unless it is recognized and

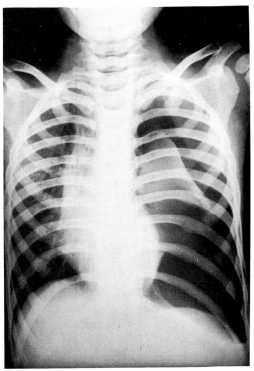

Fig. 22. Roentgenogram of chest following perforation of esophagus. There is a left pneumothorax.

treated promptly (Fig. 22). When this complication occurs, treatment consists of relief of the pyopneumothorax with an intercostal drainage tube to which moderate suction is applied. This plus gastrostomy for feeding and intensive antibiotic treatment usually is successful.

When the acute esophageal perforation is not associated with a pleural communication, gastrostomy for feeding and antibiotic therapy may suffice, provided that the perforation is small. When ingestion of contrast material outlines a large opening and the puddling of contrast material in the mediastinum, extrapleural drainage is indicated. Rarely is it helpful to attempt a direct closure of the esophageal opening, particularly when there has been an interval of several hours between perforation and treatment. In such situations infection has become established, and suturing of the opening will usually fail. Hence, in such situations extrapleural mediastinal drainage and gastrostomy offer optimal surgical therapy.

If the esophageal perforation is in the superior part of the chest and the resulting abscess is in the superior mediastinum, drainage can be established by making a low lateral incision in the neck. The dissection is made medial to the sternocleidomastoid muscle and carotid sheath, and lateral to the trachea. An esophagocutaneous fistula is common after mediastinal drainage. Such a fistula invariably closes spontaneously.

A major part of the treatment of all patients with esophageal perforation is gastrostomy, which places the esophagus at rest and promotes healing at the site of perforation. Removal of the foreign body is not undertaken until the patient has made a recovery from the acute infection. Great skill is required to locate the foreign body because of the local inflamation and granulation tissue.

ORVAR SWENSON

REFERENCES

ABLE, L. W. Tracheo-esophageal fistula without esophageal atresia. Texas J. Med., 61: 22, 1965.

CLATWORTHY, H. W., Jr. Esophageal atresia: Importance of early diagnosis and adequate treatment illustrated by a series of patients. Pediatrics, 16: 122, 1955.

DE BOER, A., and POTTS, W. J. Congenital atresia of the esophagus with tracheo-esophageal fistula. Surg. Gynec. Obstet., 104: 475, 1957.

DeMONG, C. V., GROW, J. B., and HEITZMAN, G. C. Congenital tracheo-esophageal fistula without atresia of the esophagus. Amer. Surg., 25: 156, 1959.

DESJARDINS, J. G., STEPHENS, C. A., and MOES, C. A. F. Results of surgical treatment of congenital tracheo-esophageal fistula, with a note on cine-fluorographic findings. Ann. Surg., 160: No. 1, 1964.

FERGUSON, C. C., and SCHOEMPERLEN, C. B. Congenital tracheo-esophageal fistula in an adult. Ann. Surg., 149: 582, 1959.

HAIGHT, C. Congenital atresia of the esophagus with tracheo-esophageal fistula. Ann. Surg., 120: 623, 1944.

——— Congenital tracheo-esophageal fistula without esophageal atresia. J. Thorac. Surg., 17: 600, 1948.

HAYS, D. M., and SNYDER, W. H., Jr. Results of conventional operative procedures for esophageal atresia in premature infants. Amer. J. Surg., 106: 19, 1963.

HOLDER, T. M. Transpleural versus retropleural approach for repair of tracheo-esophageal fistula. Surg. Clin. N. Amer., 44: No. 6, 1944.

——— CLOUD, D. T., LEWIS, J. E., Jr., and PILLING, G. P., IV. Esophageal atresia and tracheoesophageal fistula. Pediatrics, 34: 542, 1964.

——— McDONALD, V. G., Jr., WOOLLEY, M. M., and GROSS, R. E. The premature or critically

ill infant with esophageal atresia: Increased success in a staged approach. J. Thorac. Cardiov. Surg., 44: 344, 1962.

HOLINGER, P. H., BROWN, W. T., and MAURIZI, D. G. Endoscopic aspects of post-surgical management of congenital esophageal atresia and tracheo-esophageal fistula. J. Thorac. Cardiov. Surg., 49: No. 1, 22, 1965.

HOWARD, R., and MYERS, N. A. Esophageal atresia. A technique for elongating the upper pouch. Surgery, 58: 725, 1965.

HUMPHREYS, G. H., HOGG, B. M., and FERRER, J. Congenital atresia of esophagus. J. Thorac. Surg., 32: No. 3, 332, 1956.

——— and FERRER, J. Management of esophageal atresia. Amer. J. Surg., 107: 406, 1964.

KELLEN, D. A., and GREENLEE, H. B. Transcervical repair of H-type congenital tracheo-esophageal fistula. Ann. Surg., Vol. 162: No. 1, 1965.

KOOP, C. E., and VERHAGEN, A. D. Early management of atresia of the esophagus. Surg. Gynec. Obstet., 113: 103, 1961.

LADD, W. E. Surgical treatment of esophageal atresia and tracheo-esophageal fistula. N. Eng. J. Med., 230: 625, 1944.

——— and SWENSON, O. Esophageal atresia and tracheo-esophageal fistula. Ann. Surg., 125: 23, 1947.

LANMAN, T. H. Congenital atresia of esophagus. Arch. Surg., 41: 1060, 1940.

LEVEN, N. L. Congenital atresia of esophagus with tracheo-esophageal fistula. J. Thorac. Surg., 10: 648, 1941.

MACKENZIE, M. A Manual of Diseases of the Throat and Nose. New York, William Wood and Co., 1884, Vol. 2, p. 149.

MARTIN, L. Exposé des travaux de 1 Soc. roy. de. méd. de Marseille. Marseille, Kreuter, Legrand, Weber, 1821, p. 44.

MINNIS, J. F., Jr., BURKO, H., and BREVETTI, G. Segmental duplication of the esophagus associated with esophageal atresia and tracheo-esophageal fistula. Ann. Surg., 156: 271, 1962.

MINTON, J. P., and CLATWORTHY, H. W., Jr. Congenital esophageal atresia: A report of improved survival of infants through prompt recognition and surgical correction. Ohio Med. J., 58: No. 11, 1962.

POTTS, W. J., and IDRISS, F. Review of our experience with and without complicating fistulae. Maryland Med. J., 1960.

SCHMITZ, J. A. Ueber die formale Genese der Oesophagusmissbildungen. Virchow. Arch. path. Anat., 247: 278, 1923.

SCHNEIDER, K. M., and BECKER, J. M. The "H-type" tracheo-esophageal fistula in infants and children. Surgery, 51: No. 5, 677, 1962.

SCHULTZ, L. R., and CLATWORTHY, H. W., Jr. Esophageal strictures after anastomosis in esophageal atresia. Arch. Surg., 87: 136, 1963.

SIEBER, W. K., and GIRDANY, B. R. Tracheo-esophageal fistula without esophageal atresia—congenital and recurrent. Pediatrics, 18: 935, 1956.

SMITH, E. I. The early development of the trachea and esophagus in relation to atresia of the esophagus and tracheo-esophageal fistula. Carnegie Institution of Washington Publication 611, Contribution to Embryology, 36: 41, 1957.

SWEET, R. H. Subtotal esophagectomy with high intrathoracic esophagogastric anastomosis in treatment of extensive cicatricial obliteration of esophagus. Surg. Gynec. Obstet., 83: 417, 1946.

SWENSON, O. End-to-end anastomosis of the esophagus for esophageal atresia. Surgery, 22: 324, 1947.

——— LIPMAN, R., FISHER, J. H., and DE LUCA, F. G. Repair and complications of esophageal atresia and tracheo-esophageal fistula. N. Eng. J. Med., 267: 960, 1962.

TUQAN, N. Annular stricture of the esophagus distal to congenital tracheo-esophageal fistula. Surgery, 52: No. 2, 394, 1962.

VOGT, E. C. Congenital esophageal atresia. Amer. J. Roentgen., 22: 463, 1922.

WOOLLEY, M. M., CHINNOCK, R. F., and PAUL, R. H. Premature twins with esophageal atresia and tracheo-esophageal fistula. Acta Pediatrica, 50: 423, 1961.

30

Herniations Through the Diaphragm

CONGENITAL DIAPHRAGMATIC HERNIA: BOCHDALEK HERNIA

Congenital diaphragmatic hernia is not too uncommon. In a study in England of neonatal deaths from diaphragmatic hernia, it was estimated that the instance was 1 in 2,200 births. The type of patient seen with diaphragmatic hernia has changed considerably in the last two decades. It was common 20 to 30 years ago to see a baby several months of age or children several years of age with the so-called upside-down stomach. It was rare at that time to see a baby less than two or three days of age with a diaphragmatic hernia. It is interesting that the mortality then was 15 to 20 percent. In the last two decades, this mortality figure has risen, and this is undoubtedly related to the fact that many babies under two or three days of age are recognized as having the condition and undergo surgical correction. The precarious condition of these young infants is reflected in a higher mortality in current series compared to those published two decades ago.

ETIOLOGY

The defect in embryological development responsible for diaphragmatic hernia is probably related to diaphragmatic formation and perhaps to the growth relationship of the abdominal cavity to the chest. It is known that the diaphragm develops from several quadrants and is completed when it unites in the central tendon. Growth of the intra-abdominal organs is accelerated at about the time union of the diaphragm occurs. It has been postulated that this rapid growth creates a disparity between accommodations within the abdominal cavity and the thoracic cavity, and this may be a factor in the failure of the diaphragm segments to assemble properly and in the resulting defect in the central tendon or in the posterolateral quadrant of the structure. The instance of left-sided hernias is considerably greater than that of right-sided ones, the figure usually being four out of five on the left side. The role of the liver in buttressing the formation of the complete diaphragm may be a factor in the lower instance on the right side.

PATHOLOGY

The lesion usually is in the posterolateral quadrant of the diaphragm. The size varies from a relatively small opening to a massive defect with a narrow rim of tissue lateral and posterior to the defect. Rare cases of hernia with complete absence of one diaphragm have been reported.

The number of patients with diaphragmatic defects who have a sac covering the abdominal viscera in the chest varies from series to series. Usually less than half of the patients with Bochdalek defects have a true hernial sac.

There is a definite relationship of malrotation in patients with diaphragmatic hernia. The instance of this also varies, being as high as 30 percent in some reported series. Usually it is nearer to 10 to 15 percent, and the number with obstruction is considerably lower. Other lesions of the gastrointestinal tract, obstructive in type, occur but are rare in their association with diaphragmatic hernia.

The development of the lung on the side of the hernia is abnormal in a number of cases and perhaps to a small degree in all cases. In the study of the British Perinatal Mortality Survey in 1958 (Butler, 1962), it was found that the ipsilateral lung weighed on the average of 3.7 g and on the opposite side a little over 4 g.

Normal lung weights are dependent on total body weight. Potter gives 64 g as the average in babies weighing 3750 to 4250 g. Snyder states that the lung weights were about 30 g in a small series of patients with diaphragmatic hernia. It would seem likely that the severe respiratory defect in some newborns with diaphragmatic hernia may be related to hypoplastic lungs as well as to mechanical displacement of the respiratory system. A careful study of lung weights in relation to body weight in patients with diaphragmatic hernia is needed. Postmortem material must be evaluated in regard to pathology in the lung, which may well increase the weight of a hypoplastic lung. It is true that in the majority of instances the lung on the ipsilateral side is adequate provided it is given an opportunity to slowly expand over a week or ten days.

There are instances of accessory lung that may or may not be connected to the bronchial system. Usually they are small and separated from the normal lung. Removal is wise, for they may be the source of infection if left in place.

There is a high incidence of associated lesions in the very young patients that die without benefit of therapy, the figure being as high as 50 percent. The associated anomalies are severe in nature, such as anencephalus, Arnold-Chiari syndrome, hydrocephalus, malformations of the heart, and omphalocele. For this reason, inspection of the diaphragm is wise when repairing omphalocele.

In reviewing clinical material, the babies that survive usually are relatively free of anomalies. Severe associated malformations usually contributed largely to the demise of the infant. It is interesting to note that in rare cases, the lesion may be bilateral. Only a few such cases have been reported, and it would appear that this instance is in the realm of less than 1 percent of patients.

DIAGNOSIS
SYMPTOMS AND PHYSICAL SIGNS

The baby with a diaphragmatic hernia usually has respiratory distress, may have cyanosis, and may occasionally vomit after feedings. The baby who has no cyanosis may develop this sign after an attempt at feeding that fills the upper gastrointestinal tract and thus further embarrasses the respiratory system. It is interesting that the hernias of the foramen of Bochdalek have been observed in patients in their fifth and sixth decades. Some of these patients have had few symptoms, particularly when herniated viscera is limited to small intestine and colon. However, when the stomach herniates into the thoracic cavity, the patient usually complains of epigastric pain and occasionally of shoulder pain.

On rare occasions there may be intestinal obstruction in part of the intestinal tract involved in the hernia. Patients with this condition may be quite asymptomatic until the obstruction occurs, and then they have both the symptomatology of intestinal obstruction and respiratory embarrassment.

The baby has respiratory distress, usually with rapid respirations and varying degrees of cyanosis. The cyanosis may be intermittent and follow attempts at feeding. The clinical picture is quite distinct, and a scaphoid

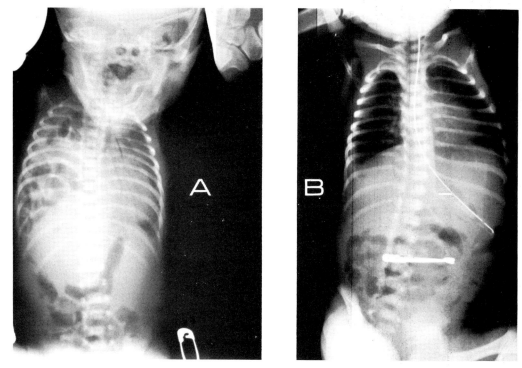

Fig. 1. A. Roentgenogram of neonate with massive right diaphragmatic hernia. B. Same patient 24 hours postoperatively. Note small residual of pneumothorax.

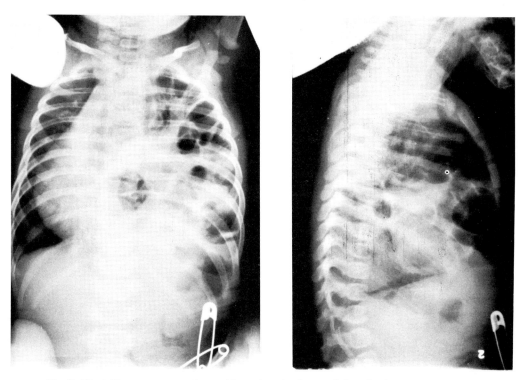

Fig. 2. Chest film, anteroposterior and lateral projection outlining diaphragmatic hernia.

abdomen smaller than the thorax usually confirms one's suspicion.

Changes in auscultation of the chest do occur, and there may be peristaltic sounds heard on the affected side. However, in small but normal babies there may be transmission of peristaltic sounds through a stethoscope applied to the chest. Displacement of the heart may be the most readily detected abnormality on physical examination. Because of these patients' small size, percussion and ausculatory signs are difficult to interpret. Therefore, we are dependent upon roentgenograms to establish the diagnosis. In most instances plain roentgenograms in the anteroposterior and lateral projections give ample evidence that a diaphragmatic hernia is present, for, in most instances, the presence of gas-filled intestine is characteristic (Figs. 1 and 2). There is an occasional situation where the baby may be afflicted with staphylococcus pneumonia and develop cystic structures within the lung field that may be indistinguishable from the air seen in intestine in the thoracic cavity. In these cases caused by infection there is usually fluid in the thoracic cavity, and this should give a clue and alert the physician and surgeon to investigate the patient further. Wherever there is the question of the presence of a staphylococcus pneumonia, or of some type of cystic disease in the lung, barium in limited amounts should be administered to the patients, and observing intestine filled with contrast material in the chest establishes the diagnosis (Fig. 3).

TREATMENT

Once the diagnosis has been made it is imperative to embark upon surgery promptly. This is particularly true for the neonate with severe respiratory difficulty and cyanosis. The mortality in this group is extremely high and probably cannot be lowered unless diagnosis and therapy becomes more prompt.

When the patient is first seen after the diagnosis has been made care should be taken not to use a mask technique for the administration of oxygen, particularly if posi-

tive pressure is to be used. The technique pemits air to be forced into the gastrointestinal system and intensifies the infants' distress. Rather, the baby should be promptly intubated and oxygen administered through the intratracheal tube. If respirations are to be assisted, care should be taken that excessive pressure is not used. Cases have been reported where a contralateral pneumothorax developed under tension and proved fatal because of its rapid encroachment on the small margin of pulmonary function these infants have. The cause was presumed to be excessive pressure during assisted respirations. This course of events is probably related to the higher compliance of the ipsilateral lung, so that any force exerted by assisted respiration is transferred mostly to the good lung. So far, no technique of assisted respiration has proven wholly successful in relieving the respiratory distress. Rather, prompt operation is the key to success.

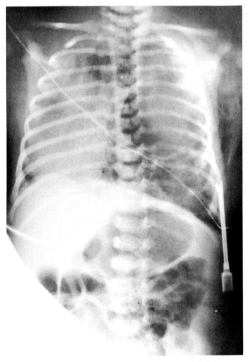

Fig. 3. Chest film of patient who had multiple congenital cysts of lung which appeared similiar to diaphragmatic hernia.

TYPE OF INCISION

OPERATIVE TECHNIQUE

There has been considerable debate about the type of incision that has the greatest advantage in a patient with diaphragmatic hernia. It would appear that in the neonate the most useful approach is through the abdomen. The reason for this is that such an approach gives the surgeon an opportunity to investigate the gastrointestinal tract and to be sure that no obstructive lesion is present.

Furthermore, repair of the diaphragmatic defect can readily be accomplished without any difficulty, since no force is necessary to bring the edges together. However, when a thoracic approach is used, closure of the diaphragm may prove to be extremely difficult because of increased intra-abdominal pressure. The third advantage of the abdominal approach is that a repair with only the skin can be utilized in those cases where the increase of intra-abdominal pressure would be prohibitive should an attempt be made to close all the layers of the abdominal wall. This is a safety measure that is associated with the abdominal approach and is denied to the surgeon when he uses the thoracic route. However, in the patient several months of age the thoracic approach has advantages. The behavior of such infants has demonstrated that the gastrointestinal tract is free of associated obstructive anomalies, thus freeing the surgeon from direct examination of the tract. In the older patient there is a second advantage to the thoracic approach. It is not infrequent to find adhesions that attach the intestine or other abdominal contents high in the thoracic cavity, and such adhesions may prove difficult to deal with when the abdominal approach is used. In the third place, the older patient, through the use of his gastrointestinal tract, has forced the abdominal cavity to become larger, and it is usually relatively simple to move the abdominal viscera out of the thoracic cavity into the abdominal cavity and to perform a repair of the diaphragmatic defect.

In the neonate a rectus muscle-splitting incision has distinct advantages. It is placed on the side where the hernia is present (Fig. 4). A muscle-retracting incision has a disadvantage should it become necessary to limit the closure to the skin. However, when a muscle-splitting incision is used there is prolapse of the abdominal contents through the deeper portions of the wound into the subcutaneous space. The first duty of the surgeon is to completely investigate the gastrointestinal tract. It may be necessary to inject saline with a syringe and fine needle into the small intestine and to demonstrate that there is no mechanical obstruction. In most instances, the patency of the gastrointestinal tract can be established without resorting to injection technique. Any abnormality, such as malrotation, should be corrected as a first step.

Occasionally it is difficult to remove the abdominal viscera from the thoracic cavity. This maneuver can be facilitated by passing a small rubber catheter up into the thoracic cavity and injecting a reasonable amount of air; this destroys the negative pressure and facilitates delivery of the abdominal contents from the chest. Care should be taken in removing the spleen. It is helpful not to do a splenectomy unless it is necessary, for there is some question about what defect in immune capabilities an infant has after splenectomy. However, at times there is an injury to the spleen or considerable congestion of the spleen so that it is fairly large, or both. In such situations one of the ways of providing more space in the abdominal cavity is to perform a splenectomy. However, this should be condemned except in cases of absolute necessity.

When there appears to be no rim of tissue in the posterolateral quadrant of the diaphragmatic defect, careful investigation should be made for a rim of tissue that can be freed from the thoracic cavity and become useful in repair of the defect. Two rows of interrupted 5-0 silk are placed, one on the

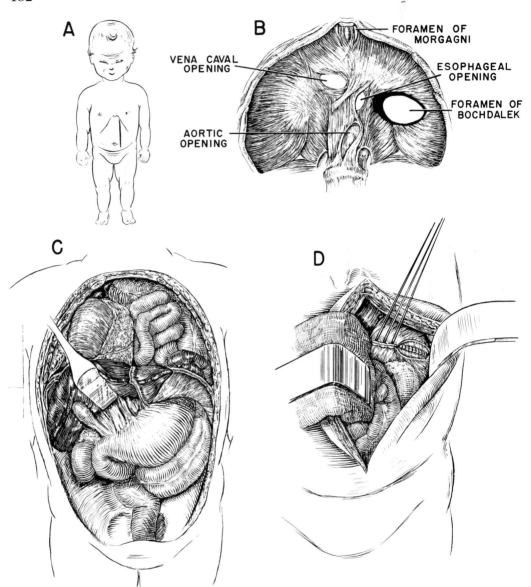

Fig. 4. Repair of left diaphragmatic hernia. A. Drawing indicating position of incision. B. Diagram of diaphragm indicating position of normal and abnormal openings. C. Drawing of left diaphragmatic hernia with small intestine and spleen in the thoracic cavity. D. Closure of diaphragmatic opening is accomplished with two rows of interrupted silk sutures, one to the pleural side and the other to the peritoneal side.

pleural side and one on the peritoneal side. These can be placed in the large defects on the pleural side first and gradually approximated and tied. This technique has the advantage that the force of bringing the defect together is distributed over the entire length of the defect. Crushing of the phrenic nerve is no longer practiced. It does not add to

survival and may actually increase the number of complications and thus give a higher mortality figure. Once the defect has been closed, an attempt is made to close the abdominal wall. It is unwise to produce a high intra-abdominal pressure by a persistent attempt to close the abdominal wall in layers. When this situation arises, and it probably

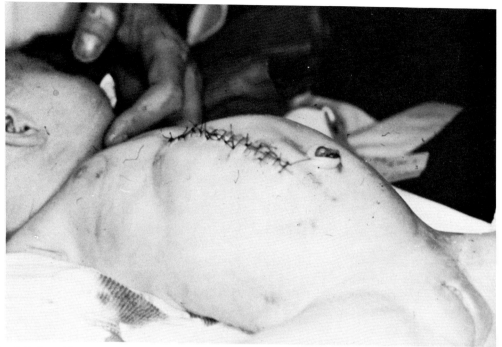

Fig. 5. Baby with a large right diaphragmatic hernia. Closure of the abdominal wall could not be accomplished. The skin was closed, and ten days later the abdominal cavity had accommodated to an extent that closure of the abdominal wall could be accomplished.

should not be encountered more than 15 percent of the time, it is wiser to free the skin extensively on both sides of the incision and to close the skin with a row of interrupted 5-0 silk sutures (Fig. 5). Adhesion formation is reduced by suturing the peritoneum to the anterior fascia on both sides of the incision. It is possible to go back 10 to 14 days after operation, when the abdominal cavity has enlarged and accommodated to the increased volume of viscera, and to perform closure of the abdominal wall in layers.

The management of the pneumothorax is debated. We have found that placing a catheter up into the thoracic cavity through the diaphragm and letting the anesthesiologist produce reasonable inspiratory pressure (not over 30 cm of water) will permit a lot of the pneumothorax to escape through the tube.

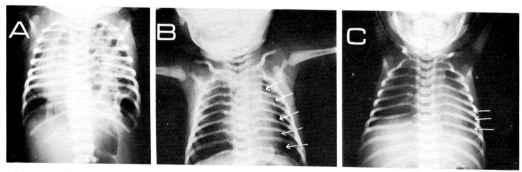

Fig. 6. A. Chest roentgenogram of infant with left diaphragmatic hernia. B. Same patient 24 hours after repair of the diaphragmatic hernia. Arrows indicate extent of pneumothorax. C. Same patient ten days later. The pneumothorax is minimal.

It should be clamped during expiratory phases to prevent reaccumulation of pneumothorax. It is not necessary to completely eliminate the pneumothorax. The expansion of the lung will take place in a gradual process and will be completed in 10 to 12 days (Fig. 6). The practice of using high suction for immediate expansion of the lung is to be condemned, for it has proven to be a dangerous procedure. Some authors favor leaving a tube in the thoracic cavity to permit expansion of the lung. In our experience this has not added to the care of the patients.

POSTOPERATIVE CARE

These patients present a complicated problem in postoperative care because of the fact that they have a defective respiratory system. They should be maintained in isolettes where temperature and humidity can be controlled and oxygen administered as needed. The important thing is to assist respiration when needed and to have blood gas analysis performed at frequent intervals so that the effectiveness of respiratory assistance can be assessed. It is the experience of some centers such as The Children's Hospital in Los Angeles that with great attention to this aspect of the postoperative care considerable improvement in survival rates can be anticipated.

CHALASIA

Chalasia is a relatively new clinical entity, described in the United States by Neuhauser and Berenberg (1947). The condition occurs in young infants. It is characterized by vomiting, and when it is severe it may be the cause of failure to gain weight or even of weight loss. Chalasia is probably more common than medical reports indicate, for, when the symptoms are mild and there is a normal weight gain, the radiographic examinations necessary to establish the diagnosis are rarely made.

Chalasia is probably related to a congenital abnormality of the hiatus and esophagogastric junction. Some believe it to be related invariably to hiatus hernia. Function of the normal esophagogastric junction is unknown. Furthermore, what structural or functional defects are the precursors of free gastric reflux into the esophagus are not understood. Vomiting and failure to gain weight beginning in the first or second week of life are the cardinal symptoms of chalasia, and on the basis of symptoms alone these infants are indistinguishable from babies with pyloric stenosis. The vomitus contains no bile. Chalasia should particularly be suspected in a baby who has a history consistent with pyloric stenosis but in whom a pyloric tumor cannot be detected by palpation. Only by fluoroscopic examination of the esophagus and stomach with barium can the reflux be observed and a diagnosis of chalasia made (Fig. 7). Radiographically, it is not possible in most instances to demonstrate any gastric mucosa above the hiatus, particularly in the early stages of the disease. Free reflux of barium from the stomach into the esophagus

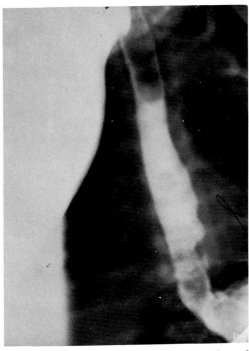

Fig. 7. Spot roentgenogram demonstrating reflux of barium through an open cardia into the esophagus. This patient has chalasia.

occurs when pressure is placed on the stomach. The mechanism of vomiting is such that, when refluxed gastric contents enter the hypopharynx, vomiting occurs. Treatment consists of thickening feedings (1:20 with farina) and maintaining the infants in upright position for an hour following each feeding. A small, well-padded chair into which the infant may be strapped is a convenient device to maintain the infant in upright position (Fig. 8).

As these children grow older, there is spontaneous improvement, and most of them will have a normal cardia when reexamined at two to three years of age. Some, however, develop reflux esophagitis and small hiatus hernia. The normally low gastric acidity of infants may account for the benign course of chalasia. Later, as acidity becomes normal, the infants are old enough to be in the upright position a good part of the time, and gravity counteracts reflux. Perhaps the few who do not progress will have high gastric acidity with the so-called ulcer diathesis. At any rate, some become problems, developing reflux esophagitis, stricture, and hiatus hernia—lesions that are resistant to treatment.

ACHALASIA

This condition, also referred to as cardiospasm, consists of what seems to be a stricture of the cardia and massive dilatation of the esophagus. In many respects, it seems comparable to the lesion seen fairly commonly in adults. A mechanical stricture does not exist, for at operation, when digital dilation is performed by means of a gastrostomy, there is no stricture. The cardia is tight but can be dilated in an infant, so that the index finger can be easily inserted. This absence of a fibrotic structure indicates that a defect in function is the basic pathology. There is some evidence in similar adult patients that there is dysfunction of the esophagus. This has not been true in two children we have studied by means of multiple balloons in the

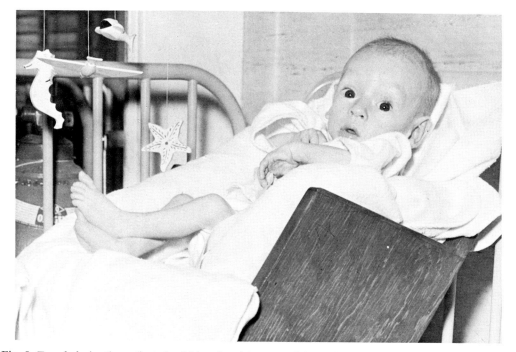

Fig. 8. For chalasia, the patient should be placed in an upright position for 30 or 40 minutes after eating, as shown here.

esophagus; both had what was considered to be normal peristalsis. Biopsy of the lower end of the esophagus contained no ganglion cells. More data are needed, but it seems that achalasia is a parasympathetic lesion with an aganglionic segment similar to Hirschsprung's disease.

DIAGNOSIS

Some children with achalasia may not develop symptoms until solids are started; others may have trouble in the first few weeks of life. Some patients may complain little of vomiting but will have a chronic cough and be underweight. A careful history will reveal a small food intake, consisting mostly of liquids, and occasional vomiting. The vomitus contains undigested food. Such cases may go undetected for years, since all attention is focused on the respiratory symptoms. A widened esophagus may be suspected from some chest roentgenograms on these children. An esophagogram outlines a massive esophagus and cardiospasm.

TREATMENT

In some cases, one or two vigorous dilations are curative (Fig. 9). A Plummer inflatable bag dilator is used, pumped to 8 pounds of pressure and maintained in position for 5 minutes. Such vigorous dilation is not without some danger of esophageal rupture, since it is effective presumably because some of the muscular layer is torn, leaving the mucosa intact. On the other hand, gentle dilations are not helpful. When two or three dilations fail to relieve the symptoms, a plastic operation to the esophageal gastric junction is indicated. The Heller operation seems to be the most effective in this condition. Under general anesthesia, with the child on the right side, a transtho-

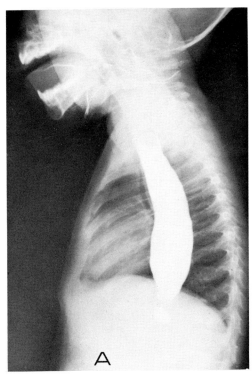
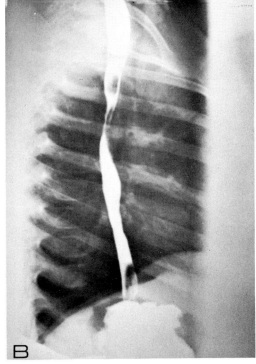

Fig. 9. A. Esophagogram of patient with achalasia. Treatment consisted of dilation on two occasions. B. Roentgenogram of same patient two years after treatment. Note normal size and configuration of the esophagus.

racic approach is made between the eighth and ninth ribs. The lung is packed away so that the lower mediastinal pleura is exposed. The pleura over the lower 5 to 6 cm of esophagus is divided, and the esophageal surface is exposed. Dissection around the esophagus is unnecessary and unwise, for damage to the vagal fibers may occur and augment esophageal dysfunction. The exact position of the cardia can be determined by passing a Miller-Abbot tube into the stomach. After inflating the balloon, the tube is

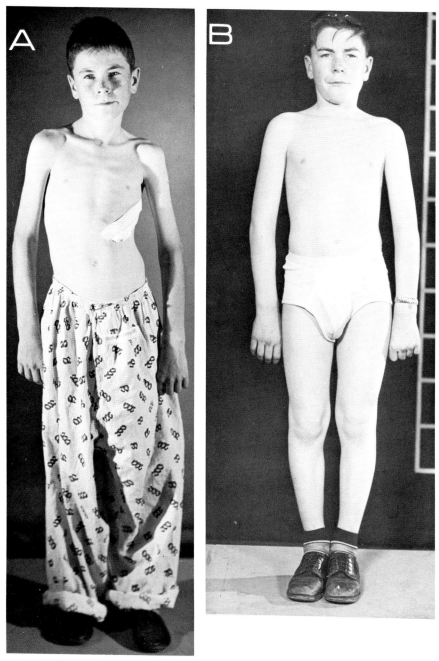

Fig. 10. A. A patient just after a Heller type of operation for achalasia. B. The patient six months after operation.

withdrawn. The balloon will impinge on the cardia and indicate its position to the surgeon. An incision about 3 cm in length is made from the stomach along the esophagus, dividing both the muscular layers and the mucosa. It has been our impression that, unless the mucosa is divided, complete relief may not be attained. The mucosa is approximated with chronic catgut interrupted sutures so that the incision, which was made parallel to the esophagus, is closed transversely, thus enlarging the lumen. The muscular coat is then approximated again transversely with interrupted 5-0 silk sutures. The pleura is also closed with interrupted silk sutures. A catheter for chest decompression is left in place through a stab wound. The incision is closed with two or three sutures of 3-0 catgut around the eighth and ninth ribs. After these are tied, the intercostal muscle layer and the subcutaneous tissue are approximated with separate rows of interrupted silk sutures. The skin is closed with a continuous 5-0 plain catgut subcuticular suture.

POSTOPERATIVE CARE

Feedings are started on the second or third postoperative day. The patients do well postoperatively. However, years later they may have recurrence of symptoms because of the development of reflux esophagitis. In the hope of preventing this, the children are made to sleep with the head of the bed elevated 4 to 6 in., and antacids are given between meals to reduce gastric acidity. The early results are good (Fig. 10).

HIATUS HERNIA

Hiatus hernia is not a common lesion; however, the treatment of the condition once stricture has developed is so difficult that it warrants considerable attention. In the past there has been considerable confusion between hiatus hernia and cardioesophageal relaxation and reflux. It is obvious that newborns and babies for some period of time reflux gastric contents into the esophagus

with burping. However, reflux that occurs spontaneously when the patient is in Trendelenburg position is considered to be abnormal after the baby is six to eight weeks of age.

ETIOLOGY

The embryology of the esophagus and stomach with the adjacent diaphragm is complicated. The stomach and esophagus develop, and at a later date the portions of the diaphragm unite to form a continuous barrier between the thoracic and abdominal cavities. It is perfectly possible for this development of the diaphragm to be delayed or defective. Under such circumstances a defect in the structure of the diaphragmatic hiatus may be such as to foster the formation of a hernia. Certainly in the cases subjected to surgical repair the hiatus is enlarged, permitting the stomach to herniate into the chest, and because of the laxness of the crura the normal sphincteric action of these structures is lost and gastroesophageal reflux is possible.

The existence of a congenital short esophagus is challenged, the shortness being attributed to the secondary changes of esophagitis, which are fibrosis and possible shortening. Such a course of events seems reasonable and is supported by serial roentgenographic examinations of a patient in whom this process seems to be documented. The fact that congenitally short esophagi have been noted shortly after birth is strong evidence that this is a congenital entity and is not invariably related to secondary esophagitis and fibrosis.

PATHOLOGY

Normally, esophageal reflux into the esophagus does not occur after the baby is several weeks of age, the process being blocked by an effective mechanism at the esophagogastric junction. This mechanism must be fairly effective in view of the fact that there is negative pressure in the thoracic cavity that is transmitted to a certain degree to the esophagus. Consequently there may be some differential in pressure between the full stomach and the empty esophagus. The nature of the mechanism that prevents reflux is a complicated one and probably consists of two parts: the intrinsic mechanism of the esophagus itself and the crura of the diaphragm, which are wrapped around the esophagus and actually serve as a pinch-cock mechanism that becomes more effective as the stomach dilates. It is questionable how frequently a hiatus hernia is present when there is gastroesophageal reflux. This association was thought to be rather unusual in the past. However, with the development of better techniques of examination, such as cinefluorography, it is becoming more common to find small hiatus hernias in association with esophagogastric reflux.

There is one other entity that should be given consideration at this time, and that is aberrant gastric mucosa in the esophagus. While it is quite common for small islands to be present, to have a large amount or a section of the esophagus lined with gastric mucosa is unusual. However, it does occur and may extend a considerable distance from the esophagogastric junction upward. This has been noted both on radiographic examination and on the basis of postmortem material.

Esophagitis is one of the serious complications of hiatus hernia. The reflux of acid fluid into the esophagus has a detrimental effect on the mucosa and promotes an inflammatory mucosal response that later may develop into ulcerations and actual fibrosis and stricture formation. To distinguish between spasm and fibrosis in narrowing of the lumen in association with reflux of esophagitis is difficult. Where actual fibrotic changes exist the lesion is rigid and similar on all phases of examination. Narrowing caused by spasm changes and such variation in caliber during an examination may enable the radiologist to surmise that the narrowing is not a fibrotic one.

It is interesting that in a small number of patients there is an association between congenital pyloric stenosis and hiatus hernia. This association is usually 1 in 10 to 15 patients, and it used to be assumed that distal obstruction played a large role in the formation of hiatus hernia. It was disappointing in the past that pyloromyotomy alone did not yield a high percentage of cures of hiatus hernia. However, it is interesting that these two relatively unusual lesions are occasionally found associated.

The actual pathology of hiatus hernia is an enlargement of the esophageal hiatus so that the effective sphincter action of the diaphragm on the esophagus no longer is effective. Undoubtedly this is a congenital malformation in infants.

SYMPTOMS

The commonest symptoms of hiatus hernia are vomiting and failure to thrive. Although occasionally one sees an infant with a hiatus hernia and vomiting who maintains a reasonable weight gain, this is exceptional. In a varying number of the patients, there is vomiting of coffee-ground or bright blood. This occurs in about one fourth of the patients. In some series the figure is more than one third of the patients. The amount of bleeding is not excessive in infants and small children. There might be flecks of bright red material in the vomitus. On occasion, there may be vomiting of a considerable amount of blood, and we have observed in one of our patients a fall of hemoglobin to 3 g following a bout of bleeding. Anemia from chronic blood loss is not common in infants, although this is common in adult patients with hiatus hernia. It is impossible to say definitely that the patients do not have pain. Some of the older patients have complained of substernal discomfort. It should be mentioned that while the vomitus may be blood-streaked or coffee-ground, it never is bile-stained. Vomitus consists of material that may be gastric in type or unchanged formula or food. These patients may appear to have pyloric stenosis. However, their vomiting

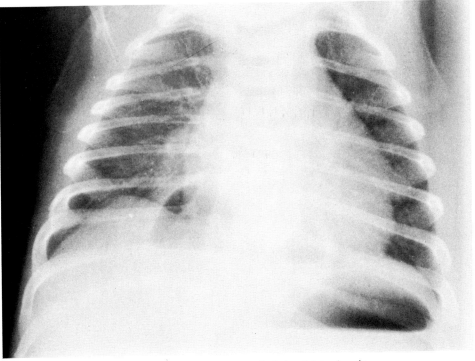

Fig. 11. Chest film. Note entrapped air in a hiatus hernia.

does not tend to be projectile, nor is there the constipation and dark urine which is so characteristic in patients with congenital pyloric stenosis. Another difference is that gastric peristaltic waves are not as common or as vigorous in hiatus hernia as in pyloric stenosis.

Failure to gain weight normally or actual weight loss is associated with the entity. Recurrent pulmonary infection may be a part of the symptomatology, particularly when night vomiting is present.

DIAGNOSIS

The diagnosis depends entirely on radiographic examination and on esophagoscopy. At times, a plain film of the chest may outline a gas bubble, which is characteristic of hiatus hernia. However, the diagnosis cannot be made with complete assurance on such plain films (Fig. 11). It is necessary to have the patient ingest barium and to make observations during swallowing. It is important to determine whether at one point there may

be an elevation of the gastric wall into the thoracic cavity. This may be transient and hard to detect. Cinefluorography films are most successful in detecting this, and consequently the diagnosis of hiatus hernia is

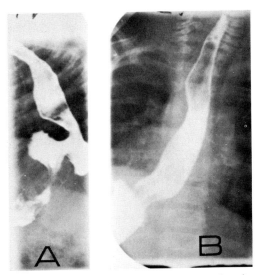

Fig. 12. A. Esophagogram of small hiatus hernia. B. Same patient several months following repair.

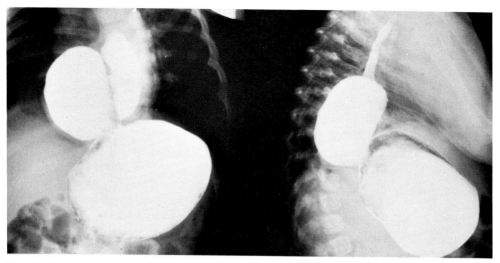

Fig. 13. Roentgenograms in the anterioposterior and lateral projection outlining a large hiatus hernia.

made more frequently when this equipment is used for the examination. During the examination it is important to make observations of esophagogastric reflux after the stomach becomes reasonably filled. No further contrast media is offered the babies. They are placed in Trendelenburg position, and pressure is applied to the abdomen and observations made about gastroesophageal reflux. It is possible to establish this diagnosis with films of the esophagus made during swallowing. However, the lesion will frequently be overlooked when the examination is limited to this technique. It is far better to observe the patient fluoroscopically while swallowing is progressing and, best of all, to have a movie made of the swallowing process, for on such films it is possible to detect a hiatus hernia that will be missed by other techniques (Figs. 12, 13, and 14).

These patients should be esophagoscoped

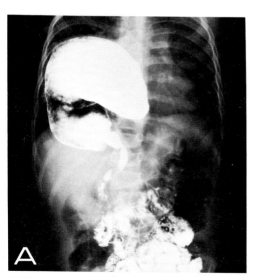
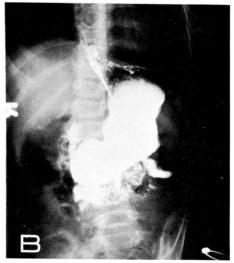

Fig. 14. A. Roentgenogram with barium in a massive hiatus hernia. The esophagus has normal length. B. Same patient six months after repair of hiatus hernia.

to determine the presence of esophagitis. When this process is well established the esophagal mucosa is reddened and edematous and bleeds easily. There may be actual ulcer formation. It is also possible to observe strictures during such examinations and to a certain extent to determine how fibrotic they are.

TREATMENT

It is generally agreed that in the very young baby with a small hiatus hernia, treatment should be conservative. This consists of keeping the patient in an upright position for a period after each feeding.

In the more resistant cases the baby should be maintained in an apparatus which places the esophagus 60° from the horizontal position during the entire 24 hours. The second part of the treatment is to thicken the feedings. Farina 1:20 is commonly used. With this therapy vomiting is usually controlled and a gain in weight is recorded. There is also evidence that the small hiatus hernia may disappear after a period of treatment. However, recently there has been some evidence presented that the number of cures of hiatus hernia by this conservative treatment is no greater than the spontaneous rate of disappearance of the lesion. It is agreed by most workers that extremely large hiatus hernias, even in babies who are doing reasonably well, should be treated by surgical repair. A patient who fails to respond to medical therapy or who has a large hernia or in whom there is beginning stricture formation should be subjected to surgical therapy. The problem in this disease is in the treatment of the patient who has a hiatus hernia plus a stricture. Here successful treatment is difficult. It is for this reason that some centers are more liberal in their indications for surgical repair of hiatus hernia. Also it is believed that there is a possibility that the small hiatus hernia that becomes less significant clinically may well be the lesion that reappears in middle and later life. This is totally unsubstantiated and should

not play a role in deciding on therapy for these patients. However, an effort to prevent stricture formation is to be commended because the treatment once this complication has developed is unpredictable.

There is one aspect of this disease that has not been studied in infants and children, and that is the relation of gastric acidity in the patients with esophagitis. We have studied a small group of patients, and it appears that over half of them do have hyperacidity, and this may be an important consideration in their treatment. Further data will have to be accumulated before it is possible to say that hyperacidity is a common associated finding in these patients and whether treatment of this will effectively prevent stricture formation.

SURGICAL REPAIR

There are a number of different methods of repairing hiatus hernia. It would appear that there are advantages to the thoracic approach as well as disadvantages, and there are also disadvantages to the abdominal approach. It is interesting that Allison (1951), who has had a large experience with this disease in adults, uses the thoracic approach but opens the diaphragm in order to fix the fundus of the stomach to the diaphragm as a part of the repair. We have utilized the thoracic approach, since this provided a better opportunity to free the esophagus, which is often shortened, and to assure that it is mobilized to such an extent that it can be brought down to the level of the diaphragmatic hiatus. The difficulty with this approach is in the patient with hyperacidity, who we believe requires vagotomy and pyloroplasty. This requires an incision through the diaphragm, and although the vagotomy can be performed with ease the pyloroplasty may present some difficulty, particularly when the duodenum is relatively fixed. It would appear that the surgeon should use the approach that has been successful in his hands, for apparently sound repairs can be achieved by either technique. In the abdominal type of repair, the hiatus is closed anterior to the esophagus. It is felt that here the structures are thicker and, despite its being a muscular structure, can be closed quite effectively. Some British surgeons have a success of about 80 to 85 percent with anterior closure. It is then the practice to tack the fundus of the stomach up on the dome of the diaphragm to help fix the structures in place.

It has been our practice to repair the lesion through a chest incision going between the fifth and sixth ribs (Fig. 15). This gives an excellent exposure, and one can identify the lesion clearly. The pleura over the esophagus is divided well up toward the hilum of the lung, providing an excellent exposure for freeing the esophagus. This exposure permits one to preserve the vagi if so desired. Our experience makes us tend more and more toward vagotomy and pyloroplasty, particularly if there is any indication of hyperacidity in the preoperative studies. We develop the hiatus, and it is usually two or three times normal size. We close it anterolaterally, and it is important to place a row of fine 5-0 or 6-0 sutures through the muscular coat of the esophagus and through the hiatus around its circumference to prevent recurrences. With this, we have found it unnecessary to tack the stomach to the peritoneal side of the diaphragm. Vagotomy can readily be performed. We then make an opening in the diaphragm and deliver the duodenum and pylorus and perform a pyloroplasty. It is important in closing the pyloroplasty that the edges should not be turned in. A row of interrupted chromic catgut sutures is placed to bring the mucosa together, and a second row of 6-0 silk is used to bring the muscular coats together. This has proved to be far more efficient functionally than when the layers are turned in. It is important to make the hiatus snug around the esophagus. It is amazing how tight this can be made without causing the patient any difficulty in swallowing. This part of the operation is important in preventing reflux (Fig. 16).

While repair of the hiatus hernia can be performed in one of several ways with a high degree of success, the treatment of the patient with an associated stricture is difficult. In the past, resection of the stricture, bringing the fundus of the stomach into the chest, has been used, and this may be successful for five or six years. However, the tendency is for reflux to recur, and with this there is reformation of a stricture. This has been our experience with the patients treated in this manner. There has been some suggestion of bringing more of the stomach into the chest and making the anastomosis higher on the esophagus in order to prevent the complication of reformation of the stricture. The problem that this poses in the small baby is that there is such an encroachment on the patient's pulmonary function that shortness of breath develops when the patient consumes normal feedings. We have had the opportunity to observe a patient for a number of years with this anatomical arrangement, and an infant feeding had to be offered every two hours in small amounts in order to prevent overdistension of the stomach and respiratory distress.

It has been the practice of Filler (1964) to resect the stricture at the time of repairing the hiatus hernia. The resection is made, and an anastomosis is performed between the stomach and the normal esophagus above the stricture. While he is well pleased with the results, the followup is short. Heimburger (1965) has reviewed a series of cases and found that with a repair of the hiatus hernia in patients with stricture there was a high incidence of stricture persistence. He now believes that an interposition operation using colon or small intestine should be used whenever the surgeon encounters a true fibrotic stricture. Our own experience and that of Rehbein (1962) has been that some of the patients with stricture will improve after repair of the hiatus hernia. This may well be related to the possibility that our improvements have been in patients who have had more spasm than fibrotic changes. Certainly there is a small number of patients

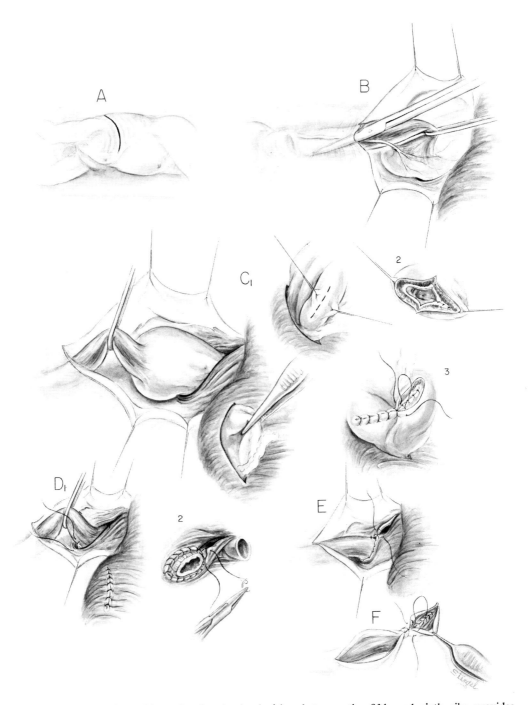

Fig. 15. Surgical repair of hiatus hernia. A. An incision between the fifth and sixth ribs provides an adequate exposure. B. When there is an associated short esophagus, it becomes necessary to mobilize the esophagus sufficiently to permit reduction of the hernia. C. 1. When a pyloroplasty is required, a small diaphragmatic incision permits the pylorus to be drawn into the field. 2. An incision through the pylorus in its long axis is made. 3. It is closed in two layers without any turn-in of tissue.

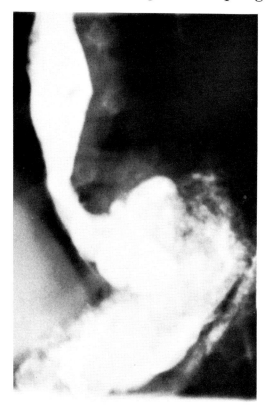

Fig. 16. Esophagram following repair of hiatus hernia.

round Y arrangement with a submucosal circumferential suture that forces the swallowed material in through the stomach yet maintains continuity of a sort of the intestine to promote circulation.

HERNIA OF THE FORAMEN OF MORGAGNI

Hernia of the foramen of Morgagni is probably more rare in the pediatric age group than hiatus hernia. A majority of patients with this lesion are encountered in middle and later life. The defect in the diaphragm is rather small and permits only a limited amount of herniation, and consequently the symptoms related to this type of hernia may be quite minor and not detected until the patient grows older. Another possible explanation might be that the lesion does not develop until later in life.

ETIOLOGY

The precise etiology of hernia of the foramen of Morgagni is debated. From an embryological standpoint it is possible for a defect to occur in the subxiphoid region as well as in the posterolateral diaphragmatic quadrant. The lesion is invariably in the midline below the xiphoid and may be a defect of attachment of the diaphragmatic structures in the midline anteriorly. A defect in the diaphragm itself in this region is a real possibility. It is believed by some that this is a traumatic lesion that occurs later in life. Even in such instances it may be that there is a congenital weakness in this area that permits the herniation to take place.

who have a persistence of the stricture who are indeed difficult to treat. One word of conservatism should be entered at this point and the value of dilation after repair of the hiatus hernia be commended. This has been successful occasionally in achieving a permanently adequate stoma of the esophagus. It would appear that one way of handling these patients is to repair the hiatus hernia and to observe the results. If the stricture persists, a series of dilations should be performed, and, if these fail, interposition operation appears to be the best solution to the problem. The actual technique of the interposition operation is important. There have been many complications reported, and Aylwin's technique is unusual in that it is a

PATHOLOGY

In all of these hernias there is a true peritoneal sac, which may be evidence that this

Fig. 15 (cont.). Surgical repair of hiatus hernia. D. 1. The esophagus is sutured to the hiatus in the diaphragm with interrupted 5-0 silk sutures. 2. The entire circumference of the esophagus is sutured to the hiatus in the manner illustrated. E. The excess size of the hiatus is reduced with interrupted 4-0 silk sutures. F. The pleura is closed over the repair.

is more of an acquired lesion than a true defect in formation of the diaphragm. The lesion is rarely associated with any other malformations. Defects in lung development have not been reported.

CLINICAL PICTURE

These patients may have few symptoms. The lesion can often be detected on plain roentgenograms of the chest by the presence of a gas bubble, usually to the right of the cardiac silhouette. There may be vomiting and slight respiratory distress associated with this lesion, particularly when all of the stomach is in the thoracic cavity. The so-called upside-down stomach is more clearly seen in the hernia of the foramen of Morgagni than in the true Bochdalek type of hernia. The stomach herniating through this defect literally turns upside down and can be seen in this position clearly when barium contrast material is fed to the patient (Fig. 17). In older patients dyspepsia may be a chief complaint: There may be substernal pain and referred pain in the shoulder. The diagnosis is often made when a roentgenographic search is made for the cause of the pain. At times the lesion may be detected on a plain roentgenogram, or at least its presence may be suspected and the lesion outlined by contrast material.

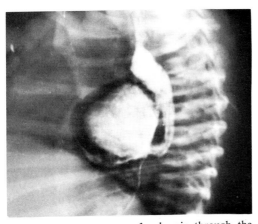

Fig. 17. Roentgenogram of a hernia through the foramen of Morgagni.

SURGICAL TREATMENT

This lesion should be treated surgically despite the paucity of symptoms, for as the patient grows older symptoms become more severe. Repair is most readily accomplished through the chest by way of a low thoracic incision. The sac is excised and the defect, being small, is closed without difficulty. These patients do not present any serious postoperative problem in care and usually make a rapid recovery.

EVENTRATION OF THE DIAPHRAGM

Eventration of the diaphragm is rare and can be divided into three types: the true congenital eventration, where there is a paucity of muscular fibers in the diaphragm and where a smooth saclike structure has replaced the normal diaphragm; a second group, where there is branchial plexus palsy and perhaps an associated phrenic nerve lesion; and a third group, where there is iatrogenic phrenic palsy caused by damage to the nerve sustained during an operative procedure. The explanation of the congenital form of the eventration is difficult. It may be caused by a congenital lesion in the phrenic nerve that has failed to properly innervate the diaphragm. Electric stimulation studies have not been performed on a sufficient number of such patients to make a conclusion reliable. There may be some other obscure congenital malformation that leads to the stretching out and loss of function.

PATHOLOGY

To understand the cardiopulmonary sequellae to eventration of the diaphragm, one must recall the behavior of the injured diaphragm during respiration. There is paradoxical movement of the diaphragm so that the normal side contracts and becomes lower. The affected side rises to a higher level in the chest. Consequently there is loss of respiratory function that probably is more telling in producing respiratory distress than the high level of the diaphragm (Fig. 18). Regardless of the etiology of the lesion, the pathology and malfunction is similar in all situations.

CLINICAL PICTURE

The patient with eventration of the diaphragm may have severe respiratory difficulty with rapid respirations and cyanosis of varying degree. It is to be recalled that respiratory function in the small baby is primarily diaphragmatic, the thoracic wall and movement of the thoracic cage playing a more insignificant role than in the adult. It is probably for this reason that a paradoxical movement of one diaphragm produces clinical symptomatology in the neonate and small infant that is not encountered in the adult with a similar lesion. This may also be a result of the fact that in the older patient there is more fixation of the mediastinal structures so that the paradoxical movement

of one diaphragm does not have such a devastating effect on the mechanical action of the patient's respiratory system. Jewett (1964) has pointed out the importance of being on the alert for iatrogenic lesions to the phrenic nerve, particularly during removal of large tumors or during pulmonary resections where there has been chronic infection and where landmarks are obscured. When diaphragmatic function is questioned it is important to test the function of the phrenic nerve by electrical stimulation to be certain that diaphragmatic function is present. The advantage of detecting the lesion during the initial operative procedure is that plication of the diaphragm can be accomplished and thus save the patient a second operation. Jewett has presented cases where it has been necessary after iatrogenic lesions to return the patient to the operating room and to perform plication of the diaphragm in order to restore effective pulmonary function. It is convenient to approach the eventration through a chest incision and to per-

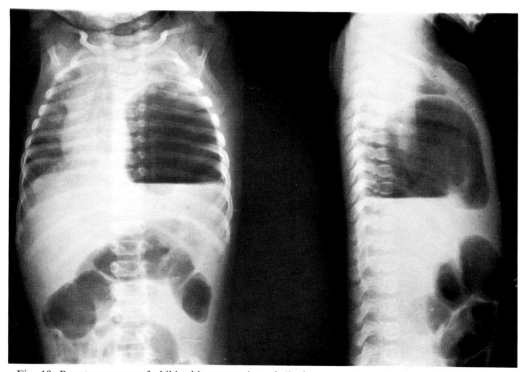

Fig. 18. Roentgenogram of child with eventration of diaphragm, anteroposterior and lateral views.

form plication of the diaphragm. The object is to connect the diaphragm to a firm division between the thoracic and abdominal cavities so that paradoxical movement is eliminated or minimized. It is recommended that a row of interrupted silk mattress sutures be placed, which everts the diaphragm into the abdominal cavity. A second or third row may be required to bring the diaphragm into a taut structure, so that paradoxical movement is largely eliminated. It is surprising to observe the beneficial effects this procedure has on patients with eventration and severe respiratory distress. The reported followup on these patients is not great; however, reasonable periods of time demonstrated the durability of results. One would predict that there would be recurrence of the eventration, and this may take place but usually does not occur within a reasonable length of time.

In some patients there may be a localized eventration on the right side which permits a part of the liver to herniate into the chest. On casual observation of the chest film, the lesion may be mistaken for an intrathoracic tumor. These are usually easy to repair.

TRAUMATIC RUPTURE OF THE DIAPHRAGM

Traumatic rupture of the diaphragm is a rare lesion, and until the last two or three decades it was not given attention clinically. In 1953, Chamberlain and Ford described traumatic rupture of the diaphragm and stated that this was no longer a rarity, for it was recorded with increasing frequency in high-speed automobile accidents. Often this lesion is associated with extensive damage, so that survival is impossible. However, case reports have been published in which the lesion has been detected and corrected surgically. Myers (1964) has recently reported two instances in children. In one case the patient suffered an automobile accident, and it was at a later date that intestinal obstruction with perforation of the stomach occurred. At postmortem examination a traumatic defect in the diaphragm was found with herniation of the stomach and small intestine into the chest. It is well known in veterinary medicine that traumatic rupture of the diaphragm occurs in dogs, and often there is survival with a later development of intestinal obstruction weeks after the original accident, when the scarring reduces the diaphragm defect and produces intestinal obstruction in the herniated part of the gastrointestinal tract. This seems to be a course of events that also takes place in children. In examining patients following extensive injury involving high-speed accidents, the possibility of rupture of the diaphragm must be given attention. Certainly during abdominal operations in severely injured patients an effort should be made to palpate the diaphragms and to prove their integrity before closing the abdomen. Closure of a diaphragm rent is not difficult.

ORVAR SWENSON

REFERENCES

ALLISON, P. R. Reflux esophagitis, sliding hiatal hernia, and the anatomy of repair. Surg. Gynec. Obstet., 92: 419, 1951.

AYLWIN, J. A. The physiological basis of reflux oesophagitis in sliding hiatal diaphragmatic hernia. Thorax, 8: 38, 1953.

BENJAMIN, H. E. Agenesis of left hemidiaphragm. J. of Thorac. Cardiov. Surg., 46: 265, 1963.

BENTLEY, G., and LISTER, J. Retrosternal hernia. Surgery, 57: 567, 1965.

BINGHAM, J. A. W. Herniation through congenital diaphragmatic defects. Brit. J. Surg., 47: 1, 1959.

BISHOP, H. C., and KOOP, C. E. Acquired eventration of the diaphragm in infancy. Pediatrics, 22: 1088, 1958.

BOCHDALEK, V. A. Einige Betrachtungen über

die Entstehung des angeborenen Zwerchfellbruches. Als beitrag zur pathologischen Anatomie der Hernien. Vjschr. prakt. Heilk., 19: 89, 1848.

BOIX-OCHOA, J., and REHBEIN, F. Oesophageal stenosis due to reflux oesophagitis. Arch. Dis. Child., 40: 197, 1965.

BONHAM-CARTER, R. E., WATERSON, D. J., and ABERDEEN, E. Hernia and eventration of the diaphragm in childhood. Lancet, 1: 656, 1962.

BURKE, J. B. Partial thoracic stomach in childhood. Brit. Med. J., 2: 787, 1959.

BUTLER, N., and CLAIRVEAUX, A. E. Congenital diaphragmatic hernia as a cause of perinatal mortality. Lancet, 1: 659, 1962.

BUTSCH, W. L., and LEAHY, L. J. A technique for the surgical treatment of congenital eventration of the diaphragm in infancy. J. Thorac. Surg., 20: 968, 1950.

CARRE, I. J. Postural treatment of children with a partial thoracic stomach ("hiatus hernia"). Arch. Dis. Child., 35: 569, 1960.

——— Pulmonary infection in children with partial thoracic stomach ("hiatus hernia"). Arch. Dis. Child., 35: 481, 1960.

CERILLI, G. J. Foramen of Bochdalek hernia cases at the Children's Hospital of Denver, Colorado. Ann. Surg., 159: 385, 1964.

CHIN, E. F., and DUCHESNE, E. R. The parasternal defect. Thorax, 10: 214, 1955.

CRAIGHEAD, C. C., and Sturg, L. H. Diaphragmatic deficiency in the retrocostoxiphoid area. Surgery, 44: 1062, 1958.

DeBORD, R. A., and GUINTA, E. J. Congenital eventration of the diaphragm. J. Thorac. Surg., 31: 731, 1956.

FILLER, R. M., RANDOLPH, J. G., and GROSS, R. E. Esophageal hiatus hernia in infants and children. J. Thorac. Cardiov. Surg., 47: 551, 1964.

FITCHETT, C. W., and TAVAREZ, V. Bilateral congenital diaphragmatic herniation. Surgery, 57: 305, 1965.

HEIMBURGER, I. L., ALFORD., W. C., Jr., WOOLER, G. H., and AYLWIN, J. A. Hiatal hernia and reflux esophagitis in children. J. Thorac. Cardiov. Surg., 50: No. 4, 463, 1965.

HOLCOMB, G. W., Jr. A new technique for repair of congenital diaphragmatic hernia with absence of the left hemidiaphragm. Surgery, 51: No. 4, 534, 1962.

HUMPHREYS, G. H., WIEDEL, P. D., BAKER, D. H., and BERDON, W. E. Esophageal hiatus hernia in infancy and childhood. Pediatrics, 36: 351, 1965.

——— FERRER, J. M., and WIEDEL, P. D. Esophageal hiatus hernia of the diaphragm. J. Thorac. Surg., 34: 749, 1957.

HUNTER, W. R. Herniation through the foramen of Morgagni. Brit. J. Surg., 47: 22, 1959.

HUSFELDT, E. Hiatus hernia in infants and adults. Great Ormand Street Journal, 6: 71, 1953.

JEWETT, T. C., Jr., and THOMSON, N. B., Jr. Iatrogenic eventration of the diaphragm in infancy. J. Thorac. Cardiov. Surg., 48: No. 5, 861, 1964.

KIRKLAND, J. A. Congenital postero-lateral diaphragmatic hernia in the adult. Brit. J. Surg., 47: 16, 1959.

MARTIN, L. W. Management of esophageal anomalies. Pediatrics, 36: 342, 1965.

MEEKER, I. A., Jr., and SNYDER, W. H., Jr. Surgical management of diaphragmatic defects in the newborn infant. Amer. J. Surg., 104: No. 2, 196, 1962.

MICHELSON, E. Congenital diaphragmatic hernia in the adult. A new technique in the closure of Bochdalek hernia. J. Thorac. Cardiov. Surg., 39: 238, 1960.

MYERS, N. A. Traumatic rupture of the diaphragm. Aust. New Zeal. J. Surg., 34: No. 2, 1964.

NEUHAUSER, E. B. D., and BERENBERG, W. Cardio-esophageal relaxation as a cause of vomiting in infants. Radiology, 48: 480, 1947.

OLSEN, A. M., HOLMAN, C. B., and HARRIS, L. E. Hiatal hernias in children: Special reference to the short esophagus. Dis. Chest, 38: 495, 1960.

POLK, H. C., Jr., and BURFORD, T. H. Hiatal hernia in infancy and childhood. Surgery, 54: 521, 1965.

POTTER, E. L. Pathology of the fetus and newborn. Chicago, Year Book Publications, 1952.

REHBEIN, F., und RÖPKE, Th. Abdominothorakale Operation der Hiatushernie beim Saugling und Kleinkind. Erfahrungen bei 50 Fällen. chir. prox. 6, E.u.H. Marseille Verlag München, 1962. Pp. 291–301.

RIKER, W. L. Congenital diaphragmatic hernia. Arch. Surg., 69: 291, 1954.

SNYDER, W. H., and GREENEY, E. M., Jr. Congenital diaphragmatic hernia, 77 consecutive cases. Surgery, 57: 576, 1965.

31

Surgical Lesions of the Heart and Great Vessels

PEDIATRIC CARDIAC SURGERY: HISTORY

Prior to 1938, cardiac surgery in childhood was limited to an occasional case of pericardiectomy for cardiac tamponade. That year the first successful ligation of a patent ductus, by R. E. Gross, initiated a rapid growth in the scope of cardiac surgery that has not yet slackened.

The history of the spectacular development of heart surgery over the past 25 years can be divided into three distinct stages: (1) extracardiac procedures, 1938–1948; (2) blind intracardiac procedures, 1948–1953; and (3) intracardiac surgery under direct vision, 1953 to the present. During the first 10 years of the development of cardiac surgery, attention was concentrated on the great vessels and their branches, and operations for correction of the patent ductus (performed by Gross, in 1938), coarctation of the aorta (by Gross and Crafoord, in 1945), and double aortic arch (by Gross, in 1945) were performed successfully. The fear of cardiac arrhythmias, hemorrhage, and infection and the lack of refined instruments and anesthesia discouraged a direct attack upon the heart. Toward the end of this era, Alfred Blalock, in 1945, and Willis J. Potts, in 1946, devised systemic-pulmonary shunts to provide greater pulmonary blood flow in patients with such conditions as the tetralogy of Fallot and tricuspid atresia.

After the war, and undoubtedly accelerated by it, advances in antibiotics, blood replacement, and anesthetic techniques and greater knowledge about cardiac arrhythmias and their management encouraged the surgeon to turn his energy toward direct attacks on intracardiac defects. While Bailey and Harkins began to perform mitral commissurotomies in adult patients, Sir Russell Brock (1948) performed blind transventricular pulmonary valvulotomies, and V. A. Bjork discovered a method for closure of ostium secundum interatrial septal defects (Bjork, et al., 1954). Many ingenious procedures were devised, but it was recognized that unless direct vision of the pathology could be attained during surgery for these congenital defects, complete and safe repair was often impossible, and many lesions were beyond the scope of these techniques.

Experimental research was then concentrated on a means of developing open heart surgery. A wide variety of channels were explored, but attention became focused on two methods, hypothermia and extracorporeal circulation and oxygenation.

Hypothermia was used clinically by Lewis (1953) and Swan (1954) for closure of the interatrial septal defects and for pulmonary valvulotomy, respectively, after the pioneer work on the subject by N. W. Bigelow. Since circulatory arrest for more than two minutes at normal temperatures usually results in irreparable brain damage, some means of safely prolonging this arrest time was mandatory. Reduction of tissue temperature reduces the metabolic rate and hence the cells' oxygen requirement. It was found that lowering body temperature to 85° F would allow a safe period of total circulatory arrest of about ten minutes. With the techniques of vena caval inflow occlusion, this would allow direct vision repair of several lesions, such as uncomplicated interatrial septal defects and pulmonary valve stenosis. Unfortunately, many congenital defects could not be repaired safely in this limited time, and the relentless ticking of the clock was not conducive to calm, deliberate surgery.

Some means of bypassing both heart and lungs had to be developed in order to permit repair of most intracardiac defects. Finally Gibbon (1954) using a pump oxygenator, and Lillehei (Lillehei, et al., 1955b) using cross circulation, performed open cardiac surgery with total cardiopulmonary bypass. The problems in temporarily pumping and oxygenating the patient's blood were myriad and resulted in a number of different systems, only a few of which have remained in use.

The pump which substitutes for the heart must allow one-way flow of the blood, of an adequate volume and with minimal damage to the blood elements. Most of the piston or diaphragm type of pumps with internal valves were difficult to care for and sterilize and resulted in excessive hemolysis and platelet destruction. More universally acceptable were the pumps with external "valves," such as the DeBakey roller-type pump and the Sigmamotor finger-type pump, both of which involve external pumping or "milking" forces or tubing that is both easily sterilized and disposable.

Oxygenation has posed more of a problem, and undoubtedly further improvement lies in the future. Among the earliest oxygenators used on patients were homologous lungs, either in the form of animal lungs or cross circulation with human beings. In the latter system a second person was used to oxygenate the venous blood of the patient. This system was reasonably efficient but involved risk to a healthy individual and was abandoned as soon as an adequate mechanical system was evolved.

Film oxygenators expose a thin film of blood to a direct stream of oxygen which efficiently oxygenates the blood and removes the carbon dioxide. Many means of filming were devised, from beads to bubbles, but only a few have proved efficient and safe. The screen-type oxygenator devised by Gibbon films the blood over a stationary screen through which oxygen flows. Disk-type oxygenators made by Bjork, and later Kay and Cross, consist of a series of rotating disks that pick up a thin film of blood in which they are partially immersed and expose it to a flow of oxygen. The bubble-type oxygenator still widely used was devised by De-Wall in 1955. Oxygen is bubbled into the venous blood, and when adequate oxygenation has occurred the bubbles are removed by an antifoam agent.

A third type of oxygenator interposes a plastic membrane between the blood and oxygen flow. Theoretically the membrane oxygenator is the most physiological and the least traumatic to the blood. However, there are still technical problems that require solution before the use of this type of equipment becomes general. Imbalance of gas exchange, difficulties with sterilization, and the large size and the high resistance to blood flow are a few of the obstacles. Although the ideal type of oxygenator has not been developed, it will probably be of this type.

A typical method of cardiopulmonary bypass using extracorporeal circulation and oxygenation is shown in Figure 1. After heparinization of the patient, large plastic catheters are inserted into the inferior and superior venae cavae through the atrial wall and into the right femoral artery. When the patient is connected to the pump oxygenator, the venous blood flows by gravity into a collecting chamber (A) and passes into the oxygenator (B). The rotating disks continually pick up a thin film of blood, which is oxygenated by a flow of 98 percent oxygen and 2 percent carbon dioxide introduced

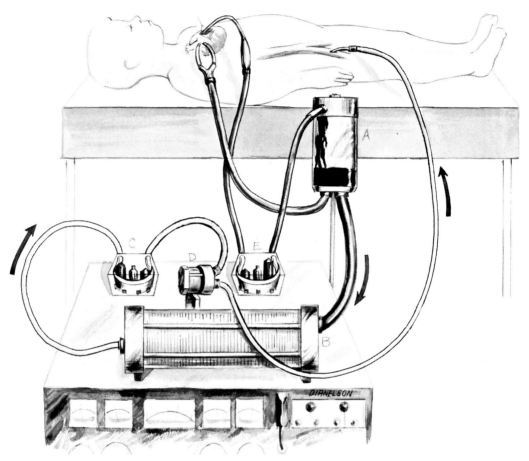

Fig. 1. Heart-lung machine. Schematic drawing of a system of extracorporeal circulation. Venous blood drains by gravity from catheters in the venae cavae into a collecting chamber. (A) It then flows through a disk oxygenator (B) and oxygenated blood is sucked out by a roller pump (C) and passed through a filter and debubbling chamber (D). From there it passes into the femoral artery cannula and perfuses the aorta and its branches by retrograde flow. Blood in the cardiac cavity is sucked up and returned to the collecting chamber through the cardiotomy suction pump (E).

through the top of the oxygenator chamber. The oxygenated blood is then sucked out of the chamber by the arterial pump (C), passes through the filter (D), and into the femoral artery. During the operation any blood in the opened heart is sucked up and returned to the venous reservoir via a cardiotomy suction pumphead. In certain cases the left atrium is vented through a catheter and the blood pumped into the reservoir. In many cases temporary cessation of coronary flow and cardiac arrest may be necessary and is obtained by cross clamping the ascending aorta.

The field of cardiac surgery is still widen-ing, and the emphasis in research is at present on cardiac transplantation and the development of mechanical devices to replace the heart. Certain congenital heart defects, such as tricuspid atresia and truncus arteriosus, will require nothing short of this for complete correction.

PATENT DUCTUS ARTERIOSUS

The first ligation of a patent ductus in 1938 by Gross focused attention on this condition, bringing better understanding of its physiology and improved methods in diagnosis.

The ductus serves a useful purpose in fetal life by helping to bypass the unused lung, but upon expansion of the lungs after birth the ductus is no longer needed. The pulmonary artery pressure drops as the arteriolar resistance decreases, and the ductus undergoes obliteration as its muscular medium contracts. This usually occurs during the first few days or weeks of life. Later anatomical closure of the ductus during the first year occasionally occurs. It is estimated that 1 in every 4,000 remains open permanently. This represents 12 percent of the various types of congenital cardiovascular defects.

DIAGNOSIS

Most children with patent ductus are asymptomatic and exceedingly active. If the flow through the ductus is large, the patient may be thin and underdeveloped and may experience some fatigue and occasionally dyspnea on exertion.

The condition is usually called to the physician's attention by the loud, continuous "machinery"-like murmur heard best at the second left interspace. The coarse thrill felt over this region was likened by one child to a "bag full of bees," by another to "Mommy's washing machine." The runoff of blood through the ductus during diastole results in a high pulse pressure, bounding pulses, and capillary pulsations visible under the fingernails. The heart is usually normal in size but may be moderately enlarged if the ductus is large and with a high flow.

Roentgenograms reveal a prominence in the pulmonary artery segment and increased vascularity of the lung fields that is due to the large pulmonary flow. The electrocardiogram most often is normal without axis shift, though at times there is a left-axis shift or a combined ventricular strain pattern. Any tendency to the right heart strain is ominous and suggests a "hypertensive ductus" with high pulmonary vascular resistance.

The diagnosis of the typical patent ductus is usually made on the physical examination, chest roentgenogram, and ECG; however, in a small percentage of cases catheterization and selective angiograms may be necessary if other lesions are suspected or if pulmonary hypertension of a severe degree is feared.

A small group of infants with patent ductus are in cardiac failure after birth and are very difficult to manage medically. If the failure is due to a huge pulmonary flow, emergency surgery is necessary to close the ductus. Some of these infants have severe pulmonary hypertension and a bidirectional shunt or even a reverse-flowing ductus. In many of these infants only a systolic murmur is heard.

PROGNOSIS

The average life expectancy of an individual with a significant patent ductus is said to be 30 years. The usual complication of a large ductus is increasing heart strain and eventual cardiac failure. In some instances pulmonary vascular resistance may rise resulting in right heart strain. A few children develop subacute bacterial endarteritis that is difficult to cure unless the ductus is obliterated. As the decades pass weakening of the adjacent vascular structures may give rise to aneurysm formation and possible rupture.

TREATMENT

Since the mortality for surgical closure of an uncomplicated patent ductus is so low, the operation is advised for all children by the time they reach three years of age. However, if an infant is in trouble because of the patent ductus earlier, emergency surgery is performed.

In the early days only ligation of the ductus was advocated, but after five or six years of experience investigators found that of several hundred collected cases of ductus ligation almost 5 percent had recurrence of the shunt or residual shunts owing to incomplete closure. Double clamping, division of the ductus between the clamps, and suture of the

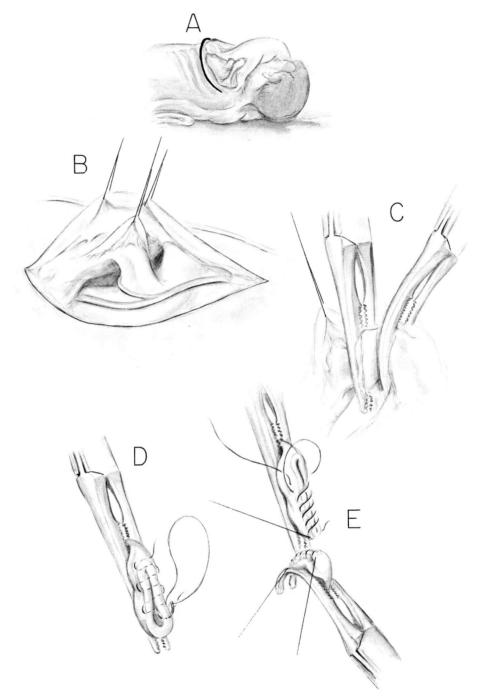

Fig. 2. Division and suture of a patent ductus arteriosus. A. Left posterolateral incision through the fourth intercostal space. B. Isolation of the ductus with retraction and preservation of the vagus and recurrent laryngeal nerves. C. Application of multitoothed clamps to each end of the ductus, which then is divided. D. Suture of aortic stump of ductus with initial layer of 5-0 silk in a vertical mattress stitch. E. Suture of pulmonary stump of ductus showing second suture layer of an over-and-over stitch.

stumps was adopted by most surgeons, with various types of clamps and techniques being used.

With the patient placed on his right side the left pleural cavity is entered through the fourth intercostal space (Fig. 2). An incision is made in the mediastinal pleura just anterior to the vagus nerve. The nerve is carefully dissected out and retracted posteriorly, exposing the recurrent laryngeal nerve as it dips around the ductus. Dissection of the loose areolar tissue down to the adventitia of the vessel is begun over the aorta and carried anteriorly across the ductus and onto the pulmonary artery, where a lappet of pericardium is encountered and retracted. Further dissection is extended around the ductus until it is well cleaned of the surrounding tissues, so that the clamps will not slip off. Multitoothed, atraumatic forceps are clamped onto the ductus at the aortic end, and the pulmonary end and the ductus is divided. The stumps are sutured with 5-0 cardiovascular silk, with an initial deep layer of continuous to-and-fro mattress stitches and returning with an over-and-over running stitch at a slightly more superficial level. A piece of Gelfoam is usually placed between the stumps, more to prevent friction between them than for hemostasis.

The mediastinal pleura is closed loosely over the area, and the chest is closed in layers with a catheter left in the pleural cavity coming out through the sixth interspace for drainage for 24 to 48 hours as indicated. The children can usually leave the hospital after seven days.

Ligation of the ductus is occasionally used in selected cases, especially in the small, critically ill infant when brevity of operation is of utmost importance. Ligatures of 2-0 silk are tied about the ductus at the pulmonary and aortic ends, and a transfixion suture is put between these if space and time permit. A long, narrow ductus is easily tied securely but is also easily clamped and divided. The large, short ductus (almost a fistula) is hard to clamp and divide but equally difficult to tie off completely and safely.

In certain cases the ductus may be short but large in diameter. One may want control of the aorta in case of hemorrhage during dissection or at the time of division and suture. The few minutes spent putting an umbilical tape about the aorta above and below the area of ductus give the surgeon peace of mind and make it possible to clamp the aorta for a short time if necessary to gain control of the situation.

If the ductus seems too short to clamp and divide in the usual manner, the aorta may be freed enough to apply the Potts-Smith clamp used in aortic-pulmonary anastomoses. The resultant lip of aorta pinched off in the clamp will gain a few vital millimeters on the aortic stump of the divided ductus.

RESULTS

At The Children's Memorial Hospital, 850 patients have had the ductus occluded, and among them there were 8 deaths. All but one of these deaths were in patients with severe pulmonary hypertension and high pulmonary vascular resistance. If the pulmonary hypertension is due to a high blood flow, the pressure in the pulmonary artery will drop when the ductus is clamped, and it is then perfectly safe to divide the ductus. If the pulmonary artery pressure rises when the ductus is occluded there is reversal of flow in the ductus, and division will result in right heart failure and death. If the pressure neither rises nor falls upon clamping the ductus, the outlook is poor. Some patients have died after division of the ductus in these circumstances, and several have survived but maintained systemic levels of pressure in their pulmonary circulation. If this type of patient is excluded from a surgical series, the mortality for patent ductus division in childhood should be less than 1 percent.

COARCTATION OF THE AORTA

It is estimated that the incidence of coarctation of the aorta is 1 in 2,000 births and constitutes 14 percent of all congenital cardiovascular anomalies.

Significant narrowing of the aorta may occur anywhere along its course. It is rare in the abdominal aorta or lower thoracic aorta but is occasionally present in the ascending aorta just above the aortic valve. Most commonly the site of narrowing is just below the origin of the left subclavian artery, at or near the region of the ductus arteriosus. The anatomical terms "preductal" and "postductal" have little clinical significance, but, in contrast, the classification into adult-type and infantile-type coarctations is of help diagnostically and in planning surgical therapy.

Most coarctations are of the adult type, with an abrupt narrowing of the aortic lumen near the site of the ductus, which may be patent but is usually obliterated. The etiology of the formation of this obstruction is not clear, although there is a plausible theory that the inherent contractile and obliterative forces in the ductus arteriosus extend to the aorta and cause the constriction.

The complex of infantile coarctation in its strictest sense includes a hypoplasia of the arch of the aorta down to the region of the ductus and a widely patent ductus arteriosus supplying blood to the aorta below the obstruction, aided by a pulmonary hypertension secondary to narrowing of the pulmonary vascular bed similar to that existing in fetal life. This gives rise to differential cyanosis, with arterial oxygen saturation normal above the obstruction but low in the lower half of the body. Patients with this type of infantile coarctation usually succumb following operation because of right heart failure secondary to closure of the ductus.

The term "infantile coarctation" has been extended to include a transitional group of infants with narrowing of a long segment of the aortic arch, some increase in the narrowing above the ductus region, and a small or closing ductus without a right-to-left shunt of blood or increased pulmonary resistance. This group can have their lesions corrected with reasonable success.

The hemodynamic results of the coarcta-

tion are a proximal hypertension and a distal hypotension with eventual formation of collateral circulation to help supply the lower aorta through enlarged intercostal arteries, internal mammary arteries, and other channels.

DIAGNOSIS

Symptoms of this lesion may be few if the obstruction is not severe and the collaterals are well developed. It is often discovered when hypertension is observed during a routine physical examination. More frequently headaches and palpitations secondary to the proximal hypertension and cramps, coldness, or weakness of the lower extremities because of poor circulation may be the presenting symptoms.

Physical examination discloses hypertension in the arms and hypotension in the legs, with absent or weak femoral pulses. A systolic murmur may be heard over the left chest, and often the hum of collateral circulation can be heard over the scapular regions. Their pulsation can be palpated and occasionally seen if they are well developed, especially in older persons.

Chest roentgenograms may reveal slight or mild left ventricular enlargement, and in patients in the second decade of life notching of the lower margin of one or more ribs may be present, caused by their erosion by the enlarged collateral channels. An esophagogram will outline a double notching in the region of the coarctation. The electrocardiogram may be normal or may show left ventricular hypertrophy. Hypertension in the right arm with lower pressure in the left may suggest a longer segment of narrowing involving the arch of the aorta.

In the straightforward case, without evidence of such other cardiac lesions as aortic stenosis or septal defects, angiograms and catheterization of the aorta are not necessary for diagnosis. With the complicated case, catheterization of the heart or aorta and retrograde or selective angiograms are helpful in outlining the site and extent of the involvement and indicating the presence of additional lesions.

PROGNOSIS

Most patients progress normally during infancy and early childhood; however, a small percentage of infants will be in severe difficulty with left heart failure shortly after birth. Many of these can be helped with good medical management permitting good collateral circulation to form and adequate heart function to develop. A few infants, however, remain in trouble despite good medical care and require early resection of the coarctation and aortic anastomosis.

As the decades pass the constant hypertension begins to take its toll of most patients with coarctation, resulting in left heart strain and eventual failure and the ever-present danger of cerebrovascular hemorrhage as the arteries become weakened by atherosclerosis. Aneurysms may form above or below the areas of narrowing, and we have observed one child who died of rupture of a distal aneurysm. Subacute bacterial endarteritis may become established at the site of narrowing.

The average life expectancy with this disease is said to be 30 years. With each succeeding decade of life there is less chance to revert the patients to normal blood pressure after operation, because of long-standing spasm and vascular changes related to their hypertension.

TREATMENT

Operative repair is advised for all patients with coarctation. The ideal age for surgery is eight to ten years, for at this age degenerative changes have not taken place in the vessels, and the aorta is of sufficient size for the anastomosis to be adequate in later years.

The technique in the ordinary case is straightforward, but there are many dangers for the unwary, such as dilated and friable intercostal arteries or an unsuspected patent ductus. These difficulties increase in direct proportion to the age of the patient.

The patient is placed with the left side up, and the chest is entered through the fourth intercostal space in the younger child. In larger individuals, the fifth rib is resected for better exposure. The aorta is dissected out above and below the area of the ligamentum arteriosum, which is doubly clamped and divided. Since there is often a lumen on one side or the other, the stumps are oversewn with 5-0 silk. After this, the dissection of the aorta above and below the coarcted area is completed, freeing enough aorta to allow coaptation of the ends after the narrowed segment is removed (Fig. 3). Dissection may be extended up the aortic arch and subclavian artery above and continued downward, with as many pairs of dilated intercostal arteries as necessary being ligated and divided.

Multitoothed, atraumatic clamps are put on the aorta above and below the narrowed area, and this portion of the aorta is excised, with the size of the lumens being matched as closely as possible. If the upper stump is short the clamp may have to be crowded up on the aortic arch, including within it the subclavian artery. The ends are brought together and usually clamped in a retaining device for easy handling. An end-to-end anastomosis of the aorta is made with over-and-over stitches of 5-0 silk. It is convenient to place two stitches close to each other at the lower end of the clamps; then the two over-and-over sutures can be brought up each side of the anastomosis, meeting at the top. The lower clamp is released, allowing blood to fill the areas of anastomosis and permit clotting in the suture holes. The upper clamp is then released, and a possible precipitous drop in blood pressure is watched for. Packing and applying pressure for a few minutes will usually stop any bleeding that might occur.

In almost all cases enough aorta can be freed to allow an anastomosis without the interposition of a graft. In only one instance have we had to use any type of graft; this was in a patient who had undergone a previ-

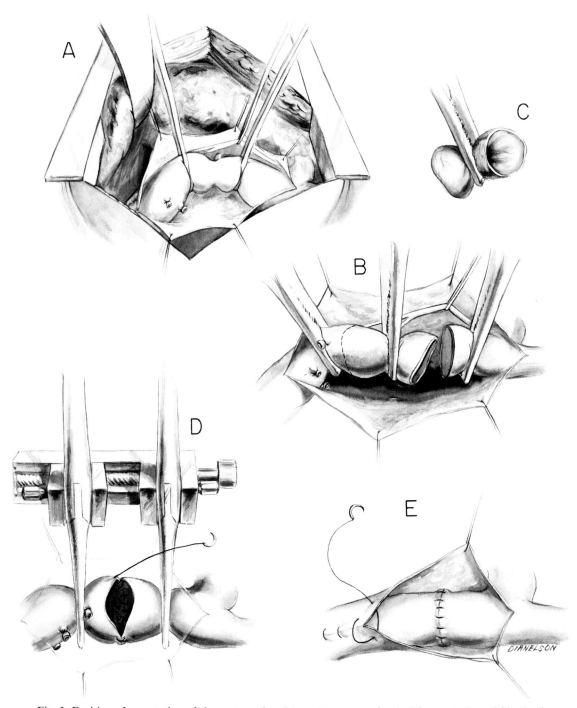

Fig. 3. Excision of coarctation of the aorta and end-to-end anastomosis. A. The aorta is mobilized, dividing and suturing the ligamentum arteriosum and as many intercostal arteries as necessary. B. Multi-toothed clamps are placed on the aorta above and below the narrow segment, which is then removed. C. Resected segment. The internal lumen is usually smaller than the outside diameter indicates. D. With the clamps held together in a vise, an end-to-end anastomosis is done using an over-and-over stitch of 5-0 silk. E. The completed anastomosis.

ous attempt at a plastic repair of a long segment coarctation.

RESULTS

In children there is usually a prompt drop in arm blood pressure to normal and the appearance of normal femoral pulses. In a series of 225 patients with resection of the coarctation of the aorta there were 9 deaths. They occurred in the group with infantile coarctation with reverse-flow ductus arteriosus. Obliterating the ductus precipitated right heart failure.

A significant residual gradient was present in two cases because of the smallness of the upper segment of aorta chosen for anastomosis. If the child is quite small at the time of operation, at least half of the circumference of the anastomosis is sutured with interrupted stitches to allow for future growth.

Another complication is the so-called post-coarctation syndrome, simulating an acute surgical abdomen with pain, tenderness, and muscle spasm. This is a result of the sudden distension of the smaller arteries in the bowel wall and mesentery. Without the external support present in the solid abdominal organs, the vessel walls may split, forming hematomas like small lead shot. Gastrointestinal hemorrhage also may occur. Mild forms of this syndrome are not uncommon, but fortunately severe attacks are quite rare.

VASCULAR RING

Vascular rings encircling the esophagus and trachea are not common, but considering the complicated embryology of that region it is amazing they do not occur more often.

During embryonic development six pairs of aortic arches, one for each gill cleft, pass from the ventral aortic sac around the pharyngeal pouch to join the dorsal aorta (Fig. 4). The third enters into the development of the carotid arteries, the fourth arch forms the arch of the aorta, and the sixth arch produces the pulmonary artery and ductus.

When the embryo reaches the 15-mm

stage the right side of the fourth aortic arch disappears, producing the normal configuration with the aorta arching to the left of the trachea and esophagus and then descending on the left side of the midline. If the left fourth arch disappears and the right persists, the configuration of the right aortic arch is seen, as frequently occurs in patients with tetralogy of Fallot. If both aortic arches persist, a double aortic arch or vascular ring encircles the trachea and esophagus (Fig. 4A). The left, or anterior, arch is usually smaller and accounts for a majority of the vascular rings. If the right, or posterior, segment of the ring is small, the surgical approach is more difficult (Fig. 4B). Fortunately, these are rare. An incomplete vascular ring is formed when there is a right aortic arch and left ligamentum arteriosum (Fig. 4C). This type is seen in about a third of the cases. Another form of incomplete vascular ring occurs when the right subclavian artery originates distal to the left subclavian artery on the descending aorta and passes upward and to the right behind the esophagus (Fig. 4D). This lesion is described as "dysphagia lusoria" and usually produces no respiratory difficulties, the symptoms being limited to esophageal compression. Rarely an anomalous left innominate or carotid artery may cross the front of the trachea, causing compression.

DIAGNOSIS

If the ring is incomplete and does not cause constriction of the trachea and esophagus, no symptoms may be present. The typical tight vascular rings, however, result in noisy respirations, inspiratory stridor, and intercostal and suprasternal retractions aggravated when respiratory infections are present and when the child is fed. A "barking" cough is heard, and pulmonary infections are frequent. Less than one third of these patients have dysphagia.

Physical examination confirms the pressure of tracheal obstruction. Laryngoscopy rules out more frequent causes of obstruc-

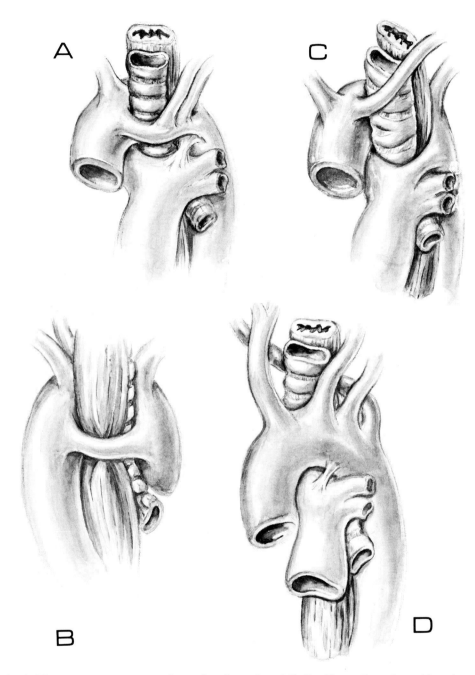

Fig. 4. The most common types of vascular rings. A and B. Double aortic arches with truly complete encirclement of esophagus and trachea. A. The most common type with the small segment anterior. B. Posterior view of a double aortic arch with the small segment behind the esophagus. C. The second most common vascular ring occurs when the aortic arch is on the right and the descending aorta is pulled over behind the esophagus by a tight ligamentum arteriosum on the left. D. "Dysphagia lusoria" with posterior esophageal compression by a right subclavian artery with anomalous origin from the descending aorta.

tion at the site of the cords or above. Esophagograms should be done on any child suspected of having this type of lesion. Anterior and posterior roentgenograms outline a mild to moderate degree of narrowing, but lateral films reveal most clearly the posterior indentation of the esophagus, "cookie bite," and narrowing of the tracheal air column. Oblique narrowing suggests an anomalous right subclavian artery. Bronchoscopy and esophagoscopy are usually superfluous but will show tracheal flattening and posterior pulsating compression of the esophagus.

TREATMENT

Patients with tight vascular rings are in trouble from birth and must be operated upon during infancy, often as an emergency. Patients having rings with less severe constrictions may go on into childhood or even adult life with some degree of symptomatology. An anomalous right subclavian artery may produce no significant dysphagia until the child is older. Operative division of the constricting ring is advised for any patient having symptoms from the tracheal or esophageal compression.

The approach may be made through a left anterolateral, submammary incision or a midline sternal-splitting incision. The ascending aorta, aortic arch, and descending aorta are dissected out and identified. All branches are encircled with tape and identified by compression and palpation of the axillary and carotid arteries. The smaller segment of the ring is divided at a point that will give maximum release of the constriction. In cases with right arch and left ligamentum arteriosum the ligamentum need only be divided. In the case of the anomalous right subclavian artery, the segment behind the esophagus can be removed between ligatures. The trachea must be completely freed of any surrounding fibrous tissue well above and below the area of constriction. Infants with severe tracheal compression pose a difficult problem in anesthesia, since the airway compression may be at or near the carina. Passing an endotra-

cheal tube beyond the obstruction may be impossible, and postoperative edema from intubation may complete the tracheal obstruction. Most of the deaths during or shortly after operation arose from this problem. One infant at The Children's Memorial Hospital had complete obstruction of the trachea at the carina postoperatively and was oxygenated for several days by inserting a small polyethylene catheter into one of the mainstem bronchi with a slow flow of humidified oxygen passing through it into one lung.

Since the trachea cartilage has formed in an abnormal shape because of the constant compression, release of the vascular ring may not relieve all of the obstruction. Some noisy respiration and barking cough may persist until growth of the trachea results in more normal cartilaginous rings and an adequate airway.

RESULTS

In the small infant in severe distress the operation may be lifesaving. Relief of symptoms in the older child will usually be complete but may take time to be accomplished. Fifty-eight children have had release of vascular rings in The Children's Memorial Hospital, with 10 deaths, or a mortality of 17 percent. Two deaths resulted from hemorrhage during and after operation. The rest died because of an inability to oxygenate them during or immediately after operation.

AORTIC STENOSIS

Aortic stenosis is defined as the presence of a gradient between the left ventricle and aorta. This stenosis may be valvular, subvalvular, supravalvular, or muscular in type. The true valvular stenosis is by far the most common. Each of the types can be corrected by surgery quite satisfactorily, except the muscular, which probably should be classified entirely separately as a "functional" subaortic stenosis and be grouped as a myopathy. Embryologically the valvular deformities occur later than the subvalvular and therefore are not commonly associated with septal defects. However, other abnormalities may be found with aortic stenosis, such as coarctation of the aorta and patent ductus arteriosus.

Symptoms accompanying aortic stenosis are uncommon in children. Likewise, the physical development of these children is usually normal, in contrast to many of the other congenital lesions. Fatigue and dyspnea are probably the most common symptoms if any are elicited. The older child may complain of chest pain. A peculiar pallor associated with dyspnea is sometimes described by the parents.

The diagnosis of aortic stenosis is usually made early because of the loud systolic murmur heard best at the second right interspace. A palpable systolic thrill and transmission of the thrill to the suprasternal notch and carotids usually accompany the murmur. The presence of an aortic click suggests valvular stenosis in contrast to a subvalvular stenosis. The roentgenograms on these children usually are normal. There is rarely heart enlargement, but a prominent aortic arch may be seen in some. The electrocardiogram is seldom normal, usually showing left ventricular hypertrophy of varying severity.

Because of the wide range of the degree of stenosis and the paucity of symptoms and findings even with a severe aortic stenosis, it is difficult to know what should be done when the diagnosis of aortic stenosis is made. A number of series have shown that about 7 percent of these young patients die suddenly, whereas a mild stenosis may be tolerated for a full life span. Even though a child with a severe stenosis may have a normal roentgenogram and a normal electrocardiogram, the electrocardiogram is usually the most sensitive index in determining the severity of aortic stenosis. Cardiac catheterization frequently must be resorted to as the final diagnostic tool to measure the gradient across the aortic valve and thereby determine the method of treatment. Probably all children who have auscultatory findings of an aortic

stenosis and who either show an abnormal electrocardiogram or have symptoms should have a cardiac catheterization.

Frequently not only can the gradient be measured but positive localization of the lesion can also be obtained. In view of the fact that the "muscular" or "functional" aortic stenosis is not satisfactorily treated with surgery nearly as often as the other types, localization is most important in selecting which lesions should be operated upon. Determination of the location and severity of the stenosis is best done by left heart catheterization retrograde through the aorta. A slow pulling back of the catheter from the body of the ventricle to the aorta with pressure tracings will indicate the location of the obstruction. Selective angiocardiograms are often quite helpful.

The treatment of aortic stenosis is to obliterate the gradient. Using extracorporeal circulation the aorta distal to the obstruction is cross-clamped, allowing the ascending aorta to be opened and the narrow area to be visualized. If the obstruction can be relieved in a matter of a few minutes, the resultant stoppage of coronary circulation is not important. However, if the aorta is to be cross-clamped for longer periods, the myocardium must be protected by coronary artery perfusion, myocardial hypothermia, or both. If the stenosis is supravalvular, we have found that the most suitable way to correct the narrowing is to insert a diamond-shaped patch into the wall of the aorta, as described by Kirklin. This patch is best placed in the area of the noncoronary sinus.

If the lesion is subvalvular, the operation is quite simple in that the valve leaflets are retracted to allow visualization of the web or membrane that lies immediately beneath the attachment of the aortic leaflets. The web or membrane is removed completely, with caution being taken not to injure the septal leaflet of the mitral valve. Since the valve above the stenotic diaphragm is usually normal, the prognosis should be more favorable than with other forms of aortic stenosis.

If the stenosis is valvular, the ideal treat-

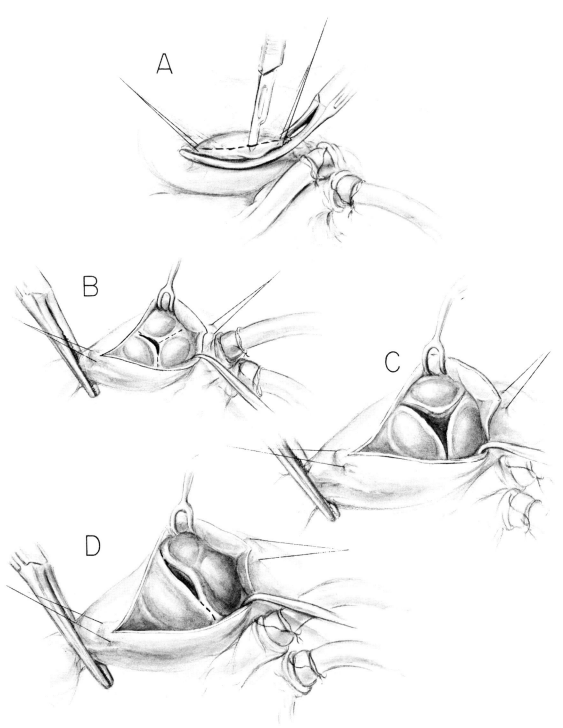

Fig. 5. Aortic valvotomy for aortic stenosis. A. With the patient on extracorporeal circulation an anterior lip of aorta is isolated with a curved multitoothed clamp and incised. B. The aorta above is cross-clamped and the curved clamp removed revealing the aortic valve. C. If the cusps are equally developed, all three commissures may be opened. D. If the cusps are malformed and eccentric, only two commissures must be opened to avoid postoperative regurgitation.

ment is to open all three commissures to the annulus. Even with a severe gradient the existing aperture of the aortic valve always seems to be larger than one anticipates. It is extremely rare to find the severe commissural fusion of the aortic leaflets that is usually seen in the congenital pulmonary valvular stenosis. Since the competence of the aortic valve is so much more critical than that of the pulmonary valve, great care and precision must be exercised when cutting the commissures of the stenotic aortic valve (Fig. 5). When three well-developed leaflets are in evidence there is no problem, but frequently there are two well-developed cusps and one triangular underdeveloped cusp that is not well supported. In such a situation it is preferable to cut two commissures, making a bicuspid valve, and to avoid the insufficiency that would be produced by freeing the unsupported miniature third leaflet. Muscular subvalvular stenosis is more difficult to deal with. Incision of the thick muscular protuberance below the aortic valve may be done through an aortotomy in larger patients. This incision may be deepened and spread to prevent constriction during systole. More complete relief of the obstruction may be obtained by the excision of a good deal of the muscle constricting the outflow. This may best be done through a combined aortotomy and left ventriculotomy approach.

Our series of 69 cases of aortic stenosis was divided into 54 valvular, 5 supravalvular, and 10 subvalvular and muscular. Of these we have had 4 deaths. The cause of 1 death was a disruption of the aortotomy because of *Staphylococcus aureus* coagulase positive bacteremia. An older patient with muscular stenosis had had a previous aortic valvolotomy and subsequently developed a severe obstruction 3 cm below the valve. The obstruction was relieved, but the boy died postoperatively with sudden onset of ventricular fibrillation.

The results of surgical treatment of aortic stenosis of the valvular and subvalvular type are generally good. Although the patients all retain some residual murmur, the gradient almost always can be alleviated. The residual murmur is probably caused by the abnormally thickened cusps that are always part of the abnormality. There is a small number of patients in whom the aortic annulus is abnormally small in addition to the valvular stenosis. In this group the gradient over the stenotic valve may be reduced somewhat but is not obliterated.

AORTIC INSUFFICIENCY

Isolated congenital aortic valvular insufficiency is an exceedingly rare lesion. We have not had the occasion to treat surgically a congenital aortic insufficiency. As mentioned before, aortic regurgitation can result from an aortic valvotomy, especially if a bicuspid valve is made into a tricuspid leaflet.

Aortic insufficiency is occasionally found associated with interventricular septal defects. The treatment of this complication is dealt with in the section on interventricular septal defects.

PULMONARY STENOSIS

Pulmonary stenosis with an intact interventricular septum is a common congenital lesion and probably about three times as common as aortic stenosis. The anomaly almost always involves the valve. However, subvalvular or infundibular stenosis with an intact septum also may be seen in a small percentage of the cases with or without associated valvular narrowing.

As in aortic stenosis symptoms may be lacking or minimal at first. Because of an intact septum better pulmonary flow can be accomplished than in those with a ventricular septal defect. This results in a higher right ventricular pressure and work load, thereby producing more severe right ventricular hypertrophy. Those younger patients who develop cardiac dilation because of extreme stenosis may become cyanotic because of a right-to-left shunt at the atrial level. The elevated right ventricular and diastolic pressure and rise in right atrial pressure blows open a patent foramen ovale. Thus, infants with severe stenosis may exhibit cyanosis in association with other evidences of right heart failure, such as heart enlargement, venous engorgement, and pulsating liver.

The prominent diagnostic feature is a loud stenotic type of systolic murmur at the second to fourth left interspace and a palpable systolic thrill with a quite pulmonic second sound. Right ventricular enlargement with a prominent pulmonary artery segment is evident on roentgenograms. The electrocardiogram shows right ventricular hypertrophy and frequently a significant P pulmonale. Cardiac catheterization shows the absence of a shunt at the ventricular level and elevated right ventricular pressures depending on the severity of the stenosis with a low pressure in the pulmonary artery. Although cardiac catheterization is not necessary to establish the diagnosis it may be used for confirmation, and also, if the right ventricular pressure is well above or below the left ventricular pressure and there is no evidence of a shunt, the possibility of a ventricular septal defect is ruled out. However, if the pressure in the two ventricles is equal, some consideration must be given during the operation to the possibility of a ventricular septal defect.

The prognosis of patients with pulmonary stenosis varies with the severity of the obstructions. Infants with severe stenosis may present with severe heart failure within the first weeks of life. Less severe valvular obstruction may produce symptoms in later childhood and adult life. The mildest stenosis may never produce symptoms. Persons with the last sort of lesion usually fall into the group with a right ventricular pressure less than 40 mm Hg. The choice of patients for pulmonary valvotomy will depend on the severity of the pressure gradient from right ventricle to pulmonary artery. Elevation of right ventricular pressure above 60 mm Hg is considered by many to be indication enough for surgery even though there may be no symptoms at the time.

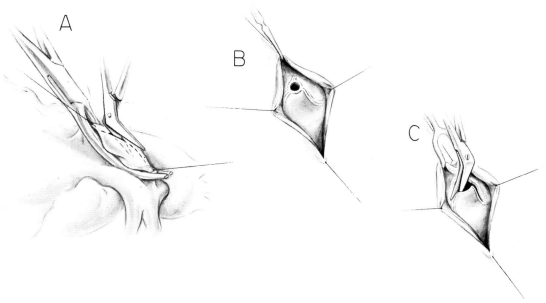

Fig. 6. Pulmonary stenosis. Technique of pulmonary valvotomy. A. An anterior lip of the main pulmonary artery is excluded with a clamp and incised. B. The clamp is removed after stopping the blood flow into the heart, and the fused valve is exposed. C. The commissures are carefully cut out to the valve ring.

Pulmonary valvotomy was one of the first successful attacks on intracardiac congenital defects. Brock developed a technique for transventricular valvotomy that is still used in some tiny, critically ill infants who cannot survive otherwise. The right ventricle and pulmonary artery are exposed through a left submammary incision. Traction stitches are taken in the ventricular wall on either side of the proposed ventricular stab wound. The valvulotome is inserted into the ventricular chamber, expandable blades are opened, and the instrument is passed into the pulmonary artery, cutting the valve on both sides.

More accurate valvotomy was obtained, however, when hypothermia (85° F) and inflow occlusion of circulation into the heart were developed. This allowed the pulmonary artery to be opened and the valve examined and its commissures opened accurately and completely. This method allows up to ten minutes of intracardiac operating time, which is adequate for uncomplicated situations. If infundibular stenosis is found or an unsuspected interventricular septal defect is discovered, more time is needed. For this reason, extracorporeal circulation is required in most cases.

After the patient is "on bypass" the aorta may be occluded to stop coronary blood flow into the right side of the heart and the pulmonary artery opened. The valve is usually dome-shaped, with all commissures fused and only a small opening left in the center. The commissures are cut and a finger passed into the ventricle to see if significant muscular obstruction is present below the valve (Fig. 6).

If subvalvular or infundibular obstruction is present, a right ventriculotomy is done to facilitate accurate removal of the fibrotic or muscular tissue without damage to the supporting structures of the tricuspid valve.

RESULTS

Transventricular valvotomies were done in the first 89 patients, with 1 death. Open valvotomy under hypothermia was employed in the next 73 cases, with 1 death. Fifty-eight patients have had valvotomies using extracorporeal circulation, with 1 death, for a total of 216 patients and a mortality of 1.3 percent.

PULMONARY INSUFFICIENCY

Pulmonary valve incompetence as an isolated congenital lesion is extremely rare. This anomaly is usually described as "idiopathic" dilation of the pulmonary artery. We have not had the occasion to operate on any of these patients, and there is very little information available concerning the long-term natural history of this abnormality.

MITRAL STENOSIS

Isolated congenital mitral stenosis without endocardial fibroelastosis is an exceedingly rare lesion. Involvement of the aorta and aortic valve as a concomitant abnormality is more common. As with other valves the clinical picture varies according to the severity of the stenosis. The primary clinical findings are those resulting from pulmonary venous obstruction evidenced by respiratory difficulties. The diagnosis is usually made by the presence of an accentuated pulmonary second sound, a prominent left atrium on the roentgenogram, and right ventricular enlargement, right-axis shift, and P pulmonale on electrocardiogram.

The prognosis for patients with congenital mitral stenosis varies directly with the severity of the obstruction. Usually the severely stenotic lesions cause death early and are seldom relieved with surgery because of the underdevelopment of the entire left heart. The less severe usually cause symptoms later and are more amenable to surgery.

Congenital mitral stenosis can be treated surgically, provided the lesion is uncomplicated. Frequently the valve is so deformed and the annulus so abnormal in those patients having severe symptoms early that little can be accomplished. In the older children with less difficulty the valve is thickened and rubbery with fusion of the commissures, so that some benefit can be obtained by incising the commissures. This requires direct vision and the aid of extracorporeal circulation.

Our series of 6 cases has a mortality of 16 percent. One child operated upon at the age of seven years has been followed for eight years and has become an active high school girl who participates in all athletics without symptoms.

MITRAL INSUFFICIENCY

Congenital mitral insufficiency as an isolated lesion is also a rare anomaly. It is more frequently seen with associated lesions, such as coarctation of the aorta, endocardial cushion defects, and ventricular septal defects. If the insufficiency is secondary to dilation of the ventricle because of an accompanying defect, the later defect should be corrected first.

In patients with isolated congenital mitral insufficiency the prognosis is determined by the severity of the incompetence. The diagnosis is made by the combination of clinical and roentgenological findings. Catheterization is usually necessary not only to confirm the diagnosis but also to further prove the absence of other lesions.

The treatment of choice is to repair the incompetent mitral valve. If the pathology is primarily a dilated annulus, an annuloplasty can be done by suturing the annulus at the commissures. However, frequently the pathology is confined to the leaflets, which are malformed or improperly attached. We have encountered on two occasions a septal aortic leaflet of the mitral valve that was merely rudimentary. The treatment of choice under the circumstances is a valve replacement. Our experience is extremely limited and confined to four Starr-Edwards valve prostheses. One was placed in a three-year-old girl who had intractable heart failure at bed rest and steroids for six months. She responded dramatically postoperatively and has remained well with full activity. The rest have done extremely well.

INTERATRIAL SEPTAL DEFECTS

Early in fetal life the interatrial septum is formed by elements of the septum primum, septum secundum, and septum intermedium. Incomplete fusion of these or deficiencies in their formation result in a defect in the septum.

Interatrial septal defects range from an obliquely patent foramen ovale, which is not rare but which is usually clinically insignificant, to a common atrium. These defects have been classified as ostium secundum defects, which are in the central part of the septum with single or fenestrated openings; sinus venosus defects, which are located high in the septum near the entry of the superior vena cava and which are frequently associated with anomalous pulmonary venous drainage; and the so-called ostium primum defect, which is usually large and adjacent to the tricuspid valve annulus, with clefts in the mitral and occasionally tricuspid valves. Although embryologists may dispute this nomenclature, it is convenient for the clinician and surgeon.

OSTIUM SECUNDUM DEFECTS

It is estimated that about 10 percent of all congenital cardiac defects are ostium secundum defects, which appear in about 1 out of every 13,500 children. The diagnosis of ostium secundum and sinus venosus defects is based on the effects of a large left-to-right shunt at the atrial level. Symptoms may be minimal, or there may be varying degrees of easy fatigability and dyspnea on exertion. Uncomplicated cases are not cyanotic. The heart is slightly to moderately enlarged, with an increased apical impulse. The systolic murmur is usually moderate in intensity and located near the second interspace to the left of the sternum. A middiastolic murmur is frequently heard at the apex. The second sound is usually widely split and fixed with respirations.

X-ray examinations show slight to moderate cardiac enlargement, prominence of the pulmonary segment and increased vascularity of the lung fields. The electrocardiogram will usually show right ventricular hyper-

trophy and often an incomplete right bundle branch block.

Cardiac catheterization is helpful in that passage of a catheter through the defect or

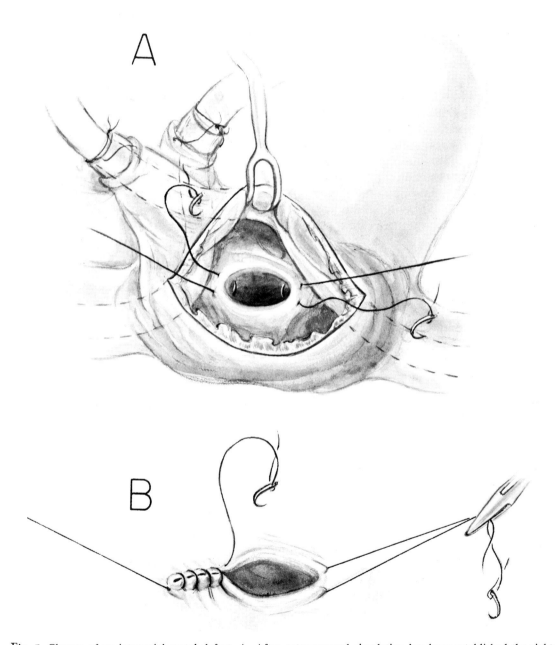

Fig. 7. Closure of an interatrial septal defect. A. After extracorporal circulation has been established the right atrium is opened and the defect identified. Stitches are placed at each end of the defect and tied. B. Traction on these will convert the circular defect to an ellipse or a slit, and over-and-over suturing will complete the closure.

a jump in oxygen saturation at the atrial level gives confirmatory evidence. It is most important to find the degree of hypertension in the pulmonary artery and to rule out other cardiac defects. Angiograms are helpful occasionally, not only to show the shunt, but also in searching for other defects.

The prognosis in infancy and childhood is good, but as the decades pass the mortality increases. Since closure of the defect at the present time carries such little risk, the mortality being 1 percent or lower, such surgery is advised if the patient is in otherwise good condition.

TREATMENT

The closure of interatrial septal defect has intrigued the surgeon for many years. Cohn, and later Bailey, devised a method of closure involving sewing an inverted dimple of atrial wall to the edges of the defect. Sondergaard (1954) used an encircling suture through the interatrial groove. Gross sutured a rubber well to the right atrium to permit fingers and instruments to be put in the atrium through the pool of blood. Lewis, in 1953, used an open technique of closure with hypothermia and inflow occlusion (Lewis and Tauffie, 1953). This was quite satisfactory for many uncomplicated cases, but it was not until extracorporeal circulation was perfected that safe and secure closure of all defects was assured.

After the patient is on extracorporeal circulatory bypass the atrium is opened with a longitudinal incision parallel to the vena cavae (Fig. 7). After the right atrium is aspirated the cardiotomy suction tip is placed in the orifice of the coronary sinus, keeping the field relatively bloodless without the need for aortic cross-clamping and cardiac arrest. If the left atrium is kept full, there is little risk of air being trapped in the left side of the heart and resulting in air embolism.

The defect usually can be closed with direct suture of over-and-over running silk. Occasionally the defect is so large that a prosthesis of a circular piece of plastic must be sutured to its rim. This is often the case when one or more pulmonary veins drain into the right atrium. The patch must then act as a tunnel under which the venous return is directed into the left atrium. Care must be taken while suturing near the vena caval orifices not to partially occlude them or divert one of them into the wrong atrium.

RESULTS

Since the period of extracorporeal circulation is short and arrest of coronary flow is unnecessary, the operative risk should be minimal. With the low pressure in the atria and less forceful contractions, recurrence of the defect should be rare.

During the period when hypothermia and inflow occlusion were used, 30 cases were operated on, with no deaths. Using cardiac bypass an additional 135 cases have had closure of their defects without any deaths.

OSTIUM PRIMUM DEFECTS

The term "ostium primum defect" has been applied to defects in the septum extending down to the atrioventricular valve tissue. The lower border consists of the adjacent mitral and tricuspid valve rings. These defects are usually larger than the secundum defect. There is usually a cleft in the mitral valve leaflet and occasionally another cleft in the tricuspid valve leaflet.

DIAGNOSIS

These defects result in the signs of a large left-to-right atrial shunt as well as evidence of mitral insufficiency of varying degree. Because of this these patients are in trouble earlier, and symptoms of dyspnea and poor exercise tolerance are much more prominent than is the case with secundum defects.

The heart is enlarged and active with a louder systolic murmur over the lower precordium than with secundum defects. The middiastolic rumble of increased flow across the tricuspid valve is prominent, and an apical systolic murmur indicates the mitral insufficiency. X-ray examination indicates an enlarged heart, prominent pulmonary artery segment, and increased vascularity of the lung fields. The electrocardiogram usually shows combined ventricular hypertrophy and incomplete right bundle branch block. Cardiac catheterization confirms the large left-to-right atrial shunt, and the catheter flips from left-to-right atrium directly.

PROGNOSIS

Since the effect of this type of defect upon the heart is more severe, the symptoms are more severe and occur earlier. The outlook is poor, and therefore surgical repair is usually indicated.

TREATMENT

The procedure of correction of ostium primum defect differs from that of secundum defects in several ways. The cleft valve or valves must be repaired by interrupted silk mattress sutures and the defect closed with a Teflon patch. The prosthesis is necessary not only because of the usually large size of the defect but also because carefully placed, interrupted sutures must be used in the lower border of the defect from the coronary sinus up to the middle of the valve annulus, since in this area lie the atrioventricular node and the bundle of His. This results in a longer operative and bypass time, increasing the operative risk and postoperative morbidity.

RESULTS

Closure of the defects is almost always secure, but repair of the valve cleft does not usually eliminate the mitral regurgitation. Reduction in the heart size is seen, with concomitant improvements in the symptoms. Eighteen patients have had ostium primum defects repaired, with one death, which was due to sudden postoperative hemorrhage caused by slipping of the ligature at the site of the atrial cannulation.

ATRIOVENTRICULAR CANAL

When the cardiac septal cushions fail to fuse a common atrioventricular canal results, with a confluent low atrial septal defect and high ventricular septal defect. The mitral and tricuspid valves cannot attach at an annulus in the center, so they form two festoons of common valve leaflets passing from one side to the other. If the interventricular septal defect is small, an ostium primum defect is simulated; however, in most of the patients the hemodynamic effects of a large atrial and ventricular shunt plus severe valvular regurgitation are so profound that survival past one year of age is rare.

DIAGNOSIS

Infants with atrioventricular canals are thin and dyspneic and soon go into heart failure. The heart is large, and there is a harsh, diffuse murmur over the lower precordium. X-ray examination shows gross cardiac enlargement involving the right atrium, right ventricle, and pulmonary outflow. Pulmonary vascularity is increased, with hilar pulsations. The electrocardiogram indicates left-axis shift and right ventricular hypertrophy in the precordial leads. Many of the children are mongoloid, and some have associated cardiac defects.

Cardiac catheterization shows a large left-to-right shunt at the atrial level, often with no further increase in oxygen saturation in the right ventricle. Pulmonary hypertension is the rule. The catheter may flip from the left atrium to the right ventricle and then to the right atrium.

PROGNOSIS

As indicated, death in infancy is common, and survival beyond five years of age is quite rare. Surgical correction would be desirable if possible.

TREATMENT

Several patients with a diagnosis of ostium primum were found to have small ventricular septal defects with separation of the valve rings. During suture of the clefts in the mitral and tricuspid valve leaflets, the annulus was sutured together with several interrupted silk mattress sutures that included a bite in the ventricular septum. After this the atrial septal portion of the defect was closed with a patch.

In patients with larger ventricular septal defects a dumbbell-shaped patch may be used, suturing one of the circular portions to close the ventricular portion of the defect, attaching the valves to the narrow portion, reconstructing the valves, and using the other circular portion of the patch to close the atrial portion of the defect. Unfortunately, the common valves frequently are deformed and deficient, and satisfactory repair is impossible.

RESULTS

Total correction of a true atrioventricular canal is infrequently attained, and the mortality is quite high. Nevertheless, attempts must be continued in an effort to solve this problem.

INTERVENTRICULAR SEPTAL DEFECTS

The ventricles are separated by the downward growth of tissue from the bulbus cordis and by the upward growth of the apical ridge of the interventricular septum. When fusion is complete, muscle forms in the septum, except for the portion closed by an extension of tissue from the fused atrioventricular cushions. This remains fibrous in nature and is called the septum membranaceum. It is in or near this area that a majority of the defects occur.

Interventricular septal defects vary greatly in size, and the size is not always indicative of the amount of blood shunted from the left ventricle to the right. Although most defects are located in or adjacent to the membranous septum, a few are located in the muscular septum, at times well down toward the apex. Many of these have a single opening on the left side of the septum but empty into the right ventricle through multiple openings between the trabeculae. Rarely there may be two separate septal defects. The most severe form of defective ventricular septum is the single ventricle.

Isolated interventricular septal defects make up approximately 20 percent of all congenital cardiac deformities. The hemodynamics depend not only on the size of the defect but also on the relative pressure in the ventricles. Lower pressure in the right ventricle will result in a large left-to-right shunt, a huge pulmonary blood flow, and left or combined ventricular hypertrophy. If there is some degree of stenosis of the outflow of the right ventricle or increased pulmonary arteriolar resistance, the right ventricular pressure rises, decreasing the shunt. This results in less pulmonary blood flow and a smaller heart.

DIAGNOSIS

Symptoms in many children may be minimal, with only mild limitation of activity and slight dyspnea with extremes of exertion. On the other hand, some infants with huge pulmonary blood flows have dyspnea at rest and frequent lower respiratory infections and may go into cardiac failure.

The large defects may give an increased apical impulse and some degree of cardiac enlargement. A loud, harsh systolic murmur and thrill are maximal at the third to the fifth interspaces to the left of the sternum. An apical diastolic rumble occurs when a large pulmonary flow results in a relative obstruction of the normal mitral valve. An accentuated pulmonary second sound indicates pulmonary hypertension.

X-ray examination shows the heart size to be normal or moderately increased with a prominent pulmonary artery segment and increased vascularity of the lung fields. Electrocardiograms in most cases indicate left or combined ventricular hypertrophy. Predominant right-side hypertrophy suggests severe pulmonary hypertension and central or peripheral obstruction.

Cardiac catheterization is necessary to confirm the diagnosis of ventricular septal defect, rule out additional anomalies, determine right-sided pressures, and estimate relative pulmonary to systemic blood flow and peripheral resistance. Usually there is a sharp rise in oxygen saturation upon entering the right ventricle. An elevation of oxygen saturation in the right atrial samples might indicate an additional atrial septal defect or a ventricular septal defect with its jet of blood directed into the atrium between tricuspid valve leaflets. Angiocardiography often helps not only in confirming the diagnosis but also in locating the septal defect.

PROGNOSIS

There is incontestable evidence that some septal defects close in early life. Most, however, remain open, and thus carry the possibility of continued heart strain and decreased exercise capacity, development of pulmonary vascular resistance, and the hazards of bacterial endocarditis.

Certain patients with large pulmonary flows with some degree of pulmonary hypertension need surgical correction. Others, in whom severe hypertension and peripheral pulmonary vascular resistance are so great that the vascularity of the peripheral lung fields is diminished, for whom ECG shows only right heart strain, and in whom there is a bidirectional shunt with some degree of peripheral arterial oxygen desaturation, are not candidates for closure of the defect. Another group of infants with large pulmonary blood flow and heart failure frequently needs operation as a lifesaving procedure.

TREATMENT

Many infants in failure due to ventricular septal defects may require surgery. Some can

be carried on medical management until they improve at about one year of age. In the others the best results have been obtained from narrowing the pulmonary artery with a band of umbilical tape or woven Teflon. The artery is approached through a short anterolateral incision in the left fourth interspace. The main pulmonary artery at its base is encircled and the band tightened until the distal arterial pressure is lowered to as near normal as possible. This requires narrowing of the lumen to one third to one fourth of its previous diameter. If the right ventricle dilates and the heart shows, the band must be loosened. If the child becomes at all cyanotic because of reversal of the shunt, the constriction is excessive.

Usually these children do well postoperatively, with the disappearance of respiratory problems and heart failure. At the age of three or four years or more the septal defect may be closed and the band removed. Frequently there is a stenosis of the artery at the site of the banding, requiring a diamond-shaped patch pericardium to enlarge the vessel adequately.

Attempts at closure of ventricular septal defects by the placement of tubes of fascia or pericardium through the defect or direct suture with a blind, closed heart technique were not successful. Only when extracorporeal circulation was perfected was safe and effective closure of the defects possible.

The approach is usually through the anterior wall of the right ventricle with the incision placed so as to avoid major coronary vessels (Fig. 8). A longitudinal incision is our usual choice, although a horizontal incision has many champions. Some of the defects can be reached through a right atriotomy, avoiding the injury to the right ventricular myocardium. In most instances, however, the exposure is superior through a right ventriculotomy.

The size of the defect and the character of the rim will dictate the method of closure. Small defects with fibrous rims are effectively closed with several figure-eight mattress stitches of 5-0 or 4-0 silk. A large de-

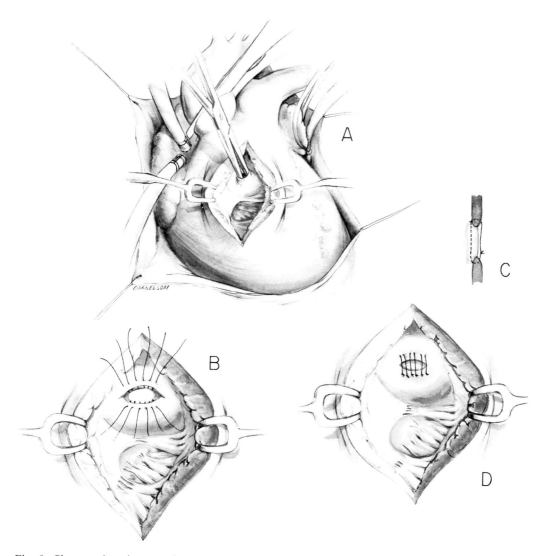

Fig. 8. Closure of an interventricular septal defect. A. Right ventriculotomy is done in a manner that will preserve the coronary vessels. Through this the defect is identified. B. Closure of a defect of moderate size using interrupted sutures passed through a Teflon felt pledget. C. Upon tying the sutures the prosthesis is forced over to the left ventricular side of the defect. D. The sutures are tied tightly, effectively closing the defect. Smaller defects can be closed by direct suture. Larger ones may require a circular patch, as shown in Figure 10.

fect, especially one with a soft muscular rim, is best closed with a Teflon felt patch because less tension on the sutures occurs during cardiac contraction. Interrupted sutures of 5-0 silk are best used in suturing the patch to the lower border of the defect where the conduction system runs. The suture is put through the patch, then along the rim of the defect parallel to the conduction fibers, and

then back through the patch. Along the upper rim the suturing may be done as an over-and-over stitch to save time.

A defect of an intermediate size or a small defect with a soft muscular rim may best be closed with a series of interrupted sutures passing through the lower edge of the defect, then through a pledget of Teflon felt and out the upper rim of the defect. When these are tied the closure is buttressed by a pledget which is forced over to the left ventricular side of the defect.

Cross-clamping of the ascending aorta produces a bloodless field and anoxic cardiac arrest. Although this maneuver is unnecessary in repair of small defects, it is often helpful in the closure of more complicated defects. Intermittent occlusion of the aorta or continuous occlusion of up to 30 minutes does not seem to produce irreversible changes in cardiac action or long-term damage to the myocardium. Several special surgical problems in certain complicated ventricular septal defects should be mentioned. At times a rather marked overriding of the aortic root into the right ventricle may be found. If there is no pulmonary stenosis or increased peripheral pulmonary vascular resistance, the only technical problem is that the suturing of the patch to close the defect must be done in a tilted plane to baffle the blood from the left ventricle to the aorta, much as is done for the tetralogy of Fallot. If there is pulmonary stenosis, it must be relieved by infundibulectomy, valvolotomy, or both, as is necessary. In true Eisenmenger's syndrome with cyanosis and decreased pulmonary flow caused by peripheral pulmonary artery obstruction, closure of the defect would be fatal.

In certain cases, prolapse of one of the leaflets of the aortic valve into the defect occurs, producing aortic insufficiency in addition to the findings of septal defect. Not only must the defect be closed, but the aorta must be opened and the redundant leaflet shortened and shored up with mattress sutures reinforced by Teflon felt pledgets to prevent the tearing through of the stitches.

Ventricular septal defects may have their flow directed between the leaflets of the tricuspid valve, producing a shunt from the left ventricle to the right atrium. This is suspected preoperatively when all signs point to a ventricular septal defect, but at catheterization the left-to-right shunt is found at the atrial level. Repair of these defects can usually be done through the right atrium, sparing the trauma of a ventriculotomy.

The extreme in size of ventricular septal defects is the single ventricle. If there is no other associated defect, it is tempting to try to divide the ventricle into left and right sides by suturing a large plastic patch midway across the common ventricle. Unfortunately, when the ventricles contract and shorten, the patch does not, resulting in a buckling and obstruction of one or the other ventricular outflow tracts.

RESULTS

The mortality that occurs with the closure of ventricular septal defects is mostly related to the degree of pulmonary hypertension. In a series of 324 repairs there were no deaths in patients with pulmonary artery pressures of 80 mm Hg or less (or four fifths of the systemic pressure). When pulmonary pressure equals systemic pressure, and especially when the pulmonary peripheral resistance reaches 8 or 9 units (normal is 3 to 4), the mortality and morbidity become rather forbidding.

Several complications may occur after the closure of ventricular septal defects. Postoperative hemorrhage, infection, and atelectasis are vexing but not usually fatal. More peculiar to the procedure are the complications of heart block and residual or recurrent septal defects. In our experience permanent complete heart block due to interruption of the bundle of His is rare, but when it does occur it may be fatal unless a pacemaker is implanted. Residual septal defects are more common, occurring in as many as 5 percent of the cases in some series. This complication is more frequent in repair of the tetralogy of Fallot and the septal defect with pulmonary stenosis, possibly because of the larger size of the defects and the obliquity of the suturing.

TETRALOGY OF FALLOT

Tetralogy of Fallot was the first cyanotic congenital heart lesion to be surgically treated. Although this combination of symptoms was mentioned in the literature earlier, it was described in detail by Fallot in 1888 and bears his name (see Fallot, 1888). In

1945 Blalock and Taussig, while working on the physiology of pulmonary hypertension, developed the subclavian pulmonary artery anastomosis, which was applied to the tetralogy at Taussig's urging and which proved successful in alleviating the cyanosis (Blalock and Taussig, 1945). Because the subclavian pulmonary artery anastomosis frequently clotted in tiny infants with small subclavian arteries, in 1946 Potts devised an aortic pulmonary anastomosis that permitted more accurate and adequate shunts in infancy (see Potts, Smith, and Gibson, 1946).

Shortly after these two initial palliative procedures, Sir Russell Brock (1948) devised his method for closed pulmonary valvotomy. This was later extended to permit excision of the obstructed infundibulum in cases of tetralogy of Fallot. It varied in popularity but was utilized by several cardiovascular surgeons to rescue seriously ill infants who would not tolerate shunt operations.

Total correction of tetralogy had to wait for development of the heart-lung machine. Once this equipment was developed, total correction became feasible. Lillehei first successfully accomplished excision of the right ventricular outflow tract and closure of the ventricular septal defect (Lillehei, et al., 1955a). This success was repeated by many.

Today, one of the major problems facing the surgeon treating tetralogy of Fallot is the takedown of shunts prior to total correction. Systemic-pulmonary shunts are not much of a problem, but the takedown of aortic-pulmonary shunts furnishes a real challenge to the surgeon. Kirklin and Devloo (1961) added a great deal to the safety of closing aortic-pulmonary shunts by developing the use of hypothermia with extracorporeal perfusion to permit closure of the aortic-pulmonary shunt from inside the pulmonary artery prior to total correction of tetralogy.

PATHOLOGY

Fallot's surgical description listed four components: (1) overriding aorta, (2) ventricular septal defect, (3) pulmonary stenosis, and (4) right ventricular hypertrophy.

Within the confines of these four changes, however, a great number of variations may exist. The tetralogy of Fallot complex exhibits variations that range from relatively simple ventricular septal defect with mild obstruction of the outflow tract of the right ventricle to marked overriding aorta with an oblique ventricular septal defect and severely deformed and obstructed infundibulum and pulmonary valve. Further studies demonstrated that the size of the pulmonary artery may vary, about one third being normal in size, one third being moderately small but capable of sustaining adequate flow to the lungs, and one third being extremely small, so that primary repair of the defect would be impaired by the lack of an adequate channel to the lungs. This last group of patients necessarily requires initial shunt operations to expand the pulmonary arterial bed and to lead to adequate enlargement of the left side of the heart prior to total correction.

DIAGNOSIS

The diagnosis of tetralogy of Fallot can be suspected in many instances by the "scratchy" systolic murmur that is heard over the precordium and the pulmonic area. Those patients also having stenosis of the pulmonary valve may be distinguished by the absence of the pulmonic second sound. The patient, of course, is cyanotic because of the right-to-left shunt across the ventricular septal defect, and children with tetralogy frequently assume a characteristic squatting posture when they tire.

Roentgenograms of the chest usually show a small heart and the absence of the pulmonary artery shadow. The pulmonary vascular markings are usually diminished. The small heart differentiates tetralogy from isolated pulmonary valvular stenosis, which usually has an enlarged heart associated with it. Electrocardiograms show right ventricular hypertrophy.

TREATMENT

Surgical therapy falls into two categories, palliative and corrective. Total correction is

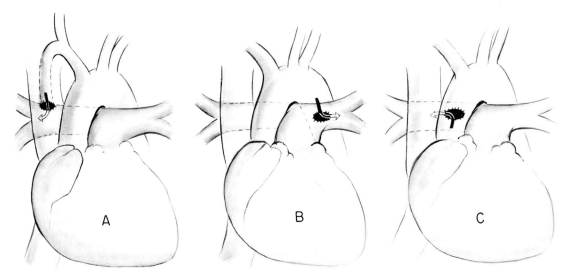

Fig. 9. Tetralogy of Fallot. Systemic pulmonary shunts commonly used in treating tetralogy of Fallot and other cases with diminished pulmonary blood flow. A. Subclavian-pulmonary anastomosis (Blalock). B. Descending aortic-pulmonary anastomosis (Potts). C. Ascending aortic-pulmonary anastomosis.

usually delayed until the child is several years old to facilitate the use of extracorporeal circulation. If the child is mildly cyanotic and only slightly handicapped, operative procedures are postponed. If, however, the infant is quite incapacitated, with a marked decrease in exercise tolerance or unconscious spells, a shunt procedure is performed to tide the patient over until corrective surgery can be done. The other indication for a preliminary systemic-pulmonary artery shunt is the presence of an underdeveloped pulmonary vascular system (Fig. 9).

The Brock procedure has been used only sparingly in my experience, on very tiny infants with small pulmonary arteries, in whom even an aortic-pulmonary anastomosis would have little chance of success. Under these circumstances, blind resection of the infundibulum was accomplished, and several of these children survived. Resection of the outflow tract was by no means complete, but it did permit enough of an increase in the blood flow to the lungs to improve peripheral oxygenation.

In 20 percent of patients with this complex there is a right aortic arch. The side on which the aorta lies determines the operative approach. A subclavian-pulmonary anastomosis is best performed on the side opposite the aortic arch, since the takeoff of the subclavian artery from the innominate gives better flow than when it comes directly off of the aorta. The aortic-pulmonary anastomosis naturally must be performed on the side of the aorta.

In the subclavian-pulmonary anastomosis, a thoracotomy is done and the subclavian artery is dissected free. The pulmonary artery is also isolated, and an end-to-side anastomosis is created between the subclavian artery and the pulmonary artery, utilizing an everting 5-0 silk suture. In the aortic-pulmonary anastomosis, the descending aorta distal to the subclavian artery is dissected free, and several intercostal arteries are divided in order to permit application of an aortic exclusion clamp. Once this is accomplished, the pulmonary artery is fixed to the side of the aorta with temporary occluding ligatures, and a side-to-side anastomosis is created between the aorta and the left main pulmonary artery.

In the Brock procedure the infundibular obstruction may be partially relieved by instrumentation, but in tetralogies it is usu-

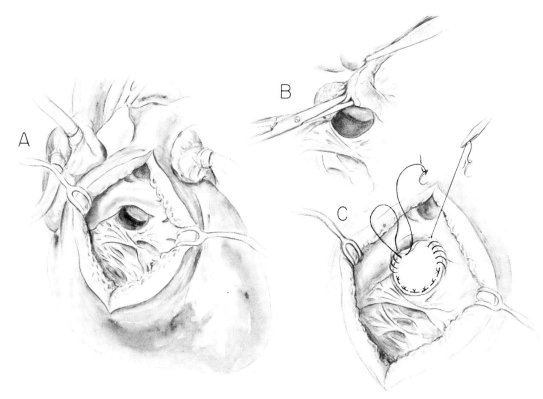

Fig. 10. Total correction of the tetralogy of Fallot. A. Right ventriculotomy shows the anatomy of tetralogy with a large interventricular septal defect, hypertrophy, and deviation of the crista supraventricularis to the right side resulting in pulmonary outflow obstruction and "overriding" of the aorta. B. The infundibular obstruction is being excised. The leaflets of the aortic valve can be seen immediately behind. C. A patch of Teflon felt is sutured to the edges of the defect.

ally necessary to do rapid blind excision of the infundibulum through a small incision in the right ventricular outflow tract. Hypothermia and inflow occlusion of the superior and inferior vena cava may facilitate this operative procedure.

TOTAL CORRECTION

The treatment of choice, whenever possible, is total correction of the defect. This is accomplished by means of extracorporeal circulation, which permits thorough excision of the obstruction in the outflow tract of the right ventricle and closure of the ventricular septal defect (Fig. 10). In all instances, closure of the ventricular septal defect required introduction of a plastic patch. We presently use Teflon felt for this purpose. Since the defect is always large and, because of the

overriding of the aorta, lies obliquely, direct suture closure is not advisable. The aortic outflow tract may be obstructed, or the sutures may tear out, leaving a residual defect and a left-to-right shunt if the pulmonary stenosis has been relieved.

An oval or round piece of Teflon felt is cut to fit the defect and sutured in place. Around the lower rim of the defect, 5-0 silk mattress stitches are taken, through the felt, into the rim of the defect, paralleling the conduction fibers, and then back through the felt. When the upper ridge of excavated crista supraventricularis is reached, a continuous suture is safe and timesaving.

Left atrial decompression is essential in these cyanotic patients, since enlarged bronchial arteries supply a good flow through the lungs. The outflow tract of the right ventricle occasionally may not be large enough after excision to relieve the obstruction adequately. If it is not, one can enlarge the outflow tract by suturing an elliptical piece of pericardium or a plastic prosthesis to the sides of the ventriculotomy to produce a larger outflow. One may obtain an estimate of the adequacy of the outflow tract by measuring relative pressures of the right ventricle and the pulmonary artery after adequate heart action is resumed.

RESULTS

The operative mortality of total correction of tetralogy of Fallot is intimately related to the size of the main pulmonary artery and the severity of infundibular stenosis, as well as to the degree of overriding of the aorta and the size and strength of the left ventricle. In general, we do shunt procedures (aortic-pulmonary or subclavian-pulmonary arterial anastomosis) as preliminary palliative operations in patients with small pulmonary arteries with severely constricted right ventricular infundibular tracts. However, although the shunts seem to promote development of the left heart and prepare it for eventual total correction, the operative mortality is compounded by the necessity for performing two operative procedures to achieve eventual total correction. This is particularly true of the aortic-pulmonary anastomoses, which require not only extracorporeal circulation but also profound hypothermia and temporary cessation of the extracorporeal perfusion to permit closure of the anastomosis.

In our series of 859 shunt procedures (aortic-pulmonary or subclavian-pulmonary) the mortality for patients over one year of age is less than 10 percent, but that for patients under one year of age remains near 20 percent, most deaths being among the neonatal group. During the past eight years 218 patients have undergone total correction of tetralogy of Fallot.

The mortality rate in primary total correction and total correction with closure of a previous subclavian-pulmonary anastomosis

runs close to 10 percent. Because of difficulties in the procedure when an aortic-pulmonary anastomosis must be closed, the mortality rate in this type of case is approximately 25 percent. This may largely be because of the selection for reoperation of patients with large shunts, aneurysms of the pulmonary artery, or increased vascular resistance in the pulmonary arteriolar bed.

Residual or recurrent ventricular septal defects are more common in the patients with tetralogy of Fallot repair, probably because of the size and obliquity of the defects. Persistent heart block is rare in these cases because the conduction mechanism dips to the left side of the septum.

TRANSPOSITION OF THE GREAT VESSELS

Transposition of the great vessels is a heart malformation in which the pulmonary artery originates from the left ventricle while the aorta originates from the right ventricle. Thus, there is complete separation of the systemic and pulmonary circulations, and consequently cyanotic blood from the vena cava returns to the peripheral arterial circulation, while oxygenated blood from the lungs returns to the pulmonary arterial cidculation. The anomaly is incompatible with life unless some communication exists between the systemic and pulmonic systems, such as interventricular septal defect, interatrial septal defect, or patent ductus arteriosus. Despite the presence of such partially compensatory lesions most patients are dead before the age of one year, although some have lived into early adulthood. This is a formidable challenge to the cardiac surgeon, since it constitutes about 40 percent of cyanotic congenital heart disease in some reported series.

The modern history of transposition probably begins with the complete description of the condition by Taussig in 1936. Shortly thereafter, attempts at its correction began, and the first partially successful operations were reported by Hanlon and Blalock (1948). They consisted of (1) the creation of atrial septal defects and (2) the creation of various venous shunts. The former procedure has since gained in popularity, not only because of its ease of performance but also because it does provide some significant palliation in very young patients. Recently, a modification of this procedure by Edwards (1949) has enhanced its efficiency, and at present a great deal of interest exists in the creation of atrial septal defects for transposition in early infancy. Albert (1955) introduced the concept of shifting the interatrial septum in order to transpose the venous circulations. Although these early attempts were unsuccessful, they stimulated a great deal of work, which culminated in the successes reported by Senning (1959) and later by Mustard (1964). At present, these approaches can be added on to the performance of an earlier Blalock-Hanlon atrial septal defect and provide the best approach currently available for total correction of selected cases of transposition. Because many patients with transpositions have pulmonary hypertension or other associated anomalies that militate against total correction, a partial correction operation introduced by Baffes (1956) is still useful for palliating most of the transpositions. Since this procedure can also be combined with the Mustard operation at a later date, it continues to be useful, although the technical difficulties encountered by some in its performance have reduced its acceptance.

A number of workers have explored the possibility of transposing the aorta and pulmonary artery directly. Bjork and Bouckaert (1954) attempted this using homografts but were unsuccessful. Murphy (1955) and his associates attempted to use the interventricular septal defect for similar purpose without success. Mustard and his associates transferred the aorta and pulmonary artery directly and added the concept of surgical transfer of one of the coronaries as well. This notion was expanded by efforts reported by Idriss (1961) and his associates and by Baffes (1960) and his associates, in which attempts were made to transfer both coro-

nary arteries. Bailey (1950) and his associates have made similar attempts. None was successful.

In patients with severe tricuspid stenosis or pulmonary valvular stenosis, shunts have been used to palliate the condition. Systemic pulmonary anastomoses have been used in those patients with severe pulmonary stenosis and low pulmonary artery pressure. The anastomosis of the superior vena cava to the pulmonary artery developed by Glenn and Patino (1954) has been used in cases with tricuspid stenosis.

PATHOLOGY

The applicability of any surgical procedure in the treatment of transposition depends on the pathology encountered. The transposition defect frequently is more complicated than mere separation of the systemic and pulmonary circulations. Superimposed on the basic transposition complex may be any of the usual other congenital heart anomalies, including valvular stenosis, coarctation of the aorta, anomalous or aberrant coronary arteries, and septal defects. Assuming that the particular transposition anomaly is not so deformed as to defy any operative intervention, the effectiveness of therapy is influenced by two added anomalies—pulmonary hypertension and ventricular septal defect. If either of these lesions is present, it greatly complicates total correction of the transposition defect.

VENTRICULAR SEPTAL DEFECT

In 147 cases studied morphologically by our group, only 51 specimens were encountered having transposition of the great vessels without ventricular septal defect. Of these, 23 (16 percent of the entire series) would have been ideal candidates for total corrective procedures. The rest had other anomalies (e.g., fetal coarctation or deformed chambers) that militated against complete therapy. Patients with ventricular septal defect, in contrast, were considered difficult to correct completely. In the absence of pulmonary valvular stenosis, most of them had pulmonary hypertension. Even those without obvious pulmonary hypertension faced the added burden of closure of the ventricular septal defect in addition to total correction of the transposition complex.

PULMONARY HYPERTENSION

Approximately one third to one half of all transpositions have increased pulmonary arterial pressure. In some this represents the natural state of the infantile lung and may eventually disappear. In others the condition is irreversible. In the symptomatic infant facing total correction of a transposition complex, however, the physiological implications of both types of pulmonary arterial hypertension are the same. There is no known way to differentiate between them before surgery. In the presence of pulmonary hypertension, therefore, total correction is not feasible at the present time.

DIAGNOSIS

Because transpositions become symptomatic early in infancy, clinical diagnosis is particularly important. The infant is cyanotic and dyspneic shortly after birth. A systolic murmur is audible over the precordium, and the heart sounds are dynamic. The heart is usually enlarged. Roentgenograms not only confirm cardiac enlargement but also usually outline an egg-shaped heart with a narrow mediastinum resulting from the anterior relationship of the aorta and the pulmonary artery. The lung fields are prominent and congested, in contrast to the other usual types of cyanotic congenital heart disease. Electrocardiographic findings vary. Signs of right ventricular hypertrophy are common. Some patients with pulmonary stenosis of pulmonary hypertension have indications of left ventricular hyperplasia. Depression of the S-T segment indicative of coronary ischemia may also be observed.

Intensely cyanotic infants with transposed great vessels but without ventricular septal defect have no distinctive murmurs. They rarely survive beyond the first few weeks of life. Diagnosis may be confirmed by venous angiography, which demonstrates the aorta originating from the right ventricle.

OPERATIVE PROCEDURES

It is difficult to conceive of a single operative procedure that would apply to all transposition complexes and their individual variations. The solutions, therefore, are multiple and take the form of both palliative and corrective operations.

PALLIATIVE OPERATIONS

Historically, three palliative operations are important because they represent early successful attempts to alleviate transposition; in addition, they still constitute the only successful approach to some more complicated forms of transposition. These operative procedures are (1) creation of an interatrial septal defect, (2) anastomosis of the right main pulmonary artery to the superior vena cava, and (3) systemic pulmonary shunts (subclavian-pulmonary and aortic-pulmonary anastomoses).

CREATION OF AN ATRIAL SEPTAL DEFECT

The most popular palliative procedure used today is the creation of an interatrial defect between the right and left atria by the excision of the posterior portion of the interatrial septum, as described by Blalock and Hanlon (1950). More recently, it has been modified by Mustard (1961). It is extremely useful as an emergency procedure in neonates who cannot tolerate more difficult or more prolonged operations. It is especially advantageous because other, more complicated corrective operations can be superimposed after the child has grown up. It also can be applied to a large number of transposition complexes likely to be encountered. A minor shortcoming is that the operator can never be precisely sure of the size of the atrial septal defect created by the original closed technique of Blalock and Hanlon. Mustard has made a significant contribution by designing a similar technique that can be performed under direct vision with hypothermia and inflow stasis by occlusion of the superior and inferior vena cava.

RIGHT MAIN PULMONARY ARTERY– SUPERIOR VENA CAVA ANASTOMOSIS

The anastomosis of the right main pulmonary artery to the superior vena cava has found its chief use in treatment of transposition complexes with tricuspid or pulmonary stenosis. The right main pulmonary artery is divided from its central trunk, and the distal end is anastomosed (end to side) to the lateral wall of the superior vena cava. The base of the superior vena cava is then ligated at its point of entry into the right atrium, and all blood from the superior vena cava is thus forced to pass through the right lung.

SYSTEMIC-PULMONARY SHUNTS

In severe pulmonary or tricuspid atresia, where pulmonary blood flow is greatly impaired (i.e., where pulmonary artery pressures are less than 20 mm Hg), the subclavian-pulmonary and aortic-pulmonary shunts may offer an opportunity for successful palliation. It is difficult to evaluate the efficacy of these procedures because in our experience they have been applied in extremely ill infants in whom unanticipated severe impairment of pulmonary blood flow has been encountered. When successfully accomplished, however, they have offered significant palliation, and they must be retained as part of the armamentarium for transposition of the great vessels.

PARTIAL VENOUS CORRECTION OF TRANSPOSITION

In 1956, Baffes devised an operative procedure for partial correction of transposition in which inferior vena cava was transferred to the left atrium by the use of a homologous or plastic graft while the right pulmonary veins were transferred to the right atrium (Baffes, 1956). Over 150 patients, ranging in age from three weeks to 15 years, have had this operation, with an operative mortality of 25 percent. Survivors have been followed for over 9 years and have showed improvement in peripheral oxygen saturation ranging from 75 percent saturation to values as high as 91 percent saturation. Improvement in exercise tolerance, growth, and development has been gratifying.

Although this operative procedure presents some difficulties in its technical performance, it is attractive because it can be accomplished without profound hypothermia or extracorporeal circulation in the majority of the transposition complexes. It can be applied in the face of pulmonary hypertension and ventricular septal defects, and even in its primary form it adds many years to those patients who survive its performance. In spite of its technical difficulties it is attractive because it may have a salutary effect upon the reactive pulmonary hypertension that might result from the profound cyanosis inherent in transposition. It also can be superimposed upon it, at a later date, either a second stage, designed by Baffes and his colleagues, or a modification of the Mustard total corrective procedure, described below. In either case, the door is open for later total correction of the transposition defect, and especially in patients in whom pulmonary hypertension or ventricular septal defects contraindicate initial performance of other total corrective procedures, this operation becomes the procedure of choice. In fact, it may be the bulwark of transposition therapy, since it may be applicable in as high as 60 percent of transposition complexes.

TOTAL CORRECTION

A great deal of time and effort has been expended to achieve total correction of transposition of the great vessels, and it is not within the scope of this section to review completely all the procedures that have been devised. They may be classified, however, into two major groups—those attempting to correct the anomaly of the aorta and pulmonary artery by repositioning them so that they emerge from the correct ventricle and those in which this anomalous relationship is accepted and attempts are made to correct the venous return to the heart. Although the former group of procedures has assiduously been attempted, no successes have been reported, and they will not be reviewed. Success has been achieved, however, by Senning and Mustard, who designed procedures for venous correction of the transposition defect.

SENNING PROCEDURE

In 1958, with the aid of extracorporeal circulation, Senning accomplished total correction of the transposition defect by shifting the atrial walls and thereby transferring the venous circulation in order to compensate for the transposition (Senning, 1959). The correction was accomplished by (1) shifting the posterior aspect of the interatrial septum and anastomosing it to the lateral rim of the ostia of the left pulmonary veins, then (2) anastomosing the posterior margin of the lateral wall of the right atrium to the anterior rim of an incision into the interatrial septum and then (3) completing a channel for the pulmonary venous flow behind the heart by anastomosing the anterior rim of the lateral incision in the right atrium to the lateral rim of the incision in the anterior aspect of the right pulmonary veins.

The first success was later repeated by Kirklin and his associates. The need to utilize profound hypothermia and cessation of the extracorporeal circulation made this operation somewhat hazardous, yet successes continued although with a high operative mortality. A method to eliminate the necessity of stopping extracorporeal circulation in the midst of the Senning operation was devised, but further work on the Senning operation was virtually aborted by development of the Mustard procedure for transferring the venous circulation in transpositions.

MUSTARD PROCEDURE

In 1964 a method for utilizing pericardium as a baffle to redirect both venous circulations across a large interatrial septal defect successfully accomplished total correction of selected cases of transposition (Mustard, 1964). Unfortunately, successes in infancy could not be accomplished, and eventually it became apparent that this operative procedure would have to be preceded by the creation of atrial septal defects in the young infants with symptomatic transpositions. Yet, within 18 months after that preliminary operation, it was possible to perform the transatrial venous redirection with reasonable expectation of success. The operative procedure consists of excising the interatrial septum and rerouting the venous return to the heart using a large patch of pericardium as a baffle. The vena caval flow goes under the patch to the left ventricle while the pulmonary venous return goes around the patch to the right ventricle. A number of cases were also attempted in patients with transposition and ventricular septal defects. The added burden of closure of the ventricular septal defects made success in these cases limited. At present this procedure represents the best method for total correction of transposition complexes. It is particularly applicable in patients without ventricular septal defects, especially those who can survive infancy by virtue of persistence of interatrial septal defect or patent ductus arteriosus. In those infants who become symptomatic early in life because of the absence of those fortuitous compensatory defects it is possible to perform a Blalock-Hanlon operation to create an atrial septal defect and follow this preliminary operation with the Mustard procedure in approximately 18 to 24 months.

TRICUSPID ATRESIA

The complex of tricuspid atresia and stenosis can range from complete atresia of the tricuspid and pulmonary valves with a rudimentary, nonfunctioning right ventricle to a mild tricuspid stenosis with a slightly hypoplastic right ventricle, with or without pulmonary stenosis.

The most striking group includes those with complete tricuspid atresia. These cases are not common, making up a small but significant percentage of infants with cyanotic heart disease.

There is no trace of the valve structures; instead, solid heart muscle separates the right atrium from the right ventricle. Venous return to the right atrium must pass through an interatrial septal defect to the left side of the heart. Blood reaches the lungs via an interventricular septal defect into the right ventricle and out to the pulmonary artery, or, if no septal defect is present, a patent ductus arteriosus provides pulmonary flow. Transposition of the great vessels may also be present as an additional defect.

DIAGNOSIS

Cyanosis is usually severe, with episodes of unconsciousness occurring in the more critically ill infants. A loud, harsh systolic murmur can be heard in the third left interspace. Cardiomegaly is rarely present, but enlargement of the liver is usually palpable. Roentgenograms of the chest reveal a heart of normal size with a rounded left border and diminished vascularity of the lung fields. Electrocardiograms show left heart strain and peaked, prominent P waves.

Cardiac catheterization and angiocardiograms will serve to confirm the diagnosis and to aid in the discovery of complicating lesions; however, in the very ill tiny infant only one procedure may be tolerated and that would best be an operative attempt to get more blood to the lungs.

PROGNOSIS

Most of the patients do not survive the first months of life, and only those with a significant flow through the right ventricle or a patent ductus can be expected to survive the first few years. In infancy, as the life-sustaining ductus closes, cyanosis deepens and unconscious spells become frequent, leading to sudden death.

TREATMENT

Because of the almost inevitable demise without surgery, immediate operation must be undertaken. Since total correction of the defect is impossible short of cardiac transplant, at the present time attempts are aimed at palliation by providing increased pulmonary flow.

The earliest operative procedure was an aortic-pulmonary shunt. This side-to-side anastomosis of the two arteries effectively increased blood flow through the lungs, and if it is of the proper size the child will lose the cyanosis and increase its exercise tolerance and life span.

In the young infant of a few days or weeks of age, the standard technique of aortic-pulmonary anastomosis using the Potts-Smith clamp may have to be modified. The moribund child may not tolerate dissection of the aorta with possible ligation of life-sustaining bronchial arteries or traction on the vessels resulting in occlusion of a small patent ductus arteriosus. It may be better to pull adjoining lips of the two vessels together into a curved, multitoothed clamp, make slits of the appropriate size in each lip, and accomplish a rapid side-to-side anastomosis with a continuous over-and-over 6-0 silk suture. Another method utilizes partial occlusion of the aorta with a curved clamp and involves fastening temporary ligatures from the pulmonary artery to the clamp to approximate the two vessels.

The length of the incision must be kept

under 5 mm in the tiny infant, which results in an opening of about 3 mm in diameter. If the shunt is smaller it will frequently close. If it is larger the child will probably soon go into heart failure.

The shunt from the superior vena cava to the right pulmonary artery not only routes more blood to the lung but also spares the right atrium the load of pushing all the systemic venous return into the left atrium. In the classical operation introduced by Glenn and Patino in 1954 the proximal right pulmonary artery is ligated and the distal stump is anastomosed to the side of the superior vena cava. Ligation of the cava as it enters the atrium forces all the return flow from the upper part of the body through the right lung. Several methods have been tried to divert right atrial blood to the left lung, but without uniform success.

This procedure gives effective palliation and is probably the preferred procedure in the older patients. Unfortunately the tiny infant a few days old, and even up to several months of age, may have very small pulmonary arteries and a consequent slow flow and resultant clotting of the anastomosis. In this age group a systemic artery–pulmonary artery shunt may be best.

The interatrial septal defect is almost always large enough to allow blood flow from right to left. In an occasional case the septal defect may be small, resulting in the damming back of venous return and a grossly enlarged liver and distended veins. Enlargement of the interatrial septal defect using a closed or open technique may be necessary.

RESULTS

Of 130 patients with tricuspid atresia operated on, all but 15 have had aortic-pulmonary anastomosis, most being done in the first six months of life. Of these there was a 20 percent immediate postoperative mortality. Late deaths brought the mortality up to 35 percent. Of the survivors a little over half can be classified as good results.

Of patients undergoing the Glenn proce-

dure, all operated upon under six months of age succumbed, but all over six months at the time of surgery have done well.

EBSTEIN'S COMPLEX

Ebstein's complex consists of a deformity of the tricuspid valve with displacement of the leaflets distally to the usual annulus of the valve. This results in gross regurgitation with right atrial enlargement and a right-to-left shunt at the atrial level. Although there is rarely anatomical pulmonary stenosis, there is functional stenosis, since it is easier for the blood to escape backward from the right ventricle during systole than to move forward.

Catheterization and selective angiocardiograms will aid in the diagnosis.

TREATMENT

Little operative benefits have been forthcoming as yet. Because of the valvular deformity, nothing reparative is effective. Replacement by a prosthetic ball valve is possible, but the suturing near the atrioventricular node often results in a permanent heart block.

Palliative procedures may be of some help, such as an anastomosis between the right pulmonary artery and right atrium. The high right atrial pressure and pumping action of the regurgitation facilitate blood flow through the right lung.

AORTIC-PULMONARY WINDOW

The aortic-pulmonary window, an opening between the ascending aorta and the main pulmonary artery, is also called the aortic septal defect. It results from the incomplete separation of the two vessels, which are formed from a common trunk. The opening may be relatively small in diameter and long, resembling a ductus arteriosus, but is usually large and short, amounting to a fistula between the two vessels.

Hemodynamically the window is identical to a patent ductus, but because of its size the pulmonary blood flow is very large, and the pulmonary artery pressure is usually equal to that of the aorta. The prognosis is worse than with a patent ductus because of the large size of the shunt.

DIAGNOSIS

Fatigability and dyspnea with exercise are often prominent symptoms. Physical findings may be identical to those found in patients with a large patent ductus. The heart is usually enlarged, and there is a loud, continuous murmur at the base of the heart, perhaps a little more to the right than in a ductus. The high pulse pressure and bounding pulses are also present. The electrocardiogram is more apt to show left or combined heart strain, and the roentgenograms of the chest show cardiac enlargement, a prominent pulmonary artery segment, and increased vascularity of the lung fields, as in a large patent ductus.

The differentiation rests with passage of a cardiac catheter from the aorta through the defect into the pulmonary artery. The catheter takes a route very different from that taken in a patent ductus. A fortuitous selective cineangiogram might also aid in the diagnosis.

TREATMENT

Since the shunt through the defect—and hence the pulmonary flow—is large, the outlook in a patient with an aortic-pulmonary window is quite poor without closure.

If the connection is long and not large in diameter it is possible to dissect apart the aorta and pulmonary artery, expose the connection and clamp, and divide and suture the stumps as one does with a patent ductus. Unfortunately, the defects are usually so large and short that this would be hazardous.

The safest approach is to have the patient on cardiopulmonary bypass with a longitudinal sternal-splitting approach. After preliminary dissection between the two vessels

the aorta can be clamped distal to the defect and the two arteries cut apart, transecting the defect. The aortic opening is closed with an over-and-over 5-0 silk suture and the clamps released. The pulmonary artery opening can then be closed at leisure.

RESULTS

Eight patients at The Children's Memorial Hospital have had closure of aortic septal defects in the manner just outlined, with excellent results. Two of these patients had been explored for a patent ductus in earlier years.

ANOMALOUS VENOUS RETURN

Anomalies of the pulmonary venous return are uncommon, but not as rare as major anomalies of the systemic venous drainage.

Persistence of a left superior vena cava is not rare and is often associated with other cardiovascular anomalies. Fortunately the vein almost invariably passes behind the left atrium and empties into the coronary sinus, so that it reaches the correct chamber and causes no functional disability. It may cause some difficulties when intracardiac defects are being repaired with the use of extracorporeal circulation. In spite of temporary occlusion of the inferior and superior vena cava a troublesome amount of blood will pass through the heart until the left superior cava is occluded.

Drainage of a vena cava into the left atrium is quite rare and results in cyanosis without murmurs or cardiac enlargement. One case of superior vena cava drainage into the left atrium has been repaired by swinging a flap of atrial wall across the mouth of the vena caval opening to divert blood to the right atrium. Inferior vena caval drainage into the left atrium is also possible.

Anomalous pulmonary venous drainage is most commonly only partial, involving one or both of the right pulmonary veins and almost invariably associated with an interatrial septal defect. The right superior vein is most often at fault, draining into the right atrium to the right of a high, sinus-venosum-type of interatrial septal defect. Occasionally the vein actually enters the superior vena cava. (The symptoms and findings are those of the interatrial septal defect. In addition, at cardiac catheterization the catheter slips easily into one or more of the pulmonary veins without traversing the septal defect.)

Correction of this condition requires the suture closure of the atrial defect in such a manner as to bring the anterior edge of the defect across the opening of the vein, diverting it into the left atrium but not obstructing the flow. At times a patch must be used to tunnel the pulmonary vein flow through the septal defect and over into the left atrium.

Total anomalous pulmonary venous drainage is less common. It presents a more difficult diagnostic problem, a high morbidity and mortality, and at times a seemingly impossible problem in surgical repair.

The veins from both lungs join in a common channel behind the heart and drain into the right atrium via systemic veins in three main methods. In the supracardiac type of drainage the pulmonary venous return passes up a vertical vein on the left and enters the innominate vein. The heart is usually enlarged, and the roentgenograms of the chest have a supracardiac bulge or "snowman" appearance.

The intracardiac type usually has the common vein emptying into the coronary sinus, and the infracardiac or infradiaphragmatic type has drainage through a long channel, traversing the diaphragm and emptying into the caval or portal venous systems. In these cases the hearts are usually small and lack the supracardiac shadow seen in the first type.

The systemic and pulmonary venous return to the right atrium intermix, and most of the flow passes through the right heart and back to the lungs. A smaller portion passes through an interatrial septal defect into the underdeveloped left side of the heart.

Because of the mixing of venous blood children with this defect will be moderately cyanotic. If there is no obstruction to pulmonary venous drainage, the pulmonary blood flow will be excessive and the vascularity on roentgenograms of the lungs will be increased. More often there is obstruction to the pulmonary vein flow, especially in the infradiaphragmatic type, resulting in pulmonary edema and increasing respiratory disease.

TREATMENT

Most patients with this lesion have increasing difficulties immediately after birth with right heart failure, pulmonary edema, and inadequate systemic circulation. Death usually occurs during the first weeks of life. An occasional patient will live beyond the first decade of life but will be severely handicapped and will have an extremely poor prognosis.

The ideal treatment is to make a large anastomosis between the common pulmonary vein and the left atrium, which lie in close approximation. This must be done with cardiopulmonary bypass. Unfortunately these neonates are in critical condition with failing right hearts, underdeveloped left hearts, and "stiff" lungs resulting from edema and vascular engorgement. The mortality for total correction in this group is essentially 100 percent at present. Partial relief may be provided by enlarging the interatrial septal communication or anastomosing the left pulmonary veins to the left atrial appendage. When the left side of the heart has developed and the child is older and in better condition, a total repair may be completed.

In the older child the right atrium may be opened, the interatrial defect enlarged if necessary, and an opening made in the back wall of the left atrium into the common pulmonary vein and a side-to-side—or, actually, a back-to-front—anastomosis made from inside the atrial cavity. In smaller children the heart may have to be moved forward and the anastomosis performed through the posterior aspect of the heart. If the left side of the heart is adequate and the anastomosis large, the vein connecting to the systemic veins may be tied off and the atrial defect closed. In doubtful cases one or both of these safety valves may be left open.

Pulmonary venous drainage into the coronary sinus may be corrected by an approach through the interatrial septal defect, removing the wall of the sinus adjacent to the left atrial cavity and thus allowing the pulmonary return flow to be directed into the left side of the heart. The decision must then be made whether or not to close the atrial defect, depending on the condition of the child and the development of the left side of the heart.

ANOMALIES OF THE CORONARY ARTERIES

A coronary artery originates from the pulmonary artery results in the perfusion of the portion of the heart supplied by that artery with hypoxic blood under lower than normal pressure. The right coronary originating from the pulmonary artery results in little incapacity, perhaps because of the lighter work load on the muscle supplied. However, if the left coronary originates from the pulmonary artery, cardiac enlargement, left heart failure, and severe incapacity result in most cases. Fortunately this anomaly is rather rare.

The infant may exhibit symptoms of paroxysmal pain (anginal) and cardiac failure and may have frequent respiratory infections. Examination reveals gross cardiac enlargement and signs of failure without heart murmurs. The enlargement is mainly left ventricular. The electrocardiogram pattern resembles that of myocardial infarction in an adult, and there is left ventricular hypertrophy.

Treatment by surgery has taken various directions. Revascularization by talc poudrage in the pericardial cavity or Vineberg's implantation of the internal mammary artery have been suggested but not extensively used. Direct anastomosis of a peripheral artery to

the detached anomalous coronary artery has been tried and proved unsuccessful.

Drainage of a major coronary artery into one of the cardiac chambers rather than into the vascular bed of the myocardium may occur. This is a rare anomaly and may be incapacitating because of the large shunt that can result. If the coronary artery drains into the left ventricle, there is predominantly a diastolic murmur with signs of aortic regurgitation. Most of the anomalous drainage enters the right heart or pulmonary artery, producing a continuous murmur suggestive of a patent ductus and signs of a left-to-right shunting of blood. It is difficult to distinguish such cases from patent ductus on the basis of physical signs alone.

The treatment of this condition is to obliterate the coronary artery involved at its origin from the aorta, its entry into the cardiac chamber, or, preferably, both. This should be done when the shunt is significant or aneurysm of the artery develops. Most cases can be operated upon without the use of cardiopulmonary bypass.

FISTULAS FROM THE SINUS OF VALSALVA

Fistulas from the sinus of Valsalva may occur as a congenital anomaly or as a result of the rupture of an aneurysm of the sinus of Valsalva. The fistula may open into the right atrium or right ventricle or, more rarely, into the left ventricle. A continuous murmur suggesting a patent ductus is heard, and signs of a left-to-right shunting of blood are present in the usual case. If the fistula enters the left ventricle, the findings mimic aortic regurgitation. Sudden onset of symptoms and murmur suggest a rupture of a previously existing aneurysm of the sinus of Valsalva. If this does not occur, a congenital fistula is more probable, especially in the younger group. Selective cineangiocardiograms with injection of the aortic root are most helpful in making the diagnosis, as they are with anomalous coronary artery drainage.

Surgical closure is usually imperative because of the large shunting of blood that occurs. The operation is done using extracorporeal circulation and obliterating the fistula. In one case of drainage into the right ventricle the tract was filled with a compressed Ivalon plug and the opening into the right ventricle tightly sutured closed. It is probably better also to go through the aorta and close to the opening in the sinus of Valsalva using hypothermia or coronary perfusion, especially if the fistula enters the left ventricle.

DISEASES OF THE PERICARDIUM

For many years the only field of endeavor of the cardiac surgeon in children was the relief of cardiac tamponade by drainage or pericardiectomy.

Acute cardiac tamponade, usually secondary to pericarditis, is a true emergency. As the effusion increases, the venous inflow to the heart is blocked more and more, producing peripheral venous distention, large liver, and edema. The heart tones are muffled and the cardiac silhouette enlarged. The output of the heart is decreased, with a lowering of blood pressure, a narrowing of pulse pressure, and a reversal of the normal variation of pressure with respiration (pulsus paradoxicus).

Pericardial aspiration must be done with care to avoid laceration of a coronary vessel, but the larger the effusion is, the less danger there may be. The tap may be done with a short beveled needle in the left fifth intercostal space 2 cm medial to the left heart border, or, in the child, it may be done from below the pericardial sac with the needle passed upward from a point just to the left of the xiphoid process. If aspiration is inadequate or the fluid reaccumulates frequently, a catheter drainage may be instituted. Rarely a window of pericardium may be removed.

Constrictive pericarditis may occasionally occur in childhood, producing chronic cardiac tamponade with the typical findings described above. Pericardiectomy must be performed, the constricting peel of scar tissue being removed from the ventricles and then from the right atrium, with special attention being paid to freeing the vena cavas.

Hemopericardium also may occur in children. One instance reported from an outlying hospital followed an insignificant chest wound from a pair of scissors. The small wound in the skin was closed to stop the brisk bleeding, and death followed in a few hours from unsuspected cardiac tamponade. Another child with an extensive mediastinal hemangioma developed sudden tamponade requiring removal of a window of pericardium to empty the blood in the pericardium into the left chest, from which it could be aspirated periodically with more safety. The same procedure was done on a patient with Cooley's anemia and spontaneous hemopericardium.

Congenital absence of all or part of the pericardium has been found in three patients. No symptoms were evident, but the appearance of the bare heart upon opening the chest was startling.

CARDIAC TUMORS

Primary cardiac tumors are very rare in children. However, rhabdomyomas and myxomas involving the chambers of the heart have been reported. Most frequently they produce obstruction to flow simulating valvular stenosis. Selective angiocardiograms in the suspected chamber will usually outline the mass. Removal of the tumor using cardiopulmonary bypass has been curative in some cases.

Tumors of the mediastinum invading the heart and pericardium are more common than primary cardiac tumors in children. Lymphomas and teratosarcomas arising in the mediastinum may become symptomatic only when they encroach on or invade the heart. Except for possible biopsy these do not represent a surgical problem, since radiation or chemotherapy is usually the only palliative therapy advisable.

CARDIA DIVERTICULA

Diverticula from the ventricles are also rare and usually accompany some degree of ectopia cordis. Atrial diverticula are discovered by chest roentgenogram. Since the relatively thin-walled diverticula enlarge during contraction of their adjoining chamber, there is inefficient emptying of blood forward into the next portion of the heart or great vessels. Poor cardiac action and heart failure results. Clots may form in these diverticula because of stagnation of blood.

Removal of the diverticula is advisable and may be done with or without cardiopulmonary bypass. If bypass is not used, the base of the diverticulum may be clamped, the excess myocardium removed, and the stump closed with silk mattress sutures and over-and-over silk stitches. In other cases it may be more advantageous to occlude the base of the sac with interrupted silk mattress sutures, remove the excess muscle, and reinforce the closure with a running suture. The use of extracorporeal circulation makes the surgical correction much simpler and safer.

One left ventricular and one left atrial diverticulum have been closed successfully by the closed technique at The Children's Memorial Hospital.

WILLIAM L. RIKER
THOMAS G. BAFFES
ARTHUR DEBOER

REFERENCES

ALBERT, H. M. Surgical correction of transposition of the great vessels. *In* Surgical Forum. Philadelphia, W. B. Saunders Co., 1955, pp. 74.

BAFFES, T. G. New method of surgical correction of transposition of the aorta and pulmonary artery. Surg. Gynec. Obstet., 102: 227, 1956.

—— et al. Surgical correction of transposition of aorta and pulmonary artery: A five year survey. J. Thorac. Cardiovasc. Surg., 40: 298, 1960.

BAILEY, C. P., et al. Experiences with the experimental surgical relief of aortic stenosis. J. Thoracic Surg., 20: 516, 1950.

BIGELOW, N. W., KLINGER, S., and WRIGHT, A. W. Primary tumors of the heart in infancy and childhood. Cancer, 7: 549, 1954.

BJORK, V. A., and BOUCKAERT, L. Complete transposition of the aorta and pulmonary artery. An experimental study of the surgical possibilities for its treatment. J. Thorac. Surg., 28: 632, 1954.

BLALOCK, A. Operative closure of the patent ductus arteriosus. Surg. Gynec. Obstet., 82: 113, 1946.

—— and HANLON, C. R. Surgical treatment of complete transposition of aorta and pulmonary artery. Surg. Gynec. Obstet., 90: 1, 1950.

—— and TAUSSIG, H. B. The surgical treatment of malformations of the heart in which there is pulmonary stenosis. J.A.M.A., 128: 189, 1945.

BROCK, R. C. Pulmonary valvulotomy for the relief of congenital stenosis; Report of 3 cases. Brit. Med. J., 1: 112, 1948.

COOLEY, J. C., and KIRKLIN, J. W. The surgical treatment of persistent common atrioventricular canal: Report of 12 cases. Proc. Staff Meet., Mayo Clinic, 31: 523, 1956.

—— and OCHSNER, A., Jr. Correction of total anomalous pulmonary venous drainage. Surgery, 42: 1014, 1957.

—— McNAMARA, D. G., and LATSON, J. R. Aortico-pulmonary septal defect: Diagnosis and surgical treatment. Surgery, 42: 101, 1957.

CRAFOORD, C., and NYLIN, G. Congenital coarctation of the aorta and its surgical treatment. J. Thorac. Surg., 14: 347, 1945.

EDWARDS, J. E., and BURCHELL, H. B. Congenital tricuspid atresia: A classification. Med. Clin. N. Amer., 33: 1177, 1949.

FALLOT, A. Contribution à l'anatomie pathologique de la maladie bleue (cyanose cardioque). Marseille-med., 25: 77, 1888.

GASUL, B. M., FELL, E. H., and CASAS, R. Diagnosis of aortic septal defect by retrograde aortography. Circulation, 4: 251, 1951.

GIBBON, J. H., Jr. *In* Discussion, *from* Warden, H. E., et al. Controlled cross-circulation for open intracardiac surgery: Phsiologic studies and results of creation and closure of ventricular septal defect. J. Thorac. Surg., 28: 343, 1954.

GIBSON, S., et al. Congenital pulmonary stenosis with intact ventricular septum. J. Dis. Child., 87: 26, 1954.

GLENN, W. W. L., and PATINO, J. F. Circulatory bypass of the right heart. 1. Preliminary observations on the direct delivery of vena caval blood into the pulmonary arterial circulation. Yale J. Biol. Med., 27: 147, 1954.

GROSS, R. E. Surgical correction for coarctation of the aorta. Surgery, 18: 673, 1945.

——— Surgical relief for tracheal obstruction from a vascular ring. New Eng. J. Med., 233: 586, 1945.

——— The patent ductus arteriosus: Observations on diagnosis and therapy in 525 surgically treated cases. Amer. J. Med., 12: 472, 1952.

——— Surgical closure of an aortic septal defect. Circulation, 5: 858, 1952.

——— Coarctation of the aorta. Circulation, 7: 757, 1953.

——— Arterial malformations which cause compression of the trachea or esophagus. Circulation, 11: 124, 1955.

——— and HUBBARD, J. P. Ligation of the patent ductus arteriosus. J.A.M.A., 118: 729, 1939.

——— et al. A method for surgical closure of interauricular septal defects. Surg. Gynec. Obstet., 96: 1, 1953.

HANLON, R. C., and BLALOCK, A. Complete transposition of the aorta and pulmonary artery. Ann. Surg., 127: 385, 1948.

IDRISS, F. S., et al. A new technique for complete correction of transposition of the great vessels. Circulation, 24: 5, 1961.

KIRKLIN, J. W., DEVLOO, R. A., and WEIDMAN, W. H. Open intracardiac repair of transposition of the great vessels. Surgery, 50: 58, 1961.

KIRKLIN, J. W. Surgical treatment of anomalous pulmonary venous connection. Proc. Staff Meet. Mayo Clinic, 28: 476, 1953.

——— DEVLOO, R. A., and WEIDMAN, W. H. Surgical treatment of ventricular septal defect. J. Thorac. Cardiov. Surg., 40: 763, 1960.

LEWIS, F. J., and TAUFFIE, M. Closure of atrial septal defects with aid of hypothermia: Experimental accomplishments and report of one successful case. Surgery, 33: 52, 1953.

——— et al. Aortic valvulotomy under direct vision during hypothermia. J. Thorac. Surg., 32: 481, 1956.

LILLEHEI, C. W., et al. Direct vision intracardiac surgical correction of the tetralogy of Fallot, pentalogy of Fallot and pulmonary atresia defects: Report of first 10 cases. Ann. Surg., 142: 418, 1955(a).

——— et al. The results of direct vision closure of ventricular septal defects in 8 patients by means of controlled cross-circulation. Surg. Gynec. Obstet., 101: 447, 1955(b).

——— et al. Surgical treatment of stenotic or regurgitant lesions of the mitral and aortic valves by direct vision utilizing a pump-oxygenator. J. Thorac. Surg., 35: 154, 1958.

McGOON, D. C., et al. The surgical treatment of endocardial cushion defects. Surgery, 46: 185, 1959.

MULLER, W. H., Jr., and DAMMANN, J. F., Jr. The treatment of certain congenital malformations of the heart by the creation of pulmonic stenosis to reduce pulmonic hypertension and excessive pulmonary blood flow. Surg. Gynec. Obstet., 95: 213, 1952.

MURPHY, T. O., et al. The results of surgical palliation in 32 patients with transposition of the great vessels. Surg. Gynec. Obstet., 101: 541, 1955.

MUSTARD, W. T. Suture ligation of the patent ductus arteriosus in infancy. Canad. Med. Ass. J., 64: 243, 1951.

——— and TRUSLER, G. A. Ventricular septal defect: An analysis of 70 cases in childhood surgically treated. Canad. J. Surg., 4: 152, 1961.

——— et al. Surgical approach to transposition of great vessels with extracorporeal circuit. Surgery, 36: 39, 1964.

——— et al. Coarctation of the aorta with special reference to the first year of life. Ann. Surg., 141: 429, 1955.

——— et al. Congenital diverticulum of the left ventricle of the heart. Canad. J. Surg., 1: 149, 1958.

——— et al. The surgical treatment of atrial septal defects in children. Canad. Med. Ass. J., 84: 138, 1961.

POTTS, W. J. Technique of resection of coarctation of the aorta with aid of new instruments. Ann. Surg., 131: 466, 1950.

——— SMITH, S., and GIBSON, S. Anastomosis of the aorta to a pulmonary artery. J.A.M.A., 132: 627, 1946.

——— et al. Diagnosis and surgical treatment of patent ductus arteriosus. Arch. Surg., 58: 612, 1949.

——— DE BOER, A., and JOHNSON, F. R. Congenital diverticulum of the left ventricle. Surgery, 33: 301, 1953.

RIKER, W. L. Anomalies of the aortic arch and their treatment. Pediat. Clin. N. Amer., 1954.

——— et al. Tricuspid stenosis and atresia complexes. J. Thorac. Cardiov. Surg., 45: 113, 1963.

ROSHE, J., and SHUMACKER, H. B., Jr. Pericardiectomy for chronic cardiac tamponade in children. Surgery, 46: 1152, 1959.

SENNING, A. Surgical correction of transposition of great vessels. Surgery, 45: 966, 1959.

SHUMACKER, H. B., Jr., and HARRIS, J. Pericardiectomy for chronic idiopathic pericarditis with massive effusion and cardiac tamponade. Surg. Gynec. Obstet., 103: 535, 1956.

SONDERGAARD, T., et al. Closure of experimentally produced atrial septal defects. Acta Chir. Scand., 107: 485, 1954.

SWAN, H., and ZEAVIN, I. Cessation of circulation in general hypothermia. Techniques of intracardiac surgery under direct vision. Ann. Surg., 139: 385, 1954.

——— BLOUNT, S. G., Jr., and VIRTUE, R. W. Direct vision suture of interatrial septial defect during hypothermia. Surgery, 38: 858, 1955.

——— WILKINSON, R. H., and BLOUNT, S. G., Jr. Visual repair of congenital aortic stenosis during hypothermia. J. Thorac. Surg., 35: 139, 1958.

TAUSSIG, H. B. Clinical and pathologic findings in congenital malformations of the heart due to defective development of right ventricle associated with tricuspid atresia or hypoplasia. Bull. Hopkins Hosp., 59: 435, 1936.

32

Umbilical Anomalies

The umbilical region is vital during fetal development, and it is understandable that a structure like the umbilicus would be the site of developmental anomalies. In the 6 mm embryo there is a communication between the yolk sac and the intestine by way of the omphalomesenteric, or vitelline, duct, and this structure traverses the umbilicus. Rapid growth of the intestine occurs, and its volume becomes greater than the abdominal cavity can accommodate. This is compensated for in the 30 mm embryo by the migration of some of the intestine into the umbilical cord. Subsequently the abdominal cavity enlarges, and in the 45 mm embryo the intestine has returned to the abdomen. Failure of adequate abdominal cavity growth may be the key factor in the persistence of intestine in the umbilical cord that results in omphalocele. Normally, the intestines return to the abdominal cavity and the vitelline duct becomes closed. If this obliteration fails to occur, a Meckel's diverticulum with several possible pathological structures results. For instance, a fistula communicating with the umbilicus and connected with a cyst situated in the tissue underneath the umbilicus can be explained by persistence of part of the vitelline duct (Fig. 1).

Under these conditions, a fibrous band

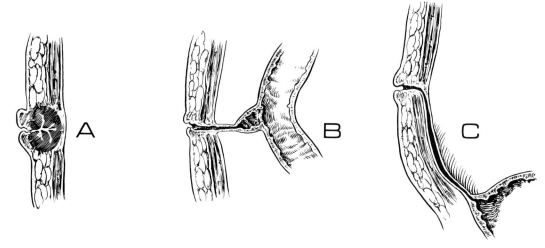

Fig. 1. A. Diagram of a fistula and cyst underneath the umbilicus. This represents a remnant of the vitelline duct. B. Diagram representing a persistent vitelline duct that communicates with a Meckel's diverticulum. C. Diagram of a urachal sinus. The structure extends from the umbilicus to the dome of the urinary bladder.

may extend between a Meckel's diverticulum and the peritoneal side of the umbilicus. Embryologically, this probably represents a vitelline duct that has become obliterated and has persisted as a solid strand of tissue. Intestinal or gastric mucosa in the umbilicus can be explained by the persistence of a bit of the vitelline duct.

Recently, attention has been called to the significance of the absence of one umbilical artery in the umbilicus. Such a finding should warn the attending doctor to be on the alert for some malformation in the neonate.

Communications between the umbilicus and the urinary bladder are harder to explain embryologically, and the explanations offered are controversial. Nevertheless, such com-

munications occur in the form of a urachal sinus. A sinus opening in the umbilicus may end blindly and may not communicate with the bladder. Occasionally, a bit of the urachus persists without communications and becomes a cyst in the abdominal wall between the umbilicus and the urinary bladder.

UMBILICAL HERNIA

As the structure composing the umbilical cord undergoes atrophy it is not surprising that in a number of infants the fascial ring is large enough for the peritoneum to protrude through it and become adjacent to the skin. When intra-abdominal pressure is in-

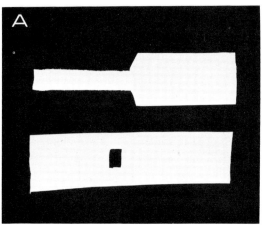

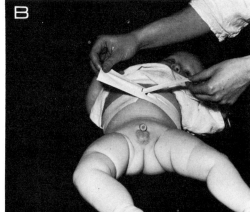

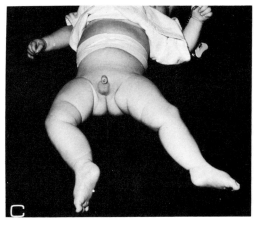

Fig. 2. A. Adhesive tape has been cut for application of keystone strapping for umbilical hernia. B. The tape has been attached and the small end threaded through. Traction on the ends compresses the umbilical hernia and brings the fascial ring together. It is advisable to paint the skin with tincture of benzoin before the strapping is applied. C. The application has been completed.

creased, the yielding peritoneum and umbilical skin protrude. In the majority of patients,
the fascial ring gradually becomes smaller,
and, when the child is several years of age,
the umbilical hernia has spontaneously corrected itself.

Studies by Sibley (1964) indicate that untreated umbilical hernias that spontaneously
disappear rarely recur at a later date. It is
difficult to determine whether strapping the
umbilicus can aid the natural umbilical closing process sufficiently to warrant the trouble
to the parents and discomfort to the baby that
this treatment involves. Infants with discomfort caused by protrusion of intestine into

the umbilical hernial sac may have relief of
their symptoms from strapping, which prevents abdominal contents from entering the
sac. Incarceration of the abdominal contents
in the sac may also be prevented. This complication is extremely rare, but it has been
observed. We have observed several incarcerated hernias in infants and children; however, none contained necrotic intestine. One
contained necrotic omentum. Mestel and
Burns (1963) have reported three incarcerated umbilical hernias, one requiring resection for gangrenous small intestine. An even
rarer complication has been rupture of the
skin with evisceration of abdominal contents.

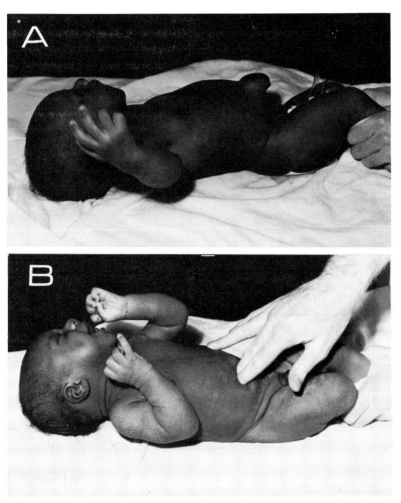

Fig. 3. A. A baby with a large umbilical hernia. B. The fascial ring at the neck of the sac admitted
two fingers. The young age of the child makes it likely that spontaneous cure will take place, despite
the large ring.

METHODS OF STRAPPING

Unless the strapping is so applied that the edges of the fascial ring are brought together, the treatment may be injurious. Such is the case when a coin or similarly rigid object is placed in the umbilicus and held in place with adhesive strapping, for the fascial ring is actually held open by such treatment. The "keystone" type of strapping is preferable and is accomplished with two pieces of 2-inch adhesive tape 6- to 8-inches long (Fig. 2). One of the pieces is prepared by cutting a 1-inch square window in the center. The other piece is trimmed from one end to the midpoint by cutting a $\frac{1}{2}$-inch strip from each side. The skin on each side of the umbilicus where the tape is to be placed is painted with tincture of benzoin. The broad end of the tape is applied lateral to the umbilicus,

leaving the narrow end free. The other tape is placed on the opposite side, leaving the window and the end beyond unattached. The narrow tongue of tape is passed through the window, the free ends of tape are pulled in opposite directions, and the umbilicus is folded inward. The traction of the tape on each side closes the fascial ring and prevents protrusion of the hernial sac. The strapping is secured by attaching the free ends of tape to the abdominal skin. Parents can manage this type of treatment after observing one application. Usually, the adhesive tape will remain in place about two weeks, after which a new application will be required. The skin of some babies becomes excoriated to such an extent that repeat strapping must be postponed for several days or the treatment abandoned.

A few umbilical hernias require surgical

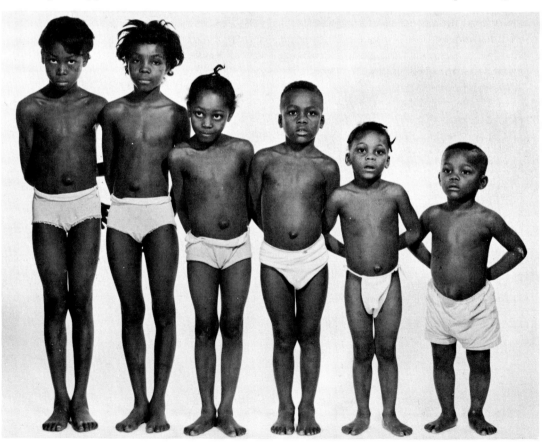

Fig. 4. Photograph of siblings with umbilical hernia. These did not tend to close as is generally the case, and some of the children required repair.

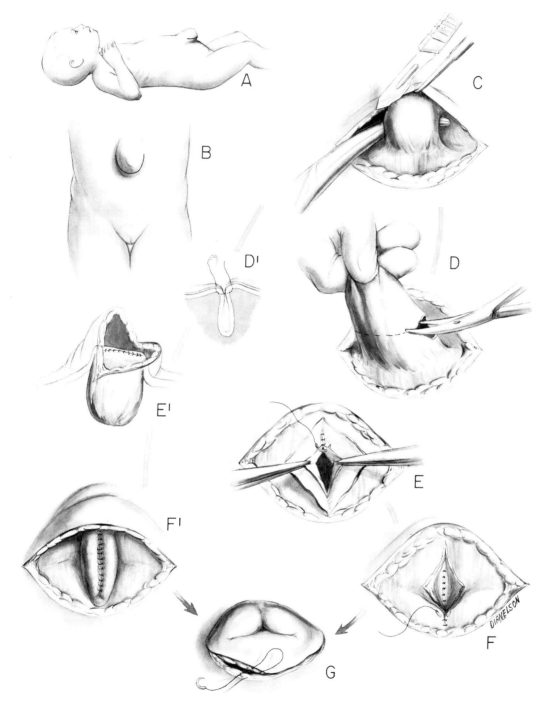

Fig. 5. Umbilical herniorrhaphy. A and B. Drawings indicating position of incision. C. The wall of the cyst has been dissected free and an instrument passed behind the sac. The skin is dissected from the sac with a scalpel. D. The top of the sac is excised. D¹. An alternate method where the unopened sac is inverted. E. The fascial ring is closed with interrupted sutures. E¹. The anterior rectus fascia at the ring is closed with interrupted silk sutures. F. The anterior rectus fascia is approximated over this defect. F¹. The closure has been completed. G. The skin is approximated with subcuticular sutures.

repair. The degree of protrusion of the hernia is not a reliable guide in selecting those that need repair; rather, the size of the fascial ring determines whether or not spontaneous correction of the hernia will occur (Fig. 3). When the ring admits the finger at ease at 6 years of age repair is indicated (Fig. 4). When the sac is large and the skin becomes very thin repair should be considered to prevent rupture of the sac. There are some infants and children with pain from an umbilical hernia that can be relieved by strapping. In such situations, when the skin cannot tolerate strapping, repair is indicated. A history or finding of incarceration that can be reduced are additional indications for repair.

UMBILICAL HERNIORRHAPHY

Techniques of repair that require excision of the umbilicus should be avoided because of the ridicule to which children without a navel may be subjected. An adequate repair can be accomplished without disturbing the umbilicus by utilizing a semicircular incision in the lower edge of the navel (Fig. 5). This provides an excellent cosmetic result, as the incision is concealed in the umbilicus. The skin is retracted with skin hooks, and the inferior and lateral surfaces of the hernial sac are separated by blunt dissection down to the rectus fascia. The cephalic side of the sac is also separated from the subcutaneous tissue, utilizing blunt dissection so that an instrument can be passed around the sac from one side to the other. The skin is then separated from the sac by scalpel dissection. It is preferable to open the sac rather than to buttonhole the skin. Consequently, the sac is frequently opened. When this is done, and particularly when the fascial ring is large, it is advisable to open the sac widely and approximate the fascial ring of the sac in a vertical plane with interrupted 4-0 silk sutures. The sac wall is then cut off and a second row of sutures placed through the rectus fascia on each side of the sac. When the fascial ring is small and the hernial sac has not been opened, the sac can be invagi-

nated and a row of interrupted 4-0 silk sutures placed through the rectus fascia on each side of the hernial defect.

Excessive separation of the rectus muscles above or below the umbilical hernia is corrected by placing additional sutures in the rectus fascia to a point beyond the separation.

Attempts to separate the peritoneum as a layer for suturing are unwise because in infants the peritoneum is so thin that tearing occurs, which makes this layer useless in the closure. Absolute hemostasis is secured before the skin incision is closed; otherwise, blood and fluid may collect, and a large protrusion of the umbilical skin may develop a few days following operation. If this occurs, aspiration is unnecessary, for absorption will

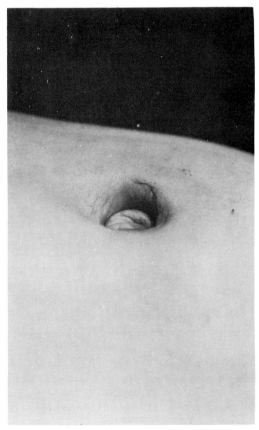

Fig. 6. Umbilicus after repair of hernia. Note normal appearance of umbilicus. The incision is inside the umbilicus.

take place over a three-to-four-week period.

The skin incision is closed with three or four subcuticular sutures of 6-0 silk. A rolled-up piece of gauze is placed in the umbilicus to hold the skin down to the fascia and to prevent accumulation of fluid in the large subcutaneous space made during the operation. Several 1-inch squares of gauze are placed over this packing and the whole dressing secured with tight adhesive taping. Twenty-four hours after operation, this dressing is removed, the incision is painted with flexible collodion, and the patient is discharged. Postoperatively, the patient is permitted some activity, including stair climbing, but rough play is prohibited for two weeks. After this period, full activity is permitted. While the navel may appear large immediately after this type of repair, the umbilicus will be essentially normal in size one year following repair (Fig. 6).

OMPHALOCELE

Omphalocele probably represents an arrest of normal development. While the details of the cause of the migration of the intestine into the yolk sac and its return into the abdominal cavity are not clearly established, omphalocele represents a failure of the return of varying portions of the intestine and other viscera into the abdominal cavity.

At birth, the sac consists of a thin translucent membrane composed of peritoneum internally, and amniotic membrane externally.

While the sac is usually intact at delivery, rupture occasionally occurs in utero or during delivery. This complication creates an emergency, and return of the intestines to the peritoneal cavity with repair of the abdominal defect should not be delayed (Fig. 7). This situation should not be confused with gastroschisis, where there is an abdominal defect beside the umbilicus. Saline-moistened gauze should be placed over the intestine and the baby encircled with a sterile towel to facilitate transportation to the op-

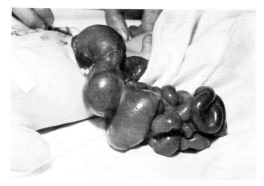

Fig. 7. Ruptured omphalocele. Repair was accomplished.

erating room. Obviously, it is a more difficult problem to repair the defect and to have the infant recover after rupture of the sac has taken place than when the sac is intact. Not only is there some contamination, but the discrepancy between the viscera and abdominal capacity may be considerable, for the exposed intestine is often considerably distended and edematous.

OPERATION

When the sac is intact and the omphalocele is small, the whole sac and abdomen is scrubbed with Zephiran-moistened gauze sponges (Fig. 8). Under a general anesthesia, the sac with the umbilical stump is removed. The abdominal cavity should be explored for other anomalies, particularly malrotation. A layered closure of the abdominal wall is performed, utilizing interrupted 4-0 or 5-0 silk sutures to the peritoneum, anterior rectus sheath, and skin.

For a large omphalocele with a wide abdominal defect, the method advocated by Ladd is advantageous. The intact omphalocele is scrubbed with six or eight Zephiran-soaked sponges, and the umbilical cord is amputated close to the sac. An incision is then made in the skin adjacent to the junction of the membranous sac and skin. The skin lateral to the defect is mobilized extensively onto the chest and around the flanks laterally. The sac membrane is removed and

the skin closed over the intestine, using interrupted silk sutures to the subcutaneous tissue and skin (Fig. 9). Gross (1940) has
modified this technique by not removing the
omphalocele sac and, after mobilization of
the skin, bringing the skin over the intact
sac. These techniques are wiser courses to
pursue when confronted with a large omphal-

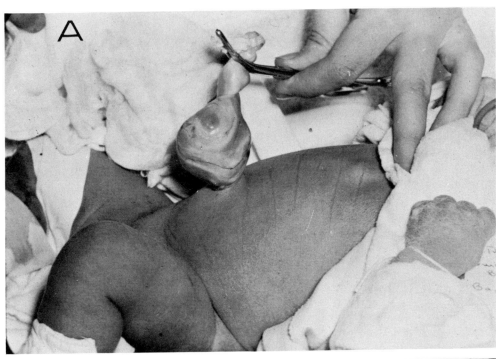

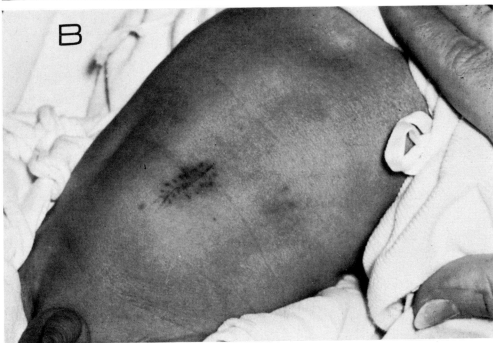

Fig. 8. A. A small omphalocele. B. Same patient ten days after repair of the umbilical lesion.

ocele than attempting a closure of the muscular and fascial layers. A layer closure may be accomplished, but the infant may succumb because of the high intra-abdominal tension produced by the suturing of the abdominal wall. Not only will such a tight closure produce elevation and limitation of dia- phragmatic movements, but also the large intraabdominal venous channels will be compressed to such an extent that swelling of the legs develops and normal venous return to the heart is dangerously reduced. These alterations in respiratory and vascular functions may cause an unnecessary death. Lewis

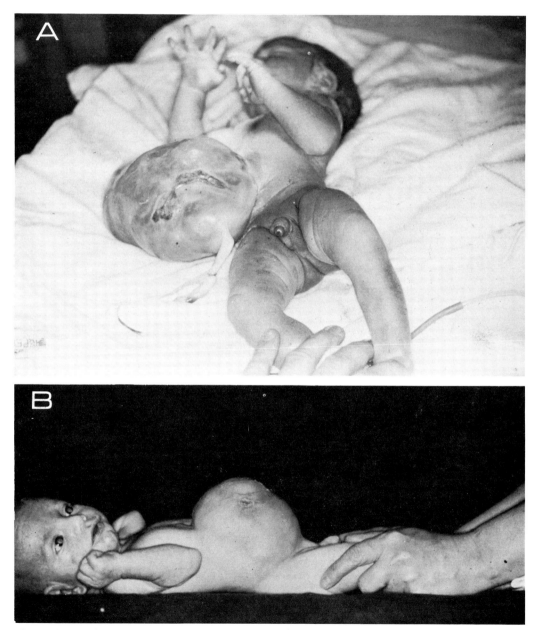

Fig. 9. A. Massive omphalocele which contained liver, spleen, and the gastrointestinal tract. B. Same patient three weeks after covering omphalocele with skin.

(1967) has suggested that manual stretching of the abdominal muscle at the time of operation gives surprising enlargement of the abdominal cavity and may convert the situation into one where the fascial and muscular layers of the abdomen can be approximated, obviating the need for troublesome secondary repairs.

Following a skin closure, there will be a massive abdominal protrusion for many months. Repair is inadvisable until this mass is easily reducible, and this rarely occurs until the child is a year or two old. At the secondary closure, two fascial layers—the posterior and anterior—can usually be developed and sutured with 4-0 interrupted silk stitches. Followups on these children reveal a sound abdominal wall that does not differ essentially from a normal one except for the absence of the umbilicus. Injection of air, creating a pneumoperitoneum, has been used successfully in these situations to enlarge the abdominal cavity prior to secondary repair. Any help that can be gained by such methods should be taken advantage of, for the technical problems confronting the surgeon during secondary repairs have been troublesome. This is particularly true when the liver is outside the abdominal musculature. The mortality has been high in our experience after secondary repairs. Grob has suggested an alternative treatment for infants with massive omphaloceles or newborns with omphaloceles who have such other lesions as severe congenital heart disease and who are poor surgical risks. This treatment consists of painting the sac with 2 percent mercurochrome daily for three days. Formation of a shrinking eschar takes place, which gradually forces the sac contents into the abdominal cavity. The disadvantage is that the process is slow, requiring about three months for completion, and eventually a surgical repair of the small remaining defect may be required. It is recommended that the child remain in the hospital for the entire period of treatment, and this an additional drawback (Fig. 10).

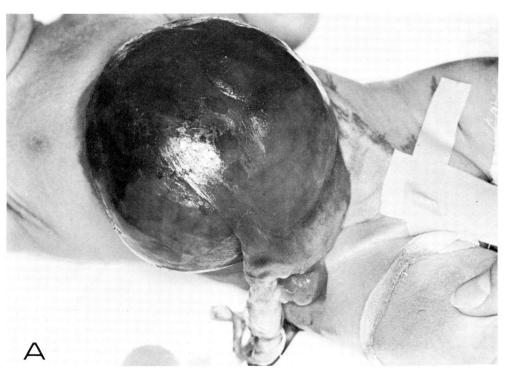

A

Fig. 10. A boy with a large omphalocele. A. The patient 24 hours after birth.

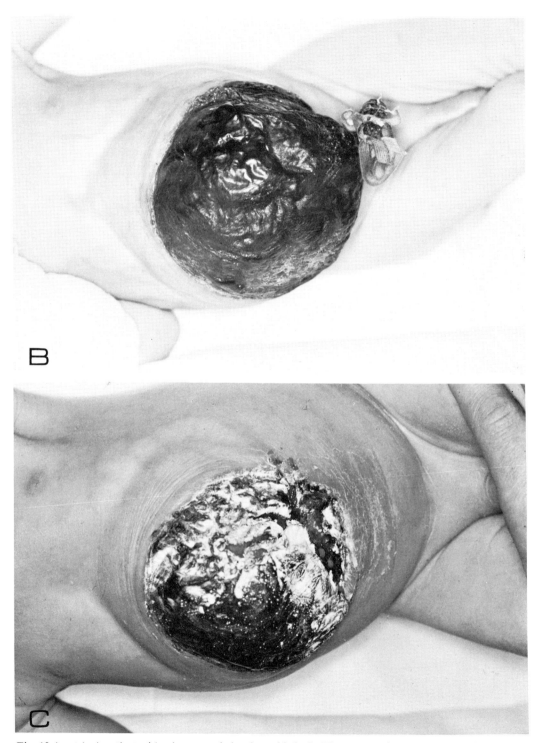

Fig. 10 (cont.). A patient with a large omphalocele at birth. B. The same patient at ten days of age. The omphalocele has been painted with 2-percent Mercurochrome. C. The patient at eight weeks.

GASTROSCHISIS

Gastroschisis is not an umbilical anomaly; rather, it is a full-thickness defect in the abdominal wall most often found adjacent to the umbilicus. Unless a careful examination is made the condition can easily be confused with ruptured omphalocele.

The embryological basis of these defects has been described by Duhamel (1963) as failure of differentiation of the lateral plate mesoderm, which produces a full-thickness

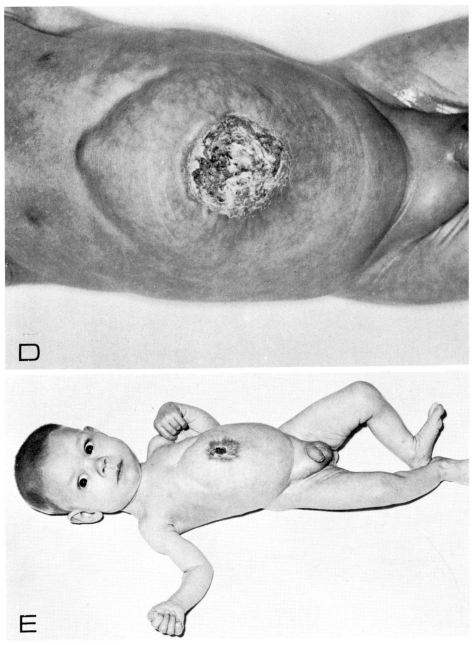

Fig. 10 (cont.). A patient with a large omphalocele at birth. D. The patient at three months. E. The patient at four months. (Figure 10, A–E, courtesy Dr. Theodor Ehrenpreis, Stockholm, Sweden.)

defect in the abdominal wall of varying sizes. A majority of these rare lesions are found on the right side of the umbilicus. They are distinguished from ruptured omphaloceles by the presence of a normal umbilicus with the usual complement of vessels and the absence of a sac or of the remnants of an omphalocele sac. The prolonged presence of the intestine in the amniotic fluid produces edema and thickening. A thick, fibrinous exudate covers the intestine and adds to their bulk. There is considerable dilation of the intestine, which is the source of the greatest difficulty in accommodating the intestine in the abdominal cavity.

TREATMENT

Return of the intestine to the abdominal cavity and closure of the abdominal wall defect should be accomplished promptly to prevent further dilation of the intestine with ingested air. The intestines and abdominal wall should be cleaned with soapy water followed by Zephiran.

The incision should be enlarged and the skin undermined to the infant's back laterally and up to the upper chest cephalad. Experience has established that intestinal function will be delayed for several days postoperatively; hence it is wise to perform a gastrostomy. A catheter inserted through the stomach into the intestine will aid in immediate partial intestinal decompression. It has been suggested that the exudate can be peeled from the intestinal surface, which reduces bulk and may speed the return of peristalsis. At times this can be accomplished. We found in one situation that all the muscular wall was being removed leaving a mucosal tube.

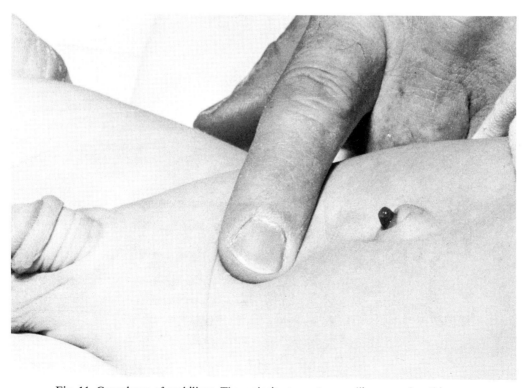

Fig. 11. Granuloma of umbilicus. The majority are not as readily exposed as this one.

This was suspected, and it proved to be the case when the removed peel was examined under the microscope after being prepared by freezing. Resection of a segment of intestine has been suggested, but it poses the problem of performing an anastomosis in chronically inflamed, edematous tissue.

The safest procedure seems to be extensive mobilization of skin, decompression of the intestine as completely as possible, and closure of the skin over the intestine. The infant is left with a large hernia that should not be closed until abdominal growth will accommodate the intestine, a process that should take place in one or two years.

Injection of air into the peritoneal cavity may help enlarge the abdominal cavity in preparation for closure of the large hernia.

Postoperatively, support must be provided for a longer period than is needed for the average abdominal operation because the thickened intestine encased in fibrinous exudate will be slow to exhibit peristalsis.

CHRONIC DRAINAGE FROM THE UMBILICUS

It is rather common to have a chronic discharge from the navel in infants. The drainage is usually a thin cloudy fluid and is sufficient to soil the child's clothing over the umbilicus. The constant presence of this moisture causes an irritation of the umbilical skin. The commonest cause of such discharge is a granuloma, composed of granulation tissue that has formed because of incomplete healing of the umbilical skin at the site of the divided cord (Fig. 11). This condition can be diagnosed by inspection, and the granuloma can be destroyed with daily silver nitrate application over a period of seven to ten days. The discharge may also be caused

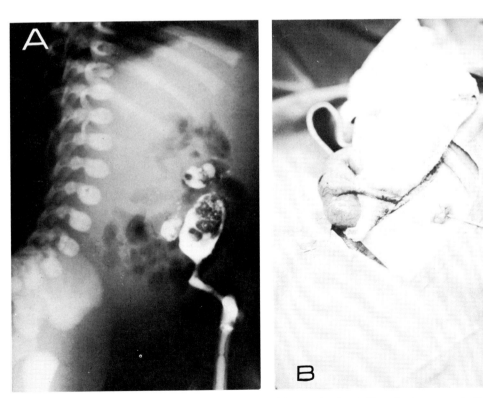

Fig. 12. A. Roentgenogram with contrast medium outlining patient's vitelline duct communicating with ileum. B. Photograph of such a lesion with probe in place. (From Lowman et al. Amer. J. Roentgenol., 70:883, 1953.)

by the persistence of intestinal mucosa, which may remain as a remnant of the vitelline duct. Usually, this is indistinguishable from a granuloma and will be destroyed by cauterization such as is used in the treatment of granulomas. Persistent drainage despite such treatment indicates that a granuloma is not the cause and should prompt an exploration of the umbilicus with a probe. If a sinus is detected, its extent and nature can be demonstrated radiographically by the injection of radiopaque material. A sinus communicating with a Meckel's diverticulum may be found that is long and narrow and that represents a persistent vitelline duct (Fig.

12). The contrast medium may reveal only a short sinus or a cyst.

Once a sinus or cyst has been demonstrated, surgical excision is indicated. A transverse incision below the umbilicus permits an adequate investigation of the tissue deep to the umbilicus (Fig. 13). By inserting a probe through the sinus, a duct or cyst is easily identified during the dissection. In all instances, the peritoneal cavity should be investigated through a paramedian incision between the rectus muscles. This permits the operator to determine whether the cyst or sinus extends by way of a fistular tract or fibrous cord to the Meckel's diverticulum. To

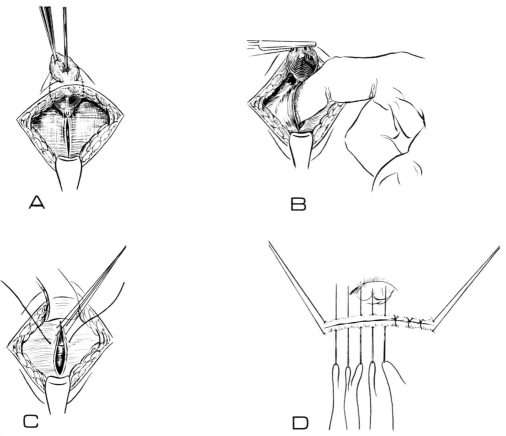

Fig. 13. Operative procedure for removal of umbilical cyst, persistent vitelline duct, and urachal sinus. A. A transverse incision is used below the umbilicus. The fascia and peritoneum are divided in the midline. B. The operator inserts his index finger and determines whether a vitelline duct or band communicates with a Meckel's diverticulum. If such structures are found, they should be removed with the Meckel's diverticulum. In the same manner, the operator can detect a urachal sinus. The cyst is removed. C. The peritoneum has been closed with interrupted black silk sutures. Diagram indicates placement of anterior sutures through the anterior rectus fascia. D. Indicates the placement of interrupted silk sutures to the skin. An alternate closure would be a subcuticular 5-0 plain catgut with collodion.

overlook such structures may lead to subsequent infection in the tract, or intestinal obstruction may be produced if the fibrous band is left in place. A small incision is adequate for the removal of an intra-abdominal band and Meckel's diverticulum.

A rare form of persistent vitelline duct is one that is large enough to permit drainage of fecal material. This condition should. be treated promptly because prolapse of intestine through the fistula is a common early complication, producing intestinal obstruction. The prolapse is difficult to reduce manually, and in most instances the infant must be submitted to operation. The danger of operating on a baby after this complication has occurred is considerably greater than that of excising an uncomplicated persistent vitelline duct. When prolapse of intestine has taken place, an operation of greater scope is required. A right rectus muscle-retracting incision is preferable, since resection is inevitable. Resection of the prolapsed nonviable intestine and of the fistula with end-to-end anastomosis is the preferred surgical treatment.

Infection in patent umbilical arteries has

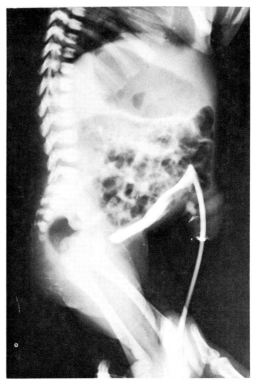

Fig. 14. Roentgenogram with contrast medium outlining patient's urachal sinus, which communicates with urinary bladder. (From Lowman, et al. Amer. J. Roentgenol., 70:883, 1953.)

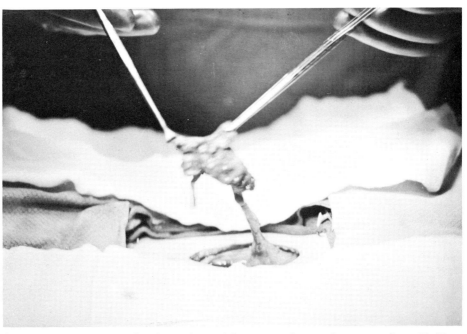

Fig. 15. Urachal cyst that has been dissected free except for attachment to urinary bladder.

been described as the cause of chronic umbilical drainage. This can be detected as tender cords running caudally and laterally. Incision and drainage is the safest course to pursue, followed by excision.

PERSISTENT URACHAL SINUS AND CYSTS

On rare occasions, the cause of chronic umbilical drainage will be a patent urachal sinus that may or may not connect with the urinary bladder. The urachal sinus is a vestigial structure and is the persistence of a sinus that in one stage of fetal development connects the bladder to the allantois. Normally, this sinus becomes obliterated and in an infant is represented as a fibrous cord. At times, patent urachal sinus may be related to atresia of the urethra, and under such circumstances the nature of the drainage is obvious. When the sinus is small and the urethra is normal, the nature of the drainage is not readily detectable.

Injection of 30-percent Diodrast into the sinus is advisable, and lateral roentgenograms of the abdomen should be made (Fig. 14). In such films, a sinus communicating with the urinary bladder can clearly be detected.

Demonstration of a urachal sinus should be followed by excision of the tract. When a large fistula is found, it is advisable to determine the adequacy of the urethra with a urethrogram.

Excision of the urachal sinus is most readily accomplished through a vertical incision below the umbilicus. With a probe in the sinus, the structure can easily be identified and traced down to the bladder, where it can be ligated with a silk suture and excised (Fig. 15). Bladder drainage with a supra-pubic catheter is unnecessary. There may be a urachal cyst located in the abdominal wall between the umbilicus and the urinary bladder. A urachal cyst remains asymptomatic unless it becomes infected, and it may be an incidental finding during an abdominal exploration. If the cyst is large, it may be palpated as a rounded smooth mass above the bladder. If the cyst is large and adjacent to the urinary bladder, a smooth mass may project into the bladder and be demonstrable in a cystogram as a filling defect in the bladder dome.

An infected urachal cyst may be the cause of repeated trouble because the true nature of the lesion is not recognized. Repeated incisions and drainage may be done for recurrent infections in the cyst. An attack of infection may destroy the lining, but this is unlikely; rather, there will be repeated infections until the true nature of the lesion is recognized and the cyst is removed.

An infected deep-seated urachal cyst may be the cause of abdominal pain and may be mistaken for acute appendicitis. It may rupture into the abdominal cavity and be the cause of generalized peritonitis. When the cyst is adjacent to the bladder, rupture may take place into the bladder, and the cyst may be converted into a diverticulum of the dome of the bladder.

Attempts to remove the cysts are inadvisable when active infection is present. Simple incision and drainage are preferable. When all infection has subsided, the cyst should be excised, and care should be taken that a minimum of rectus fascia is removed with the cyst. Unless this precaution is taken, reapproximation of the rectus sheath in the midline may be difficult or impossible.

ORVAR SWENSON

REFERENCES

BRANDON, S., and WHITEHOUSE, D. Two unusual complications of umbilical hernia in childhood. Brit. Med. J., 2: 1935, 1960.

DUHAMEL, B. Embryology of exomphalos and allied malformations. Arch. Dis. Child. 38: 142, 1963.

GROB, M. (Personal Communication)

GROSS, R. E., and BLODGETT, J. B. Omphalocele (umbilical eventration) in the Newly Born. Surg. Gynec. and Obstet. 71: 520, 1940.

HUTCHIN, P. Gastroschisis with antenatal evisceration of the entire gastrointestinal tract. Surgery, 57: 297, 1965.

LEWIS, J. E., Jr. Atlas of Infant Surgery. The C. V. Mosby Co., St. Louis, Mo. 1967.

MacLEAN, A. B. Spontaneous rupture of an umbilical hernia in an infant. Brit. J. Surg., 38: 239, 1950.

MESTEL, A. L., and BURNS, H. Incarcerated and strangulated umbilical hernias in infants and children. Clin. Pediat. (Phila.), 2: 368, 1963.

MOORE, T. C., and STOKES, G. E. Gastroschisis. Surgery, 33: 112, 1953.

RICKHAM, P. P. Rupture of exomphalos and gastroschisis. Arch. Dis. Child., 38: 138, 1963.

SIBLEY, W. L., LYNN, H. B., and HARRIS, L. E. A twenty-five year study of infantile umbilical hernia. Surgery, 55: 462, 1964.

STRANGE, S. L. Spontaneous rupture of umbilical hernia in an infant. Postgrad. Med. J., 32: 39, 1956.

33

Inguinal Hernias, Hydroceles, Undescended Testicles, and Torsion of the Testicle

Inguinal hernias and hydroceles are caused by the failure of obliteration of the processus vaginalis, which in turn is intimately related to the descent of the gonads. It is important for the understanding of the problems of hernias, hydroceles, and undescended testes to appreciate the embryological basis of the development of these anomalies.

EMBRYOLOGY

In the fifth or sixth week of gestation the gonads make their appearance on the ventromedial surface of the urogenital ridge, which bulges into the coelom as a slender structure extending caudad from the diaphragm. The trunk of the embryo rapidly elongates, resulting in an apparent shift or descent of the gonads, which at about ten weeks become situated close to the groin, and at three months they are located near the internal inguinal ring. This process is termed the internal phase of the gonadal descent. At about the third month of intrauterine life the vaginal process appears as a protrusion of the peritoneum into the ventral abdominal wall. In the male the lower pole of the testes lies near this peritoneal protrusion at the level of the internal ring. The sac evaginates through the ring, and the testes begin their phase of external descent, following the path of the gubernaculum. Between the seventh and ninth month the testes reach the scrotum pushing the vaginal sac ahead of them and protruding into its cavity. The vaginal sac normally loses communication with the peritoneal cavity shortly before or at birth as the processus vaginalis between the level of the internal ring and the upper level of the scrotum becomes a fibrous cord that is attached distally to the vaginal sac that envelops anteriorly the epididymis and the testes. The partial or complete failure of obliteration of this canal predisposes to the formation of indirect inguinal hernias or hydrocele in infancy and childhood, and it accounts for these hernias and hydroceles being classed as congenital lesions, even though they are not clinically present at birth. The processus vaginalis may fail to close completely, resulting in scrotal hernia, or it may obliterate at various levels between the abdominal cavity and the vaginal sac in the scrotum, giving rise to indirect inguinal hernias of different sizes. When the opening into the processus vaginalis is too small to admit contents of the abdominal cavity, peritoneal fluid passes through it to give rise to congenital hydroceles. The process of irregular obliteration of the processus vaginalis produces a variety of combinations of hydroceles of the tunica vaginalis, or hydroceles of the cord with and without hernias.

The stimuli to the process of normal descent of the testicle and the causes of failure of the testicle to reach the scrotum or to err in its location are not well understood. Both mechanical and hormonal factors are probably involved. The role played by the gubernaculum in the external descent of the testis is controversial. It is not clear if the gubernaculum pulls the testis into the scrotum or just prepares the way for its descent. Arey (1965) contends that the gubernaculum does not pull the testicle; rather, it prepares the way by providing space for the testicle. Around the seventh month the gubernaculum ceases to grow and shortens to about half its length; it converts into soft mucoid tissue and becomes as broad as the testes and epididymis. This process may produce dilation of the inguinal canal, and it prepares the path for the external migration of the testicle. After birth the gubernaculum atrophies.

In the female the descent of the gonads is similar to that in the male except that the external phase of descent does not exist. This is probably because the uterus is interposed between the ovarian ligament and the round ligament, which appears by the third month as a continuous cord of dense mesenchyme extending from the region of the uterus to the labia majora. A peritoneal pocket, the diverticulum of Nuck, which is related to the round ligament, corresponds to the vaginal process in the male and predisposes to the formation of inguinal hernias in the female.

ANATOMY

Understanding the anatomy of the inguinal canal and the scrotum is essential for the surgical management of hernias, hydroceles, and undescended testicles. The inguinal canal is an oblique cleft in the abdominal wall superior and medial to the inguinal ligament. It is shorter in relation to body size in infants and children than in adults. The internal ring, which is the inlet to the canal, is located in the transversalis fascia; the external ring is subcutaneous and is formed by a gap in the external oblique aponeurosis, adjacent to the pubic spine, through which emerge the spermatic cord structures in the male and the

round ligament in the female. The internal ring is superior and lateral to the external ring, providing a protective mechanism so that when there is an increase in the intraabdominal pressure the posterior wall of the canal is forced against the anterior wall, thus obliterating the space. The lowermost fibers of the internal oblique and some of the fibers of the transversus muscle arch over the internal ring to form the roof of the canal. The inferior margin of the internal oblique contributes fibers that descend along the cord to form the cremaster muscle. The cord structures rest in a deep gutter on the floor of the canal, which is formed by fibers from the inguinal ligament, the lacunar ligament, and the transversalis fascia that gives fibers intimately investing the cord structures in a layer, the internal spermatic fascia. The testicle in its descent, upon passing through the external ring acquires another coat, the external spermatic fascia, from the aponeurosis of the external oblique muscle. In this manner, the testicle and the portion of the spermatic cord outside the inguinal canal acquire their third covering.

Among the components of the spermatic cord is the vas, or ductus, deferens, which is a distinct whitish structure lying posteriorly and surrounded by the pampiniform plexus of veins. It is readily identified as a firm structure by rolling the cord between the thumb and index finger. The artery to the vas is a branch of the superior vesicle artery and is applied closely to it, while the pampiniform plexus ascends from the scrotum to the abdominal inguinal ring where it forms the spermatic veins. The internal spermatic artery, a branch of the abdominal aorta, descends anteriorly to the cord in the midst of the pampiniform plexus, while the external spermatic artery is derived from the inferior epigastric and is distributed to the elements of the spermatic sheath. The lymphatics ascend from the testicle to the lumbar and aortic glands at the renal level. The processus vaginalis, or ligament, extends from the inguinal ring superiorly, medially, and anteriorly to the cord structures and to the uppermost portion of the tunica vaginalis. The cord in the male and the round ligament in the female curve lateral and anterior to the inferior epigastric vessels.

The inguinal canal in the female is narrow and contains the round ligament and a peritoneal process that, if patent, forms the canal of Nuck.

INGUINAL HERNIA

INCIDENCE

Inguinal hernias are a common problem in infancy and childhood, being usually of the indirect type and very rarely direct. They are defined as a patent processus vaginalis that, at some time during life, contained or contains some intra-abdominal organ, such as bowel, omentum, and ovary, and so forth. With this definition we can then separate out a group of individuals who go through life with a patent processus vaginalis that is only detected at autopsy (15 to 37 percent) and that never gives rise to a clinical hernia. It is estimated from studies (Knox, 1959) done in England on the Newcastle children that about 10 out of every 1,000 children up to the age of 12 have an inguinal hernia. It is often detected before the age of 2 and is commonly noted in premature children. They are more prevalent on the right side in boys, whereas the reverse is true of girls, and they are bilateral in about one fifth of the cases.

CLINICAL DEVELOPMENT

The most common complaint that brings these children to the attention of the physician is the presence of a lump in the inguinal region that is noted by the mother or the child. The lump may vary in size and sometimes is absent; it is usually asymptomatic and only rarely associated with pain, irritability, nausea, or vomiting, unless incarceration occurs. When examining the child, it is important that the examining room and the examining hand be warm in order to prevent an overactive cremasteric reflex, which is triggered by cold drawing the testicle up in

the inguinal canal, simulating the lump of a hernia. One should ascertain at the beginning of the examination that the testicles are descended, since the lump reported by the mother may be either an undescended testicle or a testicle drawn up in the inguinal canal by the cremasteric reflex.

Often the inguinal mass that was noted by the mother has disappeared when the child is brought for examination. In these cases the examiner relies on the history from the mother and on the detection of fullness over the pubic region and an asymmetry of this area in relation to the opposite side. This may present some difficulty in infants in whom there is an abundance of suprapubic fat and also in cases of bilateral inguinal hernia. The examiner should then examine for thickening of the cord and should try and elicit the so-called silk sign. This is accomplished by placing the index finger over the cord at the pubic space and moving it from side to side over the pubic bone (Fig. 1). When the walls

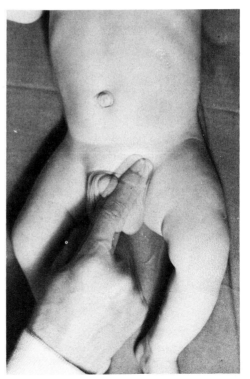

Fig. 1. Maneuver to examine thickening of the cord and detect the silk sign.

of the sac rub against each other they give a sensation similar to rubbing two layers of silk stockings. Thickening of the cord structure because of the presence of a hernial sac is easier to evaluate and is reliable. Making the child walk in the examining room or making him strain may fill the hernial sac. Occasionally, large hernias descending down and filling the scrotum may give the appearance of a large hydrocele, or the hernia may be associated with a hydrocele (Fig. 2). The two conditions may be differentiated by reducing the hernia with gentle pressure over the scrotum while the left-hand index finger is palpating the internal ring area. Transillumination is of little value in differentiating these conditions. However, an x-ray of the abdomen may be of help, provided that the hernia contains intestine, under which circumstances the intestinal air may be outlined (Fig. 3).

Exploration of the inguinal canal with the index finger through the inverted scrotal wall, as is done in the examination for hernias in

adults, is a useless maneuver in examining for hernias in infancy and childhood, for the structure's size makes it impossible for this examination to be reliable. In females an ovary may be in the sac as part of a sliding hernia (Fig. 4). Mothers will describe a bean-sized nodule in the groin in such situations. Both in girls and boys an irreducible lump in the inguinal canal may represent a hydrocele of the cord (Fig. 5). The association of a hernial sac is so prevalent in such situations that operation is advisable and should consist of excision of the hernial sac as well as of the hydrocele.

MANAGEMENT

Uncomplicated inguinal hernias are treated surgically whenever the diagnosis is made, since the risk of operating on a healthy child with a small hernia is minimal compared to the risk of treating incarceration and bowel obstruction. Whether in cases of unilateral hernia bilateral exploration should routinely be performed is the subject of controversy. A large number of publications attempting either to justify or to condemn the practice of bilateral operation for unilateral lesion have appeared in the medical literature. On the one side is the group that feels that since only a small number of children return for repair of an opposite hernia that appears later in life, routine exploration is not warranted. However, other surgeons who have performed routine bilateral explorations have detected the presence of a sac in up to three fourths of their patients. An important point is whether a very small patent vaginal process, if found, will inevitably result in a hernia. This may not be true, since a small number of patients return for repair of the new hernia on the opposite side. Furthermore, the presence of this process at bilateral exploration, which is reported as high as 60 or 70 percent under the age of two years, drops considerably in older children. Considering all aspects of the problem, no data are available that conclusively favor or condemn bilateral repair. The advocates

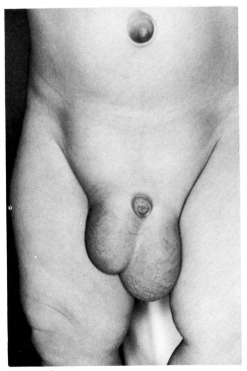

Fig. 2. Bilateral large inguinal hernias.

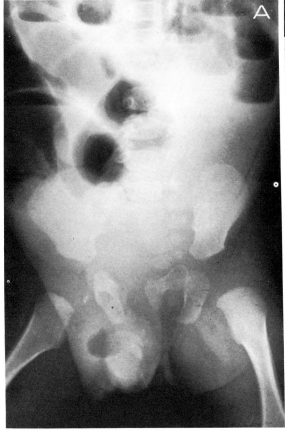
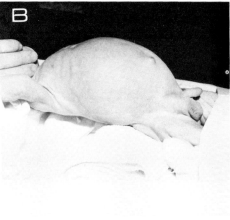

Fig. 3. A. X-ray of abdomen revealing the diagnosis of small bowel obstruction in a child caused by incarcerated inguinal hernia. B. Photograph of patient. Note distention, dehydration, and lump in the right inguinal region.

of routine bilateral repair argue that a second operation is avoided with only a slight increase in risk. Yet routine bilateral repair may result in a certain number of wound infections and iatrogenic lesions of the cord, particularly to the testicular blood supply, with no advantage to the child. Also, the lengthened operating time may increase the risk in the cases of the poorly developed child and the premature baby. It is our practice not to do routine explorations of the contralateral side. However, we do not hesitate to explore the opposite side if we were able to preoperatively detect thickening of the cord or to elicit the so-called silk sign. When the cord is thickened, it is usually caused by a hernial sac.

In the past, uncomplicated inguinal hernias in the premature child were not always treated surgically, and a truss was often used. With modern advances in the preoperative and postoperative care of the child and with modern anesthesia techniques, the risk of hernia repair of the premature child is extremely small. We, therefore, recommend repair of these hernias as soon as the diagnosis is made, so that the risk of incarceration, which is considerable in the premature child, is avoided. However, in cases of sick, debilitated premature infants, especially those having infections of the upper respiratory tract, one should be familiar with the yarn truss, so that it could be temporarily applied until the condition of the infant is more suitable for surgery (Fig. 6).

INCARCERATIONS

The most serious complication of inguinal hernias is incarceration; it occurs often and, if not properly managed, will result in dangerous if not fatal sequelae. Small bowel,

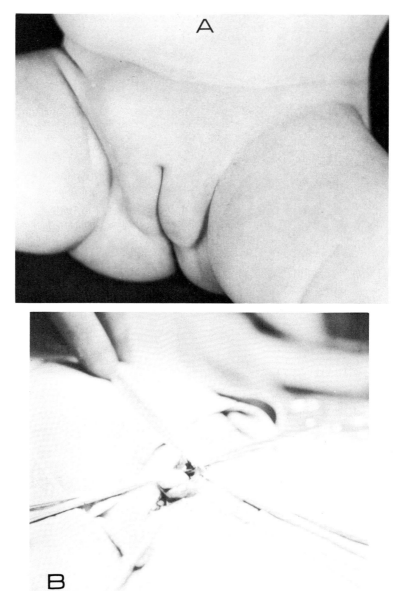

Fig. 4. A. Inguinal hernia in a girl. B. Photograph taken at surgery demonstrating the ovary in the hernial sac.

large bowel, cecum, appendix, or ovary and fallopian tube in the female may be caught inside of the hernia sac, leading to local swelling, edema, redness, pain, and tenderness. When intestine is involved progressive signs and symptoms of bowel obstruction will appear, with nausea, vomiting, abdominal distension, dehydration, and electrolyte imbalance (Fig. 3). The edema, swelling, and venous engorgement of the contents of the hernial sac increase with time, and this process may be reversed with no permanent damage provided that early treatment is instituted. However, if the situation is left uncorrected, the pressure inside the sac rises to completely obstruct the venous return, leading to strangulation of the incarcerated organs. The wall of the bowel or the ovary

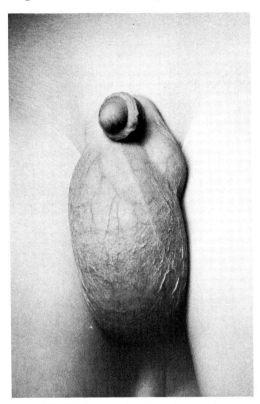

Fig. 5. Photograph of large hydrocele.

will become hemorrhagic and dark; intravascular thrombosis occurs, with loss of viability and necrosis.

TREATMENT

When the duration of incarceration is 12 hours or less, attempts at reducing the hernias should be made. This is accomplished by sedation of the child or infant with morphine, placing him in high Trendelenburg position and giving him local application of cold packs over the inguinal area to decrease the edema. Usually 2 to 3 hours of such treatment results in spontaneous reduction of the hernia. If not, gentle manual reduction is permissible. This consists of counter pressure above the internal inguinal ring with the fingers of the left hand and pressure upward with the fingers of the right hand. Forceful manual emptying of the hernial sac should be discouraged. If the reduction is successful, routine repair is advisable after a

waiting period of one to two days, so that some of the local edema subsides. If the conservative maneuvers aimed at the simple and nonforceful reduction of the incarcerated hernia are not successful after four hours, surgical repair is performed. When an ovary is suspected to be in the sac, early repair is wise, for damage due to compromise of vascular supply is common with necrosis of the gonads. Manual reduction is usually unsuccessful.

OPERATION

Routine uncomplicated hernia patients are admitted to the hospital the day before surgery. Surgery is performed the next morning after a history and physical examination, blood count, and urinalysis are made. General anesthesia is preferred, although occasionally when indicated we use local anesthesia. The patients are usually discharged from the hospital on the first postoperative day.

The fundamental aim of a hernial repair in infancy and childhood is high ligation of the sac. Plastic repair of the abdominal wall as performed in adult hernias is rarely needed.

The incision used is transverse and situated in an inguinal skin fold at a level midway between the external and internal rings. The incision varies in size with age; however, in the average size baby it measures 2 to 3 cm in length.

Figures 7A and 7B show a technique for making a straight incision by cutting the skin with a forward movement of the knife blade. The advantage of this method is to insure that the skin is cut at right angles to the surface. One or two vessels may be encountered in the subcutaneous tissue, and these are ligated with 6-0 silk ligatures. The superficial fascia, or Scarpa's fascia, may be so dense, especially in the infant, as to be mistaken for the aponeurosis of the external oblique, which is distinguished by its shiny white color and the medial and inferior distribution of its fibers. When the aponeurosis of

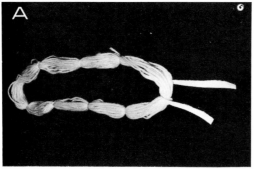

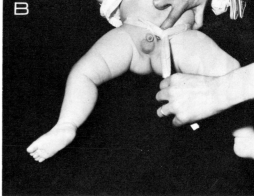

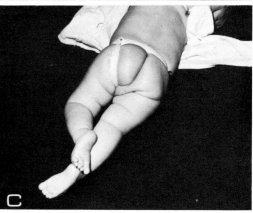

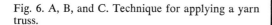

Fig. 6. A, B, and C. Technique for applying a yarn truss.

the external oblique is identified, the inexperienced surgeon may find it difficult to locate the area of the cord so as to properly place the aponeurotic incision. For this reason we teach our residents to insert a blunt instrument, such as a Kocher dissector or the blunt tip of the scissors, through the external ring and to incise into the canal the aponeurosis over the instrument that protects the cord structures and to carry the incision above the inguinal ring (Fig. 7C). Injury to the ilioinguinal nerve that runs deep to the aponeurosis of the external oblique should be avoided. The cremasteric muscle fibers enveloping the cord structures are spread with a hemostat forcep, exposing the glistening white hernial sac. When the sac is small, its rounded end is easily grasped with fine Mosquito forceps and dissected carefully from the delicate structures of the cord all the way to its neck, where properitoneal fat may be seen. The sac is ligated high with

transfixing sutures of 4-0 silk and amputated without being opened, since its walls are usually very thin and transparent enough to permit good visualization of its lumen (Figs. 7D, 7E, 7F, and 7G). Opening of the sac invites troublesome tears that quickly extend into the peritoneum. When the dissection and ligation of the sac have been accomplished high, the stump normally retracts under the internal oblique muscle. In cases of very large hernias there is no absolute need to dissect or remove the distal portion of the sac completely at the risk of oozing and bleeding from small vessels or of damage to cord structures, although in many cases complete removal can be accomplished with no risk. The sac should be transected between clamps at a level about 2 to 3 cm distal to the internal ring after positive identification of the vas and spermatic vessels, and the proximal portion should be treated as described.

In the female it is not important to dissect the sac from the round ligament. The ligament is incised between clamps, and its distal stump is ligated with 5-0 silk ligatures to prevent bleeding while the proximal stump is included with the suture ligature of the hernial sac. Sliding hernias, which are frequent in the female, are easily repaired by a series of purse-string sutures, inverting that portion of the sac with the sliding hernia.

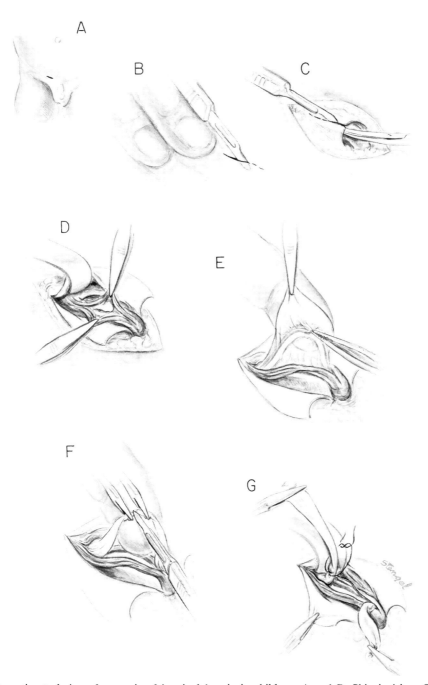

Fig. 7. Operative technique for repair of inguinal hernia in children. A and B. Skin incision. C. Opening of the external aponeurosis. D, E, and F. Dissection of the hernial sac. G. High ligation of sac with 4-0 silk.

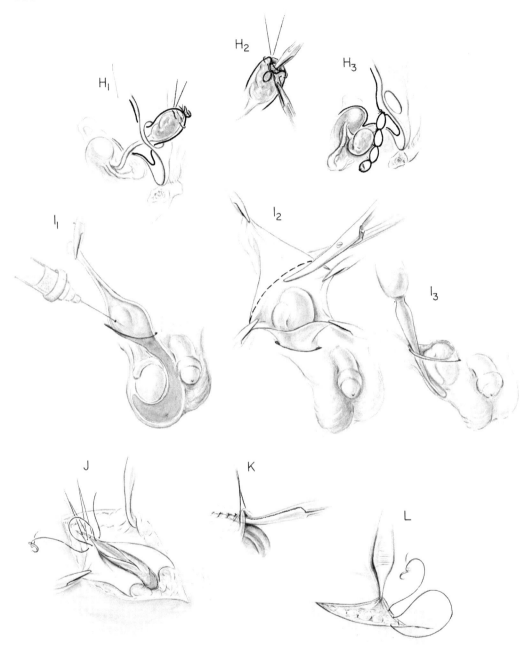

Fig. 7 (cont.). Operative technique for repair of inguinal hernia in children. H₁, H₂, and H₃. Multiple purse-string technique for sliding hernias in female. I₁, I₂, and I₃. Aspiration of hydrocele fluid and excision of a portion of the sac. J, K, and L. Closure of incision with interrupted sutures for deeper layers and continuous subcutaneous catgut sutures for the skin.

This is a far safer procedure than attempting to dissect the ovary from the sac wall, which is usually thin and tears readily, making sac closure difficult (Figs. 7H₁, 7H₂, and 7H₃).

Before closing the incision it is important

to be certain that the testicle is properly placed in the scrotum and not twisted. This is accomplished with the use of a blunt dissector to push the testicle into the scrotum. The hernial incision is closed after all the

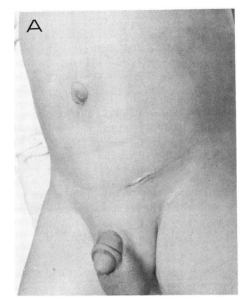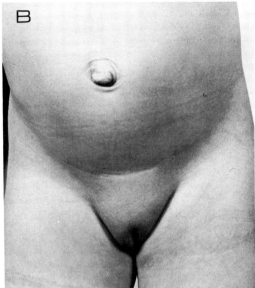

Fig. 8. A. Skin closure and collodion dressing. B. Photograph taken six months after bilateral hernia repair using transverse hernia incision in the inguinal skinfold. The scar can hardly be seen.

bleeding points have been carefully ligated with 6-0 silk ligatures. The aponeurosis of the external oblique is sutured with interrupted 4-0 silk sutures, and to make certain that the external ring is not too tight the sutures can be tied over a curved hemostat placed through the newly constructed external ring. The subcutaneous tissue is closed with 6-0 interrupted silk sutures, and the skin is closed with continuous subcuticular 5-0 plain catgut sutures and sealed with flexible collodion dressing (Fig. 8).

INCARCERATED HERNIA

When dealing with incarcerated or strangulated hernias, it is preferable not to allow the contents of the sac to return to the abdominal cavity until they are inspected. Spontaneous reduction of the hernia may occur as soon as the child is anesthetized. When this occurs, it usually means an early incarceration, and an abdominal exploration to inspect the intestines may not be necessary. The surgical technique and approach is the same for the routine hernias, although it may be more difficult because of the edema and the bleeding from local vascular conges-

tion. After the sac is identified it is opened, and its contents are examined for viability. Warm, moist compresses may be applied to these incarcerated or strangulated organs to help improve the vascularity. When viability is ascertained, the contents of the sac are returned to the peritoneal cavity. Occasionally there is need to enlarge the internal ring by incising the transversalis fascia to permit the return to the peritoneal cavity of the swollen and edematous organs. Such incisions should be made in the superior lateral portion of the internal ring. When definite necrosis is present or when there is questionable viability of these organs, they should be excised and the continuity of the intestinal tract reestablished with an end-to-end anastomosis. The hernial sac is dealt with as in uncomplicated hernia repair.

HYDROCELE

Hydroceles, which are common in early infancy, are frequently bilateral and often disappear spontaneously. The type of hydrocele encountered is influenced by the variation in location and extent of the obliterative process of the processus vaginalis. At birth, small, soft hydroceles may be present in the scrotum and are the result of delayed closure of the communication with the peritoneum. They usually disappear by one year of age. When the peritoneal opening of the processus vaginalis is too small to admit intra-abdominal organs, peritoneal fluid fills the tunica vaginalis and forms the so-called communicating hydrocele. Hydroceles may be present along the cord of the male or the round ligament in the female and are usually associated with a hernial sac.

In infants and children the source of hydrocele fluid is the peritoneal cavity. Consequently these hydroceles must not be treated by the methods used in adults.

In the adult the fluid source is the testicle and hydrocele sac. In the infant it is from the peritoneal cavity. It is important to appreciate this when treatment is undertaken.

Hydroceles are usually ovoid, soft, smooth, cystic, nontender, and of varying sizes and can be transilluminated (Fig. 5). Occasionally it is difficult to distinguish an acute hydrocele from an incarcerated hernia; absence of gastrointestinal symptoms helps in differentiating these two conditions.

MANAGEMENT

The small soft hydroceles detected at birth require no therapy since they usually disappear by one year of age; however, when an obvious hernia is associated with the hydrocele, surgical therapy is indicated. When hydroceles persist after a year of age or demonstrate marked changes in size, they should be operated upon, since these characteristics are caused by the persistence of a patent processus vaginalis. Persistent hydroceles in the pediatric age group are invariably associated with inguinal hernias; consequently the scrotal approach with excision of the hydrocele is condemned. The regular hernia incision and approach should invariably be used. While keeping the scrotum partly exposed, the lower inguinal region and scrotum are prepared. A transverse inguinal hernia incision is made, and the external

oblique aponeurosis is opened. The hernia sac is dissected and treated in a routine fashion by suture, ligature, and amputation. The surgeon should not feel obligated to remove the entire hydrocele sac at the risk of injuring the cord or causing annoying bleeding from small vessels. It is perfectly adequate to excise the easily accessible portion of the hydrocele, which can simply be exposed by pushing on the scrotum and delivering the apex of the hydrocele through the incision. Sometimes, when the hydrocele is too large, it is difficult to push it through the inlet of the scrotum, and one may resort to emptying it of most of its fluid by incising the small area exposed through the incision or by inserting a needle for drainage. Then, as much of the sac as can easily be exposed is excised, paying meticulous attention to ligation of all of the bleeding points; otherwise, the scrotum may become swollen in the postoperative period with serosanguinous fluid. There is no need to evert the edges of the hydrocele around the testicle. This should be avoided so that vascular damage to the testicle will be prevented.

Aspiration of fluid from the hydrocele through the skin of the scrotum should be discouraged. It is not only of little value but may be dangerous, since infection can be introduced in an otherwise sterile sac, or a serious complication may occur if a viscus is accidentally punctured when the mistaken diagnosis of hydrocele instead of an incarcerated hernia is made.

DIRECT HERNIA

Direct hernia is an unusual lesion in children and is difficult to differentiate preoperatively from indirect hernia. The clinical course is the same. It may be associated with disease of the collagen and can be diagnosed with some accuracy in such situations. The repair presents a problem, for the posterior wall of the canal may be partially or completely involved. Repair of the canal after the technique of Bassini, which transplants the cord superficial to the internal oblique, is sufficient to prevent recurrence and hopefully does not constrict the cord sufficiently to cause testicular atrophy.

FEMORAL HERNIA

Femoral hernia is also a rare lesion in children, usually being seen in girls 8 years of age and above. It can be suspected from the history, which usually relates the consistent presence of the inguinal lump with little change in size. On inspection the mass is lower than that of inguinal hernia, and reduction is difficult or impossible. Repair requires a lower incision than in inguinal hernia and exposure of the defect through the inguinal ligament both above and below the structure. Closure of the defect below is usually not sufficient to prevent recurrence. The defect should be repaired on both sides of the ligament, particularly above.

UNDESCENDED TESTIS

Undescended testis in infancy and childhood ranks third in frequency of the problems in the inguinal canal after hernias and hydroceles. The term "undescended testis" describes a condition in which there was arrest of the testicle in its descent, so that it never passed the external ring and reached the scrotum. It is used interchangeably with cryptorchism but should be differentiated from the term "ectopic testis," which designates a condition in which the testis has completely descended but is lodged outside the scrotum. A retractable testis is caused by a hyperactive cremasteric reflex that pulls the testicle in the inguinal canal or superficial to the external oblique aponeurosis in the pouch described by Denis-Browne. The process of testicular descent and its relationship to the formation of the processus vaginalis has been described at the beginning of the section on hernias. This descent is more apparent than actual and is probably influenced by hormonal stimulation and aided by the gubernaculum, which prepares the path for the external migration of the testicle to the scrotum. The roles played by the hormones and by the gubernaculum in the descent of the testicle are not clearly defined. Disturbance in the descent of the testicle leading to cryptorchism may be caused by mechanical factors, hormonal factors, or abnormalities of the testicle itself, so that it fails to respond to hormonal stimuli. It should be differentiated from the condition termed secondary cryptorchism, which accompanies or is produced by hypogonadism or hypopituitarism.

The undescended testis may be located in the retroperitoneal tissue anywhere between the kidney and the internal ring or in the inguinal canal and is frequently associated with a hernial sac. However, ectopic testes are outside the external inguinal ring and may be located posteriorly in the buttocks, where they may cause pain on sitting or in the perineum, the pubopenile area, the groin superficial to the external oblique aponeurosis, or the femoral canal (Fig. 9). The testicle occasionally may be completely absent (anorchism) or, rarely, duplicated (polyorchism).

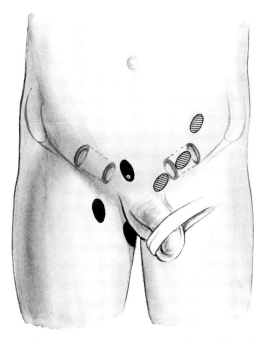

Fig. 9. Location of ectopic and undescended testicles. The locations marked in solid black represent areas of ectopic testicles.

The undescended testis is usually smaller and softer than normal, but it does not deviate from normal until about the age of 5. At this time, there appears a lag in the development of the tubules with a decrease in the activity and number of spermatogenic cells. These changes become more apparent between the ages of 9 and 10 and are very severe at puberty, with minimal or complete absence of spermatogenesis. Although the hormonal secretions of the undescended testis may be slightly decreased, they are adequate for the development of normal sex characteristics.

The incidence of undescended testes in the adult population is about 0.28 percent, while at birth in the full-term baby, it is 3.4 percent and in the premature baby it is up to 30 percent. Most of the undescended testes discovered at birth will descend spontaneously in the first year of life and bring the incidence by the age of one down to 0.66 percent. When this percentage is compared to the adult rate of occurrence, it becomes apparent that half of the testicles not descended by a year of age will be descended by adulthood. Cryptorchism is more often seen on the right side and is bilateral in about 15 percent of the cases.

Medical advice is usually sought when parents note the empty scrotum in the child (Fig. 10). It is estimated that about 80 percent of these cases are caused by a hyperactive cremasteric muscle reflex that becomes weaker as the child grows older, so that at puberty and early adulthood the testicle does not leave the scrotum. The parents' history of having noted a bulge in the scrotum when the child was placed in a warm bath strongly suggests the diagnosis of a retractile testis, and the parents can be assured that in time the testis will take its normal position without treatment.

Examination of the child for undescended testicles should be performed in a warm room, and the hands of the examiner should be warm so as not to elicit a cremasteric reflex. A small, empty, and underdeveloped

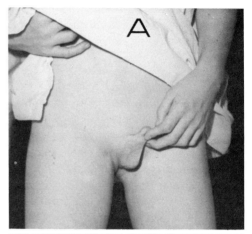

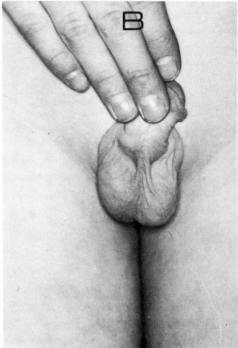

Fig. 10. A. The empty underdeveloped scrotum of undescended testicle. B. Same patient one year after orchidopexy.

scrotum and the absence of any testicular mass is diagnostic of intra-abdominal testes. Sometimes the testis can be palpated in the inguinal canal, and a gentle attempt should be made to see if the testicle will reach the scrotum. A bulge in the inguinal area may be caused by an accompanying inguinal hernia.

MANAGEMENT

The rationale for therapy in cryptorchism is based on several considerations:

1. Hernias: Since undescended testes are usually accompanied by patent processus vaginalis it is imperative that sooner or later the hernial sac be repaired and at the same time the testicle brought down into the scrotum.
2. Trauma: A testis that resides in the inguinal canal is more subject to trauma, especially when situated over the pubic bone, and it is better protected when placed in the more resilient scrotum.
3. Torsion of the spermatic cord: There is a high incidence of torsion in cryptorchism.
4. Malignancy: The chances of malignancy developing in an undescended testicle are probably higher than in a normally placed one. Therefore, orchidopexy is recommended, although there is no proof that placing the testis in the scrotum prevents the occurrence of malignant tumor. Also, because of this fear of malignancy, it is recommended that orchiectomy be performed on any intra-abominal testis that could not be brought into the scrotum after adequate surgical attempt. There are obvious advantages to having the testicle in an area where inspection is routine. Should growth take place in adult life the change can be detected early and effective therapy undertaken. Considerable growth could take place before detection if the testicle were intra-abdominal.
5. Psychological factors: The presence of an empty scrotum has a psychological impact, especially in older boys. These psychological factors provide a primary indication for orchidopexy, especially in the unilateral cases where the question of sterility is not as important as when the lesion is bilateral.
6. Sterility: Since it has been shown that spermatogenesis in the undescended testis becomes severely impaired at puberty it is imperative to place these testes in the scrotum to prevent this complication. Long followup of patients who have undergone bilateral orchidopexies before puberty between the age of 10 and 12 years demonstrated that these operations prevented sterility and resulted in a fertility rate of about 80 percent.

The age at which orchidopexy should be performed has been the subject of controversy. One group of surgeons argues that orchidopexy should be performed around the age of 5 years, since it is at that age that a lag in tubular development begins to appear on histological section of the testes. On the other hand, another group of surgeons, including ourselves, recommends that orchidopexy be delayed until 9 to 12 years of age, but definitely never past puberty. It is felt that in this older age group failure to maintain the testicle in the scrotum is less than when early operation is undertaken. More important, some testes will descend spontaneously between the ages of 5 and 10. We will continue to follow this policy unless new evidence is produced that demonstrates that the results and the fertility rate are better if the operation is performed at an earlier age than 9 to 12. What is needed is a series of biopsies on children who have biopsy and orchidopexy at 4 to 5 years of age, and when they become 12 it must be determined if early repair prevents the microscopic changes that occur when the testicle is left undescended until 12 years of age. The changes may be part of the congenital malformation and not influenced by early repair. Of course, if a hernia accompanies an undescended testicle and becomes troublesome, operation is performed at any age to repair the hernia, and the testis is brought down to the scrotum at the same time. In regard to the use of hormones, we do not believe this type of therapy has a place in the treatment of cryptorchism except when definitely indicated, such as in cases of hypopituitarism and hypogonadism.

OPERATION

The operative site is draped so that a part of the scrotum is exposed. A transverse incision in an inguinal fold is used. The dissection in the subcutaneous tissue should be done with caution in order to avoid damage to an unexpected ectopic testicle. The external ring is identified and opened after inserting a blunt instrument through the ring into the inguinal canal. Blunt dissection is used to free the external fascia above and below the incision, particularly the shelving edge of Poupart's ligament. The sac, testicle, and cord structures should be separated from the canal as a unit, and this necessitates division of some vascular bands at the tip of the sac.

The next step in the operation is to divide the posterior wall of the inguinal canal (Fig. 11). This is important, for it permits the cord structures, particularly the vas, to traverse a direct route from the posterior aspect of the bladder to the external ring, rather than traversing the longer triangular route over the deep epigastric vessels. Division of the posterior wall of the inguinal canal can be accomplished safely only after ligation and division of the deep epigastric vessels. One artery and two veins are almost invariably present, and each vessel is individually freed, ligated, and divided. The transversalis fascia can then be divided. When the testicle is intra-abdominal, there will be a hernial sac in the inguinal canal, and traction on the sac usually brings the intra-abdominal testicle into view. Opening the hernial sac exposes the testicle. The vessels and the vas deferens will be adherent on the posterior aspect of the sac, and the next step in the operation is to detach, by careful blunt dis-

section, these structures from the sac halfway between the testicle and the inguinal ring. Much annoyance can be avoided in the operation if these structures are detached without tearing the sac. When the vessels and vas have been separated from the sac, a clamp is placed across the sac and it is divided. This gives the operator control of the proximal sac and facilitates separation of the vas and the vessels from the peritoneum beyond the hernial sac. The sac is ligated with a transfixing suture at the peritoneal level.

The vas is freed by blunt dissection down to the bladder. The next step is to free the vessels up to the kidney. This is accomplished by using long ribbon retractors for exposure and blunt dissection along the vessels. There will be attachments between the vessels and the retroperitoneal tissue that can be cut during the first part of the dissection. Restricting bands close to the kidney cannot be exposed, and hence it is necessary to use blunt dissection for their division. Among the vessels in the vascular pedicle there are fibrous bands that can be identified by palpation; cutting these will elongate the vascular pedicle. This should not be resorted to unless adequate length of the pedicle cannot be achieved by any other method, for it involves considerable likelihood of damage to the vessels.

When maximum length has been attained, 2-0 silk suture on a long Keith needle is passed through the lower pole of the testicle in such a way that a good bit of the testicular capsule is included. The free end of the suture is also threaded on the needle. A curved Kelly clamp is placed on the needle so that the point is protected, and a similar clamp is used to grasp the shaft of the needle. Space for the testicle in the scrotum is now provided by blunt dissection. The clamps and attached needle are then passed into the scrotum, and the first clamp is removed, permitting the needle to be pushed through the scrotal skin. The second clamp is removed and the needle pulled through. Traction on the double suture pulls the

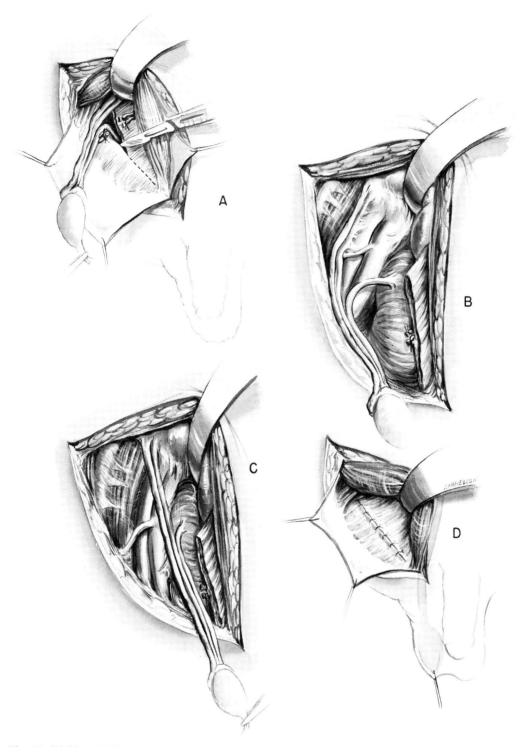

Fig. 11. Division of the posterior wall of the inguinal canal to permit a freeing of the vas and the cord structures in orchidopexy.

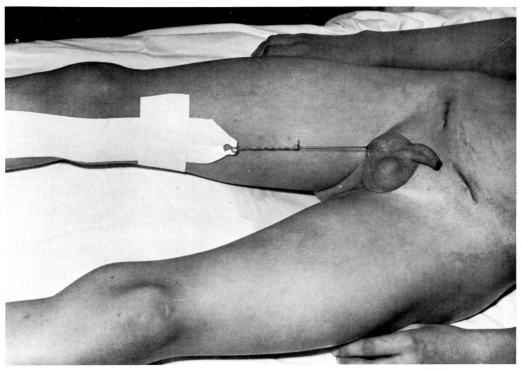

Fig. 12. Traction sutures to stabilize the testicles in the scrotal sac after orchidopexy.

testicle into the scrotum. Twisting of the cord structures as the testicle is brought into the scrotum should be prevented.

The transversalis fascia is reapproximated with interrupted 4-0 silk sutures, leaving room for the cord structures in the external ring region adjacent to the pubic spine. The internal oblique muscle and conjoined tendons are sutured to the shelving edge of Poupart's ligament, care being taken to provide space for the vessels and vas to emerge at the pubic spine.

The external oblique is approximated with interrupted silk sutures of 4-0 silk. The subcutaneous tissue is approximated with a few 6-0 silk sutures and the skin approximated with continuous subcuticular 5-0 plain catgut sutures. Collodion is painted on the wound directly.

A long piece of tape is attached to the patient's leg, and a rubber band is looped through a hole in the free end of the tape above the knee. The suture from the testicle is tied to this rubber band so that sufficient traction is supplied to maintain the testicle in the scrotum (Fig. 12). The object of this traction is not to elongate the cord structures but to overcome the tendency of the small scrotum to push the testicle back into the inguinal region. The traction should be maintained for five days and then removed. It is advisable to have the patient on complete bed rest during this period. For the first day or two after operation, sedation may be required because of pain.

When the testicle has been intra-abdominal and the efforts to provide adequate length of cord structures to place the testicle in the scrotum have been unsuccessful, a two-stage procedure is advisable. At the first operation, the testicle is brought down as far as possible into the scrotum. If the testicle fails to maintain a scrotal position—and this is usually the situation with intra-abdominal testicles—a second operative attempt is made a year or two after the initial operation. Such two-stage efforts are often rewarded by a satisfactory result.

TORSION OF THE TESTICLE AND ITS APPENDAGES

Torsion of the testis is caused by a twist of the cord interfering with the testicular circulation. Although trauma has been implicated as an etiological agent of this disease, it probably does not play as important a role as some congenital anatomical factors that predispose to the occurrence of torsion. In this respect two conditions have been noted, one is that there is some anomaly of the mesorchium, which is relatively long and with a short base, and the other is an abnormal attachment of the tunica vaginalis high on the cord. Thus, the testis is suspended inside the vaginal sac to form the so-called bell-clapper testis.

The twist of the cord can occur inside the tunica vaginalis, which is most frequently the case, but it may also occur in the extra-vaginal portion of the cord. Occasionally torsion is associated with undescended testicles. Although torsion of the testis can occur at any age, there are two peak incidence periods, one below the age of 2 years and the other between the ages of 10 and 16 years. The onset of symptoms is usually severe, with pain referred to the abdomen, the thigh, or the back and often associated with vomiting and mild shock. Upon examination, the scrotum exhibits unilateral redness, swelling, edema, and marked tenderness. The differential diagnosis includes mumps orchitis, epididymo-orchitis, hematocele, acute hydrocele, scrotal hernias, and torsion of the appendix testis. It may be difficult to differentiate torsion of the testis from acute orchitis or acute epididymo-orchitis; but these conditions are very rare in the pediatric group, so that every painful testicular swelling of sudden onset and not preceded by mumps or associated with a

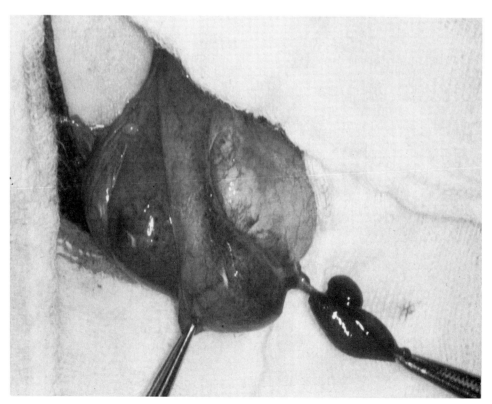

Fig. 13. Photograph demonstrating the dark hemorrhagic discoloration of the appendix testis following torsion.

previously known inguinal hernia should be considered a torsion of the testicle until proven otherwise. The signs and symptoms of torsion of the testicular appendages are not as severe as those of torsion of the testicle. The onset of pain and swelling is milder and slower and is not associated with vomiting. Occasionally one may see through the thin scrotal wall of the child a pea-sized structure, dark in color, which represents the necrotic appendix testis.

TREATMENT

The treatment of torsion is surgical and should be prompt, since the spermatogenic cells can be completely eliminated if ischemia lasts more than six hours. The surgical approach is through an inguinal hernia incision. The tunica vaginalis should be opened and the testis explored and untwisted. Every effort should be made to save the testis unless there is absolutely no evidence of return of blood supply after detorsion. The testis is then replaced into the scrotum and fixed to the inner layers of the scrotum with a few interrupted sutures. Some authors advocate fixing the opposite testicle to the scrotum to prevent future torsions; this maneuver may be wise, especially when a completely necrotic testis is found at operation. Torsion of the appendix testis could be treated conservatively, but this increases the period of the pain and one may miss an associated torsion of the testis. Therefore, surgery should be advised, and the procedure is simply excision of the appendix testis (Fig. 13).

FAROUK S. IDRISS

REFERENCES

AREY, L. B. Developmental Anatomy, 7th ed. Philadelphia, W. B. Saunders Co., 1965.

BROWNE, D. Some anatomical points in operation for undescended testicle. Lancet, 1: 460, 1933.

BURTON, C. C. The embryologic development and descent of the testis in relation to congenital hernia. Surg. Gynec. Obstet., 107: 294, 1958.

CAMPBELL, H. E. Incidence of malignant growth of undescended testicle—critical statistical study. Arch. Surg., 44: 353, 1942.

——— The incidence of malignant growth of the undescended testicle—a reply and re-evaluation. J. Urol., 81: 663, 1959.

CHARNEY, C. W., and WOLGIN, W. Cryptorchism. New York, Paul B. Hoeber, Inc., 1957.

CLATWORTHY, H. W., Jr., GILBERT, M., and CLEMENT, A. The inguinal hernia, hydrocele and undescended testicle problem in infants and children. Postgrad. Med., 22: 122, 1957.

——— and THOMPSON, A. G. Incarcerated and strangulated inguinal hernia in infants—a preventable risk. J.A.M.A., 154: 123, 1954.

CLAUSSEN, E. G. Inguinal exploration of hernia. Surgery, 44: 735, 1958.

COLODNY, A. H., and HOLDER, T. M. Rectal examination—a useful maneuver to aid in differentiating an incarcerated inguinal hernia from a hydrocele in infancy. Surgery, 53: 544, 1963.

COOPER, E. R. A. Histology of retained testes in human subject at different ages and its comparison with scrotal testes. J. Anat., 64: 5, 1929.

CRESSON, S. L. Management of hernias in infants and children. Med. Clin. N. Amer., 75: 920, 1957.

DeBOER, A. Inguinal hernia in infants and children. Arch. Surg., 75: 920, 1957.

DONOVAN, E. J. Torsion of the spermatic cord in infancy. Ann. Surg., 92: 405, 1930.

FARROW, G. A., and THOMSON, S. Incarcerated inguinal hernia in infants and children: A five-year review at The Hospital for Sick Children, Toronto, 1955 to 1959 inclusive. Canad. J. Surg., 6: 63, 1963.

GANS, S. L. Sliding inguinal hernia in female infants. Arch. Surg., 79: 109, 1959.

GILBERT, J. B. Studies in malignant testes tumors. V. Tumors developing after orchidopexy—report of 2 cases and review of 65. J. Urol., 46: 740, 1941.

——— and HAMILTON, J. B. Studies in malignant testes tumors—incidence and nature of tumors in ectopic testes. Surg. Gynec. Obstet., 71: 731, 1940.

GILBERT, M. G., and CLATWORTHY, H. W., Jr. Bilateral operations for inguinal hernia and hydrocele in infants and children. Amer. J. Dis. Child., 102: 34, 1961.

GOLDSTEIN, I. R., and POTTS, W. J. Inguinal hernia in female infants and children. Ann. Surg., 148: 819, No. 5, 1958.

GROSS, R. E. Surgical management of the undescended testicle. International Record of Medicine and General Practice Clinics, 169: 353, 1956.

———— and JEWETT, T. C., Jr. Surgical experience from 1,222 operations for undescended testes. J.A.M.A., 160: 634, 1956.

———— and REPLOGLE, R. L. Treatment of the undescended testis. Opinions gained from 1,767 operations. Postgrad. Med., No. 3, 34: 266, 1963.

HAMMERICK, L. C., and WILLIAMS, J. O. Is contralateral exploration indicated in children with unilateral inguinal hernia? Amer. J. Surg., 104: 52, 1962.

HOLCOMB, G. W., Jr. Routine bilateral inguinal hernia repair. An evaluation of the procedure in infants and children. Amer. J. Dis. Child., 109: 114, 1965.

JONES, P. Torsion of the testes and its appendages during childhood. Arch. Surg., 37: 214, 1962.

KEITH, A., SIR. Origin and nature of hernia. Brit. J. Surg., 11: 455, 1924.

KNOX, G. The incidence of inguinal hernia in Newcastle children. Arch. Dis. Child., 34: 482, 1959.

KOOP, C. E. Inguinal herniorrhaphy in infants and children. Surg. Clin. N. Amer., 37: 1675, 1957.

———— and MINOR, C. L. Observations on undescended testes (II. The technique of surgical management). Arch. Surg., 75: 898, 1957.

KRISTIANSEN, C. T., and SNYDER, W. H., Jr. Inguinal hernia in female infants and children. Western J. of Surgery, Obstet. & Gynecology, 64: 481, 1956.

LONGINO, L. A., and MARTIN, L. W. Torsion of the spermatic cord in the newborn infant. New Eng. J. Med., 253: 695, 1955.

LYNN, H. B. Hernia, hydrocele and undescended testis. Amer. J. Surg., 107: 486, No. 3, 1964.

McFARLAND, J. B. Testicular strangulation in children. Brit. J. Surg., 53: 110, 1966.

MOORE, C. R., and QUICK, W. J. The scrotum as a temperature regulator for the testes. Amer. J. Physiol., 68: 70, 1924.

OECONOMOPOULOS, C. T., and CHAMBERLAIN, J. W. Torsion of the appendix with observations as to its etiology, an analysis of 26 cases. Pediatrics, 26: 611, 1960.

PACKARD, G. B. Inguinal hernia of infancy and childhood. Arch. Surg., 86: 299, 1963.

POTTS, W. J., RIKER, W. L., and LEWIS, J. E. Treatment of inguinal hernia in infants and children. Ann. Surg., 132: 566, 1950.

RAVITCH, M. M., and HITZROT, J. M. The operations for inguinal hernia (I. Bassini, Halsted, Andrews, Ferguson; II. Halsted, Lotheissen, Hopkins Hernia). Surgery, 48: 439, 1960, and 48: 615, 1960.

RICHARDSON, W. R. Inguinal hernia of the internal genitalia in female infants and children. Amer. Surg., 29: 446, 1963.

ROBINSON, J. N., and ENGLE, E. T. Cryptorchism—pathogenesis and treatment. Pediat. Clin. N. Amer., 2: 729, 1955.

———— and ———— Some observations on the cryptorchid testis. J. Urol., 71: 726, 1954.

SCORER, C. G. Descent of the testes in the first year of life. Brit. J. Surg., 27: 374, 1955.

———— The incidence of incomplete descent of the testicle at birth. Arch. Dis. Child., 31: 198, 1956.

SHANDLING, B., and THOMSON, S. The Cheatle-Henry approach for inguinal herniotomy in infants and children—The Hospital for Sick Children, Toronto. Canad. J. Surg., 6: 484, 1963.

SNYDER, W. B., BRAYTON, D., and GREANEY, E. M. Pediatric Surgery—Undescended Testes. Chicago, The Year Book Publishers, Inc., pp. 1041–1061, 1962.

SNYDER, W. H., Jr. Inguinal hernia complicated by undescended testis. Amer. J. Surg., 90: 325, No. 2, 1955.

———— and CHAFFIN, L. Surgical management of undescended testes. J.A.M.A., 157: 129, 1955.

SOHVAL, A. R. Histopathology of cryptorchidism—Study based upon comparative histology of retained and scrotal testes from birth to maturity. Amer. J. Med., 16: 346, 1954.

SWENSON, O. Diagnosis and treatment of inguinal hernia. Pediatrics, 34: 412, 1964.

34

Neonatal Intestinal Obstruction

Obstruction of the intestinal tract of newborn infants is a common problem in pediatric surgery. In addition to those congenital anomalies resulting from abnormal embryonic development, a number of acquired lesions of the bowel may occur either in utero or during early postnatal life.

Whenever the passage of intestinal contents is blocked by an obstruction there is an increased proliferation of bacteria within the bowel lumen, with the production of toxic materials that are damaging to the mucosa and even the deeper circulation. Because of the thinness of the bowel wall and the limited defenses against invasive infections of newborn babies, the bacterial overgrowth associated with neonatal intestinal obstruction may very rapidly lead to sepsis.

There are several differences between neonatal and adult bowel obstruction which require comment. For example, the removal of all questionable bowel may seem unwise to the surgeon who only occasionally treats neonatal obstructions, and consequently compromise operations may be done which are unsuccessful. On other occasions the obstruction is not a mechanical one, and it cannot be dealt with surgically. Such an obstruction is associated with sepsis, prematurity, or other functional abnormalities. In a baby with a functional obstruction which cannot be corrected surgically, operation usually proves disastrous. Not only is considerable judgment required in the selection of the proper time to operate and of the preoperative care that may be necessary, but there are also many problems of postoperative management in the nutritional and bacteriological difficulties that may arise. It is the purpose of this chapter to discuss certain of these general considerations and to present a classification of the neonatal intestinal obstructions. The diagnosis and management of the specific lesions associated with bowel obstruction in the newborn are considered in other parts of the book.

CLASSIFICATION

For purposes of discussion, the neonatal period is considered to extend to the end of the fourth week of extrauterine life. During these early weeks anatomical congenital anomalies are responsible for the great majority of cases of bowel obstruction. About one half of the patients are found to have aganglionosis of portions of the colon. The remainder suffer from meconium ileus, from atresias of the duodenum, ileum, or jejunum, or from mechanical obstructions occurring shortly after birth. Impaired small bowel activity also results from such conditions as neonatal sepsis, cerebral injury, drugs administered to the mother during labor, drug (heroin) withdrawal reactions in the baby after delivery, congenital hypothyroidism, and prematurity. Very rarely the etiology of a serious bout of newborn intestinal obstruction remains obscure both clinically and at postmortem examination.

TABLE 1. CAUSES OF SMALL BOWEL OBSTRUCTION IN NEWBORN INFANTS

MECHANICAL

Intrinsic
  Atresia and stenosis
  Meconium ileus
    Without atresia
    With atresia or perforation
  Meconium plug syndrome
  Valvelike intestinal folds
Extrinsic
  Malrotation of intestines with midgut volvulus
  Volvulus without malrotation
    Localized
    Massive, owing to poor fixation of mesentery
  Incarcerated hernia—inguinal or internal
  Congenital peritoneal bands
  Duplications
  Meconium peritonitis
  Intussusception

NEUROGENIC

Congenital aganglionosis
  Of the rectum (short segment type)
  Of the colon (rectosigmoid, partial, total)
  Of the colon and part of the small bowel
Paralytic ileus due to cerebral injury

INFECTIOUS

Enterocolitis
  Secondary to aganglionosis or partial bowel obstruction
  Secondary to generalized sepsis
Paralytic ileus due to generalized sepsis or enteritis (pseudomonas), pneumonia, pyelonephritis, and so on
Acute peritonitis
  Secondary to perforation of the bowel
  Primary

FUNCTIONAL

Prematurity
Drugs in labor (hexamethonium or other ganglionic blocking agents)
Drug withdrawal (maternal heroin or morphine addiction)
Congenital hypothyroidism
Idiopathic

It is convenient to group the various types of neonatal small bowel obstruction into those of mechanical, neurogenic, infectious, and purely functional origin (Table 1). In patients seen late in the course of the occlusion, a combination of these factors may be present, greatly complicating the problems of diagnosis and treatment.

ETIOLOGY

There are many different causes of the various forms of neonatal bowel obstruction. They may be thought of as genetic, developmental, and accidental. The "accidental" group refers to such acute intrauterine catastrophes as fetal vascular thrombosis, volvulus, intussusception, and spontaneous perforation of the fetal intestinal tract associated with meconium peritonitis (Louw, 1959). In many of the cases genetic and acquired factors are combined—for example, the intestinal volvulus or atresia that may be associated with the meconium ileus in mucoviscidosis. It has long been recognized that the incidence of congenital anomalies is increased when there are relatives with anomalies. Other lesions appear to be purely developmental in origin. The history of maternal virus infections, hormonal administration, or toxic influences during the course of the pregnancy may relate directly to the type of lesion and to its management and prognosis.

It is fortunate that aside from duodenal atresia and meconium ileus, obstructive lesions of the small intestine in the newborn appear to be largely unrelated to genetic or developmental factors. Most of the obstructive lesions of the small bowel are apparently caused by intra-abdominal catastrophes occurring in the fetus or are the result of intestinal volvulus or sepsis in early postnatal life. These last-mentioned conditions are not usually complicated by other anomalies or by mental deficiency, and so the outlook for normal life is excellent if the primary disorder can be corrected.

In addition to the mechanical causes of neonatal bowel obstruction, severe paralytic ileus may occur for any of a number of reasons, including cerebral injury, uremia, enteric infections with Pseudomonas, and generalized sepsis of varied etiology. Occasionally a baby is encountered in whom spasm of the terminal ileum has led to intestinal obstruction in the absence of any other obvious abnormality. A plug of firm meconium in an otherwise normal intestinal tract may also lead to serious obstruction if the force of peristalsis is not sufficient to dislodge and propel the mass. Enemas may assist its expulsion, but if it is high in the tract, operative removal may be necessary. Following the clearing of the obstruction these babies usually develop normally, in distinction to those with true meconium ileus. In this condition the barium enema may be therapeutic as well as diagnostic, as emphasized by Mikity (1967).

Studies to rule out cystic fibrosis and Hirschsprung's disease (congenital aganglionosis) must be done within the first few days of life. It is well to remember that congenital aganglionosis, one of the most frequent causes of newborn bowel obstruction, extends in 3 percent of the cases to the ileocecal valve and in a very small number may be found to involve not only the colon but part or even all of the small intestine. An unusually rare condition causing defective peristalsis is the absence not of ganglion cells but of portions of the intestinal musculature. This defect of the intestinal wall may be located over only short segments of the bowel, as described by Handelsman (Handelsman, et al., 1965), or it may be more extensive, sometimes along the entire intestinal tract.

SIGNS AND SYMPTOMS

Failure to pass meconium or feces, abdominal distension, and persistent vomiting of bile are the cardinal manifestations of all forms of intestinal obstruction in the newborn infant. These signs and symptoms may occur shortly after birth, or they may be delayed for several days. The radiographic appearance of the different types of lesions and the rate at which the symptoms have appeared make an accurate preoperative diagnosis possible in most of the cases.

Congenital anomalies may be anticipated when the pregnancy has been complicated by early bleeding, hydramnios, maternal diabetes, or toxemia. Hydramnios during the pregnancy should alert the physician to the possibility of congenital obstruction of the gastrointestinal tract of a newborn infant. In a series of 74 mothers with polyhydramnios (amniotic fluid in excess of 2,000 ml) Moya and his associates (1960) found 27 percent of the infants to have severe congenital abnormalities. Six of the patients (8 percent) had anomalies in the gastrointestinal tract, and 3 of these were duodenal or high jejunal obstructions. In Clatworthy's series (Clatworthy and Lloyd, 1957) 45 percent of infants with duodenal or high jejunal atresias were born to mothers with polyhydramnios. Low ileal or colonic atresias are less likely to be associated with polyhydramnios, presumably because a greater proportion of the swallowed amniotic fluid can be absorbed into the child's circulation and thence be transferred through the placenta to the mother for excretion.

Abnormalities of the placenta also suggest the possible presence of major congenital anomalies. A *single umbilical artery* noted at the examination of the cut surface of the cord during delivery is the most common and the most diagnostic abnormality. According to Benirschke and Bourne (1960) it occurs in 1 percent of single births and in 7 percent of twin births. Stillbirths or early fetal deaths are associated with 58 percent of the cases, and major congenital anomalies are present in 30 percent or more of the survivors.

When one baby in a family has been born with a major congenital anomaly, the chances are greater than usual that another child will have the same or another abnormality. The history of an affected sibling should alert the physician to this possibility during subsequent deliveries.

The regurgitation of small amounts of mucus or gastric content is not uncommon during the first hours or days of life, particularly in premature infants. *Persistent* vomiting of yellow or green material, however, usually signifies mechanical bowel obstruction, and it should be taken seriously. Nixon (1955) states that only two babies out of a group of 4,000 delivered during a one-year period had bile-stained vomiting in the absence of an organic cause. Abdominal distension in association with bilious vomiting is almost pathognomonic of serious obstruction, but its absence should not be taken as a sign that obstruction is not present. Gaseous distension that is due to a complete occlusion may not occur if the baby vomits easily or has a relatively high obstruction, since the number of distended loops of bowel may not be sufficient to produce significant·abdominal enlargement.

Delay in the passage of true meconium is always important. According to Sherry and Kramer (1955), 94 percent of normal babies have meconium stools within 24 hours, and 99.8 percent pass meconium within 48 hours. Occasionally a baby with complete obstruction will discharge a moderate amount of light green or grey putty-like stool, and this material will be incorrectly recorded as meconium in the nurse's notes. True meconium is a dark-green, tenacious, tarlike material, while the stool of obstruction, the so-called white meconium, is firm, mucoid, and light in color. This latter material is formed by intestinal content passed before the occlusion occurred, or from desquamated bowel epithelium and mucus produced below the site of the obstruction.

PHYSICAL EXAMINATION

The physical examination of a newborn with intestinal atresia usually yields only moderate information about the site or cause of the obstruction. The high obstructions produce little distension; the lower ones are more likely to cause it. When the abdomen is excessively distended or is tympanitic and edematous, and particularly if dark discoloration of the skin is present (Fig. 1),

perforation of the bowel should be expected. Absence of the bowel sounds is an important sign of bowel devitalization or perforation, but since peristalsis sometimes continues to some degree in small babies until the onset of severe generalized peritonitis, the presence of bowel sounds does not necessarily indicate that devitalization has not occurred.

Jaundice occurs in association with high intestinal obstruction in a surprising number of infants. In the series presented by Louw (1966), 5 of 17 babies with jejunal atresia were deeply jaundiced, and 3 required exchange transfusions. Boggs and Bishop (1965) found 48 percent of a group of 48 infants with duodenal or jejunal occlusions to have total bilirubin levels (mostly indirect) of over 20 mg percent. Such hyperbilirubinemia does not seem to occur with ileal or colonic lesions to the same degree that it does in the higher bowel atresias. Inasmuch as jaundice is a sign of sepsis in the newborn, a condition that may also lead to vomiting and abdominal distension, the difficulties of diagnosis are increased when it is present.

The history of the passage of normal meconium prior to the onset of vomiting should lead to a diligent search for a diagnosis other than an atresia. It is important to look for the signs of *sepsis of the newborn:* an irregular or very low temperature, lethargy, pallor, low serum sodium, and albuminuria. Since it is exceedingly difficult to differentiate bowel atresia or volvulus with local infection from gram-negative septicemia accompanied by focal bowel necrosis, such apparently insignificant facts as the time of passage of meconium and the general course of the infant prior to the onset of vomiting may be the only clues to the proper diagnosis. One such clue is that bowel necrosis due to generalized sepsis is associated with only partial bowel obstruction for a considerable period of time, in distinction to the complete obstruction caused by atresia, which dates from birth.

Abdominal tenderness can be determined by observing the baby's face during palpation. He will usually wince or cry more vig-

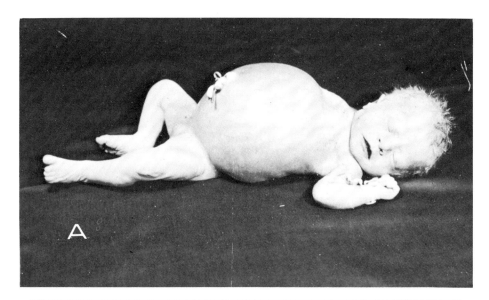

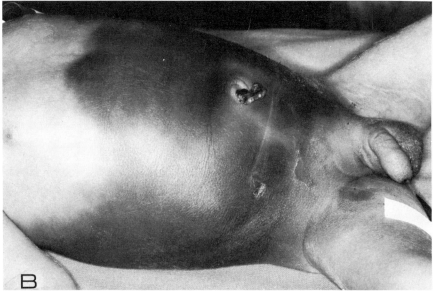

Fig. 1. A. Newborn bowel obstruction with enormous abdominal distension. B. Discoloration of the abdomen in presence of free intraperitoneal meconium.

orously if peritonitis is present. A mass is palpable in many cases of intra-abdominal sepsis. In babies it is formed by edematous loops of bowel which are adherent one to the other over a site of perforation. When the bowel sounds have been heard initially and then have disappeared completely, peritonitis and intra-abdominal sepsis are very likely to be present. Auscultation of the abdomen must always be performed at intervals in order to assess the changes which may occur. Needless to say, in a baby with evidence of one congenital abnormality other defects should always be suspected and ruled out.

RADIOGRAPHIC FINDINGS

Any baby with persistent vomiting or other signs of bowel obstruction, however

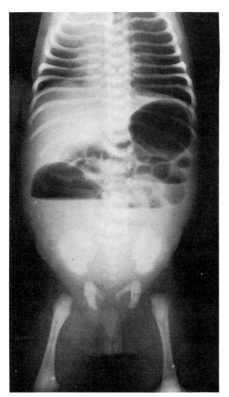

Fig. 2. Atresia of the ileum. Several air-fluid levels are present.

markings do not develop until the infant begins to stand erect, and the caliber of the normal colon is no greater, and often less, than that of the small intestine. For these reasons babies with multiple air-fluid levels should be examined by means of barium enema to determine the caliber, configuration, and position of the colon. The only possible exception to this rule is the baby with intra-peritoneal calcification (Fig. 3). In this situation, meconium peritonitis in association with an atresia of the small intestine is almost invariably present. Even here, however, the barium enema will clear the lower colon of white meconium and prove the absence of colonic obstruction, permitting the surgeon to do a small bowel anastomosis with more confidence. The contrast material should be introduced through a large-bore plastic enema tip and the neces-

slight, should be examined radiographically. Supine and upright films are required as the first step. Of great importance is the diagnosis of the *level* of the obstruction. High atresias are characterized by only a few distended loops of bowel and their associated air-fluid levels. By contrast, the radiographs of low ileal obstruction show multiple gas-filled bowel loops (Fig. 2). Duodenal obstructions, of course, are diagnosed by the characteristic "double bubble" sign.

When only a few loops of distended bowel are present, further films are unnecessary. The lack of gas along the course of the lower bowel testifies to a complete occlusion of the upper intestinal tract, which must be relieved by operation. If there are multiple air-fluid levels, however, the obstruction may lie in either the lower small intestine or the colon. It is extremely difficult in infants to determine whether a given gas shadow is that of distended ileum or of colon. The haustral

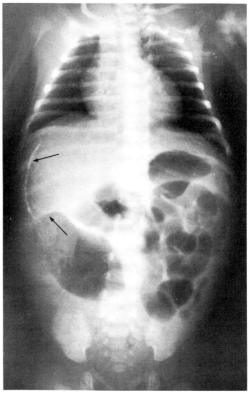

Fig. 3. Meconium peritonitis with atresia of the ileum. Resection and anastomosis were successfully performed.

sary pressure produced only by gravity, not by injection through a syringe.

Most babies with low bowel obstruction will be found to have congenital aganglionosis (Hirschsprung's disease), not small bowel atresia. Because the operative approach to the two abnormalities is entirely different, the barium enema is essential to determine whether mechanical obstruction or aganglionosis is the proper diagnosis.

It is perhaps not generally appreciated that a normal colon x-ray pattern usually indicates the absence of neonatal small bowel obstruction, while an irregular small-caliber colon is a sign of congenital obstruction above the ileocecal valve. The reason for this is that the colon ordinarily fills progressively with meconium and dilates to its normal size during late fetal life, while the "unused" colon associated with small bowel obstructions does not distend, remaining small in caliber and often having an irregular course. This sign is not reliable if stools have been passed prior to the onset of the obstruction: Small bowel stenosis rather than atresia may have permitted sufficient meconium to enter the colon to dilate it during intrauterine life. A normal colon is also present when the obstruction has developed in extrauterine life, as occurs, for example, in neonatal volvulus.

If the functional causes of paralytic ileus in the newborn (prematurity, hypothyroidism, meconium plug syndrome, drugs given the mother) have been ruled out, the probable diagnosis when the colon appears normal is congenital aganglionosis. The contrast radiographs in aganglionosis do not reveal proximal dilatation with sufficient consistency to establish the diagnosis in the first few days of life. At times the colon may remain normal in appearance for many weeks or months. In addition, rectal spasm may suggest the diagnosis of Hirschsprung's disease in patients subsequently proved to have normal ganglion cells on histological examination. It is for this reason that a rectal biopsy

and frozen section examination should always be done before an operation for apparent low small bowel obstruction in the newborn when the colon appears normal by barium enema.

PATHOPHYSIOLOGY OF NEONATAL BOWEL OBSTRUCTION

Whatever the cause of newborn bowel obstruction, a characteristic series of events occurs. Vomiting is common to all forms of obstruction, since the gastrointestinal tract cannot empty its accumulating secretions. If vomiting develops early, the stomach may remain undistended; when the vomiting reflex is less well developed, enormous gastric dilation and intestinal distension may occur. The fluid lost from the stomach is highly acid after the first eight hours of life (pH 1.0 to 3.0), with a high content of chloride. When the intestinal content is regurgitated (as evidenced by a change of the suction drainage to a greenish hue), sodium, bicarbonate, and potassium are lost in larger quantities, with an associated rapid decrease in their serum concentrations.

In addition to obvious loss from the stomach by vomiting or gastric aspiration, large "third space" fluid collections occur within the intestinal lumen and peritoneal space. Because the baby's water reserves are low (total body water in a 3-kg baby is about 2,200 ml)* this combination of fluid loss and sequestration leads to serious dehydration. Low blood volume, serum hypotonicity, and circulatory collapse are the inevitable results of untreated bowel obstruction. Rapid dehydration with circulatory collapse is most marked in the babies with "closed-loop" obstruction, since the accompanying venous obstruction leads to excessive fluid transudation and blood loss into both the bowel lumen and the peritoneal cavity. The amount of fluid lost by gastric aspiration in cases of duodenal atresia is not great, and so unop-

---

* Human fetal body water at 10 weeks' gestation is 94 percent of the body weight, decreasing to 70 to 80 percent at term. Extracellular body water constitutes 38 to 43 percent at term.

erated and untreated babies with this condition may live for many days. Infants with low colonic obstruction may become dehydrated soon after birth, but some of them also survive for prolonged periods of time as the result of relatively normal secretion–absorption ratios along the course of the intestinal tract.

Distension of the bowel eventually leads to decompensation of both its propulsive and its absorptive activities. There is venous engorgement of the mucosa, and bacterial overgrowth occurs in the stagnant intestinal content. The defective circulation and absorption of bacterial toxins lead to devitalization of the bowel wall. The smooth muscle is overstretched, thinned, and ischemic. The mucosal capillary circulation is diminished by the increasing intraluminal pressure, and areas of necrosis appear which are rapidly invaded by bacteria. This is particularly true with volvulus, in which the secretions are trapped within the closed bowel loop. Low colonic occlusion also leads to a similar "closed-loop" obstruction when there is a competent ileocecal valve, since the air and fluid which mass in the colon cannot escape by retrograde flow. Bowel necrosis and bacterial invasion of the peritoneal cavity are the usual result of prolonged obstruction. If the obstruction of the bowel is not complete, as in uncomplicated small bowel stenosis, rectal aganglionosis, and anorectal atresia with fistula formation, such bowel devitalization does not immediately occur but bacterial overgrowth may still develop and lead to an acute or chronic enterocolitis which interferes with the baby's growth and development.

The pattern of electrolyte deficits can be predicted only partially from the known site of the obstructive lesion. High obstructions lead to large chloride and potassium losses, with resulting severe metabolic alkalosis. Lower lesions produce more marked losses of sodium in addition to losses of the other electrolytes. Low serum sodium and chloride values and a normal potassium concentration are the usual findings, particularly when dextrose in water has been used to rehydrate the patient. Despite obvious dehydration, the blood urea nitrogen is usually normal unless sepsis is present. A raised blood urea nitrogen in association with a persistently low serum sodium is almost always indicative of sepsis in small babies without other evidence of renal disease.

BACTERIAL INFECTION AND INTESTINAL SURGERY

Bacterial infection is a constant threat to newborn infants. This danger is increased in infants with bowel obstruction for several reasons. The stasis of bowel contents leads to marked overgrowth of bacteria within the bowel lumen, and devitalization of the mucosa caused by capillary obliteration increases the probability of their penetration into the bowel wall. Bacterial endotoxins, which further impair the mucosal circulation and permit extension of the infection into deeper portions of the bowel wall, are produced by many organisms. The intestinal lymphatics are invaded, and seeding of the bloodstream may occur.

The newborn baby swallows air with his first breath and often ingests material during his passage through the birth canal. Air usually appears in the lower colon within four hours of birth. This progress of the swallowed air is accompanied by a similar progression of infectious organisms.

The bacterial content of the small intestine is variable, but the counts are normally very low in infants and children. Cultures of the small bowel in adults, on the other hand, are usually positive for both aerobic and anaerobic organisms, as shown by Bornside, Welsh, and Cohn (1966), who have studied the flora of the small intestine in a group of 50 adults without primary intestinal disease. Only 20 percent of the specimens from the jejunum and 28 percent of those from the ileum were sterile. These bacterial counts are several orders of magnitude lower than they are in the colon. In children the enterobacteria are usually absent in the small intestine, but when stasis occurs, the number of organisms rises very rapidly.

Aside from phagocytosis, the baby's main defenses against bacterial infection are the immune globulins acquired by passive transfer from the mother and those which are manufactured in response to invasive infection. Newborns, particularly the small ones, do not have efficient cellular phagocytic mechanisms. According to Gluck and Silverman (1957), phagocytosis is ineffective in premature infants and progresses only slowly in efficiency in relation to increases in the birth weight. Since many babies with bowel occlusion are premature or are infants of low birth weight, defective polymorphonuclear phagocytosis can be expected to be detrimental to their control of infection.

The most important humoral factor against infection during early neonatal life is the I_gG or 7S gamma globulin with a molecular weight of 165,000 which comes from the maternal circulation. The high molecular weight I_gM (19S) immunoglobulin is not transmitted across the placenta. This latter globulin appears to be responsible for antibody activity against the somatic "O" antigen of several gram-negative organisms, including *Escherichia coli, Klebsiella, Aerobacter,* and the *Salmonella* group, and so these intestinal bacteria are likely to be more dangerous to the newborn infant than they are to larger babies. Contrary to previous teaching, I_gM globulin can be manufactured at birth in both premature and full-term infants; however, significant amounts do not appear before three to five days of life, the time when babies are usually brought to operation for neonatal intestinal obstruction.

Weakness of the phagocytic mechanisms and deficient quantities of I_gM gamma globulins place newborn babies at high risk from infection. The stresses of anesthesia and operation also appear to depress the body's resistance, since infants with signs of mild sepsis or early pneumonia may succumb rapidly to overwhelming infection after surgical procedures of reasonable length. Hypovolemia

and anemia further reduce the body's resistance to infection. For these reasons adequate transfusion at the time of operation, and the substitution when possible of local for general anesthesia, may increase the chance for survival of desperately ill babies with newborn bowel obstruction.

Antibiotics should be used in infants after all intestinal surgical procedures requiring bowel transections. This is not prophylactic therapy, since there can be no doubt that organisms are present in the bowel lumen and also within the tissues of the mucosa. The bacteria are spilled at operation and are included in the suture line of a bowel anastomosis. Proper antibiotic therapy can reduce the proliferation of these organisms until healing has occurred or the normal body defenses have been mobilized. In general it is best to use bactericidal drugs for this purpose rather than the tetracyclines, which have only a bacteriostatic effect.

Cultures of the peritoneal fluid should be made both at the time of opening of the abdomen *and just prior to its closure.* Within 12 hours the possibility of spillage infection can be determined, and at 24 to 36 hours sensitivity studies can be obtained to guide subsequent antibiotic therapy.

The organisms encountered both preoperatively and postoperatively in sepsis of the newborn are *E. coli,* the *Klebsiella* group, *Aerobacter aerogenes, Pseudomonas aeruginosa,* and occasionally *Proteus vulgaris* and enterococci. These are organisms which require the high molecular weight I_gM gamma globulin for their control. In modern times antibiotic therapy has slowly evolved into a reasonably satisfactory plan of attack which can offset to some extent the deficiencies of this material in relation to the baby's protective mechanisms. Sensitivity measurements are of importance to determine which of the antibiotics are best suited to control the organisms encountered.

Escherichia coli, Aerobacter aerogenes, Klebsiella, and *Proteus vulgaris* are usually sensitive to kanamycin and nalidixic acid.

Polymyxin B is the drug of choice for Pseudomonas. We have been impressed with the combination of Polymyxin B with cephalothin (Keflin) in the treatment of serious Pseudomonas infections and have not found it detrimental to the kidney or other metabolic functions in small babies. Penicillin is usually combined with one or another of these drugs in the treatment of newborns after surgical procedures. It does protect against infection with the enterococci and some Proteus organisms, and it may control postoperative pulmonary infections. It should not be used alone. The extensive clinical studies of Gluck, Wood, and Fousek (1966) have revealed, on the basis of sensitivity testing, that penicillin has only about 1 chance in 14 of being effective against the organisms responsible for neonatal sepsis.

It is our current practice to treat newborn infants postoperatively with penicillin, 150,-000 units, and kanamycin, 15 mg per kg in 3 divided doses daily, and then to change to other antibiotics as indicated by the results of sensitivity studies of cultured organisms. It appears possible that the use of Kantrex may encourage Pseudomonas infection in some hospitals, and many surgical units have therefore returned to the use of streptomycin (20 mg/kg) in association with penicillin. The dangers of auditory damage appear to be insignificant when streptomycin is used for no more than five days in the newborn infant. If the signs of sepsis appear, repeated blood, urine, throat, and stool cultures should be done. Failing a positive blood culture, the predominance of *Aerobacter aerogenes* in the stool calls for kanamycin therapy, while Pseudomonas infection should be treated with Polymyxin B (2.5 mg/kg) and cephalothin (50 mg/kg) in 2 to 3 divided doses. Other organisms are dealt with as they appear. This specific antibiotic therapy should be continued for a minimum of seven days, in contrast to the initial course of antibiotics, which should be stopped, in the absence of septic complications on the fifth postoperative day.

MASSIVE BOWEL RESECTION IN INFANCY

ADAPTIVE PROCESSES

The problems of inadequate digestion and absorption arise postoperatively in the treatment of many forms of neonatal intestinal obstruction. It may be necessary in some cases to resect considerable amounts of devitalized bowel, and on other occasions the intestine may already be abnormally short because of the congenital defect. Although conservation of healthy bowel is the ideal goal of surgical treatment, defectively functioning bowel must not be left behind in an effort to conserve length, for this may result in poor recovery of intestinal peristalsis, poor healing of an intestinal anastomosis, or even perforation of a remaining nonviable portion of the bowel.

When midgut volvulus is present, the proximal and distal ends of the bowel may be marginally viable. It is sometimes possible to save a considerable amount of bowel by resecting the obviously nonviable central portions, following which an anastomosis is made between the questionable areas. The worst disease having been removed, the child's condition can be stabilized with blood and plasma during the next 24 hours, at which time a "second look" operation may reveal that the bowel has regained its color or that it has become necessary to resect more of it in order to secure a safe anastomosis.

Estimates of the amount of bowel required for nutrition and growth have been continually revised downward during the past 20 years. Improved parenteral therapy and the availability of antibiotics have increased the survival rate of infants with extensive bowel resections who might otherwise have died. It is now known that the intestines will usually hypertrophy and elongate when massive intestinal resections have been performed. The outcome depends on the maintenance of the patient on special feeding mixtures and parental fluid therapy until the enlargement of the remaining bowel has occurred.

Louw (1959) states that the small bowel is about 250 cm (100 inches) in length at birth. Obviously there is great variability in this figure from baby to baby. In his review of massive resections of the bowel in infancy, MacMahon (1966) observed that the infant's intestinal tract is about half the length of the adult intestine and that it grows an additional 30 percent during the first year of life. Since the small intestine in adults varies in length from 10 feet (340 cm) to 28 feet (863 cm), a baby's intestine may be expected to be 150 to 400 cm long during early neonatal life.

Many conditions requiring bowel resection in infancy have already produced an abnormally short intestine. This is particularly true of the intestinal atresias, which are thought to arise from volvulus or other causes of vascular impairment to the fetal intestine. The subsequent absorption of the sterile infarcted segment necessarily results in shortening of the bowel, which is further increased by resection of the atretic ends. It is important, therefore, to measure the amount of bowel *remaining* at the close of the surgical procedure rather than the amount which has had to be resected. Reports are now appearing of the successful treatment of infants in whom only 28 to 36 cm of the small intestine remained after resection. Patients with such small amounts of bowel can be carried through only if meticulous attention is paid to the details of postoperative parenteral and oral feeding.

Following resection of a portion of the small intestine the lumen increases in diameter, the valvulae conniventes and villi become hypertrophied, and the remaining bowel grows somewhat in length. These changes do not occur following simple division and anastomosis of the intestine. Loran and Crocker (1963) postulated the secretion of an intestinal growth hormone after bowel resection and have demonstrated in rats that the lower ileum may be the site of its release. In a newborn infant reported by MacMahon (1966), 20 cm of jejunum remaining after massive resection had increased in length to 45.5 cm eight months later. The elongation of the bowel is never as striking as the increase in the absorptive surface area which results from mucosal hypertrophy and widening of the lumen. Flint (1912) demonstrated increases up to 400 percent in the absorptive surface area of the intestines of dogs after extensive bowel resections but found that growth in the length of the bowel did not contribute significantly to this adaptive change.

Most authors agree that preservation of the ileocecal valve is important to survival after massive bowel resections. Kremer and his colleagues (1954) found that the combined loss of the entire ileum and the ileocecal valve leads to increasing inanition and fluid loss in dogs and that preservation of the valve is associated with improved nutrition and survival rates. Stahlgren and associates (1962) have reaffirmed these findings. Although Wilkinson (Wilkinson et al., 1963) has shown that dilation and hypertrophy of the remaining bowel and prolongation of the intestinal transit time develop in humans whether or not the ileocecal valve remains intact, both experimentally and clinically the function of the ileocecal valve appears to be of great importance in the maintenance of nutrition after massive bowel resection. Every effort should be made to save the valve, but its preservation must not be attempted when the terminal ileum or cecum is of questionable viability.

The best results of massive resection are obtained in those patients in whom a portion of the jejunum and a portion of the ileum are left intact, together with a functioning ileocecal valve. Next are patients with jejunum and ileum in whom the valve has had to be removed. Survival is better with ileum than jejunum if one or the other portion of the bowel must be sacrificed, and the problem is almost insurmountable if less than 50 cm of jejunum alone remains. This is particularly true if the colon is not available for anastomosis, as occurs when aganglionosis

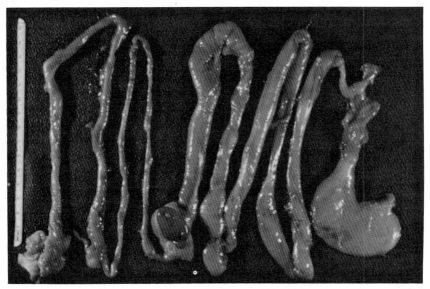

Fig. 4. Aganglionosis extending to the jejunum. It is very difficult to salvage this congenital disorder.

has involved the entire colon and ileum up to the middle portion of the small bowel (Fig. 4).

PATTERNS OF NUTRITIONAL LOSS

Immediately after massive bowel resection, rapid transit and a decreased resorptive surface of the bowel lead to increased losses of fluid. After a period of adjustment, such compensatory mechanisms as delayed gastric emptying, slowing of intestinal peristalsis, and enlargement of the remaining bowel occur. These produce relatively normal transit times and fluid absorption. The degree of fluid, electrolyte, and nutritional loss from the shortened bowel depends on the amount of bowel remaining and on the types and amounts of nutrients which are ingested. Evidence that increased gastric secretion follows massive small bowel resection has been provided by Reul (1966) and others. In some cases the resulting acidity of the small bowel content further impairs the nutritional efficiency of the remaining shortened intestine.

FATS

The ability to utilize fat is markedly altered by massive resection. While fat digestion occurs in the jejunum through the action of the pancreatic and intestinal lipases, its absorption in the form of fatty acids takes place mainly in the ileum through the intestinal lymphatics. When these fatty acids are not absorbed, they increase in the feces and appear to lead to a diarrhea which further interferes with digestion of the carbohydrates and proteins. For this reason it is generally agreed that the diet of a patient with decreased bowel should be low in neutral fat. It has long been recognized that premature babies utilize olive oil and soybean oil more effectively than butterfat. These materials have been recommended for patients with the short bowel syndrome. Recently, formulas containing medium-chain triglycerides have been made available to provide the calories associated with normal fat intake without the production of steatorrhea. The medium-chain triglycerides,* which contain 8 to 10 carbon atoms as opposed to the 16- to 18-

* Available from the Mead Johnson Company as Product 7010-X (MCT oil) or in a powdered formula marketed as Portagen.

carbon fatty acids derived from ordinary dietary fat, are rapidly absorbed directly into the portal venous system, rather than into the intestinal lymphatics. They do not produce diarrhea and appear to be utilized in the body's metabolic pool for the production of growth and energy.

CARBOHYDRATES

Carbohydrate utilization is impaired by massive bowel resection. The absorption of both xylose and labeled glucose was found to be decreased by about one half in a patient reported by Winawer and his associates (1966). These findings persisted for more than nine months after the resection. Unlike fat, however, equivalent percentages of the ingested glucose are absorbed as the dietary dosage is increased, and diarrhea does not result. This favorable absorption does not necessarily apply to the disaccharides. According to Dahlqvist (1962), lactose is absorbed in the duodenum and upper jejunum, maltose in the jejunum and upper ileum, and sucrose in the distal jejunum and ileum. Hydrolysis of these sugars is incomplete in the intestinal lumen and continues in the cells of the mucous membrane. In recent years a loss of the ability to digest the disaccharides has been noted to persist for weeks or months after a bout of infectious diarrhea in some infants. These infants fail to thrive and continue to have diarrhea on a regular formula despite the elimination of the infectious agent. Removal of sucrose and other disaccharides from the diet of such infants has resulted in renewed weight gain and subsidence of the diarrhea. A similar series of events often follows the relief of prolonged intestinal obstruction or the enterocolitis of Hirschsprung's disease in small infants. Deficiencies of the specific enzymes for disaccharide digestion in these cases have now been demonstrated by intestinal biopsy studies, and improvement in weight gain and decrease in the diarrhea on monosaccharide (dextrose or fructose) formulas have been found to occur.

PROTEIN

Protein digestion and absorption are decreased following massive bowel resection, but the recovery is quite rapid. Within a few weeks the infants are able to absorb 60 to 80 percent of the ingested protein, as long as diarrhea is controlled by a low-fat monosaccharide formula. Too rapid increases in the dietary fat followed by diarrhea in such infants may actually lower the protein absorption and produce a negative nitrogen balance even after weeks of satisfactory weight gain. Both of Pilling's cases were unable to gain weight until the dietary fat had been reduced to 1 to 2 percent of the caloric intake (Pilling and Cresson, 1957). The use of protein hydrolysates has not been found to be of great value, despite the logic of their use.

VITAMINS AND MINERALS

Since the fat-soluble vitamins are poorly absorbed by the short intestinal tract, the intake of vitamins A and D should be increased to several times their normal amounts. Although vitamin K absorption is undoubtedly reduced, hypoprothrombinemia is not usually encountered. Vitamin B_{12} is absorbed in the ileum, and so it must be replaced parenterally when the distal small bowel has been completely removed. Iron deficits may also be expected to occur. Calcium deficiency is a real problem, particularly in the infants with steatorrhea, in whom hypocalcemic tetany frequently develops. Magnesium absorption is reduced in some cases, and clinical signs and symptoms of its deficiency have already been reported.

FLUIDS AND ELECTROLYTES

The fluid management of patients with massive resections can be very trying. It is necessary to support these infants not only with fluid and electrolytes but also by means of carbohydrate and protein administration. The former nutrient can be given as 10 percent dextrose in water, but this material has the disadvantage of causing sclerosis and thrombosis of the veins. For long-term management, therefore, 5 percent dextrose solutions are used. Blood and plasma can be given to supply nitrogen for growth and should be used freely. They may have to be used daily to prevent anemia and starvation hypoproteinemia. Edema about the eyes and in the extremities is a late sign of such starvation. The total serum proteins may fall terminally, but generally these are reasonably well maintained at the expense of the general body development.

A technique developed at the University of Pennsylvania (Wilmore and Dudrick, 1968) has recently been shown to permit normal growth and weight gain in infants fed exclusively by the intravenous route. A #24 polyvinyl catheter is inserted into the external jugular vein and passed into the superior vena cava. Its proximal end is then drawn subcutaneously to a stab wound in the posterior parietal area of the scalp in order to decrease the chance of infection. By infusing a 25 percent glucose solution and 5 percent protein hydrolysate solution at a slow steady rate with an infusion pump and by giving vitamins, trace metals, and small amounts of plasma at intervals, the entire nutritional needs of the baby can be satisfied parenterally. To protect the site of entry of the catheter from infection, the use of an occlusive dressing and antibiotic oint-

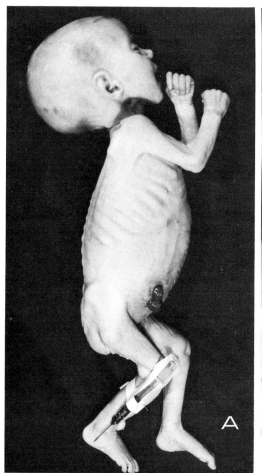 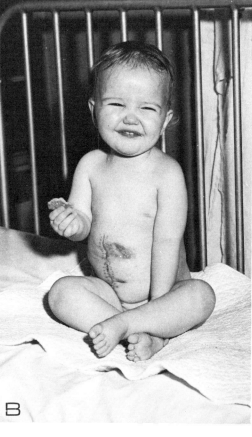

Fig. 5. A. Failure to thrive after ileostomy for total colonic aganglionosis. A previous transverse colostomy had been unsuccessful. B. The same patient at the age of 16 months after prolonged fluid therapy.

ments can be used. The infused material should be filtered through a 0.22 μ millipore unit.

THE MALABSORPTION SYNDROME

It is impossible to predict the electrolyte deficits to be expected with the malabsorption syndrome. Measurement of fecal electrolytes in ileostomy or stool collections should be done on several occasions in order to establish the pattern of loss. Frequent measurement of the serum electrolytes is important to the provision of correct replacement therapy, since it has been found that attempts to replace completely the measured losses from the intestinal tract usually lead to hypernatremia and hyperkalemia. It is well to remember that sodium, chloride, and potassium are ordinarily lost in the feces and

that their total replacement in babies with diarrhea may overload the infants' ability to utilize or excrete them.

If vomiting or diarrhea occurs on feeding, the oral intake must be dropped back or discontinued. It is then gradually increased again until full tolerance is reached. Substitution diets, which include carbohydrates as dextrose and fats as medium-chain triglycerides, should be tried when the diarrhea persists. The weight gain after massive resections is always slow, and it may require three to six months for a baby to regain his birth weight. Such slow development is necessarily discouraging, but on occasion we have been gratified to see a normal baby develop from a weak, thin infant after several months of careful therapy (Fig. 5).

WILLIAM L. DONNELLAN

REFERENCES

ALTEMEIER, W. A., and SMITH, R. T. Immunologic aspects of resistance in early life. Pediat. Clin. N. Amer., 12: 663, 1965.

BENIRSCHKE, K., and BOURNE, G. L. The incidence and prognostic implication of congenital absence of one umbilical artery. Amer. J. Obstet. Gynec., 79: 251, 1960.

BERNSTEIN, J., and BROWN, A. K. Sepsis and jaundice in early infancy. Pediatrics, 29: 873, 1962.

BOGGS, T. R., Jr., and BISHOP, H. Neonatal hyperbilirubinemia associated with high obstruction of the small bowel. J. Pediat., 66: 349, 1965.

BORNSIDE, G. H., WELSH, J. S., and COHN, I., Jr. Bacterial flora of the human small intestine. J.A.M.A., 196: 1125, 1966.

CHING, N. P. H., and BALLINGER, W. F., II. Perforation of the colon secondary to the meconium plug syndrome. Arch. Surg., 90: 65, 1965.

CLATWORTHY, H. W., Jr., SALEEBY, R., and LIVINGOOD, C. Extensive bowel resection in young dogs: Its effect on growth and development. Surgery, 32: 341, 1952.

———— and LLOYD, J. R. Intestinal obstruction of congenital origin. A study of diagnosis and management in one hundred sixty-three cases. Arch. Surg., 75: 880, 1957.

COBRINIK, R. W., HOOD, R. T., Jr., and CHUSID, E. The effect of maternal narcotic addiction on the newborn infant; Review of literature and report of 22 cases. Pediatrics, 24: 288, 1959.

CORDONNIER, J. K., and IZANT, R. J., Jr. Meconium ileus equivalent. Surgery, 54: 667, 1963.

CRAIG, W. S. Vomiting in the early days of life. Arch. Dis. Child., 36: 451, 1961.

DAHLQVIST, A. The intestinal disaccharidases and disaccharide intolerance. Gastroenterology, 43: 694, 1962.

EICHENWALD, H. F., and SHINENFIELD, H. R. Rational use of antibiotics. Amer. J. Surg., 107: 518, 1964.

ELLIS, D. G., and CLATWORTHY, H. W., Jr. The meconium plug syndrome revisited. J. Pediat. Surg., 1: 54, 1966.

FLINT, J. M. The effect of extensive resection of the small intestine. Bull. Hopkins Hosp., 23: 127, 1912.

FRIMANN-DAHL, J., LIND, J., and WEGELIUS, C. Roentgen investigations of the neonatal gaseous content of the intestinal tract. Acta Radiol., 41: 256, 1954.

GLUCK, L., and SILVERMAN, W. A. Phagocytosis in premature infants. Pediatrics, 20: 951, 1957.

———— WOOD, H. F., and FOUSEK, M. D. Septicemia of the newborn. Pediat. Clin. N. Amer. 13: 1131, 1966.

GROB, M. Intestinal obstruction in the newborn infant. Arch. Dis. Child., 35: 40, 1960.

HALLUM, J. L., and HATCHUEL, W. L. F. Congenital paralytic ileus in a premature baby as a complication of hexamethonium bromide therapy for toxemia of pregnancy. Arch. Dis. Child., 29: 354, 1954.

HANDELSMAN, J. C., BLOODWELL, R., BENDER, H., and HARTMANN, W. An unusual cause of neonatal intestinal obstruction: Congenital absence of the duodenal musculature. Surgery, 58: 1022, 1965.

HOLSCLAW, D. S., ECKSTEIN, H. B., and NIXON, H. H. Meconium ileus; A 20 year review of 109 cases. Amer. J. Dis. Child., 109: 101, 1965.

KREMER, A. J., LINNER, J. H., and NELSON, C. H. An experimental evaluation of the nutritional importance of proximal and distal small intestine. Ann. Surg., 140: 439, 1954.

KOLB, E. Kombination von oesophagus Atresie, duodenaler Stenose, Anus Atresie mit multicystischer Niere. Helv. Paediat. Acta, 18: 240, 1963.

LLOYD, J. R., and CLATWORTHY, H. W., Jr. Hydramnios as an aid to early diagnosis of congenital obstruction of the alimentary tract. A study of the maternal and fetal factors. Pediatrics, 21: 903, 1958.

LORAN, M. R., and CROCKER, T. T. Population dynamics of intestinal epithelia in the rat two months after partial resection of the ileum. J. Cell. Biol., 19: 285, 1963.

LOUW, J. H. Jejunoileal atresia and stenosis. J. Pediat. Surg., 1: 8, 1966.

——— Congenital intestinal atresia and stenosis in the newborn. Observations on its pathogenesis and treatment. Ann. Roy. Coll. Surg. Eng., 25: 209, 1959.

LOWREY, G. H., et al. Early diagnostic criteria of congenital hypothyroidism. A comprehensive study of forty-nine cretins. J. Dis. Child., 96: 131, 1958.

LUND, R. H. Recurrent small bowel volvulus in the newborn infant. J. Pediat., 57: 217, 1960.

MACMAHON, R. A. Massive resection of intestine in infancy. Aust. New Zeal. J. Surg., 35: 202, 1966.

MIKITY, V. G., HODGMAN, J. E., and PACIULLI, J. Meconium blockage syndrome. Radiology, 88: 740, 1967.

MOYA, F., APGAR, V., JAMES, L. S., and BERRIEN, C. Hydramnios and congenital anomalies. Study of a series of seventy-four patients. J.A.M.A., 173: 1552, 1960.

NIXON, H. H. Intestinal obstruction in the newborn. Arch. Dis. Child., 30: 13, 1955.

NYHAN, W. L., and FOUSEK, M. D. Septicemia of the newborn. Pediatrics, 22: 268, 1958.

PILLING, G. P., and CRESSON, S. L. Massive resection of the small intestine in the neonatal period. Report of two successful cases and review of the literature. Pediatrics, 19: 940, 1957.

POTTS, W. J. Pediatric Surgery. J.A.M.A., 157: 627, 1955.

PROUTY, M., BRUSKEWITZ, H. W., and SCHWEI, G. P. Intussusception in a newborn infant. J. Pediat., 34: 487, 1949.

RACHELSON, M. H., JERNIGAN, J. P., and

JACKSON, W. F. Intussusception in the newborn infant with spontaneous expulsion of the intussusceptum. J. Pediat., 47: 87, 1955.

RACK, F. J., and CROUCH, W. L. Functional intestinal obstruction in the premature newborn infant. J. Pediat., 40: 579, 1952.

REUL, G. J., and ELLISON, E. H. Effect of seventy-five percent distal small bowel resection on gastric secretion. Amer. J. Surg., 111: 772, 1966.

RICKMAN, P. P. Peritonitis in the neonatal period. Arch. Dis. Child., 30: 23, 1955.

ROBBIN, L. The length of the large and the small intestine in young children. Amer. J. Dis. Child., 19: 370, 1920.

SANTULLI, T. V. Intestinal obstruction in the newborn infant. J. Pediat., 44: 317, 1954.

SCHAFFER, A. J., and OPPENHEIMER, E. H. Pseudomonas (pyocyaneus) infection of the gastrointestinal tract of infants and children. Southern Med. J., 41: 460, 1948.

SHERRY, S. N., and KRAMER, I. The time of passage of the first stool and first urine by the newborn infant. J. Pediat., 46: 158, 1955.

SIEBER, W. K., and GIRDANY, B. R. Functional intestinal obstruction in newborn infants with morphologically normal gastrointestinal tracts. Surgery, 53: 357, 1963.

SMITH, B., and CLATWORTHY, H. W., Jr. Meconium peritonitis; Prognostic significance. Pediatrics, 27: 967, 1961.

STAHLGREN, L. H., UMANA, G., ROY, R., and DONNELLY, J. A study of intestinal absorption in dogs following massive small intestine resection and insertion of an antiperistaltic segment. Ann. Surg., 156: 483, 1962.

STRAUSS, J. Fluid and electrolyte composition of the fetus and the newborn. Pediat. Clin. N. Amer., 13: 1077, 1966.

THOMSON, J. The volume and acidity of the gastric contents in the unfed newborn infant. Arch. Dis. Child., 26: 558, 1951.

WEINSTEIN, L., and KLAINER, A. S. Management of emergencies: Septic shock-pathogenesis and treatment. New Eng. J. Med., 274: 950, 1966.

WILKINSON, A. W., HUGHES, E. A., and TOMS, D. A. Massive resection of the small intestine in infancy. Brit. J. Surg., 50: 715, 1963.

WILMORE, D. W., and DUDRICK, S. J. Growth and development of an infant receiving all nutrients exclusively by vein. J.A.M.A., 203: 860, 1968.

WINAWER, S. J., et al. Successful management of massive small-bowel resection based on assessment of absorption defects and nutritional needs. New Eng. J. Med., 274: 72, 1966.

ZACHARY, R. B. Meconium and fecal plugs in the newborn. Arch. Dis. Child., 32: 22, 1957.

ZURIER, R. B., CAMPBELL, R. G., HASHIM, S. A., and VAN ITALLIE, T. B. Use of medium-chain triglyceride in management of patients with massive resection of the small intestine. New Eng. J. Med., 274: 490, 1966.

35

Pyloric Stenosis and Other Lesions of the Stomach

HYPERTROPHIC PYLORIC STENOSIS

Congenital hypertrophic pyloric stenosis is the most common pathology requiring abdominal surgery during the first six months of life. The incidence of the lesion is given by various authors as 1 in 200 to 500 births. The most reliable studies are those by Wallgren (1946), and it is his opinion, based on the large group of normal neonates whom he examined radiographically, that the occurrence is about 1 in 200. Although the lesion may be detected this frequently by careful radiographic examination, some of these patients may well fail to have sufficient obstruction to require surgical relief.

The history of pyloric stenosis is fascinating. Blair (1717) describes what one can accept as being a case of pyloric stenosis. Osler called attention to the report of Beardsley (1788) describing the clinical course and postmortem examination of a patient with congenital hypertrophic pyloric stenosis. However, it was Hirschsprung in 1887 who described the condition and established the disease as a distinct clinical entity. It is interesting that in his writings no consideration of therapy was given. The treatment began with gastroenterostomy. At first, the Murphy button was used, but it proved unsuccessful. Later, various surgeons including Willie Meyer performed gastroenterostomies with sutures, which proved more successful. However, the mortality remained high, and other methods of treatment were explored. Loreta in 1887 described his experience, in three cases of pyloric obstruction, with dilation through a stomach incision. Nicoll in 1910 applied this method to infants and was fairly successful. Pyloroplasty was reported by Dent in 1904 utilizing the methods of Heineke and Mikulicz. Approximating the hypertrophied, thickened muscle with sutures proved virtually impossible. Fredet (1910) in Paris performed the pyloromyotomy without opening the mucosa and attempted to sew the musculature in the opposite direction. This proved fairly successful. However, in this publication he still felt that gastroenterostomy had a definite place in the treatment of this disease. Weber in 1910 reported operations on two children using essentially Fredet's technique. In 1912 Conrad Ramstedt (1912) reported the operation essentially as it is performed today—that is, the musculature was split and spread apart to permit the mucosa to bulge, and there was no attempt at suturing.

ETIOLOGY

So far investigation has failed to substantiate the etiology of this disease. The fact that it does occur with some familial association, appearing in more than one sibling and occasionally in both twins, raises the possibility of its being dependent upon a genetic factor. So far, such a relationship has not been established.

There have been studies that indicate that there might be a ganglionic defect in infants with pyloric stenosis. However, these findings have not been corroborated and consequently cannot be completely accepted. It would appear that studies of ganglion cells under these circumstances must be accepted with some caution because of the fact that there is considerable edema and compression, which may distort structures histologically and make the identification of cells more difficult. Furthermore, in the neonate the ganglion cells are immature and more difficult to identify than in a one-year-old child.

PATHOLOGY

Histological study of this lesion indicates hypertrophy and an increase in the number of circular fibers. Initially, there is no evidence of inflammation, but later there is some mucosal edema and round cell infiltration, and these changes may play a role in the onset or intensification of symptoms. Wollstein (1922) has studied the changes in the pylorus after pyloromyotomy. Healing takes place in the serosa and submucosa but not in the muscular layer, for they remain separated. At the point of pyloromyotomy, the wall consists of adjacent mucosa and peritoneum. There is a gradual softening and decrease in the size of the tumor, and in about two years it returns essentially to a normal pyloric consistency and thickness. It is interesting to note that this regression does not occur unless a pyloromyotomy has been performed, for in patients treated by gastro-enterostomy, where the pylorus is left undisturbed, persistence of the tumor was found 10 years or more postoperatively.

The time of onset of hypertrophy in the pylorus is variable; it has been found in newborn infants as well as in premature infants. The tumor may develop quite rapidly. Patients have been explored at birth for malrotation without having any appreciable hypertrophy of the pylorus noted. Ten days later, because of projectile vomiting and the palpation of a pyloric tumor, pyloromyotomy has been undertaken and a fully developed, thickened, typical lesion found. Radiographic studies with contrast material corroborated this observation.

DIAGNOSIS

In the baby with pyloric stenosis, there may be a history of its occurrence in other siblings. Families of four and five children have been reported where all have had this disease. In a number of families, the mother or father were treated for the disease in their infancy. Occasionally, the disease is encountered in the premature. Twins have been reported in whom the disease has occurred in both infants and in other instances in only one of the pair. In a series of 1,120 patients reported by Benson (1964), 36 infants were premature and there were 22 sets of twins. In this group 5 sets of twins all required pyloromyotomy. In the total series, eight fathers and six mothers had undergone surgery for pyloric stenosis in infancy. The preponderance of the disease in the male is well established and usually is given at the rate of 3 or 4 to 1. Another accepted dictum is that the disease has a tendency to occur in the first-born male; however, this is challenged to a certain extent by Lynn (1960), who found that only 28 percent of the cases in his series were in the first born.

Infants who develop this disease are usually normal at birth and have no gastrointestinal symptoms for a week or more. However, there is a definite group that has mild vomiting or at least spitting up from birth, and the size of this group is given as high as 15 percent in some reports. Usually, the onset of the vomiting is at a peak during the third week of life. The vomiting begins as regurgitation and becomes projectile. It is characteristic, being of such force that the vomitus is carried 2 to 3 feet from the infant. Invariably, the vomitus is not bile-stained. It may contain flecks of bright red blood and on occasion be coffee-ground in appearance. This is presumably caused by chronic gastritis, which may be associated with the disease.

Rarely, the bleeding may be of sufficient severity to require emergency transfusion.

Characteristically, these infants tend to be constipated, which is a definite change in their normal bowel pattern. They also tend to urinate smaller amounts and a more concentrated urine that is darker in color than the normal. In a small percentage of patients there will be an associated jaundice. This may reach the level of 18 to 20 mEq of bilirubin. Usually, exchange transfusion is not required. The cause of this associated jaundice, which disappears with correction of the pyloric obstruction, has not been established. Enlarged lymph nodes, angulation of the common duct because of the peculiar position of the pylorus, and edema with a malpositioned ampulla of Vater may be appreciable factors in the production of the jaundice, which is of the obstructive type.

The weight charts of these babies will first demonstrate failure to gain weight and then weight loss. Twenty-five to 30 years ago it was not unusual to have patients admitted to the hospital in emaciated condition from prolonged vomiting. Today, physicians are so aware of this condition that such neglected cases are practically nonexistent. The diagnosis is usually made promptly with a 7- to 10-day history of vomiting.

PHYSICAL FINDINGS

Two decades ago patients with this disease often came to surgery after considerable weight loss (Fig. 1). The average infant today with congenital hypertrophic pyloric stenosis is mildly to moderately dehydrated, and on observing the patient, particularly during feedings, there will be visible gastric waves, especially if there has been a perceptible weight loss. These peristaltic waves can be observed most consistently after feeding and before vomiting and emptying of the stomach has occurred. They originate in the left upper quadrant and progress to and beyond the midline. This finding is interesting but should not be taken as conclusive evidence of pyloric obstruction, for such waves may be observed in a number of conditions where the pylorus is essentially normal. This

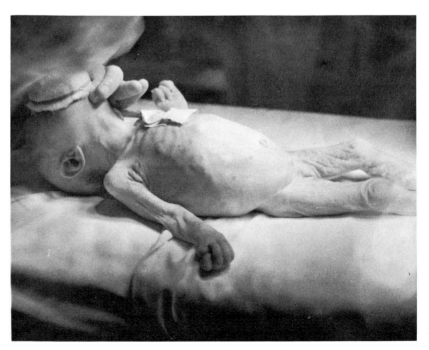

Fig. 1. Photograph of a baby seen some years ago. Note the evidence of weight loss. Infants with this degree of emaciation were common two decades ago. Today, they are virtually never seen.

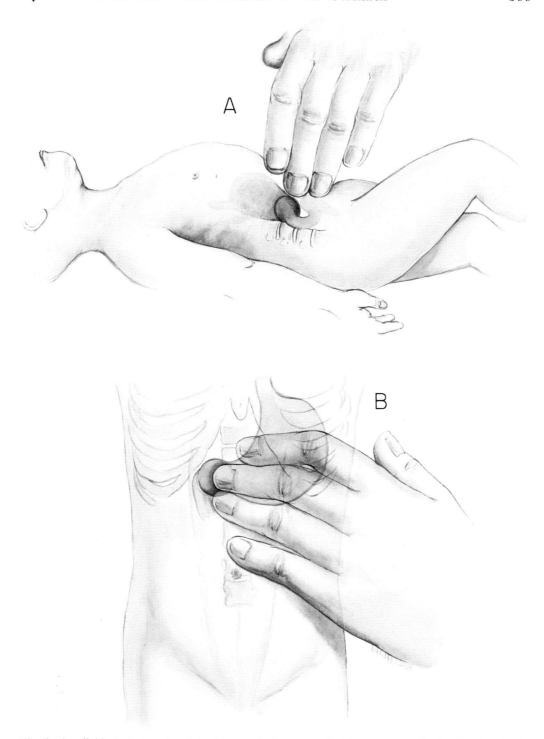

Fig. 2. A reliable technique for detecting a pyloric tumor. A. The tumor can be impinged upon the posterior abdominal wall by palpating directly downward through the abdominal wall. B. The examiner is using his left hand and detecting the tumor with the tips of his second, third, and fourth fingers.

is particularly true in some patients who vomit because of intracranial lesions.

The diagnosis can be established by palpation of the tumor in the epigastrium (Fig. 2). Depending on the experience of the examiner, from 70 to 90 percent of the patients will be found to exhibit this tumor. The mass is unique in that it is practically impossible for any normal organ or other pathological condition to be mistaken for it. It is oblong, smooth, and hard, being 1 to 2 cm in size and located in the epigastrium slightly to the right of the midline. An essential prerequisite for successful palpation of the tumor is the realization that a period of examination lasting 10 to 15 minutes is often required to detect the tumor. These infants are tense, and a feeding or a sugar nipple may induce sufficient abdominal relaxation for an adequate examination. Inability to detect a tumor may be due to the presence of an overdistended stomach that fills the epigastrium and protects the tumor from the examiner's fingers. Ideally, the best opportunity to detect the mass occurs immediately following vomiting, when the stomach is empty. On occasion it may be necessary to empty the stomach by inserting a fairly large gastric tube, deflating the stomach and thus giving favorable conditions for palpation of the tumor. Failure to detect the tumor may be the result of faulty technique. It is customary to examine the baby from his right side, pushing downward and upward with the index and middle fingers lateral to the rectus muscle in the right upper quadrant. While the tumor can frequently be detected by this technique, failure to find it may be due to the tumor being pushed upward against the soft abdominal structure and thus escaping detection. The tumor's being pushed out of the way can be prevented by palpating down through the rectus muscle so that the hypertrophied pylorus is engaged between the examiner's fingers and the firm posterior abdominal wall. Some find it more convenient to conduct the examination from the patient's left side and to place the left hand on the abdomen so that the second,

third, and fourth fingers are to the right of the midline above the umbilicus. The palm and proximal portions of the finger push the rectus muscles downward, leaving the tips of the fingers free to detect the tumor. It is surprising how superficial the tumor may be in some instances. Therefore, the examiner should exert a minimal amount of pressure initially to insure against failure to detect the superficial tumor. However, most frequently the tumor is deep, and with steady increase in pressure the baby will relax and permit the deep palpation necessary to outline the tumor. When the hard, oblong, rounded object is detected with the fingertips, it can be rolled under the fingers and a positive identification of a pyloric tumor made. It is essential to identify the tumor on at least two separate examinations before committing the patient to operation. Provided that this dictum is followed the surgeon should never be in the embarrassing position of exploring an infant and exposing a normal pylorus.

In the small percentage of infants with this disease in whom the tumor is not palpable, roentgenographic examination is required for diagnosis. It should be appreciated that this is a difficult examination, and mistakes

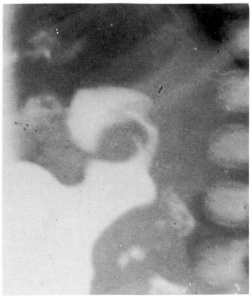

Fig. 3. Roentgenogram depicting the elongated narrow canal which is pathognomonic of congenital pyloric stenosis.

can be made, particularly if the radiologist is unfamiliar with the condition (Fig. 3). A thin mixture of barium is used to facilitate the outlining of the narrow pyloric canal. The esophagus should be studied to exclude strictures or chalasia. In pyloric stenosis the canal is narrowed and elongated, and this is the most important finding in establishing the diagnosis. It may be difficult at times to have sufficient barium in the canal to outline it on the fluoroscopic screen or on spot films. As the barium enters the duodenum, the cervix-like protrusion into the duodenum may be outlined, and this is a second observation that is a dependable aid in establishing the diagnosis. Retention of barium in the stomach is not of diagnostic value, for it occurs in many normal infants. Obviously, rapid gastric emptying excludes the diagnosis.

DIFFERENTIAL DIAGNOSIS

Chalasia or persistent cardioesophageal relaxation may stimulate pyloric stenosis, for it occurs in the same age group. Vomiting is a predominant feature of chalasia, and weight loss may occur. By a careful study of the esophagus and the stomach, the diagnosis of chalasia can be definitely excluded. Vomiting may be the initial symptom in a host of conditions, and the absence of a pyloric tumor or negative roentgenograms will differentiate these conditions from pyloric stenosis. Intracranial hemorrhages or other central nervous system lesions may produce projectile vomiting. In patients without a pyloric tumor and with a negative roentgen examination, lumbar puncture or subdural taps may clarify the problem. Occasionally, an unexpected renal lesion producing an elevated blood urea nitrogen may be the cause of vomiting, and, therefore, in obscure cases it is important to have a blood urea nitrogen determination to exclude renal damage as the cause of vomiting. Infants with duodenal obstruction generally vomit bile-stained material, and this symptom separates them from patients with pyloric stenosis.

Recently, pyloric obstructions caused by mucosal diaphragms have been reported, and these have been classified by some authors as pyloric atresia. In such patients the diagnosis should be established by roentgen examination, and obviously a probable tumor is not present. As these occur in newborns, it is additional warning to the physician that the diagnosis of hypertrophic pyloric stenosis is unlikely.

In a recent paper 17 newborns with pyloric atresia were found in the literature, with 12 survivors.

PREOPERATIVE PREPARATION

Today, the problem of preparing these patients for operation is less complicated than previously. Approximately one third enter the hospital with mild dehydration, which can be corrected without resorting to parenteral fluids. In these patients there is still a lumen, and, although curds will not pass through, clear liquids usually are retained. The oral feedings are usually equal mixtures of 5 percent dextrose and water and normal saline. Other regimes alternate feedings, one glucose and water and the other normal saline. Provided that these are given in reasonable volumes of 2 to 3 ounces at intervals of 2 to 3 hours, they are usually retained, and they support the patient's hydration and correct whatever dehydration is present.

In these patients with mild dehydration, there are minor derangements of electrolytes, with slight depressions of chlorides and a tendency for an elevated CO_2, indicating some alkalosis. In the more severely dehydrated patients there may be profound alterations in the electrolyte pattern, with moderate to severe alkalosis. The dehydrated patients with varying degrees of alkalosis can be treated intelligently only after blood determinations of serum carbon dioxide, and chlorides, sodium, and potassium are made. While these analyses are being made by the laboratory, intravenous hydration is started with a solution composed of equal parts of 5 percent glucose and normal saline. Usually the alkalosis and depressed chlorides can

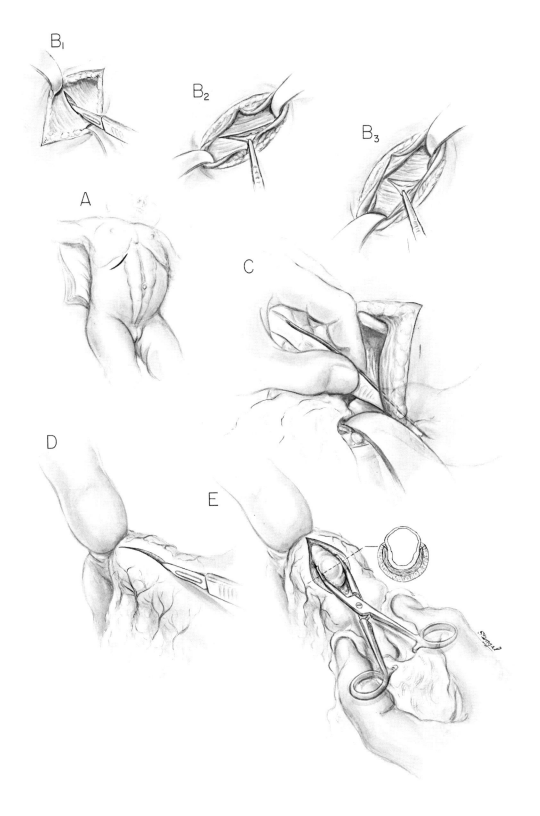

be treated successfully with saline. In the past there has been some question about the need for substances other than sodium chloride, particularly if the blood sodium becomes elevated. In such situations, calcium chloride or ammonium chloride have been recommended. The need for this is indeed rare; in such situations hypokalemic alkalosis should be searched for, and this will often prove to be the cause of the resistant alkalosis. Patients with a satisfactory urinary output may be given potassium chloride with salutary results. Resistant alkalosis in these situations will rapidly disappear, and normal electrolytes will be achieved in 24 hours. It should be stressed that pyloromyotomy is not an emergency operation, and it is advisable to completely correct the electrolyte imbalance before embarking upon surgery. This can invariably be accomplished in two or three days, and delay of this magnitude is acceptable in the treatment of this condition. On the rare occasion when the patient has been vomiting coffee-ground material, a significant anemia may be present and may require blood transfusion prior to operation. In severely dehydrated and emaciated patients, measurements of blood volume may be helpful in encouraging adequate replacement with blood and plasma before undertaking operation.

TREATMENT

There still persists in some parts of Europe a tendency to treat these patients without operation. This program consists of refeeding after each vomiting. This form of therapy requires hospitalization for weeks and maintains the baby in poor nutritional condition during an essential growth and development period. Furthermore, the mortality is higher than for surgical therapy and consequently should be abandoned. Several decades ago local anesthesia was used to accomplish pyloromyotomy. There may be an occasional extremely ill patient who requires operation under local anesthesia. However, some authorities contend that all patients should be subjected to general anesthesia. Aspiration during induction of anesthesia can be reduced by inserting a gastric tube and permitting it to drain the stomach as completely as possible before the anesthetic is administered. Deflating the distended stomach has the additional advantage of making induction more rapid by permitting complete diaphragmatic excursion. Furthermore, the operation is facilitated by making the pylorus easier to deliver and by minimizing gastric regurgitation during operative manipulation of the stomach.

OPERATION

When surgical treatment of pyloric stenosis was first attempted, gastroenterostomy was the operation performed. The high mortality rate prompted surgeons to consider other methods. A pyloroplasty was proposed, with transverse suturing of the longitudinal pyloric incision. This was found to be virtually impossible because of the thickened pyloric musculature. Consequently, the incision through the pyloric musculature was left open, with results far superior to procedures such as gastroenterostomy.

The Ramstedt pyloromyotomy is now universally used. To prevent evisceration and to permit early discharge of the patient, a grid-

Fig. 4 (opposite page). Ramstedt pyloromyotomy. A. The drawing indicates the position of the incision 1 to 2 cm below the costal margin and lateral to the rectus muscle. B_1. Opening the external oblique musculature in the course of its fibers. B_2. The internal oblique fibers are divided. B_3. The transversalis, transversalis fascia, and peritoneum are opened as one layer. C. With the use of retractors, the liver is pulled upward out of the way. The intestines are packed away inferiorly. A smooth forcep is inserted through the wound to grasp the dilated stomach. D. The index finger is placed against the duodenal end of the tumor. The incision through the serosa is made with a scalpel, only the serosa being opened at the abdominal end. The incision may be deeper as the gastric side of the tumor is approached. E. With the use of small curved clamps or special clamps, the musculature is pried apart until the mucosa balloons up to the level of or above the pyloric musculature. Care is taken to open the duodenal end of the pylorus musculature completely.

iron incision in the right upper quadrant was recommended by Robertson (1940). It is a matter of historical interest that when extremely emaciated patients were treated evisceration was the commonest cause of postoperative deaths. This led to the development of the gridiron incision some decades ago. A transverse incision over the right rectus muscle and division of the anterior rectus fascia vertically, splitting the muscles vertically and dividing the posterior fascia and peritoneum in a transverse plane, is acceptable. We have found that the gridiron incision heals more kindly, and consequently this is our choice.

The incision is placed parallel to and 1 to 2 cm below the right costal margin (Fig. 4). The incision must be well lateral, so that the rectus muscle is avoided. The external oblique fibers are separated as they extend laterally and upward. The internal oblique fibers, which extend obliquely downward and laterally, are then divided along one of the white lines to avoid bleeding. The transversalis and peritoneum are divided as one layer in the transverse plane. A small hook retractor is used at the medial angle of the incision. Two narrow ribbon retractors are used, one to hold the liver upward and the other to hold the intestine downward. The antrum of the stomach can then usually be visualized, grasped with smooth forceps, and partially delivered through the incision. The antrum is then grasped between the fingers, gauze being used to prevent slipping, and the pyloric tumor is delivered by traction. This maneuver is preferable to grasping the tumor directly with some type of forcep. A recent suggestion has been made to inflate the stomach with air at this point to make it more accessible.

After the tumor is delivered, the operator places his left index finger against the duodenal end of the tumor. An incision is made through the serosa along the anterior superior avascular portion of the pylorus. At the duodenal end, this incision must be through the serosa only; in the midportion of the tumor, it is convenient and safe to make the incision deeper. A hemostat can be inserted in the midportion of the incision and spread, splitting the pyloric musculature. The tumor edges are spread apart, first at the antral end, then toward the duodenal end until the mucosa is freed and bulges to the serosal surface of the pylorus, filling the space between the separated musculature. It is important to make sure that the muscle fibers of the pylorus are completely separated at the duodenal end of the tumor and to avoid

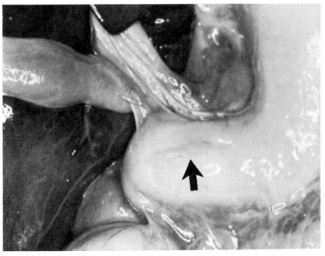

Fig. 5. Photograph of a pylorus three months after pyloromyotomy. Note how smoothly the peritoneum has healed over the defect (arrow). There is no musculature in the defect, the mucosa being adjacent to the peritoneal surface. There were no adhesions. This child died of an acute infection.

perforating the mucosa at this point where the duodenal mucosa folds over the tumor for 2 or 3 mm on account of the cervix-like projection of the tumor into the duodenal lumen. The fibers are carefully separated at the duodenal end, spreading with the fine pointed hemostat. A satisfactory separation at the duodenal end is achieved when the pyloric ring of muscles is entirely broken. This is determined by palpating the duodenal edge of the tumor. An opening in the duodenal mucosa may be detected if the area is carefully wiped with gauze and the sponge observed for bile staining. Usually, the perforations are obvious, for the mucosa tends to become everted and form a rounded protrusion. If a perforation is found, the mucosa can be closed with two or three interrupted 5-0 chromic catgut sutures. As an additional precaution, omenum should be tacked over the area. Such infants should be maintained on gastric suction for 48 hours after operation. No further precautions are necessary.

The pylorus and stomach are then returned to the abdominal cavity. Attempts to control bleeding from the pyloric incision are unnecessary. Most of the bleeding is the result of venous engorgement, as the stomach and pylorus are held outside the abdomen through a small incision. Once they are returned to normal position, the bleeding becomes insignificant.

The abdominal incision is closed with interrupted 5-0 silk sutures to the peritoneum, internal and external oblique, and subcutaneous tissue. The skin is approximated with a continuous 5-0 plain catgut subcuticular suture and painted with collodion (Fig. 5).

The gastric tube is removed, and 1 ounce of 5 percent glucose water is offered 4 hours after operation and repeated at 2-hour intervals. If this mixture is retained for six feedings, an ounce of diluted evaporated milk formula is given at 2-hour intervals. If six feedings of this milk are retained, the infant is gradually changed to a full formula over a 36-hour period.

Regurgitation is expected in 50 percent of the babies and is not an indication for altera-tion of the feeding schedule. If the baby vomits a large amount, oral feedings are discontinued for 12 hours, and parenteral fluids are supplied. Following this period, the same regimen used immediately after operation is started. The babies are discharged as soon as they are taking and retaining an adequate formula, which usually is three to five days after the operation.

If the pyloromyotomy has not been complete, the baby will have persistent vomiting. Reoperation should be delayed for four to six days to make sure the persistent vomiting is not the result of edema. Furthermore, the status of the pyloric canal should be investigated through barium contrast studies before reoperation. We have never actually observed such a patient, and we base our statement on reported cases. In a series of over 100 infants, there has been no postoperative mortality.

DUPLICATION OF THE STOMACH AND DUODENUM

Although the most common location of duplication in the intestinal tract is in the terminal ileum, this malformation also occurs both in the duodenum and stomach. Usually, the gastric duplications are without symptoms and are detected on abdominal examination or during radiographic gastrointestinal studies (Fig. 6). Tumor masses are usually oblong, firm, smooth, and movable. The duplications are usually smaller and not movable, as they are partially retroperitoneal. They occur most commonly on the pancreatic side of the duodenum. Furthermore, the duodenal duplications may encroach on the adjacent intestinal lumen and produce varying degrees of obstruction. While the outline of a smooth-feeling mass in the stomach may suggest the diagnosis of a gastric duplication, in the duodenum a duplication can hardly be differentiated from other lesions producing obstruction.

The treatment of a duplication depends upon its location. If a gastric duplication is

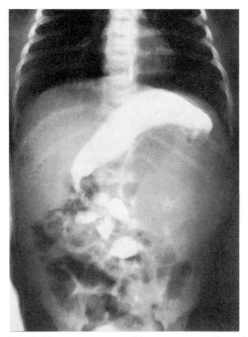

Fig. 6. Roentgenogram with contrast medium in stomach. The normal gastric outline is distorted by a space-filling mass which proved to be gastric duplication. (Courtesy of Dr. William K. Sieber.)

located along the greater curvature of the stomach, no obstruction is produced. In this situation, partial excision of the diaphragm between the two structures is possible. The presence of acid-producing mucosa is of no consequence in this location and will not result in the complications that can occur when gastric mucosa is left in place in other parts of the intestinal tract.

The incision through which the diaphragm is excised preferably is made through the duplication. The diaphragm should then be opened and excised so that the two lumens are converted into one large, smooth cavity. As the blood supply is abundant, the trimmed edge should be carefully sewed over with a continuous chromic catgut suture to minimize blood loss in the postoperative period. The opening is closed with a continuous Connell suture of 4-0 chromic catgut and reinforced with interrupted Halsted sutures of 5-0 silk.

In the pylorus or duodenum a duplication may produce some obstruction. The anatomic arrangement of duplications is such that there is a blood supply that also supplies the adjacent gastrointestinal segment. Therefore, resections of duplications are usually not feasible without resecting the contiguous segment of the gastrointestinal tract. Such a resection of a duplication is possible in the pyloric end of the stomach by utilizing the routine subtotal gastrectomy technique. Resection of the duodenal duplication is unwise when the adjacent duodenum contains the ampulla of Vater, for removing the adjacent duodenum may damage the common and pancreatic ducts. Rather than risk trauma to these important structures, the safer procedure of opening the diaphragm between the two structures is preferable. The duodenal incision should be made longitudinally and closed transversely with a Connell suture of 4-0 chromic catgut, reinforced with interrupted 5-0 silk Halsted sutures as a safeguard against producing any obstruction.

This procedure has the theoretical disadvantage of leaving gastric mucosa in the duodenum. However, since the duodenal contents are alkaline, any acid secretion should be readily neutralized and ulceration thus prevented.

Postoperatively these patients should be on gastric tube suction until peristalsis has returned, usually in 24 hours or less. The tube can then be removed and fluid in small amounts given orally. If this fluid is tolerated, nourishing liquids can be added, and a diet appropriate to the age of the patient can be ordered 24 hours after nourishing fluids are started. The patients are allowed out of bed as soon as gastric suction is dispensed with and are discharged six or seven days after operation, provided that there are no complications.

FOREIGN BODIES IN THE STOMACH AND DUODENUM

Most ingested foreign bodies will pass quickly through the stomach. However, some will require several days to pass through the pylorus. When a foreign body is not recovered in the stool 78 hours after being

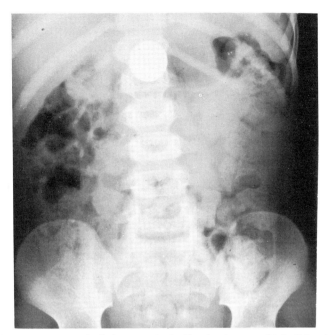

Fig. 7. Abdominal roentgenogram depicting a coin in the duodenum which did not move beyond this position. Operation demonstrated duodenal bands partially obstructing the duodenum.

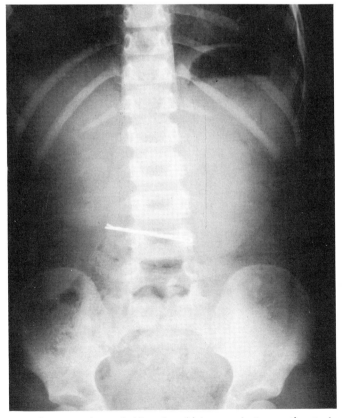

Fig. 8. Roentgenogram demonstrating a bobby pin which proved at operation to be in the duodenum proximal to the ligament of Treitz.

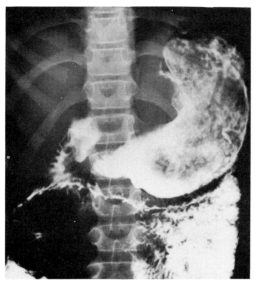

Fig. 9. Roentgenogram with contrast material in the stomach outlining a trichobezoar in the stomach.

ingested, roentgenograms are advisable to determine the position of the foreign body. If abdominal films do not locate it, a chest film is advisable to determine whether it is in the esophagus. Once a foreign body has entered the stomach, passage is practically assured

through the rest of the intestine unless there is a congenital stenosis that blocks the foreign body (Fig. 7). The object that most commonly fails to pass through the intestinal tract is a bobby pin, which is likely to become lodged in the duodenum proximal to the ligament of Treitz (Fig. 8). As long as the foreign body remains in the stomach, it can move about, and there is no danger of perforation of the stomach wall. When a foreign body is not recovered in the stool and when a roentgenogram shows the object in the upper abdomen, repeat films should be made once or twice a week. If two films prove that the foreign body has remained in the same position, surgical removal is indicated. When a long foreign body is in a transverse position, overlying the vertebral bodies with one end to the left and pointing slightly cephalad, the object is probably in the fourth part of the duodenum and is unable to negotiate the sharp turn into the jejunum. As the duodenum is a retroperitoneal structure, its wall is relatively fixed. Thus, the wall cannot escape from the pressure of a foreign body, and perforation can occur. The use of powerful small magnets that can be passed into the

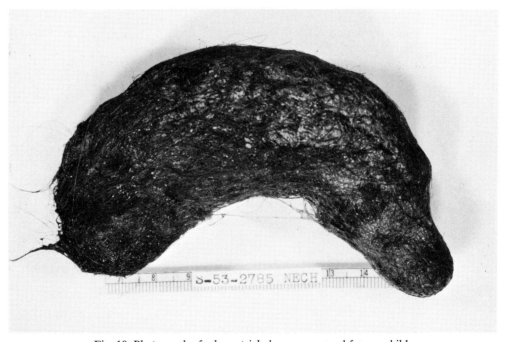

Fig. 10. Photograph of a large trichobezoar removed from a child.

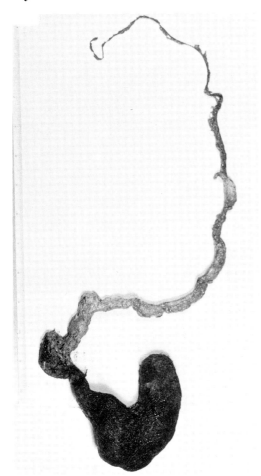

Fig. 11. A trichobezoar with a long projection which extended into the small intestine.

toneal abscess develops that is best drained through a kidney incision. The abscess will be found to contain the foreign body, and it should be located and removed. A duodenal fistula does not persist. Once a foreign body has passed through the duodenum, a swift journey through the remainder of the intestinal tract is assured. Occasionally, an open safety pin or a sharply pointed object may lodge in the rectum and require digital removal.

TRICHOBEZOAR

It is rare to encounter a stomach hairball in children, yet some seemingly normal children develop a habit of eating hair. If sufficient hair is ingested to collect in the stomach, the children give a history of actually cutting their own hair and ingesting it. Trichobezoar, which is a collection of hair

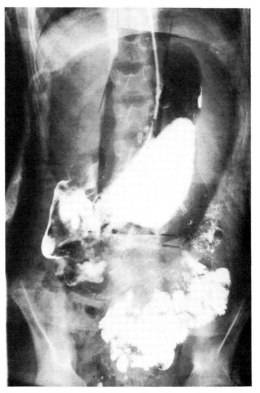

Fig. 12. Abdominal film of patient with massive gastric dilation. The situation was not corrected until the cast was removed.

stomach may be tried as a method of removing appropriate metal objects from the stomach. This technique is particularly useful in removing bobby pins.

Removal should be performed through a right rectus muscle-retracting incision. The second portion of the duodenum is opened, a clamp inserted into the duodenum, and the foreign body removed. If the foreign body is pushed into the jejunum, a second small opening may be required for its removal. The duodenal incision should be closed transversely with a Connell suture of 5-0 chromic catgut reinforced with an interrupted 6-0 silk Halsted suture. When perforation of the duodenum occurs, there may be a transient peritoneal irritation, and a retroperi-

A

B

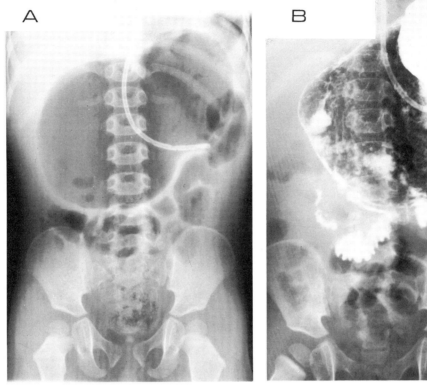

Fig. 13. A. Abdominal film outlining gastric dilation. B. Contrast material established the diagnosis of volvulus of the stomach.

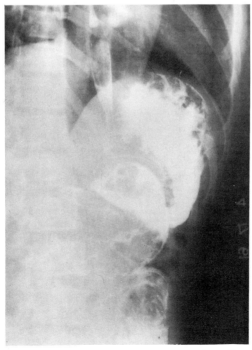

Fig. 14. Contrast material in the stomach outlines chronic gastritis.

and vegetable fibers, on abdominal palpation is an oblong mass firm in consistency and conforming to the gastric outline. There may be secondary masses in the duodenum, and even in the jejunum, anchored by strands of hair to the gastric hairball.

The symptom is failure to gain weight or actual weight loss. Although the appetite is poor, the children appear well, and there is usually no significant vomiting. The diagnosis may be suspected on palpation of a large oblong mass conforming to the stomach outline. Smaller bezoars may be diagnosed when a gastrointestinal series is made in an attempt to determine the cause of weight loss or for identification of an epigastric mass (Fig. 9). During the fluoroscopic examinations, careful observations of the duodenum and jejunum should be made to determine whether secondary masses are present.

Removal of a trichobezoar is simple and can be performed through a left rectus mus-

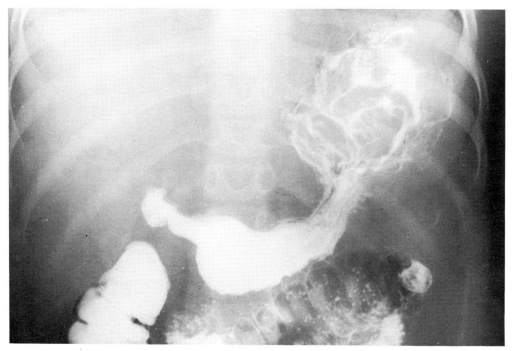

Fig. 15. Barium in the stomach makes identification of the large embryonal sarcoma of the stomach possible.

cle-retracting incision. The operative field is carefully isolated with several saline-moistened packs, and a generous opening is made in the stomach. The hairball may then be grasped and easily removed unless there are secondary collections in the duodenum and in the jejunum (Fig. 10). In such situations, secondary openings into the duodenum or jejunum may be required. The incisions should be closed transversely with a Connell suture of 5-0 chromic catgut and a second layer of interrupted 6-0 silk Halsted sutures (Fig. 11). Gastric suction is necessary only until peristalsis returns. When the tube is removed, oral feedings are given, and a full diet is usually tolerated 36 to 48 hours after operation.

It is advisable that the parents be warned about the child's habit of swallowing hair. If the parents are on guard, recurrence is rare. When such warning is not sufficient, the children should be seen by child-guidance pediatricians for a study of the possible cause of the hair-eating habit.

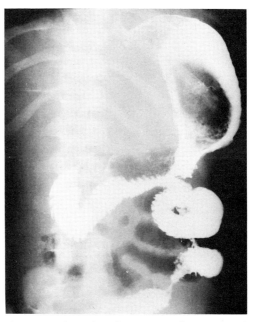

Fig. 16. A large lymphosarcoma of the stomach outlined by the barium.

GASTRIC DILATION

Acute gastric dilation is not uncommon and may take place in the postoperative period. A severe form has been reported in patients in casts, particularly following spinal fusion; it has been referred to as the cast syndrome and may be the cause of death unless promptly treated. The diagnosis is established with roentgenograms. Gastric aspiration should be attempted. When this fails, the only effective treatment is to remove the cast (Fig. 12).

VOLVULUS OF THE STOMACH

Volvulus of the stomach is a rare condition that may be confused with acute gastric dilation. When the dilation persists after tube decompression has been accomplished, this rare entity should be considered. The diagnosis is established by barium studies and by exploration (Fig. 13).

HYPERTROPHIC GASTRITIS

We have seen three patients with hypertrophic gastritis and with massive gastric bleeding. The diagnosis can be established with contrast material in the stomach (Fig. 14). The lesion was so extensive in one patient that a total resection was required to remove the lesion. In the second patient a nine-tenths resection of the stomach was required. Both children, who were in their early teens, maintained normal nutrition with no further bleeding episodes. No etiological factors could be elicited in these patients.

TUMORS OF THE STOMACH

Adenomas have been reported, some becoming considerable in size. One patient has been seen at The Children's Memorial Hospital with an embryonal sarcoma of the stomach (Fig. 15).

LYMPHOSARCOMA

Lymphosarcomas are rare (Fig. 16). The symptoms are general, with loss of weight and some abdominal pain. There is usually some bleeding from these lesions, which contributes to an anemia that is not unusual in these patients. The stools tend to be guaiac positive. Resections with postoperative radiation may be curative.

The treatment may be supplemented with Cytoxan, with some prolongation of life.

ORVAR SWENSON

REFERENCES

ARIAS, I., SCHORR, J. B., and FRAAD, L. M. Clinical conference—congenital hypertrophic pyloric stenosis with jaundice. Pediatrics, 24: No. 2, 1959.

BEARDSLEY, H. Congenital pyloric stenosis of the pylorus. *In* Cases and Observations by the Medical Society of New Haven. New Haven, 1788, F. Meigs, pp. 81.

BENSON, C. D., and ALPERN, E. B. Pre-operative and post-operative cases of congenital pyloric stenosis. Arch. Surg., 75: 877, 1957.

BENSON, C. D., and LLOYD, J. R. Infantile pyloric stenosis (a review of 1,120 cases), Amer. J. Surg., 107: 429, 1964.

BILL, A. H., Jr., HOFFMAN, H. C., and SKINNER, A. L. The use of a transverse incision over the liver and of pre-operative potassium in the case of hypertrophic pyloric stenosis. Amer. J. Surg., 106: 511, 1963.

BLAIR, P. An account of the dissection of a child, communicated in a letter to Doctor Brook Taylor, R.S. Secr. Philosophical Transactions, 30: 631, 1717.

BURMEISTER, Lt. R. E., and HAMILTON, H. B. Infantile hypertrophic pyloric stenosis in four siblings. Amer. J. Dis. Child., 108: 617, 1964.

DENT, C. On congenital hypertrophic stenosis of the pylorus. Brit. J. Child. Dis., 1: 16, 1904.

DINEEN, J. P., and REDO, F. S. Pyloric obstruction due to mucosal diaphragm. Surgery, 53: No. 5, 674, 1963.

FORBES, G. B., and ERGANIAN, J. A. Parenteral administration of ammonium chloride for alkalosis of congenital hypertrophic pyloric stenosis. Amer. J. Dis. Child., 72: 649, 1946.

FREDET, P., and GUILLEMOT, L. La stenose du pylore par hypertrophie musculaire chez les hourissons. Ann. Gynec. Obstet., 67: 604, 1910.

GAILEY, A. A. H. Congenital hypertrophic pyloric stenosis. Brit. Med. J., 1: 100, 1948.

GELLIS, S. S., ed. In Year Book of Pediatrics, 1956–1957. Chicago, Year Book Publishers, Inc., 1956, p. 198.

LONGINO, L. A., HENDREN, W. H., III, and OWINGS, R. S. Congenital hypertrophic pyloric stenosis. Amer. J. Surg., 101: No. 5, 605, 1961.

LYNN, H. B. The mechanism of pyloric stenosis and its relationship to the pre-operative preparation. Arch. Surg., 81: 453, 1960.

MARTIN, J. W., and SIEBENTHAL, B. J. Jaundice due to hypertrophic pyloric stenosis. J. Pediat., 47: 95, 1955.

MEEKER, C. S., and DeNICOLA, R. R. Hypertrophic pyloric stenosis in a newborn infant. J. Pediat., 33: 94, 1948.

METRAKOS, J. D. Congenital hypertrophic pyloric stenosis in twins. Arch. Dis. Child., 28: 351, 1953.

NICOLL, J. Congenital hypertrophic stenosis of the pylorus with special reference to its treatment. Practitioner, 85: 659, 1910.

OLNICK, H. M., and WEENS, H. S. Roentgen manifestations of infantile hypertrophic pyloric stenosis. J. Pediat., 34: 720, 1949.

RAMSTEDT, C. Zur Operation der angeborenen Pylorusstenose. Med. Klin., 8: 1702, 1912.

RAVITCH, M. M. The story of pyloric stenosis. Surgery, 48: No. 6, 1117, 1960.

RHEA, W. G., Jr., HEADRICK, J. R., and STEPHENSON, S. E., Jr. Hypertrophic pyloric stenosis with jaundice. Surgery, 51: 687, 1962.

RHEINLANDER, H. F., and SWENSON, O. The diagnosis and management of congenital hypertrophic pyloric stenosis. J. Pediat., 41: 314, 1952.

ROBERTSON, D. E. Congenital pyloric stenosis. Ann. Surg., 112: 687, 1940.

SCHUSTER, S. R., and COLODNY, A. H. A useful maneuver to simplify pyloromyotomy for hypertrophic pyloric stenosis. Surgery, 55: No. 5, 735, 1964.

SCHWARTS, D. R., and WIRKA, H. W. (Ten second abstracts.) Brief statements of the author's views or conclusions. J. Bone Jt. Surg., 46-A: 1549, 1964.

SLIM, M. S., BITAR, J. G., and IDRISS, H. Hypertrophy of the pyloric mucosa: A rare case of congenital pyloric obstruction. Amer. J. Dis. Child., 107: 636, 1964

WALLGREN, A. Preclinical stage of infantile hypertrophic pyloric stenosis. Amer. J. Dis. Child., 72: 371, 1946.

WEBER, W. Ueber einen Technische neuerung bei der Operation der pylorus Stenose des Säuglings. Berlin Klin. Wschr., 47: 763, 1910.

WOLLSTEIN, M. Healing of hypertrophic stenosis after Fredet-Ramstedt operation. Amer. J. Dis. Child., 23: 510, 1922.

36

Malrotation and Other Lesions of the Duodenum

Malrotation is a common cause of duodenal obstruction in the neonate and infant. The symptomatology and operative correction of this failure of rotation is best appreciated when there is a complete understanding of the arrested embryological process which produces this clinical entity. Because of the high instance of volvulus associated with malrotation in the neonate, there is urgency in the detection and treatment of this malformation in order to prevent deaths from gangrene of the bowel and to prevent having survivors with precarious nutrition because of deficient intestinal length. Ladd (1932) was one of the first to appreciate the true nature of this malformation and its relation to the symptoms of duodenal obstruction. He proposed the form of therapy which is widely used today. In England Dott (1923) made similar studies and came to conclusions that did not vary greatly from those of Ladd.

EMBRYOLOGY

A great deal of work has been done to elucidate the change of position of the intestinal tract during embryological development. Mall (1898), Frazer and Robbins (1915), and Snyder and Chaffin (1954) have contributed to the understanding of the normal embryological steps in the positioning of the small and large intestine. Snyder and Chaffin have divided the process into two steps. They first traced the movement of the duodenojejunal segment and then that of the cecocolic loop. Prior to their work attention was centered on the movement of the cecum and large intestine. While this latter study has prior interest to the surgeon, understanding of the movement of the jejunum and duodenum is essential for full appreciation of what occurs during the process in which the intestine reaches its normal position. In the 5-mm embryo, or about the fourth week, the intestinal tract is represented by a straight line structure. It starts to elongate and forms a forward loop that begins to prolapse into yolk stalk or umbilical cord. The mesenteric artery arises from a midpoint in the abdominal cavity to maintain the intestinal blood supply. The midgut is considered to be the duodenum, jejunum, and ileum, and the colon to its midtransverse portion. The hindgut is the colon beyond the midpoint of the transverse large intestine. Understanding of the process of rotation can be aided by a visual demonstration with a simple piece of apparatus. Snyder and Chaffin have suggested that one have a loop of cord attached at both ends to a board and a red wire to the middle of this loop fastened to the board at a midpoint between the ends of the cord loop. With this apparatus steps in the rotation can be dynamically observed. The initial position of this loop is comparable to the situation of the intestine in the 5-mm embryo which is in about the fourth week of embryonic life. In the fifth week, in which there is about a 10-mm embryo, the developing right liver and left umbilical vein have served to push down and to the right the duodeno-jejunal loop. One can demonstrate this in the simple apparatus by pushing the upper part of the loop downward and to the right. At the end of this stage the duodenojejunal segment is to the right of the mesenteric artery. In the 25- or 30-mm embryo, this rotation of the duodenojejunal loop has progressed and the duodenum has migrated to beneath or inferior to the mesenteric artery. Thus at the end of the first stage of rotation as outlined by Frazer and Robbins, the duodeno-jejunal loop lies caudal to the artery. The duodenojejunal loop rotation is completed with the duodenum becoming attached to the left of the artery, thus completing a rotation of the upper limb of the midgut to about 270 degrees in a counterclockwise direction. At this stage, there is a return of intestine to the abdominal cavity. However, some remains within the cord.

In order to complete the understanding of the embryological process of rotation, it is now well to consider what happens to the distal loop, the cecocecal portion. This part remains within the cord for a longer period than the proximal intestine. In the 10-mm embryo the cecocolic loop has moved to a position from beneath the mesenteric artery to the left side of the artery, thus completing 90 degrees of counterclockwise rotation. This relationship of the loop to the artery remains the same until the embryo is about 35 or 40 mm in length. The cecocolic loop then returns to the abdominal cavity and begins migrating above the artery in a counterclockwise movement. The cecum now assumes a position of about 180 degrees from the initial position inferior to the mesenteric artery. It is arrestive development in this position that is the commonest finding in malrotation. The completion of the process is visualized by having the cecum descend and become attached in the right lower quadrant.

An important additional step to complete the normal process consists of attachment of mesentery over a wide segment of the posterior abdominal wall. This extends as a line from the upper quadrant beyond the ligament of Treitz to the cecum in the right lower quadrant. This broad mesenteric attachment is a normal deterrent to volvulus of the midgut. It is understandable in incomplete rotation with the cecum fixed in the left upper quadrant that this final embryological development fails to take place, and that consequently the mesenteric attachment to the posterior abdominal wall is limited to the superior mesenteric artery. This limited attachment forms a small pedicle about which volvulus can readily take place.

After reviewing the series of events that finalizes the position of the intestine within the abdominal cavity one can understand that while there is the common form of malrotation most frequently encountered, there may be all variations of arrest. This fact accounts for the variety of anatomical findings encountered during the surgical treatment of duodenal obstruction and volvulus of the midgut. Unless the surgeon is completely conversant with all aspects of rotation, he will fail to appreciate this important point; unless he finds the classic situation of malrotation, he may fail to recognize that variations of anatomical findings are not uncommon and should be recognized, for they also produce symptomatology.

PATHOLOGY

The classic malrotation described by Ladd had the cecum attached in the right upper quadrant, with inevitable bands across the duodenum, which produced obstruction. While these bands may be tight enough with malrotation to produce duodenal obstruction, in other situations the obstruction is not of sufficient severity to produce symptoms unless there is volvulus of the midgut which pulls the cecum tightly toward the midline and accentuates the obstruction across the duodenum. The variation of anatomical findings is so great that it is unwise to attempt to place the cases into definite types. Rather, it is important to appreciate that arrest of rotation may occur at any point, and consequently a great variety of pathological anatomical situations may be encountered. It is well to remember that in some cases the cecum need not be attached to the posterior abdominal wall in the right quadrant, but may actually be free with a mesentery. In these situations, duodenal obstruction does not occur until volvulus of the midgut has taken place. Obstruction is produced by the drawing of the duodenum around the mesentery, producing mechanical obstruction. The most lethal aspect of this clinical syndrome is volvulus of the midgut. The infant can tolerate the duodenal obstruction for a number of days. The volvulus may lead to necrosis of intestine within the first two days of life. Consequently, there is urgency in the detection and treatment of this group of patients. Twisting of the mesentery produces first venous occlusion which can be as damaging to the tissue as arterial occlusion. Not only is there lack of proper oxygenation under these circumstances, but there is also considerable distension of the vascular spaces from vascular engorgement due to venous obstruction. If the volvulus progresses, arterial occlusion can occur as well, and when this happens, necrosis is inevitable.

CLINICAL BEHAVIOR

In the majority of instances, the infant with malrotation will have symptoms within the first few days of life. There are a small number of patients who have partial obstructions of the duodenum which may not become obvious for several days or weeks after birth. The type of duodenal obstruction which occurs with midgut volvulus may not manifest itself for weeks or months after birth. The common symptom in all of these patients is vomiting, and in the vast majority the vomitus is bile-stained. This is in comparison to the patient with pyloric obstruction where the ampulla of Vater is below the obstruction and the vomitus does not contain bile. Abdominal distension is not a common finding due to the fact that in the majority of instances in the neonate the duodenal obstruc-

tion is a prominent part of the pathology. Hence there is very little air, if any, in the small intestine beyond the duodenum. There may be some upper abdominal distension as the result of the dilation of the stomach and first portion of the duodenum. Tenderness is not a common finding but may be present particularly when the blood supply to the intestine is involved. In patients with volvulus there may be varying degrees of abdominal distension. The presence of blood in the vomitus or in the stool is a signal of an acute emergency since this signifies that there is venous obstruction and escape of blood through the mucosal wall into the lumen of the intestine. This is an indication for immediate operation.

DIAGNOSIS

In the neonate or the small infant child who has bile-stained vomitus, with or with-

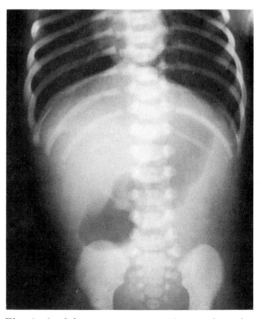

Fig. 1. A plain roentgenogram of a newborn infant with duodenal obstruction. There are two gas bubbles. The upper and left-sided one represents air in the stomach; the bubble in the right lower quadrant represents the dilated duodenum. The plain roentgenograms will be identical, whether the duodenal obstruction is due to malrotation, annular pancreas, or atresia.

out abdominal distension, there is urgent need for flat and upright abdominal films. Air is an excellent contrast medium. Consequently, in most instances, it is not necessary to add contrast material to the gastrointestinal tract in order to outline the stomach and upper part of the gastrointestinal tract. In the upright films there are characteristically two gas bubbles, the major one being primarily to the left of the midline and representing the air bubble in the dilated stomach. There is often a fluid level in the upright film. The second bubble is usually smaller, to the right of the midline and somewhat below the large gastric bubble, and is contained in the dilated duodenum (Fig. 1). This situation forms the classic double bubble sign of duodenal obstruction. Usually there is a small amount of air, if any, beyond the duodenum.

In the patient with incomplete duodenal obstruction, there may be considerable air beyond the duodenum, and the presence of the double bubble sign is obscured by this fact and also by the fact that distension of the upper intestinal tract may be rather mini-

mal. It is in these situations where the patient has vomiting and failure to gain weight that the possibility of partial duodenal obstruction must be appreciated. The diagnosis cannot be accomplished without contrast material in the gastrointestinal tract outlining the partial obstruction of the duodenum. This type constitutes a small percentage of the total number of cases of duodenal obstruction (Fig. 2).

It is a matter of conjecture in most instances as to the nature of the mechanical obstruction. The finding of duodenal obstruction is a clear-cut indication for surgical intervention. It is unnecessary prior to operation to define the precise pathology producing the duodenal obstruction. An adjunct in the diagnosis is the performance of a barium enema and demonstration of malposition of the cecum. In the small neonate, this may be hard to appreciate since distances are limited. The use of barium enema to locate the position of the cecum is particularly useful in the older child with a question of malrotation with partial duodenal obstruction.

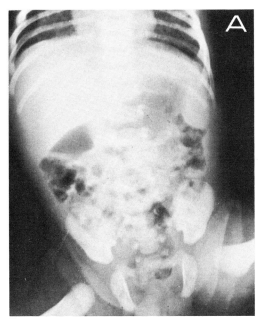 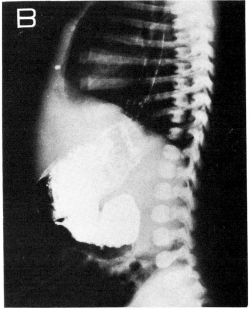

Fig. 2. Partial duodenal obstruction. A. A plain film demonstrates no detectable deviation from normal. B. With barium as the contrast medium, a partial duodenal obstruction is clearly outlined.

TREATMENT

Since duodenal obstruction is associated with midgut volvulus in a perceptible percentage of the cases, it is important to deal with this form of intestinal obstruction promptly. This is particularly true if there is any blood in the vomitus or in the stool. Fortunately, in most of such cases the child is not beyond two or three days of age when the lesion is suspected and the diagnosis made. Up to 36 or 48 hours after birth, unless vomiting has been unusual in volume, there is little if any distortion of electrolytes. Consequently, correction of hydration is simple and can be accomplished with considerable rapidity. Particularly in patients beyond 48 hours of age it is well to determine electrolytes to be sure that they are reasonably within normal range before proceeding with operation. When derangements are found, it is wise to begin correction before operation is undertaken. Exception to this may be made if there are indications of midgut volvulus.

The use of local anesthesia was advocated in the past particularly when the surgeon was faced with an extremely ill child. However, with the advancement of the technique of administering general anesthesia to the neonate, the need for use of local anesthesia has diminished. It is now a rare situation in which anything can be gained by the use of local anesthesia. It is well to remember that even with the use of local anesthesia, the onset of shock cannot be eliminated, although it may be somewhat delayed. Consequently, in most patients it is wise to use a general anesthetic so that the operation can be accomplished with a minimum of time loss, and so that an adequate examination and correction of the pathology found can be accomplished. It is important to have a fair-sized nasogastric tube in place prior to the induction of anesthesia so that the stomach and duodenum will be collapsed as completely as possible. The second value of this tube is that it can be passed down through the duodenum into the jejunum in order to eliminate the possibility of a diaphragm as a second obstructive lesion associated with malrotation in a small percentage of the cases.

OPERATIVE TECHNIQUE

The incision used by most surgeons is a right rectus muscle-retracting incision. It has the advantage of providing good exposure and is less time consuming than the transverse incision. Some surgeons prefer the transverse incision, believing that there is better healing postoperatively with this type of division of the abdominal wall. An indication of volvulus and malrotation is the absence of obvious colon as the peritoneal cavity is entered. Rather than try to deliver part of the intestine and thus examine the pathology involved, it is better to remove all of the intestine from the abdominal cavity onto warm moistened sponges or into a plastic bag in order to gain a true appreciation of the relationship of the mesentery of the intestine to the posterior abdominal wall, and thus to detect any degree of volvulus. This also gives good exposure to the attached cecum in malrotation and offers the best opportunity to free the cecum as well as to detect and correct any volvulus. Usually, the correction is a counterclockwise derotation of the intestine on its mesenteric attachment to the posterior abdominal wall. The first step is to correct any volvulus, thus having as early a return as possible of normal vascular flow through the intestine (Fig. 3). The second step is to detach the cecum completely from its position in the right upper quadrant, freeing the cecum and first portion of the colon so that they can be placed in the left upper quadrant. This procedure avoids the return of adhesions across the duodenum. The third step is to make sure that the duodenum traverses a straight course on the right side of the abdomen. This may be difficult to accomplish in some situations due to the fact that the blood supply to the duodenum may be partially endangered by such a procedure. However, in most instances it is possible with careful dissection to free the duodenum, to prevent its sharp kinking to the left, and to have it traverse a straight course down the right side of the abdominal cavity. This is an extremely important part of the Ladd procedure which perhaps was not stressed in his description in the literature but was forcefully taught to students at the

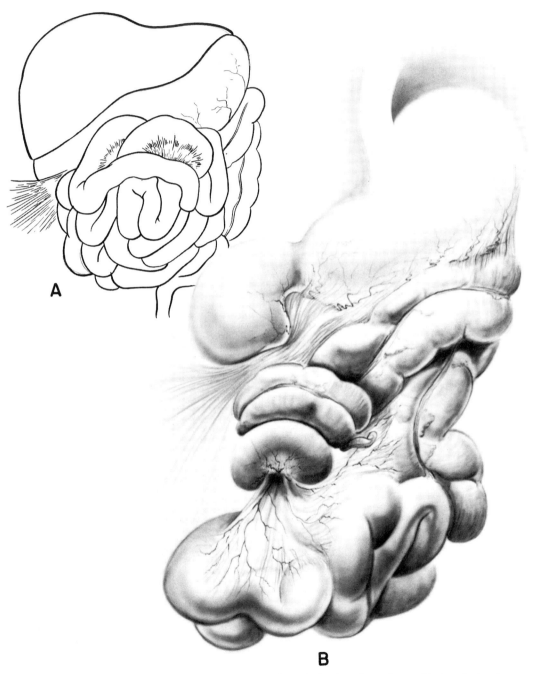

Fig. 3. Malrotation and midgut volvulus. A. Drawing of the intestine when midgut volvulus has occurred. Note that the right colon is below and covered by the small intestine. B. Exposure of the volvulus. The duodenum and cecum are twisted around the vascular pedicle of the intestine.

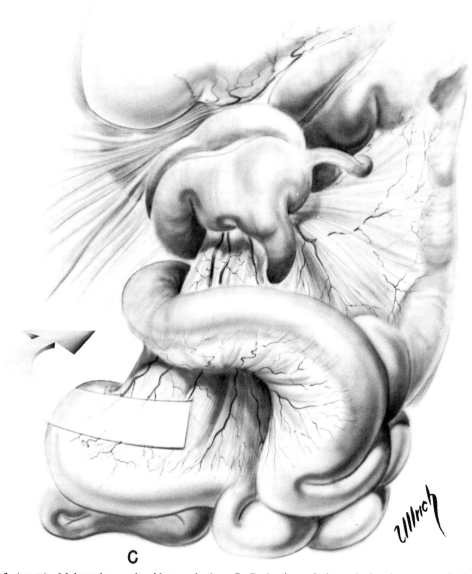

C

Fig. 3 (cont.). Malrotation and midgut volvulus. C. Reduction of the volvulus by counterclockwise twisting. There may be as many as three complete turns.

operating table. The last and very important maneuver is to pass a catheter down through the duodenum into the jejunum to assure that a second lesion such as a diaphragm in the duodenum is not present. This lesion has proven disastrous when overlooked. Should such a lesion be found the duodenum must be opened and the diaphragm adequately excised to ensure a good lumen. It is convenient to pass the gastric tube down into the duodenum and into the jejunum. On the other hand, should the operator fail to pass the tube down through the duodenum into the small intestine, he must not hesitate either to perform an opening into the stomach (thus passing the tube down), or better still,

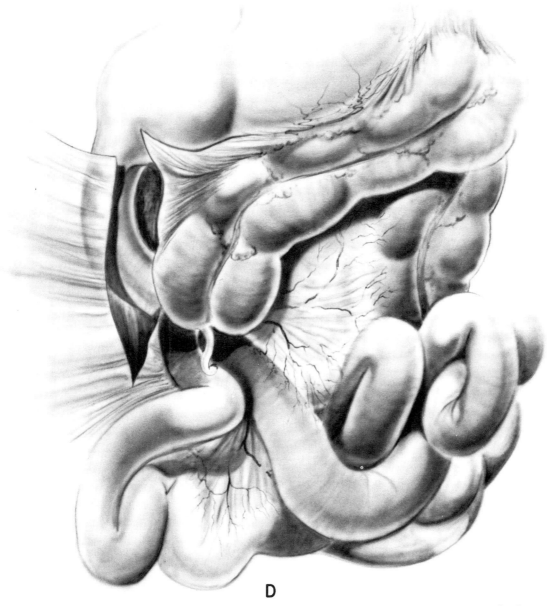

D

Fig. 3 (cont.). Malrotation and midgut volvulus. D. Detachment of the cecum for placement in the left upper quadrant. The operation is incomplete unless this step is taken.

to open the dilated duodenum and make sure that there is no intrinsic obstruction present.

Another important point is either to perform appendectomy during operation or to be certain that the parents are made aware of the fact that the child's appendix occupies an abnormal position. Removal of the appendix can be accomplished. However, oc-

casionally there are complications from this operation, and unless the baby is in excellent condition it is wise not to extend the operation by performing appendectomy.

We have found it unnecessary to perform gastrostomy. It is an added hazard to the patient as well as a prolongation of the operation. The use of a nasogastric tube has

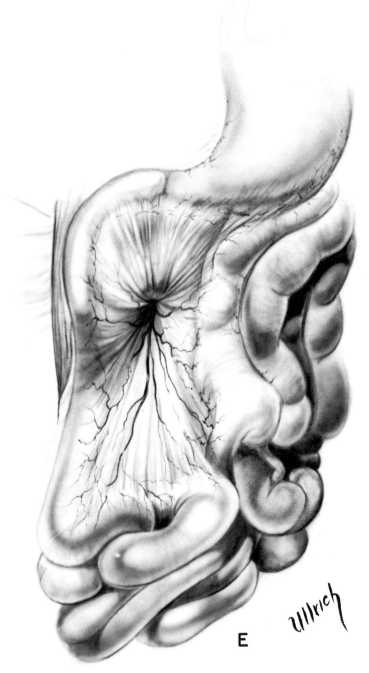

E

Fig. 3 (cont.). Malrotation and midgut volvulus. E. The duodenum has been mobilized. It now runs an unobstructed course down the right side of the abdomen.

been effective in our experience and obviates the necessity of extending the operation by performing a gastrostomy and subjecting the patient to the complications of this additional procedure.

POSTOPERATIVE CARE

There is a tendency in some of these patients to have a delay of intestinal function for 48 to 72 hours. Consequently, it is important to have the infant on nasogastric suction to prevent distension of the stomach and first portion of the duodenum. Overhydration of the patient during this period is dangerous and must be guarded against by frequent weighing. The patient's weight should have a slight decrease to account for the inevitable metabolism which occurs during the nonfeeding periods. Calculation of maintenance doses of fluid and electrolytes is important during this period of postoperative care. We have found the surface area method the best, and we give fluid on the basis of 1,200 ml per square meter of body surface per 24 hours.

In the patient with some delay in functioning, plain roentgenograms of the abdomen are useful in assessing the passage of air beyond the duodenum. If there is a good amount of gas beyond the duodenum into the small intestine, there is likelihood that effective alimentation will soon follow. On the other hand, when there is no intestinal gas pattern beyond the duodenum, there is an indication of persistence of obstruction which should not be treated complacently

for a long period of time. It is well to realize that unless the baby begins to aliment seven to ten days after initial operation, serious consideration should be given to reexploration to determine the cause of failure of intestinal function.

INTRINSIC DUODENAL OBSTRUCTION

The embryology of intrinsic duodenal obstruction can best be appreciated by a review of the changes which normally occur in the formation of the intestine. Early in the development of the intestinal tract, the intestine is a solid cord. The lumen is eventually made by the formation and coalescence of vacuoles in this solid tissue. An arrest of this process could result in atresia or in an inadequate lumen (stenosis).

It is important to appreciate that the obstruction may be a diaphragm which may prolapse a considerable distance into the continuing intestine due to the peristaltic pressures from above (Fig. 4). There have been situations where the duodenojejunos-

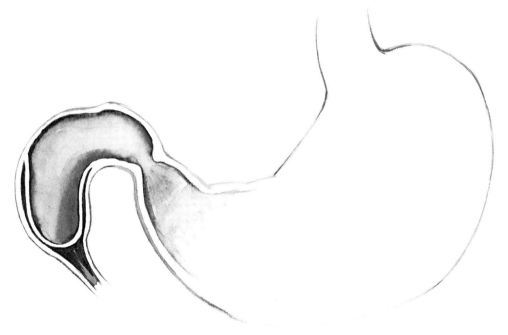

Fig. 4. Outline drawing indicating an obstructing duodenal diaphragm which has prolapsed for a considerable distance.

tomy has been made below the attachment of the diaphragm and has failed to relieve the obstruction.

DIAGNOSIS

Atresia of the duodenum is a rare entity. The symptoms are similar to those seen in annular pancreas or malrotation when these lesions produce virtually complete obstruction (Fig. 5). Atresia is most common in the duodenum beyond the ampulla of Vater, and therefore the vomitus generally contains bile. The diagnosis of duodenal atresia is suggested by early and persistent bile-stained vomiting in the newborn and by abdominal distension limited to the upper abdomen. Gastic peristaltic waves may be observed in the epigastrium moving from left to right. Duodenal waves may be observed in the right upper quadrant progressing from the upper right to the lower part of the abdomen. Meconium may be scanty,

and its microscopic examination will fail to reveal cornified epithelial cells when the lesion is an atresia. The diagnosis of complete duodenal obstruction can be made from a plain abdominal roentgenogram, for characteristically there will be a large gas bubble in the left upper quadrant outlining the dilated stomach, and a second and smaller bubble will be present in the right upper quadrant outlining the dilated portion of the duodenum. There will be no gas pattern beyond the dilated duodenum (Figs. 6 and 7).

Stenosis presents a different clinical picture from atresia. In stenosis, there may be only occasional vomiting. The infant eats poorly, gains weight slowly, and appears chronically ill. Numerous formula changes are often prescribed on the assumption that the baby has a feeding problem. Scanty stools indicate that the infant does not have pancreatic fibrosis. An erroneous diagnosis of celiac syndrome is frequently made. A positive diagnosis of duodenal stenosis or

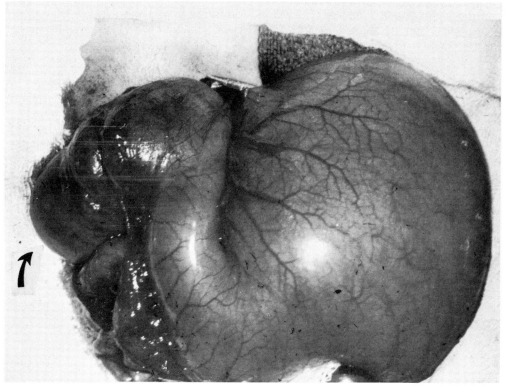

Fig. 5. Atresia of the duodenum (arrow). Note the dilation of stomach and duodenum which ends abruptly at the atresia.

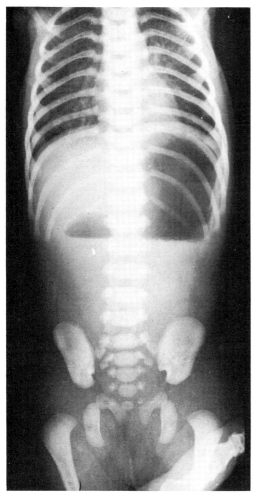

Fig. 6. Plain roentgenogram of abdomen. This neonate proved to have atresia of the duodenum.

atresia can be made by a roentgen gastrointestinal study. This will outline a dilated stomach and duodenum with a narrowing in the midportion of the duodenum and a delayed passage of the contrast medium into the jejunum.

OPERATION

A newborn infant with duodenal atresia has little dehydration or electrolyte imbalance 24 hours after birth and requires little preoperative therapy. Beyond this period, there is progressively more dehydration and excessive chloride loss, and operation is profitably delayed until these changes are

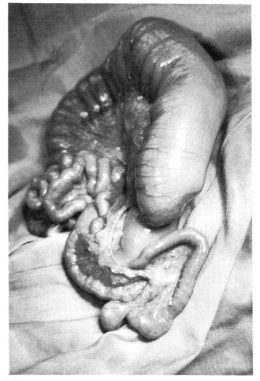

Fig. 7. Photograph of duodenal atresia. Same patient as in Figure 6. The duodenum was unattached and the atresia was in its distal portion.

corrected. The exploration is performed through an upper right rectus muscle-retracting incision or transverse incision. When the duodenum is exposed, it will be dilated and will end blindly in the second or third portion. A dissection to identify the narrowed duodenum beyond the atresia is not warranted. Instead the proximal loop of jejunum is identified in preparation for a retrocolic side-to-side duodenojejunostomy (Fig. 8).

An opening is made in the mesocolon, and the edges of this opening are secured to the duodenum with interrupted sutures of 6-0 silk in such a fashion that an adequate area of dilated duodenum is available for the side-to-side anastomosis with the loop of jejunum placed in an isoperistaltic position.

There remains a space between the mesocolon and the jejunal mesentery through which intestine could prolapse and become the site of intestinal obstruction. This complication is prevented by placing continuous

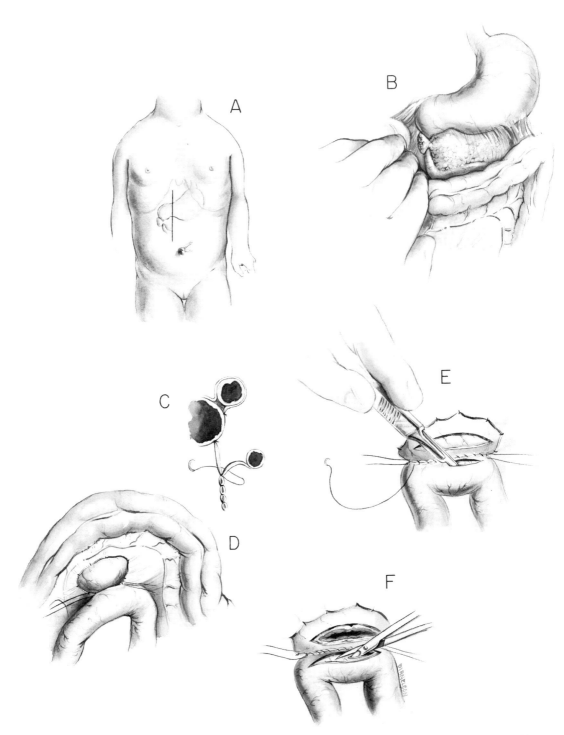

Fig. 8. Rectocolic side-to-side duodenojunostomy. A. Outline drawing indicating position of incision. B. The pathology is exposed and found to be an annular pancreas. C. An opening has been made in the mesocolon and the edges attached to the dilated duodenum. Before the anesthesia is started, the defect in the mesentery is closed. If this is left until the anastomosis is completed, there will be great difficulty in achieving this closure. D. A loop of proximal jejunum is brought to and attached to the dilated duodenum with two traction sutures. E. A continuous 6–0 silk Cushing suture approximates the serosal surfaces of the two structures, and a cut is made through the muscular coats in preparation for the anastomosis. F. The mucosa is opened with scissors.

626

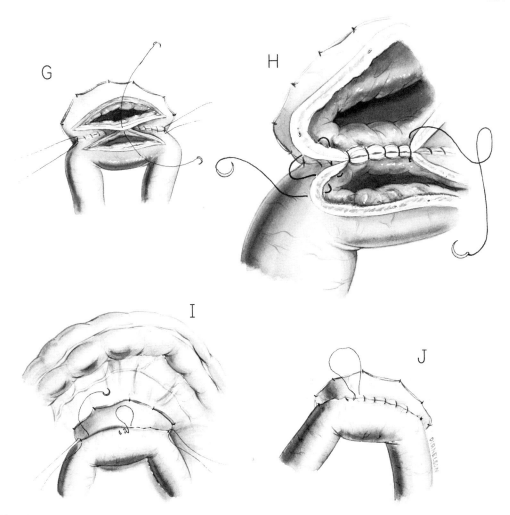

Fig. 8 (cont.). Rectocolic side-to-side duodenojunostomy. G. The inner continuous suture of 5–0 chromic catgut is started. H. Details of the suture placed to turn the edges in. This is after the method of Connell. I, J. The anastomosis is completed with a continuous 6–0 silk suture to bring the sero-muscular coats together to complete the anastomosis.

5-0 chromic catgut sutures to obliterate the space. Care must be taken to avoid placing these sutures through mesenteric vessels; otherwise, troublesome bleeding may occur, and the blood supply to the anastomosis may be endangered. The anastomosis should be about 1 inch in length. It is convenient to start the anastomosis by placing two sutures through the duodenum and jejunum at the ends of the projected anastomosis to hold the structures in position for suturing. No enterostomy clamps are used. A continuous 6-0 silk suture is placed as a posterior layer. The duodenum and jejunum are then opened $\frac{1}{8}$ inch from the silk suture line. The serosa and muscular coats are cut with the scalpel, and the mucosa is cut with plastic scissors. An over-and-over suture of 5-0 chromic catgut is then started on the posterior side in the middle of the incision. This over-and-over suture is continued until the angle is reached, at which point the suture is placed after the method of Connell to ensure that the edges are inverted. A second suture is begun at the midpoint posteriorly and progresses around the other angle. The two sutures should meet at the midpoint of the anterior side and be tied. The advantage of beginning and ending the catgut suture in the middle is elimination of the necessity for having knots at the angles, which are the weakest points of the anastomosis. It is important to remember that the chief function of the inner catgut suture is to turn in the cut edge of the intestine and to produce hemostasis. Only by placing the suture through the entire intestinal wall can hemostasis be ensured. The anterior row of sutures is then placed, using a continuous 5-0 silk Cushing suture. To strengthen the angles, they are reinforced with one or two interrupted silk sutures. Patency of the anastomosis is tested by pushing intestinal contents through the new opening.

Postoperatively, nasogastric suction is maintained until peristalses are detectable and there is no bile-stained return in the gastric tube. Small, frequent glucose and water feedings are then given. The feedings are changed to formulas as soon as they are tolerated. When intestinal function is slow to return, a plain film of the abdomen will determine whether gas is progressing beyond the anastomosis.

ANNULAR PANCREAS

One of the rarest causes of duodenal obstruction is an anomalous ringlike distribution of pancreatic tissue around the second portion of the duodenum (Fig. 9). The exact cause of this anomaly is undetermined, but the following embryological explanation seems reasonable.

Initially, the pancreas forms from two buds, one extending dorsally from the duodenum and the other extending ventrally from the duodenum. Normally, the ventral bud is rotated dorsally because of unequal growth of the duodenum, and it fuses with the dorsal bud which comprises the major portion of the pancreas. The smaller ventral bud eventually becomes the head of the pancreas. Some embryologists believe that the ventral portion is paired and that failure of the pairs to unite may be a factor in the pro-

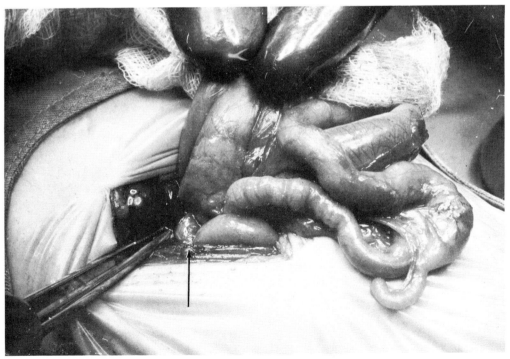

Fig. 9. Annular pancreas. The arrow points to the constricting ring of pancreatic tissue. Note the duodenal dilatation above the ring.

duction of a constricting ring of pancreatic tissue around the duodenum.

Histological examination of the pancreatic ring reveals it to be normal in cell composition. There is some variation in the duct arrangement in the ring, but generally there is an accessory duct extending around the duodenum to the right, either going into the main duct or having a separate opening into the common duct.

There may be compression of the common duct by the pancreatic tissue, and jaundice may be an early and predominant symptom. More commonly, some degree of duodenal obstruction is produced. This may be severe and produce vomiting shortly after birth. The vomitus is bile-stained unless there is an unusual anatomical arrangement with the compression around the duodenum at the level of the ampulla of Vater. The duodenal obstruction may be so slight that symptoms do not develop until the patient is an adult.

If the duodenal obstruction is fairly complete, the infant will vomit shortly after birth, and the abdominal distension will be limited to the epigastrium. Active gastric and duodenal waves may be observed. Roentgen films in such instances will demonstrate a dilated stomach and duodenum with little if any air in the intestine. If the obstruction is less complete the child may not vomit. Instead, there will be a failure to gain weight, and the clinical situation will be that of a feeding problem. In such patients, the diagnosis of duodenal obstruction can be made only radiographically with contrast medium in the duodenum. The barium will outline duodenal compression which may not differ greatly from the scarring produced by duodenal ulcer, but the young age of the patient will make the diagnosis of ulcer unlikely.

OPERATION

If the history, physical findings, and roentgenological examination indicate annular pancreas, an exploratory laparotomy is justified. Finding a dilated duodenum with a con-stricting ring of pancreatic tissue confirms the diagnosis.

A retrocolic duodenojejunostomy (Fig. 9) as described for duodenal atresia is a safer and more effective procedure than a direct attack on the constricting ring of pancreatic tissue. When the pancreatic ring is cut, the mortality is high because of acute pancreatitis and the formation of fistulas. The duct which drains a part of the pancreatic ring may be divided or damaged, and this can be the direct cause of fatal pancreatitis. Consequently, a duodenojejunostomy is preferred.

Postoperatively, the patients progress satisfactorily. Perhaps as these children are followed for long periods of time some evidences of pancreatic disease may develop. So far, such complications have not occurred in our experience. It is now known that about 30 percent of patients with duodenal obstruction also have Down's syndrome.

DUODENAL ULCER

This rare lesion of childhood is the cause of three distinct clinical situations: (1) In the newborn, there may be a large duodenal ulcer with massive bleeding. (2) During infancy, there may be perforation. (3) In older

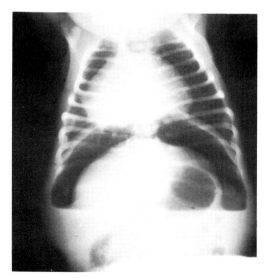

Fig. 10. Roentgenogram of infant with a perforated duodenal ulcer.

children, there may be pain which is similar to the ulcer dyspepsia of adults. The etiology of this third form is probably similar to that thought to be the cause of duodenal ulcers in adults. There seems to be hyperacidity, and the children are tense with easily detected emotional problems.

In the newborn and in infants, the situation is more complicated, for hyperacidity is not a constant finding. The association of ulcers, both duodenal and gastric, with burns (so-called Curling's ulcers) is well known.

Central nervous lesions may produce ulcers, and these may occur after successful surgical intervention for central nervous system malformations or tumor (Cushing's ulcer).

In newborn infants, hematemesis suggests duodenal ulcer, and the patients should be carefully observed. In most instances, the bleeding will subside, and the cause is probably some obscure and transient defect in the blood-clotting mechanism. If the bleeding is profuse and persistent, duodenal ulcer must be considered. Unfortunately, these

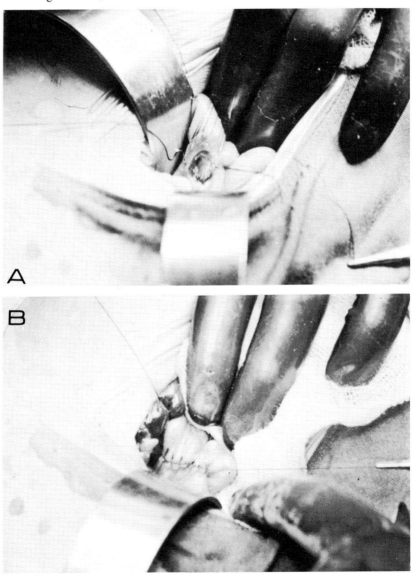

Fig. 11. A. A large anterior duodenal ulcer. B. It was possible to close this without endangering the duodenal lumen.

ulcers are difficult to demonstrate radiographically, probably due to the shallow craters and the absence of reaction in the surrounding tissue. Despite the lack of confirmatory radiographic evidence, surgical intervention is indicated if there is persistent and severe hematemesis. While these babies are being observed, a cannula should be inserted into a vein and blood made available for transfusion. Prior to exploration, it is advisable to bring the patient to the most favorable conditions possible with transfusions. Exploration should include opening of the duodenum, for it may be possible to palpate the ulcer through the duodenal wall. Ligation of the bleeding points is preferable to subtotal gastric resection providing it is accompanied with vagotomy and pyloroplasty.

Perforated ulcers occur during infancy as well as during childhood. Usually, there are no preceding symptoms. There is an abrupt onset of vomiting, and the abdominal findings, while less dramatic in children than in adults, are suggestive enough to prompt an upright abdominal roentgenogram. The presence of air under the diaphragm confirms the diagnosis (Fig. 10). In small infants, the abdominal signs may consist only of mild spasm and some abdominal tenderness.

The treatment of perforation in infants is identical with the treatment in adults. Gastric suction is instituted, and parenteral fluids are administered. For the operation, a right rectus muscle-retracting incision is preferred to the more time-consuming transverse incision. The duodenum is usually quite firm around the perforation so that the duodenal wall cannot be approximated to close the opening. Omentum can be held in place with several silk sutures, and the opening can be closed in this way without impinging on the duodenal lumen (Fig. 11).

Postoperatively, these infants can have the gastric tube removed and can be started on glucose feedings as soon as active peristalses have returned. Usually, these children have no further gastric difficulties.

Chronic duodenal ulcers are also encountered in children, and the symptoms are much like those in adults. Usually, there is hyperacidity. Bleeding and perforation may occur, though far less frequently in older children than in infants. There is a less concise history of postprandial pain than in adults. Occasionally, the chronic ulcers are difficult to demonstrate radiographically. However, the resulting scarring of the duodenum is usually detected (Fig. 12).

As in adults, children with ulcers have a history of epigastric pain interspersed with periods of freedom from discomfort. During acute episodes, there may be a high degree of duodenal obstruction because of acute inflammation around the ulcer. Usually, this subsides on conservative treatment consisting of gastric suction followed by a Sippy regimen, but scarring may eventually develop and require surgical attention.

Medical treatment is difficult at home. The child soon feels well and will no longer follow the diet or stay on complete bed rest. Furthermore, the emotional problems which

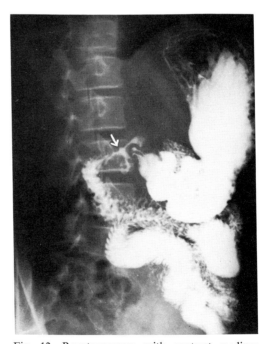

Fig. 12. Roentgenogram with contrast medium demonstrating a chronic duodenal ulcer. The patient was a boy nine years of age who had had symptoms for three years. He received medical treatment and remained in good health during the five years after this roentgenogram was made.

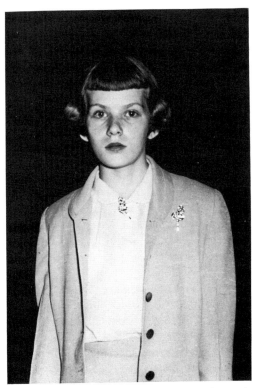

Fig. 13. A girl five years after subtotal gastric resection, Polya type. Her growth and development have been normal.

usually are associated with this type of ulcer are present to aggravate the situation. For these reasons, adequate medical care can be provided only by hospitalization of the child for three or four weeks. This hospital treatment is effective, but when the child returns home to full activity there is likely to be recurrence.

Surgical treatment has not been used except in children with severe bleeding or pyloric obstruction. One reason for this conservative attitude of physicians and surgeons is a limited knowledge concerning the fate of a child following subtotal gastrectomy (Fig. 13). Normal growth and development after subtotal gastric resection have taken place in a small number of patients followed for periods up to five years. Consequently, in children whose symptoms cannot be controlled medically or in those with repeated bouts of bleeding or with pyloric obstruction, subtotal gastric resection is indicated.

We have used vagotomy and pyloroplasty with satisfactory results in patients with duodenal ulcers which have bled excessively. Some of these patients had been on cortisone, and bleeding had required more than one complete replacement of the child's blood volume. Benson and Lloyd have used hemigastrectomy with vagotomy with satisfactory results.

ORVAR SWENSON

REFERENCES

BENSON, C. D., and LLOYD, J. R. Duodenal obstruction of congenital origin. Amer. J. Surg., 101: 610, 1961.

BLOUGH, J. B., and SMITH, P. D., Jr. Malrotation of midgut associated with absence of superior mesenteric vein outflow. Amer. J. Surg., 108: 409, 1964.

DOTT, N. M. Anomalies in intestinal rotation: Their embryology and surgical aspects with report of five cases. Brit. J. Surg., 11: 251, 1923.

ESTRADA, R. L. Anomalies of Intestinal Rotation and Fixation. Springfield, Ill., Charles C Thomas, Publisher, 1958, p. 1.

FRAZER, J. E., and ROBBINS, J. H. On factors concerned in causing rotation of intestine in man. J. Anat. Physiol., 50: 75, 1915.

HIS, W. Anatomie menschlicher Embryomen.

Leipzig, Verlag Von F.C.W. Vogel, 1880–1885, Part III, p. 12.

KEITH, A. Human Embryology and Morphology, 5th ed. Baltimore, William Wood and Co., 1933, pp. 321 and 326.

LADD, W. E. Congenital obstructions of the duodenum in children. New Eng. J. Med., 206: 277, 1932.

——— Surgical diseases of the alimentary tract in infants. New Eng. J. Med., 215: 705, 1936.

MALL, F. P. Development of the human intestine and its position in the adult. Bull. Hopkins Hosp., 9: 197, 1898.

McINTOSH, R., and DONOVAN, E. J. Disturbances in rotation of the intestinal tract. Amer. J. Dis. Child., 57: 116, 1939.

PERNKOPF, E. Development of the form of the

stomach and intestinal canal in man. Z. Anat., 77: 1, 1925.

RICKHAM, P. P. Intestinal obstruction in the neonatal period. Brit. J. Clin. Pract., 11: 833, 1957.

SALZBERG, A. M., and MARTIN, C. J. Intestinal malrotation in infancy and childhood. Amer. J. Surg., 101: 105, 1961.

SCHULTZ, L. R., LASHER, E. P., and BILL, A. H., Jr. Abnormalities of rotation of the bowel. Amer. J. Surg., 101: 128, 1961.

SNYDER, W. H., Jr., and CHAFFIN, L. Embryology and pathology of the intestinal tract: Presentation of 40 cases of malrotation. Ann. Surg., 140: 368, 1954.

37

Small Bowel Atresia and Stenosis

Atresia of the jejunum or ileum is an uncommon condition, occurring once in from 10,000 to 20,000 births. Unlike the congenital occlusions of the esophagus, duodenum, or anorectal area, atretic lesions affecting the small bowel are not commonly associated with other defects, and most of the babies are of normal birth weight. It would seem, therefore, that their prognosis for life and normal development should be excellent. Yet in 1941 Ladd and Gross could report only 9 survivors out of 52 patients, and even in 1963, Handlesman and his colleagues found a 20 to 30 percent mortality rate in treated patients. In untreated patients, death usually occurs within four to eight days from perforation of the distended bowel, sepsis, or dehydration.

ETIOLOGY

The etiology of the jejunal and ileal atresias may be different from that of other portions of the gastrointestinal tract. The theory of Tandler that the occlusion results from excessive epithelial plugging of the embryonic intestinal tract during the solid stage of its development has been accepted by many students of this disorder, but Lynn and Espinas (1959) do not confirm that such epithelial overgrowth occurs along most of the intestinal tract. While the formation of a solid cord of cells is usual in the duodenum during the fifth to eighth week of fetal life, this normal occlusion of the intestinal tract rarely occurs to any significant extent in the remainder of the bowel. Heaping-up of the entoderm (epithelium) does occur just prior to the elongation of bowel which begins quite suddenly during the fifth week of intrauterine life, and it is conceivable that the heaped-up entodermal cells might go on to complete occlusion of the intestinal lumen or that they might induce the formation of a stenotic ring or frank atresia in some of the cases. Other theories of the etiology of the atresias, however, appear more likely to be correct.

The vascular theory, which originated over 100 years ago, has been found to be a more satisfactory explanation for the wide variety of abnormalities which occur in the atretic bowel. Current opinion holds that the jejunoileal, the colonic, and perhaps even the duodenal atresias usually result *from interruption of the blood supply* to these portions of the bowel during embryonic life. The cause may be a thrombosis or embolus of one or more feeding vessels, a kinking or occlusion of the vessels during the rotation of the mesentery, or some form of catastrophic accident such as a volvulus, an intussusception, or a herniation of the bowel through a constricting opening. In support of this theory is the frequent finding of mummified intussusceptions, persistent areas of volvulus, wide gaps between the bowel ends, defects of the mesentery, and the presence of an atretic bowel end within the tight ring of a small omphalocele. The decreased total length of bowel and the shortened mesentery are also facts which are better explained by the catastrophic or vascular accident theory.

Louw and Barnard (1955), and other authors, have produced bowel atresias in puppies in utero which are entirely similar to the human variety, by ligating the mesenteric vessels or by producing an obstructive volvulus of the intestinal tract. Louw (1966) has pointed out that there is an abnormal vascular pattern about the blind ends of the bowel in nearly 50 percent of the cases, and that defects in the mesentery occur at the

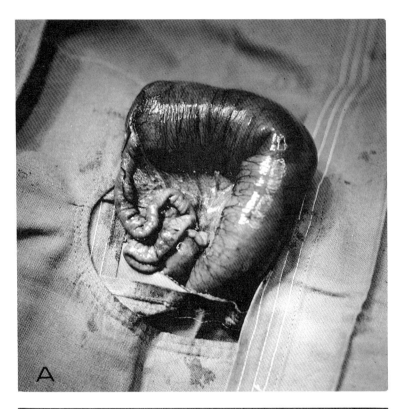

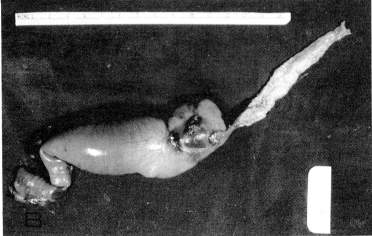

Fig. 1. Atresia of small bowel. A. Note discoloration of enormously dilated proximal bowel in jejunal atresia. B. Necrosis with impending perforation in ileal atresia.

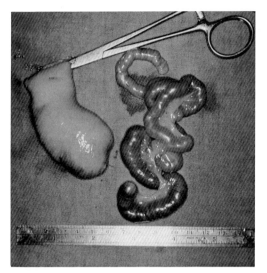

Fig. 2. Complete gap between bowel ends. Poor blood supply is present on each side of the defect.

atretic area in fully two thirds. The rarity of other associated birth defects and the fact that bile, squamous epithelium, and hair are found distal to the occlusion in more than half of the cases also support the concept that damage has occurred to the bowel late in the course of fetal development. Microscopic

sections often reveal areas of necrosis, foreign body granulomas, and calcification about the site of the atresia, further confirming the concept that intrauterine bowel necrosis has occurred. In such instances the atresia has quite obviously resulted from sterile necrosis and absorption of nonviable areas of the bowel and mesentery which have been deprived of their blood supply in utero.

The vascular theory of small bowel atresia is an important one because it emphasizes the need for wide resection of the atretic bowel. Better healing and earlier restoration of bowel function are more likely to occur when wide resection is accomplished prior to the making of an anastomosis, since the blood supply is better and the bowel is less distended away from the site of the atresia (Fig. 1). Nixon (1960) has demonstrated, in addition, that although the dilated bowel segment is able to contract, its peristalsis is not coordinated and is ineffective for propulsion. The narrowing of the bowel from the large proximal loop to the small distal end at the site of the anastomosis is a further impediment to effective intestinal func-

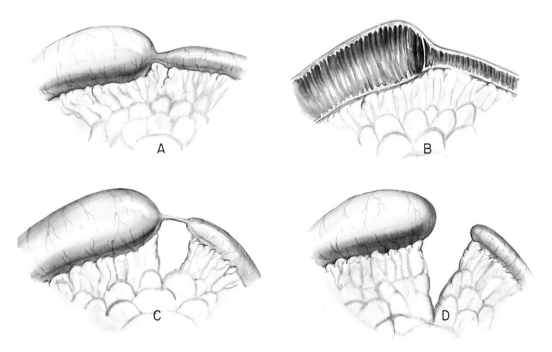

Fig. 3. A through D. Types of intestinal atresia and stenosis.

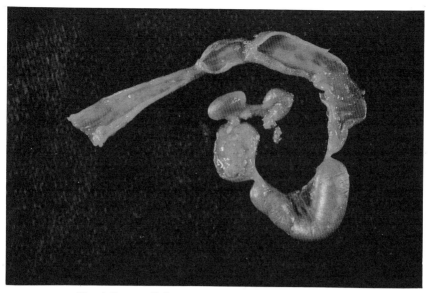

Fig. 4. Sausage-link appearance seen in multiple atresias.

tion. Persistent obstruction is frequent despite patency of the anastomosis when the dilated portion is not resected. Better results are obtained by wide resection of the dilated portion of the proximal bowel than by the performance of direct anastomosis of the blind ends without resection. The preservation of bowel length at the expense of a poorly functioning anastomosis has little to recommend it.

PATHOLOGY

Pathologically the area of simple atresia is characterized by enormous dilatation of the bowel proximal to the obstruction and by smallness of the distal end. In some cases, an external continuity of the tract is present, while in others a wide gap exists between the occluded ends (Fig. 2). Louw (1966) distinguishes four types of intrinsic occlusions. Stenosis and atresias of three different configurations are found to occur (Fig. 3). The mesentery about the atresia is often defective in the last two groups, and in more than one half of all of the cases it is not well fixed to the posterior abdominal wall and is therefore excessively mobile.

Marked fibrous adhesions or calcified

granulomas about the site of the atresia indicate intrauterine perforation of the bowel with the development of sterile peritonitis. This is *meconium peritonitis,* which may be indicated radiographically by extensive intra-

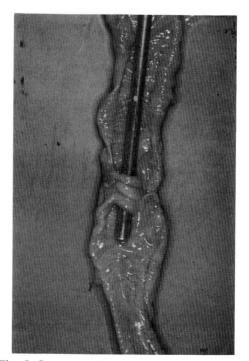

Fig. 5. Septum causing nearly total small bowel obstruction.

abdominal calcification, and is not infrequently associated with the jejunoileal atresias. It is not necessarily a sign of meconium ileus or of cystic fibrosis of the pancreas. Multiple atresias are present in from 15 to 20 percent of the cases. The affected portions of the bowel are sometimes separated by constricted areas to give a sausage link appearance (Fig. 4). Necrosis with septic peritonitis is present in about one fourth of the patients at the time of operation. In the series of Pollock and Bergin (1961), 7 of 26 infants with jejunal atresia and 14 of 33 with ileal atresia had meconium peritonitis, intestinal gangrene, perforation, or small areas of necrosis in the distended bowel at the time of operation.

Microscopic examination reveals mucosal atrophy and poor muscular development in many of the specimens, particularly in the upper dilated segment. Occasionally these mural abnormalities also extend below the atresia. Ulceration of the mucosa is frequently seen. Sometimes there are folds of fibromuscular tissue below the atresia which partially or totally obstruct the lumen of the distal segment (Fig. 5). To avoid a postoperative disaster, these folds should always be expected to be present, and therefore complete evaluation of the patency of the entire bowel must be made before the anastomosis is accomplished. Old areas of necrosis with microscopic calcification are not uncommon in the histological sections of narrowed areas.

DIAGNOSIS

Babies with jejunal or ileal atresias are usually admitted to surgical units on the second or third day of life. Failure to pass normal meconium, increasing abdominal distension, and persistent vomiting of bile-stained mucus are common to all forms of bowel obstruction and are easily recognized by the nursery attendants. These symptoms call for immediate radiographic examinations. Supine and upright views reveal the presence of dilated bowel and the approximate site of the lesion. Two or three enlarged loops indicate an occlusion in the upper jejunum (Fig. 6), while many air-fluid levels are likely to be present in the lower obstructions

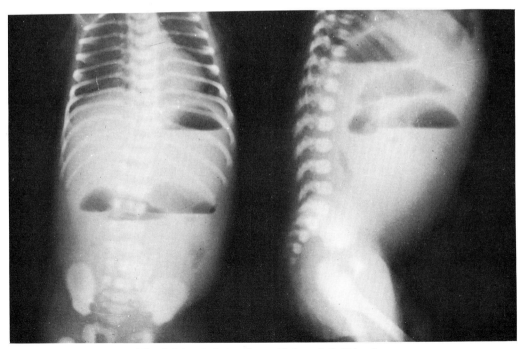

Fig. 6. Jejunal obstruction, with few air-fluid levels.

(Fig. 7). If multiple loops of dilated bowel are found, a barium enema examination must be done to identify whether or not the lesion is in the colon. In cases of small bowel atresia the colon is characteristically narrow, shortened, and unused—the so-called microcolon.

One of the most difficult problems in dealing with neonatal intestinal obstruction is to decide whether or not strangulation of the bowel is present. If there is inflammation within the peritoneal cavity the abdomen is distended and tender, as evidenced by straining and crying when palpation is attempted. Localization of the tenderness is difficult to elicit, however, and any masses which may be present are often obscured by the distension. Changes in the bowel sounds are of importance, since serious peritonitis usually leads eventually to complete ileus and disappearance of the sounds. The general condition of the infant is of the greatest importance. A flat temperature curve, a pulse rate between 120 and 160 per minute, respirations of 35 to 60, good skin turgor, absence

of shiny skin or dilated veins over the abdomen, and a good Moro reflex and cry are indications that sepsis or advanced bowel necrosis are probably not present. On the other hand, lethargy, poor muscle tone, a pale or lavender color of the skin accompanied by cyanosis of the hands and feet, absence of the femoral pulses, tachycardia, fever or hypothermia, and a shiny distended abdomen with absent bowel sounds are signs that a serious intra-abdominal catastrophe has occurred.

It is not possible to identify the presence of strangulated bowel on radiographic examination unless a gas pattern appears in the mesenteric vessels. Free air under the diaphragm is a sign of perforation of some portion of the gastrointestinal tract. This sign is less likely to occur with the atresias than with other abdominal catastrophes, since the areas of necrosis develop slowly and are usually sealed by fibrinous adhesions at the time of the perforation. The presence of a mass indicating the site of perforation may some-

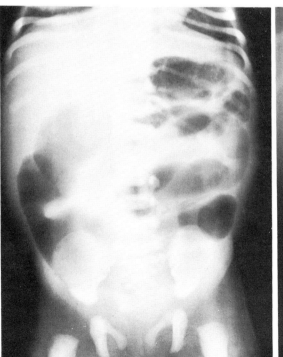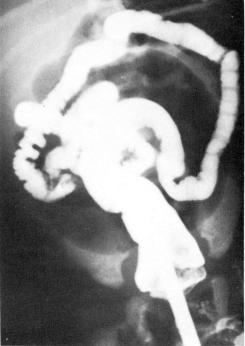

Fig. 7. Many air-fluid levels indicate obstruction in the ileum or below it. The microcolon (right) is characteristic of congenital small bowel obstruction.

times be inferred from absence of bowel markings in a localized area.

LABORATORY STUDIES

Hemoconcentration is usually present, particularly when severe dehydration has occurred, so that the hemoglobin level may be as high as 24 g percent. The white blood count is not of great value in the immediate newborn period, since it is already about 25,000 at birth and has a differential count which is similar to that in the adult. Unless the white count is greater than 25,000, therefore, it cannot be used to differentiate septic peritonitis from other conditions during the first few days of life. Persistence of polymorphonuclear predominance and elevation of the total count above 25,000 are very significant after the first week of life. Other important signs of sepsis in newborns are jaundice, low serum sodium, a raised BUN, increasing anemia without obvious blood loss, and a prolonged prothrombin time.

GENERAL CONSIDERATIONS IN TREATMENT

Following radiological confirmation of the diagnosis of intestinal obstruction and the determination of its probable level, the best time for operation must be decided upon. In many of the cases immediate operation is unwise. There is usually excessive distension which can be relieved to some extent by gastric drainage prior to operation. Pneumonia may have occurred as the result of aspiration, and sepsis is not unusual in small babies with bowel obstruction. Dehydration, electrolyte disturbances, and inadequate circulation usually develop to a significant degree only after the first 48 hours of life, but they then progress rapidly. Since these conditions are aggravated by anesthesia and operative manipulations, their treatment should be commenced before the operation, rather than after it. A period of 12 to 24 hours may be of value both in establishing a correct preoperative diagnosis and in improving the infant's condition. Further distension is prevented by a high oxygen environment and gastric suction; pneumonia is treated by frequent pharyngeal or endotracheal aspiration and antibiotics. Cultures of the blood, pharynx, and urine should be done prior to the first dose of antibiotic in order to rule out the possibility of sepsis and to determine the predominant organisms which are likely to give trouble during the postoperative period.

Although immediate surgical intervention is not always wise, uncomplicated small bowel obstruction in a reasonably healthy baby should be treated by operation as soon as the diagnosis is confirmed and baseline studies have been obtained. Delay results in further distension and devitalization of the proximal bowel, particularly at the site of the occlusion. In addition, all intestinal obstructions lead to progressive bacterial growth in the area of stasis, resulting in the production of excessive amounts of toxins and further complicating the treatment as time goes on.

It is essential to determine as soon as possible whether vascular impairment of the bowel or peritonitis are present, and in very sick babies, to decide the best time for operation. It must be admitted that the distinction between nonstrangulated obstruction, gangrenous bowel, and generalized peritonitis is difficult to make. Certainly air under the diaphragm indicates free perforation of the bowel, a complication which demands immediate surgical intervention. On the other hand, a jaundiced baby with low serum sodium, raised BUN, and other signs of sepsis should probably be treated vigorously with plasma and antibiotics and observed *from hour to hour* while the specific diagnosis is being made. This course is particularly indicated when small amounts of stool or gas continue to be passed per rectum, signifying the presence of only partial bowel obstruction. Intestinal volvulus usually leads to early intestinal devitalization. Consequently blood in the vomitus or stool is an indication for immediate operation. In general, the tendency should be to early operation rather than to prolonged delay, providing that the infant is in reasonably satisfactory condition to undergo the stresses of anesthesia and operation, and that the diagnosis of a mechanical lesion requiring surgical intervention has been made.

PREOPERATIVE TREATMENT

Because of the natural hypervolemia at birth, signs of dehydration are not usually noticed in newborns for several days unless the vomiting is severe or considerable third space losses are present. In the uncomplicated cases no special preoperative preparation is required. A chest x-ray, baseline serum electrolytes for comparison with the postoperative values, and the blood count and urinalysis are all that are required following radiographic confirmation of the presence of mechanical obstruction. Gastric drainage by means of an indwelling plastic catheter is mandatory to prevent aspiration pneumonia and to decompress the stomach prior to the operation. A high-oxygen environment may decrease the abdominal distension to some degree and improve the condition of any marginal bowel which may be present. Because of the probability of bacterial contamination at operation, antibiotics are indicated. Intramuscular penicillin, 50,-000 units, and kanamycin, 5 mg per kg every eight hours (total dose 15 to 20 mg per kg per day), are safe and effective drugs in the newborn period.

If there is pneumonia (usually in the right upper lobe), if the initial serum sodium is low, or if the baby is very lethargic and pale, serious infection is probably present. Under these conditions a delay of 12 to 24 hours may improve the chances for survival. Blood or plasma should be given during this time in amounts necessary to raise the venous pressure to 12 to 15 cm of water (usually about 10 to 20 cc per pound of body weight).

Jaundice in the infant with bowel obstruction introduces another problem. It has long been recognized that bilirubin levels in excess of 20 mg percent are associated with a significant incidence of damage to the nervous system. Kernicterus is more common in the smaller infants with hyperbilirubinemia. At The Children's Memorial Hospital we have attempted in surgical cases to individualize the treatment of infants with elevated bilirubin levels, permitting the value to rise to 25 and even 30 mg percent in some of the larger babies before exchange transfusions are performed. It is the *rate of increase of the indirect bilirubin* which appears to be of most significance. If the total bilirubin has reached 18 to 20 mg percent by the end of 48 hours, for example, it is likely to go higher before it tapers off at the fifth day. Under these circumstances referral to an exchange transfusion team is definitely indicated. On the other hand, a less rapid rise which is not associated with hemolysis is probably of less significance. Since hyperbilirubinemia due to the hemolytic processes is more likely to produce kernicterus than that due to other causes, it seems to us that if the jaundice is not due to hemolysis, an exchange transfusion added to the stress of abdominal operation may be more dangerous to the infant than the possibility of brain damage from hyperbilirubinemia. In most of the cases associated with bowel atresia the total bilirubin levels have risen to 18 to 22 mg percent and have then receded without exchange transfusions after a few days. If the indirect bilirubin rises above 17 mg percent, or if the infant is a small premature, the advisability of exchange transfusion is reconsidered.

OPERATION

In very small babies, or in those with peritonitis due to perforation, local anesthesia has the advantage of causing far less metabolic disturbance than general anesthesia, and it may increase the chance for survival. One half percent Xylocaine may be used in dosages of up to 0.5 ml per kg. The larger babies are too vigorous for satisfactory management under local anesthesia, and endotracheal halothane is preferred.

The best incision for adequate abdominal exploration in infants, we believe, is a right rectus retracting paramedian incision centered in the midabdomen. This incision can easily be extended upward or downward as necessary. On incision of the peritoneum a small amount of fluid usually exudes. If it is cloudy, a perforation or a volvulus of the bowel must be suspected. When the fluid is blood-tinged, severe vascular occlusion is probable, and the presence of strangulated bowel may be anticipated.

In all problems of newborn bowel obstruction *complete evisceration of the bowel is mandatory*. All of the bowel must be inspected, from the ligament of Treitz to the sigmoid colon. The incision must be large enough so that this inspection of the bowel can be accomplished gently but rapidly. A small incision hinders the delivery of the bowel and increases the probability of excessive traction on the mesentery, with the possibility that some of the mesenteric vessels may be avulsed from the bowel.

The dilated proximal bowel is friable and very vascular. It may be necrotic. The dilatation extends proximally for varying distances. When the atresia is in the proximal jejunum, a large dilated sausage-shaped bowel will be seen to emerge from under the mesentery of the ligament of Treitz. Since the distal bowel is unused, it is small, and therefore the proximal and distal ends of the bowel when prepared for anastomosis are always very unequal in size no matter where the atresia is located.

The amount of bowel which can safely be discarded in the newborn period has not definitely been determined. The normal newborn has about 150 to 250 cm of small intestine, and it is estimated that at least 60 percent of this amount can safely be removed. It is of great importance to preserve the ileocecal valve in bowel resections if at all possible, since postoperative nutrition is much better maintained if a functional valve is in place. When the colon is normal and the ileocecal valve is retained, perfectly adequate growth can be expected if 90 cm of

small bowel remains after resection. The prospects for normal growth are better if the middle part of the small bowel is removed, so that a portion of jejunum and a portion of ileum are left to perform their normally different functions.

In uncomplicated jejunoileal atresias, it is seldom necessary to remove more than 40 cm of bowel. The majority of the resected segment should be from the proximal dilated bowel, since the propulsive function and the blood supply become progressively better as the ligament of Treitz is approached. Removal of 20 to 30 cm of proximal jejunum and 3 to 5 cm of the distal bowel will usually ensure as good healing and function of the anastomosis as can be expected.

A serious problem arises when multiple atretic areas are found, as occurs in about 10 percent of the cases. It is definitely preferable to perform one anastomosis rather than to make several. In general, if 50 cm (2 feet) of jejunum and ileum can be preserved and the ileocecal valve is intact, adequate growth can be expected with careful nutritional management, and the remaining bowel will elongate and enlarge as time goes on. Since multiple atresias are probably the result of an intrauterine volvulus, and they are usually confined to a specific area of the bowel, it is best to remove them all en masse and to unite the ends of the bowel by a single anastomosis unless this procedure requires the sacrifice of considerable normal intestine which might be safely preserved.

The actual technique of the operation is detailed in Figure 8. After location of the atresia, the bowel content is gently milked from above into the dilated segment, and a fine Kocher clamp is applied across healthy bowel at a right angle, to give the smallest possible circumference of the proximal end. The dilated segment is then removed, the mesentery being sectioned as close to the bowel wall as possible, in order to guard against damage to the mesenteric vessels of the distal segment. The sectioned vessels are ligated with 6-0 silk. The distal bowel is searched for further intrinsic obstruction by the injection of air or saline into the bowel through a tiny needle. It is then prepared for anastomosis by placing a Kocher clamp across it at a 45 degree angle with the apex at the mesentery, about 5 cm from the site of the atresia. This maneuver provides a greater circumference of the small distal end, so that it is more easily approximated to the large upper end. When the discrepancy in size is very great, the distal bowel can be blown up by a gentle saline injection. In this way it can be made larger prior to the application of the clamp. A cut on the antimesenteric side can also be used to increase the

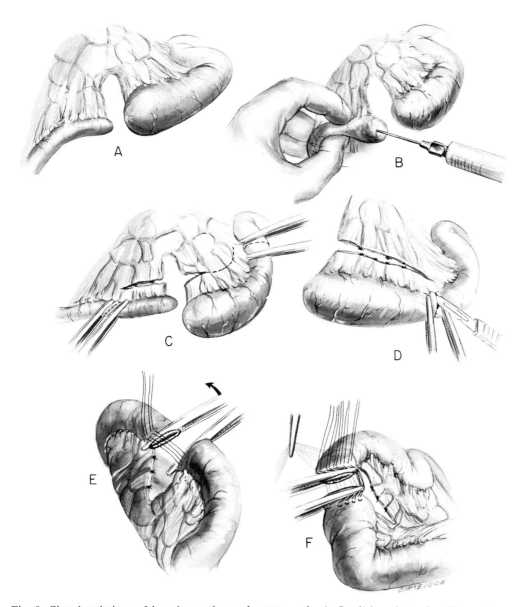

Fig. 8. Closed technique of bowel resection and anastomosis. A. Small bowel atresia with gap in mesentery. B. Dilation of the distal end with saline. C and D. Resection of the bulbous proximal and the smaller distal ends between Kocher clamps. E. Halsted sutures placed anteriorly. F. The loops of the sutures are put over the ends of the clamps when the posterior row is placed, in order to facilitate removal of the clamps without opening the bowel.

circumference, but this method necessitates the use of an open anastomosis rather than the closed aseptic type.

After resection of the bowel which is to be discarded, a one-layer aseptic anastomosis is made with 6-0 silk by the insertion of interrupted Halsted sutures (Fig. 8). The mesentery is closed with similar suture material, care being taken not to encircle or pierce any of the mesenteric vessels. Both sides of the mesentery must be closed to avoid leaving exposed irregular edges which may become the basis for adhesion formation and subsequent mechanical obstruction. As the bowel is returned to the abdomen, it should be arranged so that the possibility of postoperative volvulus or kinking is avoided as much as possible. The colon should usually lie in an anterior and superior position in the abdomen, with the ileocecal region in the right midabdomen opposite the umbilicus. Closure of the abdomen in layers

using interrupted 5-0 silk is completed with a 5-0 catgut running subcuticular suture, and the wound is covered with a thin layer of collodion.

Resection with end-to-end anastomosis is now advocated by many surgeons. Benson (1960), Louw (1966), Swenson and Fisher (1960), and several other students of intestinal atresia have published their results with this technique. Some authors use the Mikulicz procedure or methods which leave a safety vent at or below the anastomosis. Gross (1963) has long advocated the Mikulicz enterostomy, in which, after resection of the atresia, the limbs of the bowel are united in a side-to-side manner and brought out as a double-barreled stoma. When the resulting spur is crushed by a special clamp 5 to 10 days after the procedure, bowel transit is reestablished, and the resulting fistula can be removed by a minor operation. The advantage of this method is that it avoids the

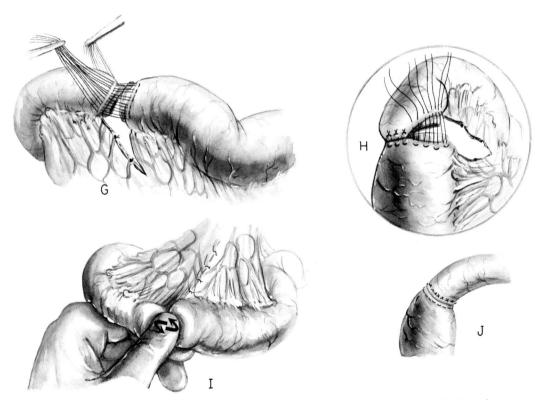

Fig. 8 (cont.). Closed technique of bowel resection and anastomosis. G. Drawing up the bowel ends. H. Bowel inversion produced by Halsted sutures. I. Rolling the anastomosis to be sure the bowel is not sutured shut. J. The completed anastomosis.

catastrophic effects of distal obstruction upon a primary anastomosis. On the other hand, it requires two operations, the fluid losses from the stoma may be difficult to manage, and in some of the cases the peristalsis returns only slowly, perhaps because of the serositis which necessarily occurs in the exposed ends of the bowel.

Side-to-side anastomoses are tempting, since they are easy to accomplish, but they have been given up because so frequently the proximal end has dilated to form a large, partially obstructed stagnant pocket. Serious nutritional deficits result from bacterial overgrowth in this pocket. The resulting blind-loop syndrome can be cured by resection and end-to-end anastomosis.

End-to-side anastomosis, with the distal bowel being brought out as an enterostomy, has been used increasingly since its description by Bishop and Koop in 1957 (Fig. 9). It has several advantages, among them the ease of making an anastomosis between segments of bowel which are greatly disparate in size, the probability that at least some of the intestinal content will progress into the distal bowel, and the presence of a safety vent in case the activity of the narrowed distal bowel remains sluggish. The resulting fistula is closed by a minor procedure when the intestine has regained its function. In our opinion, the end-to-side vented anastomosis is the method of choice for the treatment of intestinal atresia when it appears to be unsafe to accomplish a primary end-to-end anastomosis.

POSTOPERATIVE CARE

The postoperative care includes continuation of the antibiotics, intravenous fluids con-

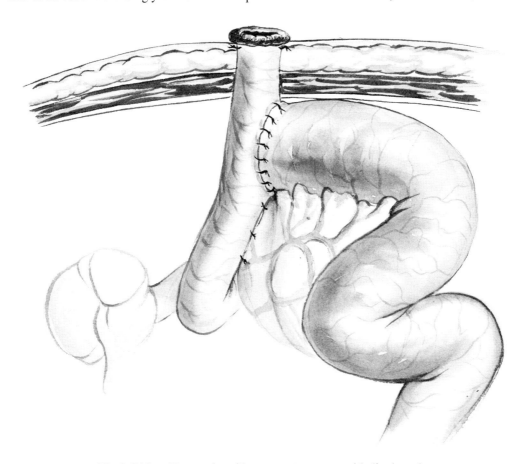

Fig. 9. Bishop-Koop end-to-side enteroenterostomy with distal venting.

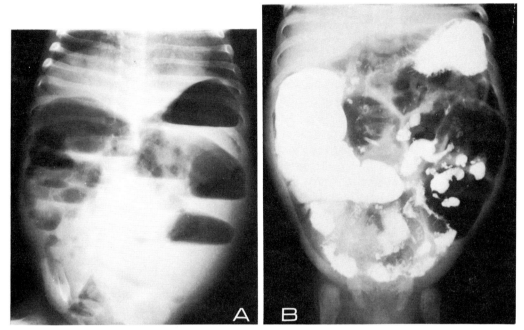

Fig. 10. A. Symptoms of intestinal stenosis occur later in infancy. B. The proximal bowel may become enormously dilated.

taining salt at the rate of 1,100 to 1,500 ml per M² per day, and also nasogastric suction by a small plastic indwelling catheter until the returned fluid has been free of bile for 24 hours and the infant has passed one or more stools. Cautious feedings of glucose water are begun at the rate of $\frac{1}{2}$ ounce every hour, and the baby is rapidly advanced to full formula feeding within 2 to 3 days.

COMPLICATIONS

The complications of surgery for small bowel atresia are many. Pulmonary difficul-

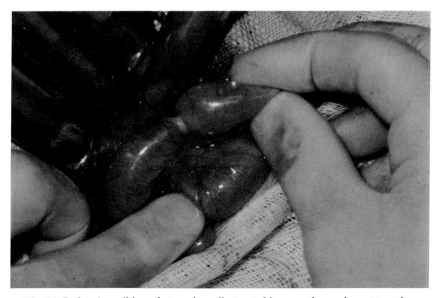

Fig. 11. Isolated small bowel stenosis easily treated by resection and anastomosis.

ties are frequent, partly because of the vomiting and aspiration which may occur post-operatively. They are treated by pharyngeal suctioning, antibiotics, and humidification. Mild wound infections are not uncommon, but these usually clear up well with warm soaks. When leakage at the anastomosis occurs, it becomes evident four to five days post-operatively and produces local or general peritonitis. A new intestinal obstruction almost always develops, and there is usually formation of a fistula to the wound. This disaster is managed by continuing the naso-gastric suction and by culture of the resulting wound infection so that a change to more specific antibiotic therapy can be accomplished. Early reoperation after treatment with antibiotics and blood is wise because of the serious infection which develops in the obstructed area. When free anastomotic leaks develop it is rare to salvage the baby either by operation or conservative management, but operation has the advantage that the anastomosis can be brought out as double-barreled ileostomy or jejunostomy, preventing further peritoneal contamination and often relieving the obstruction which inevitably develops.

If serious diarrhea develops when full-strength formulas are administered, the baby should be managed by special monosaccharide low-fat feedings as outlined in Chapter 34.

PROGNOSIS

The prognosis of jejunoileal atresia has been improving steadily. Louw (1966) treated 33 patients between 1955 and 1965 and had only 3 deaths, a survival rate of 91 percent. In his last 26 cases the survival rate was 96 percent. Swenson and Fisher in 1960 reported an 82 percent survival in 11 infants treated by resection and primary end-to-end anastomosis as did Benson and his colleagues in 1960. The percentage of survivals in large centers in the United States remains at between 60 to 80 percent. This percentage can undoubtedly be improved by attention to the details of surgical procedure which have been emphasized by experienced authors.

STENOSIS OF THE SMALL INTESTINE

Small bowel stenosis is less common, and the symptoms associated with it are usually later in onset than those associated with atresia. The vomiting is not as severe, and the abdomen is not usually grossly distended. Poor feeding and slow weight gain are the cardinal manifestations. Chronic diarrhea with the clinical picture of malabsorption may occur. The diagnosis is made by upper gastrointestinal contrast studies (Fig. 10), and the treatment is excision of the stenotic area followed by end-to-end anastomosis (Fig. 11). The outcome of such surgical therapy is excellent. Excision of a stenosing intraluminal web without resection of the entire segment has not always had good results, and it should not be done in an attempt to simplify the operation.

WILLIAM L. DONNELLAN

REFERENCES

BARNARD, C. N., and LOUW, J. H. The genesis of intestinal atresia. Minn. Med. 39: 745, 1956.
BARONOFSKY, I. D. Primary end-to-end anastomosis for congenital atresia of the small bowel. Surgery, 30: 841, 1951.
BAY-NIELSEN, H., and MOUTZOURIS, C. Intestinal atresia; 47 consecutive cases. Danish Med. Bull., 10: 71, 1963.
BENSON, C. D., LLOYD, J. R., and SMITH, J. D. Resection and primary anastomosis in the management of stenosis and atresia of the jejunum and ileum. Pediatrics, 26: 265, 1960.

BISHOP, H. C., and KOOP, C. E. Management of meconium ileus. Ann. Surg., 145: 410, 1957.

BOGGS, T. R., Jr., and BISHOP, H. Neonatal hyperbilirubinemia associated with high obstruction of the small bowel. J. Pediat., 66: 349, 1965.

CLATWORTHY, H. W., Jr., and LLOYD, J. R. Intestinal obstruction of congenital origin. A study of diagnosis and management in one hundred sixty-three cases. Arch. Surg. (Chicago), 75: 880, 1957.

CLAWSON, D. K. Side-to-side intestinal anastomosis complicated by ulceration, dilatation and anemia: A physiologically unsound procedure. Surgery, 34: 254, 1953.

DICKINSON, S. J. Origin of intestinal atresia of newborn. J.A.M.A., 190: 119, 1964.

ECKSTEIN, H. B. Weights of children with major congenital abnormalities of the intestinal tract. Arch. Dis. Child, 38: 173, 1963.

EVANS, C. H. Atresias of the gastrointestinal tract. Int. Abstr. Surg., 92: 1, 1951.

FOCKENS, P. Ein operativ geheilter Fall von kongenitaler Dündarmatresie. Zbl. Chir., 38: 532, 1911.

GHERARDI, G. J., and FISHER, J. H. Atresia of the small intestine produced by intussusception in utero. New Eng. J. Med., 264: 229, 1961.

GROB, M. Intestinal obstruction in the newborn infant. Arch. Dis. Child., 35: 40, 1960.

HANDLESMAN, J. C., ABRAMS, S., and CORRY, R. J. Improvement of therapy for congenital jejunoileal atresia. Surg. Gynec. Obstet., 117: 691, 1963.

HARRIS, R. C., LUCEY, J. F., and MacLEAN, J. R. Kernicterus in premature infants associated with low concentration of bilirubin in the plasma. Pediatrics, 21: 875, 1958.

HOLSCLAW, D. S., ECKSTEIN, H. B., and NIXON, H. H. Meconium ileus. A 20 year review of 109 cases. Amer. J. Dis. Child., 109: 101, 1965.

JOHNSON, F. P. The development of the mucous membrane of the esophagus, stomach and small intestine in the human embryo. Amer. J. Anat., 10: 521, 1910.

KREMEN, A. J., LINNER, J. H., and NELSON, C. H. An experimental evaluation of the nutritional importance of proximal and distal small intestine. Ann. Surg., 140: 439, 1954.

LADD, W. E., and GROSS, R. E. Abdominal Surgery of Infancy and Childhood. Philadelphia, W. B. Saunders Co., 1941, p. 41.

LLOYD, J. R., and CLATWORTHY, H. W. Hydramnios as an aid to the early diagnosis of congenital obstruction of the alimentary tract. A study of the maternal and fetal factors. Pediatrics, 21: 903, 1958.

LOUW, J. H. Jejunoileal atresia and stenosis. J. Pediat. Surg., 1: 8, 1966.

———— and BARNARD, C. N. Congenital intestinal atresia, observations on its origin and treatment. Lancet, 2: 1065, 1955.

LYNN, H. B., and ESPINAS, E. E. Intestinal atresia: An attempt to relate location to embryologic processes. Arch. Surg. (Chicago), 79: 357, 1959.

McKAY, R. J., Jr. Current status of use of exchange transfusion in newborn infants. Pediatrics, 33: 763, 1964.

NIXON, H. H. Experimental study of propulsion in isolated small intestine and applications to surgery in newborn. Ann. Roy. Coll. Surg. Eng., 27: 105, 1960.

———— Intestinal obstruction in the newborn. Arch. Dis. Child., 30: 13, 1955.

PARKKULAINEN, K. V. Simple low small bowel obstruction. Arch. Dis. Child., 38: 124, 1963.

PHELAN, J. T., LEMMER, K. E., and McDONOUGH, K. B. Jejunoileal atresia and stenosis. Surgery, 46: 430, 1959.

PILLING, G. P., and CRESSEN, S. L. Massive resection of the small intestine in the neonatal period; report of two successful cases and review of the literature. Pediatrics, 19: 940, 1957.

POLLOCK, W. F., and BERGIN, W. F. Management of intestinal atresia at the Los Angeles Children's Hospital. Amer. J. Surg., 102: 202, 1961.

RANDOLPH, J. G., ZOLLINGER, R. M., Jr., and GROSS, R. E. Mikulicz resection in infants and children: A 20 year survey of 196 patients. Ann. Surg., 158: 481, 1963.

REILLY, R. W., and KIRSNER, J. B. The blind loop syndrome. Gastroenterology, 37: 491, 1959.

RICHARDSON, W. R. The role and management of enterostomy in intestinal obstruction in infants. Amer. J. Surg., 106: 581, 1963.

SANTULLI, T. V., and BLANC, W. A. Congenital atresia of the intestine. Pathogenesis and treatment. Ann. Surg., 154: 939, 1961.

SCOTT, J. E. S. Intestinal obstruction in the newborn associated with peritonitis. Arch. Dis. Child., 38: 120, 1963.

SWAIN, V. A. J., PEONIDES, A., and YOUNG, W. F. Prognosis after resection of small bowel in the newborn. Arch. Dis. Child., 38: 103, 1963.

SWENSON, O., and DAVIDSON, F. Z. Similarities of mechanical intestinal obstruction and aganglionic megacolon in the newborn infant. New Eng. J. Med., 262: 64, 1960.

———— and FISHER, J. H. Small bowel atresia: Treatment by resection and primary aseptic anastomosis. Surgery, 47: 823, 1960.

TANDLER, J. Zur Entwicklungsgeschichte des menschlichen Duodenum in Frühen Embryonalstadien. Morphol. Jahrb., 29: 187, 1900.

38

Meckel's Diverticulum

A Meckel's diverticulum is the most common congenital abnormality of the intestines. This anomaly was described in detail by Meckel in 1808, but it had been noted previously by other authors. Its clinical importance lies in the fact that its lining may contain gastric mucosa rather than the mucosa of the ileum from which it arises. Acid-pepsin digestive juices are often formed by the aberrant gastric mucosa in sufficient quantity to cause ulceration of the contiguous ileal mucosa, with resultant hemorrhage. In addition the diverticulum may invert and become the leading point of an intussusception. Sometimes (but in our experience very rarely) it becomes obstructed and inflamed in much the same manner as appendicitis. It is curious that these catastrophes are not unusually common, in view of the fact that a Meckel's diverticulum is present in 2 percent of all individuals.

EMBRYOLOGY

During the earliest stages of life the primitive gut is formed by the differentiation of entodermal cells from the inner cell mass within the cystlike blastocoele of the developing ovum. These entodermal cells form a circular pattern, the *yolk sac*, which is separated from another cavity in the blastocoele, the *amnion*, by the embryonic disc. This latter structure is composed of cells which differentiate into the mesoderm, or investing cell layer, and the ectoderm, which is destined to form the skin and its related appendages.

Soon after the formation of the yolk sac and amnion both of these structures are invested by supporting cells, or *mesenchyme*, which is derived from the mesodermal layer (Fig. 1).

About the third week of life differential growth of the embryonic disc results in a folding of the body about the yolk sac. The ectoderm with its investing somatopleure grows somewhat more rapidly than the entoderm, and both grow much more rapidly than the cells of the yolk sac. The result is a progressive narrowing of the neck of the yolk sac and an infolding of the body about the foregut, midgut, and hindgut of the gastrointestinal tract (Fig. 2). That portion of the yolk sac which remains in association with the body stalk (proximal portion of the umbilical cord) is eventually called the *"omphalomesenteric duct,"* since it runs from the umbilicus to the midgut, ending on the antimesenteric border of the small intestine about two feet above the ileocecal valve. In most of the cases this primitive remnant atrophies and disappears, leaving the intestine free of any attachment to the umbilicus. Occasionally a cord or even an open duct may remain, and more often (in 2 percent of individuals) a Meckel's diverticulum is present at the site of the original connection of the yolk sac with the primitive gut.

PATHOLOGY

Meckel's diverticula arise on the antimesenteric border of the lower ileum. While

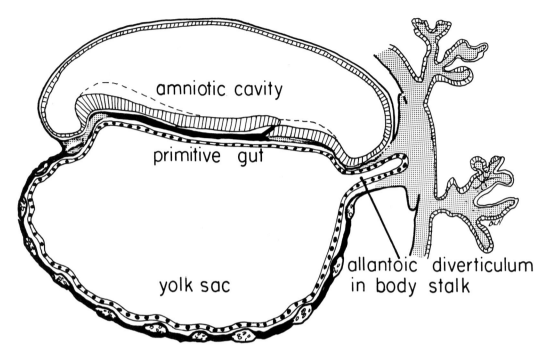

Fig. 1. Amnion and yolk sac in early embryo. The mesenchyme begins to invest these structures.

diverticula lying within the mesentery have been reported, it is very rare for them to be found there, and in most of the cases it can be shown that an antimesenteric diverticulum has simply been folded over and held by a peritoneal overgrowth. This point is of some importance surgically since the intramesenteric diverticulum requires a different type of excision than does the usual type.

The *blood supply* of the diverticulum is derived from the vitelline arteries—paired vessels which run on each side of the mesentery to surround the vitelline duct and ramify on the yolk sac. It is believed that the left vitelline artery normally atrophies and that the right goes on to form the superior mesenteric artery. When vitelline remnants such as a Meckel's diverticulum or an om-

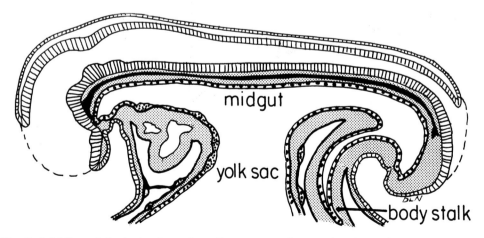

Fig. 2. Infolding of the body about the yolk sac to produce a closed anterior abdominal wall.

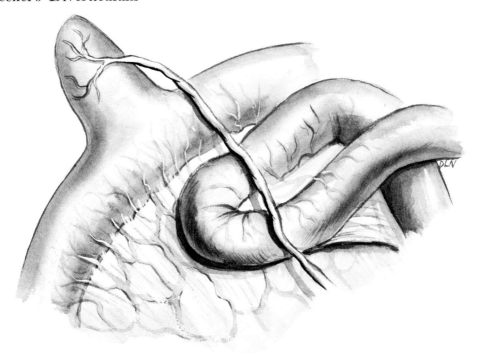

Fig. 3. The mesodiverticular band (persistent right vitelline artery separated from the mesentery) may lead to small bowel herniation and obstruction.

phalomesenteric duct persist, they are sup- plied by the right vitelline artery, which arises as an end-artery from the superior mesenteric. Occasionally this vessel is sepa- rated from the main portion of the mesentery as a mesodiverticular band, and bowel may become trapped beneath it to produce intes- tinal obstruction (Fig. 3).

Heterotopic tissue is present in about 50 percent of Meckel's diverticula. In 148 spec- imens reported by Rutherford and Akers (1966), 57 percent of the surgical specimens had heterotopic tissue, as compared to an in- cidence of only 6 percent in those diverticula which were discovered at autopsy. The types of aberrant tissue and the number of cases in which they appeared were as follows:

Gastric mucosa	51
Pancreatic tissue	10
Colonic mucosa	2
Jejunal mucosa	1
Duodenal mucosa	1

The number of specimens containing two or more types of heterotopic tissue is not men-

tioned by Rutherford and Akers, but such multiplicity appears to be infrequent. Car- cinoid tumors, which have been reported very occasionally in Meckel's diverticula,

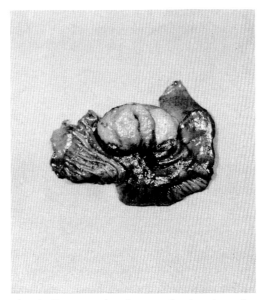

Fig. 4. Deep peptic ulcer at the junction of a Meckel's diverticulum with the ileum.

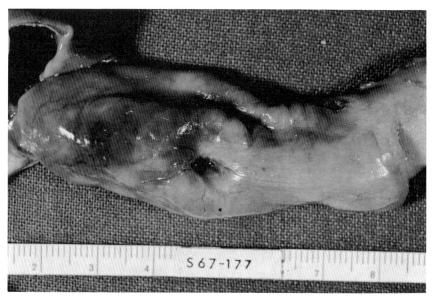

Fig. 5. Inversion of a Meckel's diverticulum to produce an intussusception, which has been reduced.

are responsible for most of the cases of malignant change.

A common complication of Meckel's diverticulum is the development of a peptic ulcer at the junction of the gastric and ileal mucosa (Fig. 4). The ulcers are deep, and significant bleeding occurs by erosion of a major artery in the intestinal wall. Like most intestinal bleeding, it is usually self-limited because of the reduction of arterial pressure and the contractility of the splanchnic vessels. The crater of the ulcer fills with blood, and the vessel is occluded by a clot which goes on to organization. Digestion of the clot may occur after the initial cessation of bleeding, with resultant secondary hemorrhage when the arterial pressure returns to normal.

Intestinal obstruction is the second most

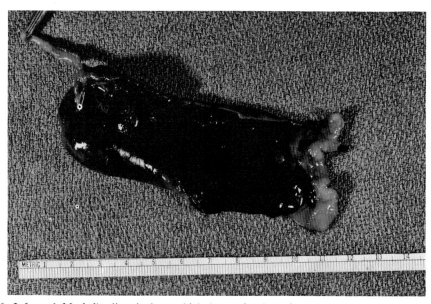

Fig. 6. Infarcted Meckel's diverticulum which has twisted on its omphalomesenteric connection.

common complication. It occurs as the result of fixation of the tip of the diverticulum by a vitelloumbilical band (obliterated omphalomesenteric duct), inflammatory adhesions resulting from perforation, inversion of the diverticulum to produce an intussusception (Fig. 5), herniation of bowel beneath a mesodiverticular band (or a free vitelline artery), and incarceration of the diverticulum in a hernia. The latter complication, the so-called Littre's hernia, is a rare occurrence. Intussusception of the proximal small intestine into a widely patent persistent omphalomesenteric duct has also been recorded.

Inflammation unrelated to peptic ulceration is a very rare complication of Meckel's diverticulum. It is often taught that the surgeon should search for an inflamed Meckel's diverticulum when the appendix in a suspected case of appendicitis has been found to be normal. True suppurative Meckel's diverticulitis, however, is rare. The diverticulum is usually wider at its base that at its tip, and therefore it does not become obstructed and inflamed as does the appendix. Ruther-

ford and Akers describe only 4 cases in a 25-year experience. It is true, however, that the base of the diverticulum may perforate as the result of peptic ulceration or that it

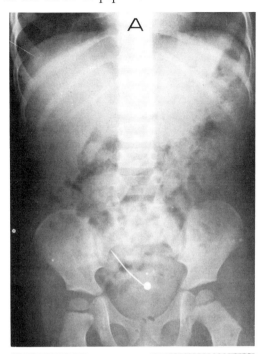

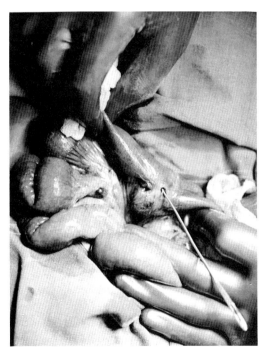

Fig. 7. Perforated peptic ulcer at the base of a Meckel's diverticulum.

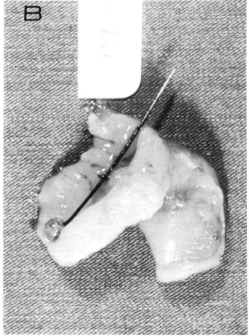

Fig. 8. A. Pin which failed to progress in the intestinal tract. B. The pin is held by a Meckel's diverticulum.

may become infarcted by twisting about a vitelloumbilical band. These events may produce the symptoms of appendicitis (Fig. 6).

Perforation with generalized peritonitis is rare. It might be expected that this occurrence would be more frequent, since the diverticulum lies quite free in the peritoneal cavity. The cause of perforation, however, is the peptic ulcer which almost invariably lies in the ileum at the lower border of the diverticulum (Fig. 7). The accompanying inflammation usually leads to the walling off of a localized abscess before the perforation is complete. Obstruction due to abscess formation is more likely to occur than free perforation with generalized peritonitis. In the reported series there has been no special predilection for perforation in any particular age group.

An interesting complication of Meckel's diverticulum is the incarceration of a foreign body within the sac. We have encountered a child with a needle trapped in the diverticulum. Whenever a foreign body does not progress in the midabdomen, this possibility should be considered (Fig. 8).

SIGNS AND SYMPTOMS

Rectal bleeding is the most common presenting symptom. In a collective review of 1,605 cases of Meckel's diverticulum Moses (1947) found that 30.9 percent of the cases presented in this manner. The bleeding is usually severe, and symptoms of shock are not unusual. The admitting hemoglobin level in most series averages about 7.5 percent, with values as high as 11.6 g percent and as low as 3.5 g percent in the individual case. According to Rutherford and Akers, anemia due to *occult* bleeding is rare in Meckel's diverticulum. In 40 percent of the cases previous frank rectal bleeding was recorded, but in all but 2 cases the symptom which finally led to operation was a single discrete episode of bleeding. Bright red bleeding with clots is less frequent than dark red blood. Tarry stools alone occur even less frequently. Often, however, a mixture of all three types is noted during the course of the bleeding episode. The blood loss is likely to be relatively more severe and the hematocrit less in infants under 2 years of age than it is in older children. Boys are more often affected than girls, in the ratio of three to one.

Pain, except for peristaltic cramps, is not a common feature of the bleeding Meckel's diverticulum. While there may be slight tenderness in the midabdomen just below and to the right of the umbilicus, this sign is not a reliable one. In the presence of obstruction, strangulation, or intussusception, the pain is more likely to be generalized.

The signs of *intestinal obstruction* are present in about 20 percent of the cases. Abdominal distension, green vomitus, and generalized abdominal pain are the usual manifestations. A mass may or may not be palpable. If present it signifies either intussusception or an inflammation about a perforated diverticulum. A child of more than 12 months of age who has sharp rectal bleeding followed by the signs of intestinal obstruction probably has a Meckel's diverticulum as the leading point of an intussusception.

In summary, the signs of a symptomatic Meckel's diverticulum are those of rectal bleeding, intestinal obstruction or peritonitis, and intussusception. Occasionally all of these are combined. The bleeding is usually massive and single, and it ceases spontaneously. Very occasionally exsanguination can occur, as reported by Rutherford (1966). There may be a history of previous episodes of bleeding. Chronic blood loss leading to hypochromic anemia, however, is rare. The intestinal obstruction is due to an intussusception in most of the cases, an edematous or inverted diverticulum acting as the leading point. In the rest it is caused either by a herniation, volvulus, or perforation of a peptic ulcer at the base of the diverticulum which goes on to local abscess formation with subsequent obstruction. Pain occurs in less than 25 percent of the cases. When present its etiology is about equally divided between the abdominal cramps associated with bleeding and the pain which is produced by one of the obstructive complications.

LABORATORY FINDINGS

Anemia associated with bleeding from a Meckel's diverticulum is usually moderate to severe. Over 60 percent of the patients have a hemoglobin level less than 8 g percent on admission. In the series of Rutherford and Akers the admitting hemoglobin level of infants under 2 years of age averaged 6.6 g percent, compared to 8.8 g percent in older children. The anemia is usually normochromic in nature, since chronic bleeding from the diverticulum does not often occur.

Leukocytosis is usually found. In the presence of a bleeding diverticular ulcer it is mild and represents moderate inflammation about the ulcer. If an abscess or a strangulating obstruction is present, the white count is almost always elevated above 20,000.

Blood in the stools is common. There is no characteristic finding. Red clots within the stools, dark red blood coating the stools, and tarry stools have all been recorded. According to Jewett and Butsch (1959), the stools should be studied for occult blood in all children with unexplained crampy abdominal pain. If the association of cramps and bleeding can be demonstrated, the diagnosis of Meckel's diverticulum can be made. In our experience this association usually indicates a *surgical* lesion, but not necessarily a Meckel's diverticulum.

Radiographic findings are those of the complications of the diverticulum, which itself is rarely visualized by contrast studies. Intussusception, intestinal obstruction, and only very occasionally intraperitoneal free air are the positive x-ray findings, but quite clearly these can be produced by many other lesions of the gastrointestinal tract.

DIFFERENTIAL DIAGNOSIS

Meckel's diverticulum has been called "the abdominal masquerader" by Jewett and Butsch. It produces symptoms as the result of its complications, each of which has its own characteristic symptom complex. For this reason the diagnosis is rarely made prior to operation. According to C. W. Mayo, (1933) "Meckel's diverticulum is frequently suspected, often looked for, and seldom found." This dictum is a good one.

In the presence of intestinal obstruction or worsening signs of peritonitis, abdominal exploration is indicated. Here there is no difficulty in making the decision to operate if the requisite surgical indications are present. If a Meckel's diverticulum is found to be the cause of the condition, it should be dealt with. Unexplained rectal bleeding, however, presents a more complicated problem.

Exploratory operations to find the source of intestinal bleeding when adequate preoperative investigations have been performed are just as likely not to reveal the source of the bleeding as they are to do so. In a group of 801 patients studied by Shandling (1965), 61 infants and children were subjected to abdominal exploration after the performance of unrevealing contrast radiographic examinations, proctosigmoidoscopy, and coagulation studies. In 31 of these children no source of bleeding could be identified at operation (Fig. 5). Exactly similar statistics are provided by Spencer (1964). In her series of 476 cases of gastrointestinal hemorrhage, the source of bleeding was found in only 14 of 28 patients explored. In all series the *usual* abnormality causing significant rectal bleeding of obscure origin is a Meckel's diverticulum with associated peptic ulceration, but it should be emphasized that this lesion is found in only one third of the children coming to exploratory operation.

The first step in making the diagnosis of a bleeding Meckel's diverticulum is to determine what is significant rectal bleeding. A distinct fall in the hemoglobin content to below 9.0 g percent should be present. By eliminating the anal fissure, which produces only slight streaking on the stools, 9 out of 10 of the cases are disposed of. Proctoscopy will reveal some cases of inflammatory mucosal bleeding, whether of infectious or idiopathic etiology. Of the remaining possible causes, polyps only occasionally cause severe bleeding, and esophageal varices or peptic ulceration can usually be demonstrated by radiographic examination of the upper gastrointestinal tract. When the above studies are nonrevealing, the patient has one chance in three of having a bleeding Meckel's diverticulum.

MANAGEMENT OF BLEEDING THOUGHT TO BE DUE TO MECKEL'S DIVERTICULUM

Since the bleeding from a Meckel's diverticulum usually ceases spontaneously, the condition is not an emergency. The child with rectal bleeding is put to bed, and an intravenous route is established. Plasma or blood transfusions (10 ml per pound) will help to stabilize the vital signs, if it is thought necessary to do so, but these should not be used routinely. A Levin tube in the stomach serves to rule out esophageal bleeding. In most of the cases continued bleeding is manifested by the frequent discharge of bloody stools, mild to severe abdominal cramps, and a rising pulse rate. The hemoglobin falls progressively if plasma is given to maintain the blood pressure. Usually the rectal bleeding ceases, and the hemoglobin stabilizes at about 8.0 g percent.

It is our practice not to explore the abdomen for rectal bleeding until the following conditions have been met:

(1) Fall in hemoglobin to below 6.0 g percent.

(2) Negative proctosigmoidoscopy and barium enema.

(3) Negative upper gastrointestinal series.

(4) Normal hemogram and coagulation studies.

(5) Recurrence of rectal bleeding on at least one occasion to a hemoglobin level below 8.0 g percent.

Children tolerate reduction of the hemoglobin content to 6.0 g percent rather well.

If the level falls below this figure, or if transfusions equivalent to 50 percent of the blood volume are required to maintain an adequate circulation, emergency conditions exist. *Before undertaking an exploratory laparotomy the surgeon must assure himself that the lower colon is not the source of the bleeding, and that esophageal varices are not present.*

When the bleeding ceases and the hemoglobin level remains above 8.0 g percent, it is our opinion that nothing need be done other than a complete radiographic and medical investigation. If a serious lesion is present it will be revealed radiographically, or it will cause renewed bleeding. The child should be examined at one- to two-week intervals for a time, with emphasis on the hematocrit and the presence of occult blood in the stools. If occult bleeding continues, repeat radiographic studies and a hemogram are indicated at the end of the month.

When operation seems necessary, *restoration of the blood volume and hemoglobin are of utmost importance.* Bowel anastomoses heal poorly in the presence of anemia or hypovolemia. It may be necessary to use packed cells to restore the hemoglobin content if a great deal of plasma has been used prior to operation to support the circulation. Retransfusion of whole blood in the amount of 10 ml per pound of body weight can be safely accomplished within 2 hours in all cases, and the remainder is given during and after the operation.

OPERATIVE TECHNIQUE

A McBurney type incision is adequate for the surgical treatment of most cases of Meckel's diverticulum. If necessary it can be extended transversely across the rectus sheaths. Some surgeons prefer to use a right rectus muscle-retracting incision, since it provides greater freedom for abdominal exploration if a diverticulum is not present. The bleeding diverticulum is usually found to be free of adhesions, and it can be drawn into the wound quite easily. Intussusception and perforated diverticula can also be brought out by a McBurney incision in most of the cases.

It is best to locate the cecum first and then to draw out the ileocecal junction. By following the small bowel proximally the surgeon will find diverticulum lying on its antimesenteric border about 18 to 36 inches from the ileocecal valve. The bleeding diverticulum may have slight inflammation of its serosa, or it may be moderately edematous and thickened at its base. A bluish color within the bowel distal to it testifies to the presence of blood in the intestinal lumen.

A bleeding diverticulum should be excised rather widely because it almost invariably contains gastric mucosa which must not be left behind. A wide "V" excision leaving the mesenteric border of the ileum is satisfactory if care is taken to excise the ulcer, which is always outside the area of gastric mucosa. Occasionally a formal small bowel resection and anastomosis are required. In both cases a one-layer anastomosis with 5-0 silk can be done over the clamps, or a two-layer open

anastomosis is accomplished. In children the latter is best done with 5-0 chromic catgut for the mucosa and 5-0 or 6-0 silk Halsted sutures to the seromuscular layer.

The asymptomatic Meckel's diverticulum found incidentally at operation for some other condition can be transected at its base, followed by an oblique two-layer closure, since less than 10 percent of these diverticula contain aberrant types of mucosa. In most cases, however, it is still preferable to perform a standard type of excision and closure as illustrated in Figure 9.

When perforation with local abscess formation is present, the entire complex should be excised. Healthy bowel is selected on both sides of the inflammatory process and is transected between clamps. The diverticulum is sufficiently far from the ileocecal valve that an excellent blood supply remains at both ends of the bowel to be anastomosed. It is important to visualize the vessels at the root of the mesentery while the bowel is being removed. A rather shallow excision of

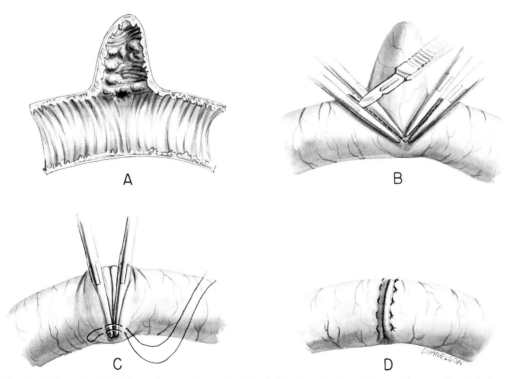

A   B

C   D

Fig. 9. A through D. Wide wedge excision of a Meckel's diverticulum. Closure by aseptic technique.

mesentery about the inflammatory mass can usually be accomplished safely.

If a Meckel's diverticulum is found to be the leading point of an intussusception, the invagination should be reduced in the usual way (see Ch. 42). If complete reduction is possible the decision must be made whether or not resection of the diverticulum is a safe procedure. Often the bowel about it is somewhat blue, edematous, and even friable. Under these conditions incision into it is unsafe. It should be returned to the abdomen and viewed again after it has been incubated there for about 10 minutes. Usually a pinkish-violet color will have returned to the affected segment and the mesenteric vessels about it will be pulsating. This type of bowel can be safely left in place, but removal of the diverticulum is unwise.

If the bowel fails to regain color and peristalsis and the mesenteric vessels are not pulsating, two courses are possible. The abdomen may be closed and the patient followed carefully for signs of intestinal gangrene. This is a dangerous procedure. It is surgically sound, and far safer, to accomplish resection of the affected segment. Usually healthy bowel is present several inches above the ileocecal valve and one or more feet above the diverticulum. It is divided and anastomosed between clamps. (This sequence of events is rare, since bowel which is strangulated in an intussusception usually cannot be reduced. If reduction of the intussusception is difficult, the procedure should be abandoned and a resection and anastomosis of healthy bowel to the terminal ileum or to the transverse colon should be done instead.)

The Mikulicz exteriorization procedure is recommended by some authors as a satisfactory method for the treatment of strangulation obstructions associated with a Meckel's diverticulum. It is our opinion that it is safer to accomplish a definitive procedure at the first operation. In desperate cases of perforation with generalized peritonitis the affected segments of bowel should be excised between clamps, and if an anastomosis appears impossible, the upper end of the bowel can be brought out as an end ileostomy. Under these conditions the lower end can be safely oversewn and dropped back into the abdomen, or it can be brought through the abdominal wall just below the skin. The child is then treated with massive antibiotic therapy [we prefer the bactericidal drugs, polymyxin B, cephalothin (Keflin), and kanamycin in appropriate doses] together with frequent transfusions of blood and plasma as required to maintain the venous pressure between 13 and 15 cm of water. When herniation or volvulus are produced by adhesions related to a Meckel's diverticulum the bowel should be reduced and the band and the diverticulum removed.

POSTOPERATIVE COMPLICATIONS

The complications of operation for Meckel's diverticulum are infrequent. They are those of any intestinal procedure—wound abscesses, evisceration, postoperative bowel obstruction, pulmonary problems including atelectasis and pneumonia, septicemia, shock, and the development of fecal fistulas. The last usually result from attempts to anastomose unhealthy bowel ends after resection for an associated intussusception.

PROGNOSIS

Most series record mortality rates of 2 to 8 percent for symptomatic Meckel's diverticula. Many of the deaths result from delay in diagnosis and the development of advanced peritonitis with hypovolemia before surgical consultation is obtained. It is rare for a patient to be lost from bleeding alone, despite the fact that severe hemorrhagic shock is not infrequently encountered.

SUMMARY

Meckel's diverticulum occurs in about 2 percent of the population. Symptoms are most frequent in the 6- to 24-month age group. They are produced by complications of the lesion which derive from the presence of ectopic gastric or pancreatic mucosa. Occasionally an intussusception occurs by inversion of a normal diverticulum into the intestinal lumen, and sometimes persistence of the attachment of the diverticulum or its arterial supply to the umbilicus leads to bowel obstruction by herniation or a volvulus. The most common complication is bleeding from an associated peptic ulceration of the bowel contiguous to the gastric mucosa of the diverticulum. Unless strict criteria are adhered to, abdominal exploration for the presence of a bleeding Meckel's diverticulum will be unrewarding in 50 to 70 percent of the cases.

WILLIAM L. DONNELLAN

REFERENCES

BENSON, C. D., and LINKNER, L. M. The surgical complications of Meckel's diverticulum in infants and children; an analysis of sixty cases. Arch. Surg., 73: 393, 1956.

FREDERICK, P. L., and JOHNSON, E. T. Meckel's diverticulum in childhood; a review of 73 cases. Postgrad. Med., 34: 341, 1963.

JEWETT, T. C., Jr., and BUTSCH, W. L. Meckel's diverticulum: The abdominal masquerader. Surgery, 46: 440, 1959.

KIESEWETTER, W. B. Meckel's diverticulum in children. Arch. Surg., 75: 914, 1957.

LONGINO, L. A., and HOLDER, T. M. Rectal bleeding in infants and children. Pediat. Clin. N. Amer., 6: 1153, 1959.

MAYO, C. W. Meckel's diverticulum. Proc. Staff Meet. Mayo Clin., 8: 230, 1933.

McPARLAND, F. A., and KIESEWETTER, W. B.

Meckel's diverticulum in childhood. Surg., Gynec. Obstet., 106: 11, 1958.

MOSES, W. R. Meckel's diverticulum; Report of two unusual cases. New Eng. J. Med., 230: 118, 1947.

MOSKOVITZ, W. S., HUGHES, C. W., and BOWERS, W. F. Meckel's diverticulum; Varied surgical manifestations in twenty cases. Arch. Surg. (Chicago), 81: 36, 1960.

RUTHERFORD, R. B., and AKERS, D. R. Meckel's diverticulum: A review of 148 pediatric patients, with special reference to the pattern of bleeding and to mesodiverticular vascular bands. Surgery, 59: 618, 1966.

SHANDLING, B. Laparotomy for rectal bleeding. Pediatrics, 35: 787, 1965.

SPENCER, R. Gastrointestinal hemorrhage in infancy and childhood: 476 cases. Surgery, 55: 718, 1964.

39

Uncommon Forms of Neonatal Small Bowel Obstruction

Intestinal atresias or stenosis, meconium ileus, and aganglionosis of the intestinal tract are the most common causes of intestinal obstruction in early infancy. Volvulus of the bowel and sepsis are less frequent but important causes of neonatal obstruction. Other abnormalities causing obstruction are intussusception, internal hernias, congenital bands, acute appendicitis, and defective peristalsis in bowel which contains apparently normal ganglion cells. The last condition may result from intrinsic defects of the bowel musculature or its innervation, or from such medical conditions as congenital hypothyroidism, prematurity, or the treatment of the mother with ganglionic blocking drugs during late pregnancy and delivery.

INTESTINAL VOLVULUS IN THE NEWBORN INFANT

Volvulus of one or more loops of bowel is an importont though infrequent cause of neonatal intestinal obstruction. Because of the venous occlusion which occurs when the mesentery is twisted tightly on itself, a serious compromise of the circulation occurs. Volvulus usually results in bowel necrosis, shock, and early death.

PATHOLOGY

It should be emphasized that malrotation of the intestinal tract is not necessarily as-sociated with neonatal volvulus. Malrotation is more likely to cause duodenal obstruction in the newborn period. If the duodenal obstruction is not severe, a massive midgut volvulus may subsequently occur as the result of associated abnormalities of fixation of the small bowel mesentery to the posterior abdominal wall. In most of the reported series of neonatal volvulus, malrotation is one of the common associated abnormalities, although meconium ileus or intestinal atresia may also be related to the production of a volvulus. The association of intestinal atresia and volvulus has been emphasized by Louw (1966), who states that redundancy of the mesentery of the small intestine is present in more than half of babies coming to operation for intestinal atresia. Conversely, atresia should be expected to be present in a proportion of the cases of volvulus. It is for this reason that the patency of the entire bowel must be confirmed after reduction of the volvulus. Persistence of the omphalomesenteric duct and the presence of duplications, intestinal polyps, or mesenteric cysts may occasionally lead to volvulus by acting as points of rotation of the bowel mesentery. While massive venous engorgement with mucosal congestion and bleeding is usual in the affected portion of the bowel, sometimes the arterial supply is also cut off at the time of the occlusion. The bowel in such cases is white, collapsed, and aperistaltic. In most of the cases it is distended, dark purple in color, and friable (Fig. 1). Micro-

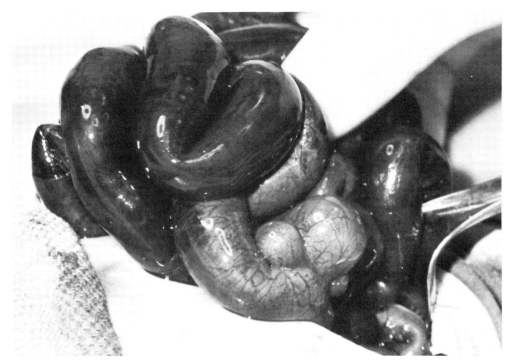

Fig. 1. Massive midgut volvulus with devitalization of bowel.

scopically, there is venous congestion, mucosal necrosis, and hemorrhage into all layers of the intestinal wall.

mesentery, or of lesions of the bowel or mesentery which produce trapping of the loop in a twisted position.

ETIOLOGY

The common etiologic factor in intestinal volvulus is *poor fixation or excessive redundancy* of the mesentery. In most of the cases of massive midgut volvulus the mesentery is unfixed to the posterior abdominal wall, and the cecum and ileum rotate freely on the narrowed mesenteric base which is formed only by the width of the superior mesenteric vessels (Fig. 2). The Christmas tree deformity, named from the resemblance of the small bowel to the decorations on a Christmas tree, is associated with high jejunal atresia and a defective proximal mesentery. The distal small bowel curls about the feeding mesenteric vessels in such cases and is therefore easily rotated en masse to produce complete vascular and intestinal occlusion. More localized forms of volvulus are the result of redundancy of only a portion of the

DIAGNOSIS

The characteristic symptoms of intestinal volvulus in the newborn are those of progressive high intestinal obstruction: feeding difficulties, episodic emesis, and finally the vomiting of bile-stained material. The infants are usually past the second day of life. Bright blood or clots may be passed per rectum, since the intestinal lumen often remains patent during the initial stages of mucosal venous congestion and bleeding. Abdominal distension is less than with most other forms of neonatal occlusion because the obstruction is generally high in the abdomen, often at the ligament of Treitz. Passage of normal meconium has usually occurred prior to the onset of the obstruction, except in those patients with an associated atresia or other congenital obstructive lesion.

With massive volvulus the signs of shock

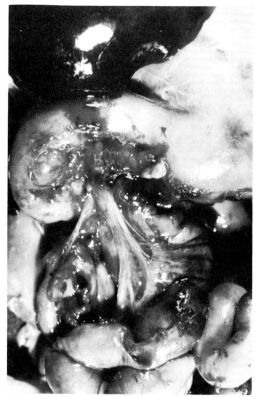

Fig. 2. Narrowed mesenteric base as a cause of volvulus.

fluid levels are present, and the appearance is easily confused with that of obstruction due to an intussusception or an internal hernia.

TREATMENT

Operative treatment requires inspection of the entire gastrointestinal tract from the stomach to the sigmoid colon in order to locate multiple kinking or the presence of intrinsic obstructions. There may be cloudy fluid within the peritoneal cavity, the result of transudation of chyle due to prolonged venous and lymphatic obstruction in the absence of necrosis. A bloody serous effusion is present when bowel infarction has occurred. In our experience there is no specific type of rotation of the bowel. One or more clockwise twists through 360 degrees have usually occurred. It is best to draw all the bowel outside the abdomen early in the procedure and then to replace it progressively, beginning with the jejunum at the ligament of Treitz and ending with the cecum and ileocecal junction. When multiple areas of intrinsic obstruction are also present, the

develop early in the course of the disease, death occurring in from 24 to 36 hours in some of the patients. In some of the cases the symptoms are relatively slow in their development, and the diagnosis of bowel obstruction is made only after several days of observation. Fever, tachycardia, an elevated white count with polymorphonuclear leukocytosis, a distended abdomen, absence of the bowel sounds, and the passage of blood in the stools are symptoms which indicate that intestinal strangulation has occurred.

The roentgenograms usually reveal a high intestinal obstruction, with little gas in the lower abdomen (Fig. 3). In an infant who was previously well, this appearance is almost pathognomonic of a massive volvulus of the intestine about a completely unfixed mesentery. This is particularly true if blood has been passed per rectum. When the volvulus is more localized, increased numbers of air

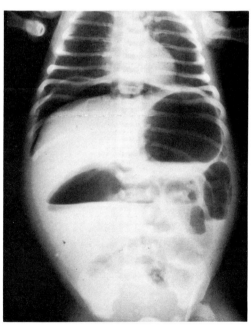

Fig. 3. Malrotation with volvulus. Free air under the diaphragm indicates bowel necrosis and perforation.

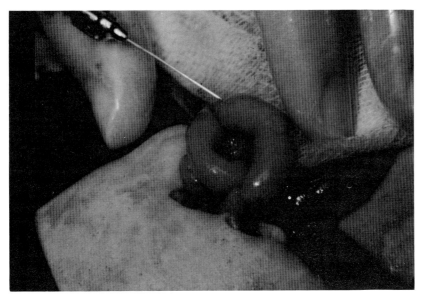

Fig. 4. Injection of saline into the bowel below an obstruction in order to prove the patency of the entire intestinal tract.

lower ones are often not visible, because distension does not occur below the first point of occlusion. For this reason the proximal bowel must be dilated with saline or with air which is then followed through to the cecum (Fig. 4).

In the Christmas tree type of deformity,

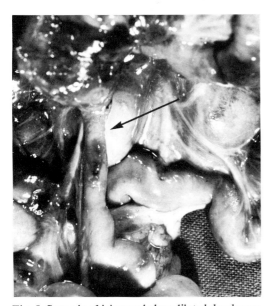

Fig. 5. Stenosis of jejunum below dilated duodenum in Christmas tree deformity.

there is no fixation of the mesentery at all; the narrow base is formed by the mesenteric vessels alone. In such cases a narrowing or an atresia of the upper jejunum is often present (Fig. 5), for the condition probably results from a proximal intestinal vascular catastrophe during middle fetal life. The integrity of the duodenum and of the entire bowel must be confirmed in all cases of neonatal volvulus before the abdomen is closed.

Bowel resection, followed by a closed one-layer silk anastomosis (Ch. 37), is necessary in many of the cases of volvulus. Removal of more than 100 cm of small bowel in neonatal life has been followed by recovery. It is important to ensure good function of the anastomosis by resecting all bowel which appears of questionable viability. Retention of the upper jejunum and the ileocecal valve makes a satisfactory outcome more likely to occur. When the viability of these areas is in doubt they may sometimes be saved by the performance of a primary anastomosis in marginally viable bowel, after resection of the obviously necrotic portions. The anastomosis is inspected in 24 hours by reopening the abdomen under local or general anesthesia. In some of the cases the remaining bowel will have become pink and healthy looking. If it has not done so, the questionable bowel must be resected back to areas of good bleeding. This may leave the infant with insufficient bowel to survive, but every effort has been made to conserve whatever viable bowel was present at the original operation.

MECONIUM PERITONITIS

Perforation of the intestinal tract prior to birth produces a sterile meconium peritonitis. The meconium causes an inflammatory and granulomatous response of the peritoneal surfaces which leads to the formation of dense fibrous adhesions. Loops of bowel are matted to each other and to the abdominal wall. The calcification which occurs in these meconium granulomas and the adhesions is visible in abdominal roentgenographs throughout the abdomen (Fig. 6).

The term "meconium peritonitis" should not be confused with that of "meconium ileus." The former implies only an intrauterine perforation of the fetal intestinal tract, and it may or may not be associated with abnormalities of the meconium. In a series of 25 operated patients with meconium peritonitis, Smith and Clatworthy (1961) found 10 (40 percent) to have fibrocystic disease of the pancreas with meconium ileus. The usual figure in other series of cases is about 50 percent. Because of the frequent coexistence of meconium peritonitis and fibrocystic disease of the pancreas, these two conditions are considered together in the discussion of meconium ileus (Ch. 40). The prognosis of infants with meconium peritonitis is not hopeless. Much depends on the cause of the condition and the amount of bowel which must be resected in order to form a satisfactory anastomosis. In patients with fibrocystic disease the outlook is not good (Ch. 40). Without this added difficulty, resection of 50 percent of the small intestine produces little nutritional deficit. Removal of 75 percent of the small bowel is still compatible with survival, providing that 50 cm of the small bowel is present, that portions of the jejunum and the ileum are included, and that the ileocecal valve is retained. The nutritional management and the operative procedures for infants requiring massive bowel resection have been described elsewhere in this volume (Ch. 34).

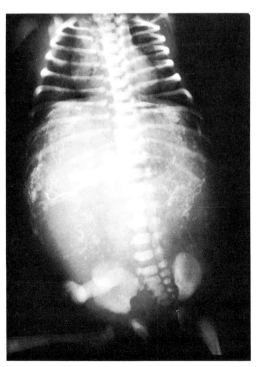

Fig. 6. Extensive intra-abdominal calcification in a case of meconium peritonitis.

ACUTE APPENDICITIS

Acute appendicitis in infants is discussed in Chapter 51. This disorder has been almost uniformly lethal during the newborn period, though it is theoretically amenable to cure. The cardinal manifestations are irritability, vomiting, abdominal distension, fever, and right lower quadrant mass. The finding of acute appendicitis in a newborn infant should lead to a search for an obstructing lesion below it, such as extensive aganglionosis of the colon.

BACTERIAL SEPSIS AND INTESTINAL OBSTRUCTION IN INFANTS

A most difficult problem in diagnosis is presented when acute abdominal symptoms develop in an infant with sepsis. It must be determined whether the abnormality is functional or organic, and if it is organic, whether or not surgical intervention is required. In some of the cases the initial findings are those of mechanical bowel obstruction—vomiting and abdominal distension with fluid levels in the upright radiograph. In other infants a sharp bout of rectal bleeding may have occurred. Although operation often appears to be necessary to relieve the obstruction or to control the bleeding, surgical therapy in such cases is usually disastrous. The resistance of the infant is further lowered and its death is hastened by operative intervention. When true organic changes such as perforation of bowel or complete intestinal obstruction are caused by metastatic bacterial infection in infancy a successful outcome is unlikely, but with modern antibiotic therapy the situation is not entirely hopeless.

The usual organisms causing newborn and infant sepsis today are *Pseudomonas aeruginosa, E. coli, Staphylococcus aureus,* the *Klebsiella* group, *Aerobacter aerogenes,* and the streptococci. The bloodstream invasion of these organisms leads to their rapid dissemination to all parts of the body, and to one or more of the signs of sepsis of obscure origin—poor feeding, generalized weakness, irregular or low temperature, convulsive twitching, jaundice, diarrhea, vomiting with ileus and abdominal distension, poor weight gain, fullness of the fontanelles, lesions of the skin, pyuria, and eventually an abnormal respiratory pattern, with cardiac irregularities and hypotension finally leading to cardiac arrest. Some of the manifestations are identical to those of the surgical obstructive disorders, while others indicate the general nature of the septic process. The correct diagnosis requires careful consideration of all of the signs and symptoms which may be present.

The abdominal symptoms and pathological changes in the intestinal tract depend to a great extent on the invading organism which is present. The association of *Pseudomonas* septicemia and enteritis with paralytic ileus has been described by Schaffer and Oppen-

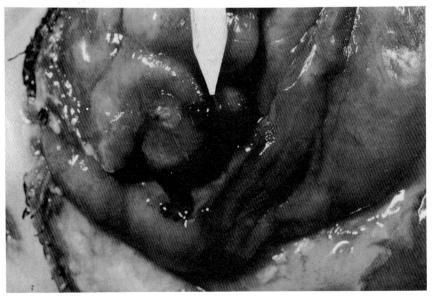

Fig. 7. Focal necrotic lesions of bowel occurring in *Pseudomonas* sepsis.

heimer (1948). We have recently demonstrated that *Pseudomonas* produces cessation of peristalsis within 24 hours after the introduction of the organisms into the ureter of an experimental animal. Since some of the strains of *Pseudomonas* manufacture hydrogen cyanide as well as other endotoxins in their metabolic processes, paralysis of smooth muscle activity may result from absorption of these toxins into the transmural lymphatics from the lumen of an infected ureter or from the bowel. When the intestine is directly involved by *Pseudomonas* bacterial invasion, multiple nonsuppurative necrobiotic lesions develop as the result of spreading arteriolar involvement. These dry gangrenous lesions are focally distributed to both the small and large bowel. After prolonged illness or surgical intervention they may go on to perforation (Fig. 7).

Organisms other than *Pseudomonas* do not usually cause intestinal paralysis or other conditions which appear to require surgical intervention. *E. coli* and *Klebsiella* enteritis in young infants are manifested by a watery greenish diarrhea. Superficial ulcerative changes in the intestinal mucosa are the only pathological findings. There is usually only slight inflammatory reaction, and obstruction or bleeding are uncommon. Pseudomembranous enterocolitis due to the staphylococci is rare in infants, in whom pneumonia, pyelonephritis, and septicemic collapse are more common occurrences during *Staphylococcus* infections. *Shigella dysenteriae* causes superficial mucosal inflammation and necrosis which results in fever and the passage of a mucoid stool containing gross or occult blood. Perforation with obstruction is rare with this organism, but abdominal distension and ileus may occasionally occur. The bleeding is not commonly sufficient to suggest the need for surgical consultation.

The treatment of bowel disorders in association with obvious signs of sepsis should be expectant. In distinction to a volvulus or a spontaneous perforation of the bowel, some rectal discharge of gas and fluid feces usually continues, indicating that the obstruction is only partial. When this sign is present, a program of watchful waiting is justified. Contrast studies of the small intestine with Gastrografin may reveal that the obstruction is not complete. This material is mildly irritating to the intestinal tract, and it passes much more easily than does barium. The absence of complete blockage to its passage rules out closed-loop obstructions, but does not by itself indicate whether bowel necrosis or walled-off perforations of the intestinal tract are present.

Cultures of the stool, blood, urine, and cerebrospinal fluid should be obtained, followed by the administration of massive antibiotic therapy with parenteral drugs active against wide ranges of gram-negative bacteria. These include Polymyxin B (2.5 mg per kg), kanamycin (Kantrex, 15 mg per kg), and cephalothin (Keflin, 50 mg per kg), all of which are well tolerated by newborn infants. Reevaluation from hour to hour is essential. Monitoring of the central venous pressure is of great value in the management of the fluid therapy, since large quantities of plasma and blood (up to twice the expected blood volume) are often necessary to maintain the circulation. Repeated x-ray examination may reveal passage of gas or Gastrografin along the bowel in favorable cases, or the presence of free air as the result of perforation in unfavorable ones. When and if the abdominal findings localize in the form of an abscess, surgical drainage should be performed. In our experience early operation at the time of generalized sepsis has usually resulted in the infant's demise.

NEONATAL INTUSSUSCEPTION

Intussusception has been described occasionally in newborns. The rarity of the condition prior to the age of three months is rather remarkable, since the mesentery in newborns is often thin and lax, and the peristalsis is vigorous. Perhaps it is the thinness of the bowel wall which prevents an irreducible progression of bowel invagination.

The lymphoid hyperplasia of adenovirus infections, recently held to be causally related to intussusception in older infants, is uncommon in newborns, and this may also be a factor in the rarity of the condition in this age group. In a collective review of 26 cases of neonatal intussusception, Talwalker (1962) described vomiting and the passage of blood in the stools as almost invariably present. Pain evidenced by screaming occurred in 4 of the 26 cases. A mass was palpable in 6 cases. The symptoms occurred during the first two days of life in over one half of these patients, and within one week in 85 percent of them. At operation simple reduction was possible in 9 patients, and resection was necessary in 12. The association of a polyp in 1 case and of other congenital lesions of the abdomen in several other patients indicates the need for careful examination of the entire bowel whenever newborn intussusception is encountered. The passage of the intussusceptum per rectum has been described by Rachelson and his colleagues (1955) and by others, but complete intestinal obstruction usually follows this event and operation is almost invariably required.

INTERNAL HERNIAS

Internal hernias within the abdomen have been discussed by Zimmerman and Laufman (1953). There are two main forms—the massive hernias occurring into preformed intra-abdominal cul-de-sacs, and small herniations through defects in the small bowel or transverse colon mesentery. The massive hernias into preformed spaces occur at many sites. They may be paraduodenal, pericecal, within the sigmoid mesocolon, or within the lesser sac or supravesical folds. The usual case is found to have almost the entire small bowel lying within the hernia sac (Fig. 8). The clinical picture is one of bilious vomiting, abdominal pain, and often diarrhea resulting from partial bowel obstruction. Distension is not usually seen because the obstruction begins in the proximal intestine in most of the cases, and the remainder of the small bowel is compressed into the herniation. Smaller herniations through defects in the mesentery are more likely to cause distension and to become gangrenous than are the massive hernias, because the usual narrow opening in the mesentery compresses the entering bowel

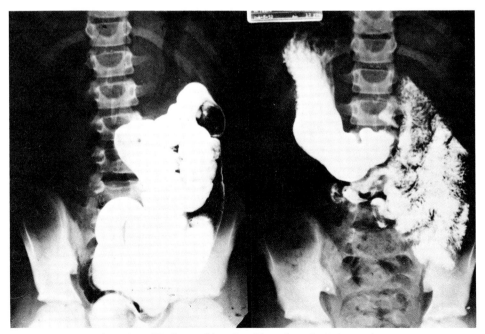

Fig. 8 A and B. Internal hernia without intestinal obstruction.

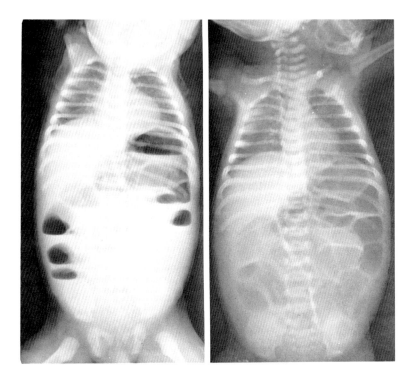

Fig. 9. A and B. Localized internal hernia producing complete small bowel obstruction.

against its sharp unyielding margins (Fig. 9). Strangulation is evidenced by the signs of vascular collapse, the passage of blood per rectum, and the development of peritonitis. At operation the entire small bowel must be drawn out of the abdomen. Reduction of the hernia with or without resection is necessary for recovery. In both forms of congenital hernia the opening in the sac must be closed by suture to prevent recurrences.

CONGENITAL PERITONEAL BANDS

Intestinal obstruction by congenital peritoneal bands is rare in newborns. Unless there is an obvious herniation beneath a tense band, or a volvulus of bowel about a persistent omphalomesenteric duct, the finding of slight distension above a band of peritoneum does not permit the surgeon to abandon his search for the true cause of the dis-

tension. If the preoperative barium enema is normal, the probability is great that an unrecognized aganglionosis is present. We have admitted several infants with severe enterocolitis due to Hirschsprung's disease following an operation in which congenital bands were said to have been lysed. Other infants have proved to have peritonitis as the cause of an obstruction. It is essential that a solution of the mechanical or infectious problem which is causing the obstruction be achieved at the first operation, for most babies do not survive a second one if the obstruction persists. It is therefore poor practice to perform simply the lysis of bands which are not clearly causing strangulation obstruction, since the primary problem may thereby be missed. The bowel must be eviscerated and a careful search made for the true cause of the disorder. This may require the frozen section for the diagnosis of congenital aganglionosis by means of extra-mucosal biopsy of the recto-sigmoid musculature.

FUNCTIONAL INTESTINAL OBSTRUCTION IN NEWBORN INFANTS

When mechanical, neurogenic, or infectious factors have been ruled out as the cause of neonatal intestinal obstruction, a functional origin for defective peristalsis must be suspected. Because the progression of material through the intestinal tract requires a nicely coordinated series of muscular events, it should not be surprising that an immature tract, or one affected by certain drugs or metabolic deficits, might fail to function in a normal manner.

The most obvious abnormality associated with functional intestinal obstruction is prematurity. Sieber and Gardany (1963) reported seven infants with functional obstruction who had no other specific pathological findings. Five of the infants were premature, weighing between 3 pounds and 4 pounds, 15 ounces. All seven infants presented with emesis and abdominal distension. Four of them had not passed meconium, while three had appeared to be entirely normal until three to ten days of life. There was no evidence of sepsis at the time of onset of the obstruction, and ganglion cells were present throughout the intestinal tract in all of them. In the three cases in which detailed histories were given, the total white blood counts were normal. Prostigmine, Pituitrin, and Ilopan all failed to elicit peristaltic activity.

Since six of the seven infants died 24 hours to 7 days after operation, five of them with *Proteus vulgaris* in the postmortem blood cultures, the role of infection cannot be entirely ruled out. The one surviving infant, weighing 3 pounds, 15 ounces at birth, however, had no drainage from an ileostomy despite drug stimulation for 10 days after operation, and then it had normal stools. No evidence of sepsis developed during the recovery period.

The experience of Sieber and Gardany suggests that small infants with low intestinal obstruction should be studied exhaustively for the cause of their obstruction before being subjected to operation. Nasogastric suction, a high oxygen atmosphere, and intravenous fluid therapy with daily plasma will improve the condition of these babies while the necessary investigations are performed. These should include cultures of the nasopharynx, urine, rectum, and cerebrospinal fluid; the barium enema examination; a rectal biopsy; serum electrolyte and BUN determinations; examination for other abnormalities such as hypothyroidism or possible drug toxicity; and repeated white blood counts to rule out the possibility of sepsis. Antibiotics are contraindicated during this time. In our experience they have masked progressive bacterial infection on several occasions, and they appear to have set the stage for *Pseudomonas* infection with organisms derived from the hospital environment.

Hallum and Hatchuel (1954) described paralytic ileus in a premature baby as a complication of hexamethonium therapy of the mother for toxemia of pregnancy, but there are few subsequent reports of neonatal ileus as the result of drugs administered to the mother during labor. A well-known disorder in this regard, however, is the onset of narcotic withdrawal symptoms in babies born to addicted mothers. Heroin withdrawal in babies results in hyperirritability, vomiting of all feedings, diarrhea, and fever. According to Sussman (1963), swaddling, demand feedings, and fluid therapy are sufficient to control the symptoms. Maternal methamphetamine addiction, in distinction to opiate addiction, does not cause withdrawal symptoms in newborn babies.

Congenital hypothyroidism is usually associated with obstinate constipation. Although this may occasionally progress in small infants to nearly complete obstruction of the lower intestinal tract—usually the colon—by hard inspissated fecal material, the full picture of intestinal obstruction is rarely present. In a study by Lowrey and his associates (1958) of 49 patients with congenital hypothyroidism, severe constipation during infancy was present in 45, but the onset was delayed for several weeks after birth in most of the patients. Feeding difficulties, however, were recorded in more than half of them. Vomiting was a prominent symptom in only 1 infant in the entire group. If a firm diagnosis of hypothyroidism can be made, relief of the constipation is achieved by the administration of desiccated thyroid and repeated colonic irrigations to remove the inspissated feces.

A syndrome of intestinal malfunction without histologically apparent abnormalities of the ganglion cells has recently been given the designation "pseudo-Hirschsprung's disease." Since biochemical changes within the intestinal wall are known to be present in true Hirschsprung's disease, specific enzyme defects may perhaps be responsible for cases of defective peristalsis in which the ganglion cells have been histologically normal. This condition may occur during early childhood after apparently normal development during infancy, or it may occur shortly after birth in otherwise normal infants who fail to develop adequate peristalsis. In some of the cases extra-abdominal infections appear to precipitate episodes of paralytic ileus which eventually lead to death. We have encountered three of these patients, all of whom died of unrelieved intestinal obstruction despite recognized forms of therapy.

OPERATIVE TREATMENT

If exhaustive studies do not reveal a cause for persistent obstipation in a newborn infant as outlined in Chapter 34, operation is indicated. If no cause is found after extensive abdominal exploration, and the rectal biopsy reveals the presence of ganglion cells, the surgeon is in a difficult position. When a rectal biopsy has not been done, an extramucosal muscle biopsy (Ch. 45) should be done in the most distal part of the colon which can be reached from an abdominal exposure. This biopsy is studied at once by frozen section examination. If ganglion cells are present, one must then decide whether to close the abdomen or to do an enterostomy.

Spasm of the terminal ileum and ileocecal valve has been found to be the only lesion responsible for newborn obstruction in a small number of infants. If such a condition is discovered and collapsed bowel is seen below an area of bowel dilatation a temporary ileostomy is fashioned just above the apparent level of the obstruction. Subsequently both limbs of the ileostomy must be irrigated to remove accumulated meconium. If bowel function returns and there is satisfactory weight gain, the ileostomy is closed by resection and anastomosis, provided that adequate peristaltic function of the distal bowel has been proved by the normal evacuation of contrast material from the colon following a barium enema examination.

WILLIAM L. DONNELLAN
ORVAR SWENSON

REFERENCES

BERNSTEIN, J., and BROWN, A. K. Sepsis and jaundice in early infancy. Pediatrics, 29: 873, 1962.
CLATWORTHY, H. W., Jr., and LLOYD, J. R. Intestinal obstruction of congenital origin. Arch. Surg., 75: 880, 1957.
COBRINIK, R. W., HOOD, R. T., Jr., and CHUSID, E. The effect of maternal narcotic addiction on the newborn infant, review of literature and report of 22 cases. Pediatrics, 24: 288, 1959.

GROB, M. Intestinal obstruction in the newborn infant. Arch. Dis. Child., 35: 40, 1960.
HALLUM, T. L., and HATCHUEL, W. L. F. Congenital paralytic ileus in a premature baby as a complication of hexamethonium bromide therapy for toxemia of pregnancy. Arch. Dis. Child., 29: 354, 1954.
LOAW, J. H. Jejunoileal stenosis and atresia. J. Pediat. Surg., 1: 8, 1966.

LOWREY, G. H. et al. Early diagnostic criteria of congenital hypothyroidism; a comprehensive study of forty-nine cretins. Amer. J. Dis. Child., 96: 131, 1958.

LUND, R. H. Recurrent small-bowel volvulus in the newborn infant. J. Pediat., 57: 217, 1960.

McNEILL, J. P., and VOTTELER, T. Meconium peritonitis. Amer. Surgeon, 21: 472, 1955.

PILLING, G. P., IV, and CRESSON, S. L. Massive resection of the small intestine in the neonatal period. Pediatrics, 19: 940, 1957.

RACHELSON, M. H., TERRIGAN, J. P., and JACKSON, W. F. Intussusception in newborn infant. J. Pediat., 47: 87, 1955.

RACK, F. J., and CROUCH, W. L. Functional intestinal obstruction in the premature newborn infant. J. Pediat., 40: 579, 1952.

RICKHAM, P. P. Peritonitis in the neonatal period. Arch. Dis. Child., 30: 23, 1955.

SANTULLI, T. V. Intestinal obstruction in the newborn infant. J. Pediat., 44: 317, 1954.

SCHAFFER, A. J., and OPPENHEIMER, E. H.

Pseudomonas (pyocyaneus) infection of the gastrointestinal tract of infants and children. S. Med. J., 41: 460, 1948.

SIEBER, W. K., and GIRDANY, B. R. Functional intestinal obstruction in newborn infants with morphologically normal gastrointestinal tracts. Surgery, 53: 357, 1963.

SMITH, B., and CLATWORTHY, H. W., Jr. Meconium peritonitis: Prognostic significance. Pediatrics, 27: 967, 1961.

SNYDER, W. H., and CHAFFIN, L. Embryology and pathology of the intestinal tract: Presentation of 40 cases of malrotation. Ann. Surg., 140: 368, 1954.

SUSSMAN, S. Narcotic and methamphetamine use during pregnancy; effect on newborn infants. Amer. J. Dis. Child., 106: 325, 1963.

TALWALKER, V. C. Intussusception in the newborn. Arch. Dis. Child., 37: 203, 1962.

ZIMMERMAN, L. M., and LAUFMAN, H. Intraabdominal hernias due to developmental and rotational anomalies. Amer. Surg., 138: 82, 1953.

40

Meconium Ileus and Peritonitis

MECONIUM ILEUS

Surgeons become involved with patients with pancreatic fibrosis for a number of reasons, the chief one being the curious form of intestinal obstruction which is present in about 15 percent of neonates with this generalized glandular disease. In 1905, Landsteiner, who later defined the blood groups accurately, described pancreatic fibrosis. Farber (1944) became interested in the disease and predicted that the patient with meconium ileus would develop pulmonary symptoms, which is common in patients with pancreatic fibrosis. It was Farber who proposed the term "mucoviscidosis," a designation which emphasizes the diffuse nature of the disease.

ETIOLOGY

Genetic studies have demonstrated that the gene is carried by the male and that about one fourth of the offspring will have this disease. Consequently, it is important in taking the history to determine if there have been siblings with pancreatic fibrosis. If this is so, one must be on the alert for the early signs of the disease in newborn siblings.

PATHOLOGY

The pathology is primarily in the pancreas. It consists of a widening of the ducts due to inspissated eosinophilic material and increasing fibrosis. At several years of age the pancreas is reduced in size, and there are rounded lobules consisting of fibrous and edipose tissue and cystic tissue in the center. In the intestine, the mucus-producing cells are enlarged and abnormal in contour. The sweat glands produce sodium chloride in excess, which is the basis of a widely used diagnostic test. The patient is induced to perspire by thermal methods, collection of the perspiration is made, and analysis for sodium and chloride is determined. Normal chloride in perspiration is 60 mEq or less. Often with this disease, the values may be well over 100 mEq.

Many glands, such as the submaxillary, are enlarged and abnormal. The parotid glands produce an abnormal secretion but are not enlarged. Patients with pancreatic fibrosis have a number of other lesions that have become apparent as duration of survival is lengthened. Cholesteatoma has been reported in these patients, again, perhaps related to abnormal secretions. Nasal polyps are common, and there are frequently hepatic lesions which may be related to the disease itself or to the malnourished state many of these patients reach. With the liver lesions there may be portal hypertension and esophageal varices with enlargement of the spleen and hypersplenism. Chronic myocarditis has been described in patients who survive for long periods of time. One of the long recognized external features of this disease is pulmonary osteopathy. Club fingers may be the finding which leads to an investigation and establishment of the diagnosis in an older child. Rectal prolapse has been reported and is difficult to treat.

The surgeon is chiefly involved because of the neonatal obstruction which is observed in about 15 percent of the patients with cystic fibrosis. It was originally postulated that patients with meconium ileus presented the most severe form of the pancreatic lesion, a concept based on the premise that the inspissated meconium was related directly to the defect in the pancreatic secretions. This was doubted by some workers, and in 1946, Glanzmann suggested that inspissation of meconium might be due to abnormal mucus production. This was the first suggestion that perhaps the meconium itself was abnormal due to its composition rather than to the lack of enzyme produced by the pancreas. Zuelzer and Newton (1949) studied a group of patients and demonstrated that the severity of the pancreatic lesion was not related to the clinical entity of meconium ileus. They showed that some of the patients with this disease who had had lesions in the pancreas of greatest severity and died within the first few weeks of life had not exhibited intestinal symptoms during the neonatal period. Buchanan and Rapoport in 1952 detected increased protein and abnormal mucoprotein in the meconium of patients with meconium ileus. The meconium in patients with cystic fibrosis has characteristics on immunological testing which are specific for this disease.

Perhaps one of the most effective screening tests will be the development of a method for the detection of abnormal mucoproteins in the meconium of patients with meconium ileus and pancreatic fibrosis. Schwachman and his associates (1956) have alluded to a new test which consists of adding 20 percent trichloracetic acid to a water extract of meconium. In normal patients there is no precipitation. In patients with meconium ileus there is a definite precipitation. The refinements of this test may lead to a reliable screening test which can be used in the first few days of life, a period when other diagnostic tests are limited in their accuracy.

More recently, Arey (1954) has illustrated abnormalities in the glands of the intestine of the patient with meconium ileus. It now appears that the inspissation of meconium is more related to the abnormal nature of the meconium than to the defect in the pancreatic exocrine substances.

In patients with meconium ileus there may be intrauterine intestinal perforation with development of meconium peritonitis. This may be widespread or limited in scope. Perforation may be healed so that at birth intestinal function is not seriously hampered. The meconium peritonitis is chemical rather than bacterial and elicits calcification in the peritoneal cavity. The calcification may be extensive, lining the peritoneum, or in large flat plaques. It may occur in the intestinal wall. This is probably related to ulceration and perforation of the mucosa with the appearance of meconium in the intestinal wall. In these instances, the calcification tends to be more globular than flat, as in the peritoneum.

There may be extensive necrosis associated with meconium ileus of the intestine, and this may lead to atresias and stenosis of the small intestine.

CLINICAL PRESENTATION

Fifteen percent of all neonates who appear with intestinal obstruction will prove to have meconium ileus. On superficial observation, the patient with meconium ileus does not appear different from any neonate with intestinal obstruction (Fig. 1). However, as the baby is observed, there may be visible dilated loops of intestine. These do not appear different from those seen in other forms of intestinal obstruction. However, on palpation of the abdomen these loops of intestine are filled with a doughy material which can actually be indented. These neonates will vomit bile-stained material and have abdominal distension and a history of failure to pass meconium. The most valuable aid in diagnosis

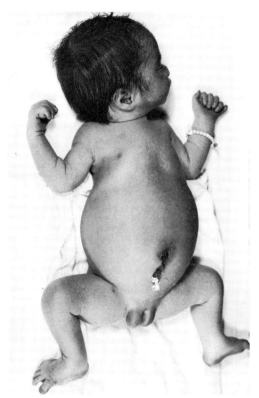

Fig. 1. Photograph of a patient with meconium ileus who developed the usual abdominal distension.

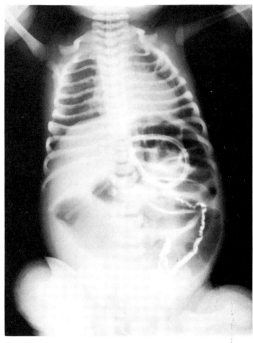

Fig. 2. Upright abdominal film which failed to outline fluid levels. The small unused colon is partially outlined with barium.

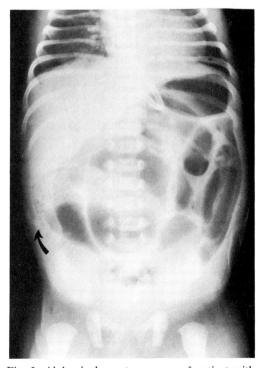

Fig. 3. Abdominal roentgenogram of patient with meconium ileus. Note the coarse granular appearance in the right side of the abdomen above the arrow.

is the flat and upright films of the abdomen. These demonstrate dilated loops of intestine. Rarely are there fluid levels, and their absence is one of the reliable features that leads the radiologist to suspect that the intestinal obstruction is due to inspissated meconium (Fig. 2).

Neuhauser (1944) has described in plain films of the abdomen a granular appearance of meconium in the intestine (Fig. 3). This is postulated to be due to the admixture of bubbles of air in the abnormal meconium. A barium enema will demonstrate a micro-colon and will help to clear out the inspissated material in the small, unused colon.

Establishment of a more firm diagnosis is not of value at this point. The thermal inducement of perspiration for sweat tests is not reliable the first few days. Indeed there is some danger associated with the tests, for the patient with this disease does not withstand heat and perspiration as well as normal individuals. Heat stroke is known as a cause of death in affected children.

Duodenal intubation for studies of pancreatic enzymes is difficult to perform at this age and particularly in patients with intestinal obstruction. Consequently it is not wise to pursue diagnostic tests beyond x-ray examination. Testing of the meconium for

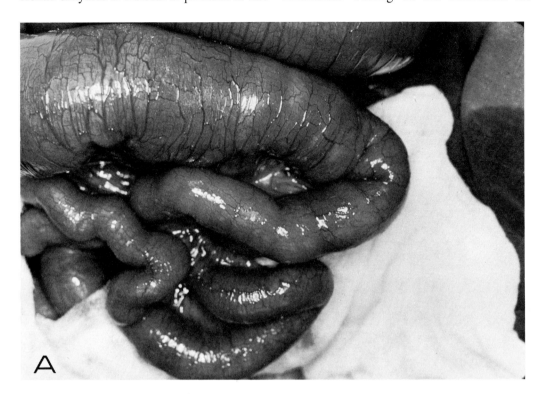

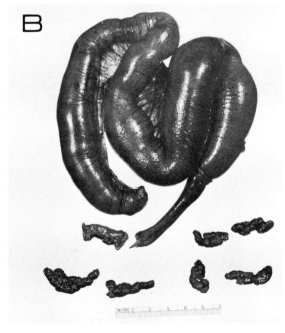

Fig. 4. A. Photograph of intestine in meconium ileus. Note there is a gradual transition from fairly massively dilated intestine to a narrow distal segment. B. Photograph of resected specimen and some of the inspissated meconium from the narrow distal intestine.

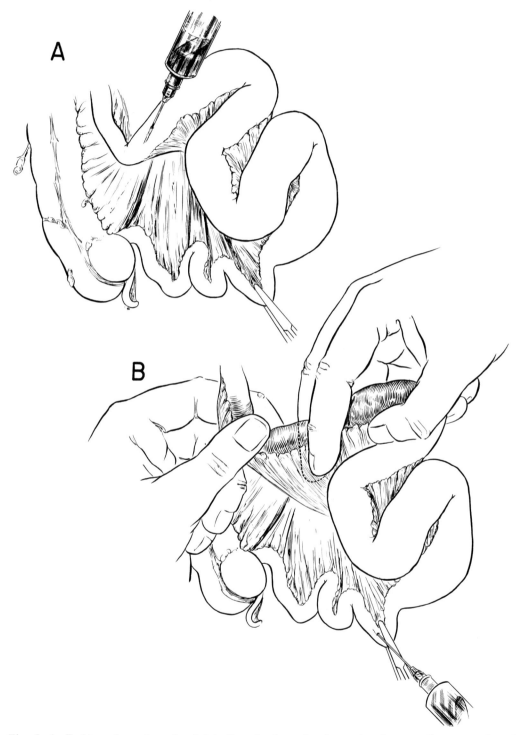

Fig. 5. A. End-to-end anastomosis of intestine. A clamp has been placed across the narrow bowel. Mineral oil is injected into the dilated bowel. B. The thick meconium is milked down into the dilated segment and a section 10 to 15 cm in length is resected. Hydrogen peroxide is injected into the narrow distal segment.

trypsin is not accurate since absence of trypsin may occur in other disease states where intestinal obstruction is a part of the clinical situation.

TREATMENT

Fluid replacement must first be made to return the patient to normal hydration. Electrolyte replenishment based on determinations of the amount of the various elements in the blood are prerequisites to therapy. The use of a nasogastric tube to prevent aspiration of vomitus is important. It is advisable to give enemas. In some instances in which the inspissation does not extend high in the intestinal tract, an enema will relieve the obstruction and obviate the necessity for

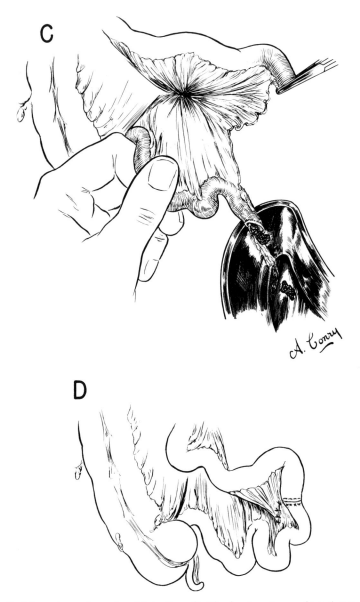

Fig. 5 (cont.). End-to-end anastomosis of intestine. C. The hard casts are forced out of the distal segment by the hydrogen peroxide. D. The end-to-end anastomosis is made with one row of interrupted Halsted sutures.

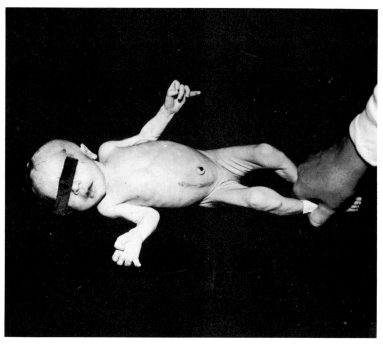

Fig. 6. Meconium ileus. A patient 10 days after resection and end-to-end anastomosis. This child died at two years of age from chronic pulmonary disease.

abdominal exploration. The composition of the enema is of importance; 0.5 percent hydrogen peroxide with Mucomist, which is N-acetylcysteine, has wide popularity. However, the hydrogen peroxide deactivates the acetylcysteine and makes this combination ill-advised. Hydrogen peroxide must be used with caution, for it has been proven that oxygen bubbles in the bloodstream may be dangerous. Most of this caution is based on experimental rather than clinical work. Nevertheless the warning should be heeded, and the concentration of the hydrogen peroxide should be 0.25 percent or less. It is also prudent to limit the volume of hydrogen peroxide solution and the vigor of the irrigation. One should be careful not to give pancreatic enzymes, for patients who are vomiting may inhale some of these agents, which may be injurious to the pulmonary system. Once these measures have failed to relieve the intestinal obstruction, operation offers the only solution. The type of operation to be performed varies from clinic to clinic. Some

years ago we advocated that the bowel be opened and irrigated with dilute solutions of peroxide and then actually to resect the dilated portion (which probably would never function well from a peristaltic standpoint) (Fig. 4). Intestinal continuity was restored with direct end-to-end anastomosis of the intestine (Fig. 5). This has been tested in a number of clinics and found fairly satisfactory (Fig. 6). A patient with aganglionosis of the entire colon and terminal ileum presented an identical gross appearance to that observed in meconium ileus. It was not until the resected specimen was studied by the pathologist that the correct diagnosis was established. This experience has established the routine in our hospital to have a frozen section made of the resected specimen to eliminate the possible diagnosis of aganglionosis.

Gross (1953) has suggested that a Mikulicz resection be performed. The advantage of this operation is that there is less manipulation of the intestine, so catheters can be passed up and down postoperatively and irrigating fluids used to dislodge the meconium and to restore intestinal function. This procedure has proved satisfactory in several centers. A modification has been suggested by Bishop (1957). The ileum proximal to a resection of the dilated segment is anastomosed to the side of the small intestine below the resection. A stump of distal ileum is left beyond the anastomosis and exteriorized. It is thought that there will be less fluid loss with this arrangement, and it has proved quite successful in some centers. Other workers who have studied the various methods believe there is no great difference in result with the various surgical methods. The advantage of the primary resection with end-to-end anastomosis is that one operation rather than two is involved. The problem of fluid and electrolyte loss from a high ileostomy is obviated. Our procedure is to open the abdomen and milk the meconium as much as possible into the dilated segment of the small intestine. The bowel is then resected. The intestine both proximal and distal to the resected specimen is opened, catheters are introduced, and with mild solutions of hydrogen peroxide the segments are cleared of meconium. Once this is achieved, an end-to-end anastomosis is performed either with a two-layer anastomosis or preferably with one silk layer.

POSTOPERATIVE CARE

Patients with meconium ileus have many complications postoperatively, and in most series there is a 60 to 70 percent mortality in the first postoperative month. This may be related to complications intra-abdominally, or there may be overwhelming pulmonary infection early in the postoperative period. The patients must be observed carefully for mechanical obstruction, but most important, they must be treated to prevent pulmonary complications. This consists of the use of mist aerosol to loosen pulmonary secretions and of judicious use of antibiotics to prevent infection. Usually, as the babies are followed, a rotation of antibiotics is offered so that resistant strains of bacteria will not flourish and overwhelm the patient. Pancreatic enzymes which are lacking are substituted in the diet. This is an important part of their care. Postural drainage is important, particularly in older patients as a part of the pulmonary hygiene which prevents recurrent infection.

MECONIUM ILEUS EQUIVALENT

In the last few years it has become evident that inspissation of intestinal contents may recur months or years after successful treatment in the neonatal period. In most instances, medical therapy should be utilized to treat this form of intestinal obstruction. Preferably, therapy should be started before obstruction becomes established. These patients will develop abdominal pain and vomiting and scanty stools. At this point, vigorous treatment with enemas should be instituted, and in most instances this will prevent obstruction and obviate the necessity of operation.

Another complication postoperatively is the formation of impactions in the intestine well above the rectum. Usually, these are in the cecum and may become quite large and so adherent to the mucosa that surgical removal is the only feasible method of treatment. Occasionally, intussusception is a complication of this disease and must be ruled out when there is evidence of intestinal obstruction in the patient with previous meconium ileus.

While many surgeons are quite discouraged in the treatment of these patients, reports, such as those by Schwachman, et al., relating that 20 patients have survived after meconium ileus, give new encouragement to surgeons and should prompt them to be more aggressive in the treatment of this disease. There are a small number of patients who can be salvaged and will survive as healthy individuals.

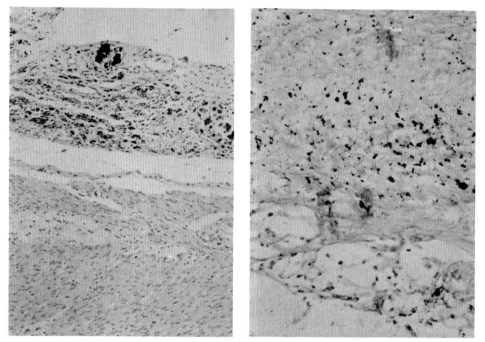

Fig. 7. A. Photomicrograph of peritoneum illustrating the severe chronic inflammation and fibrosis. B. An iron stain indicating the amount of iron in the chronic reaction in the peritoneal cavity.

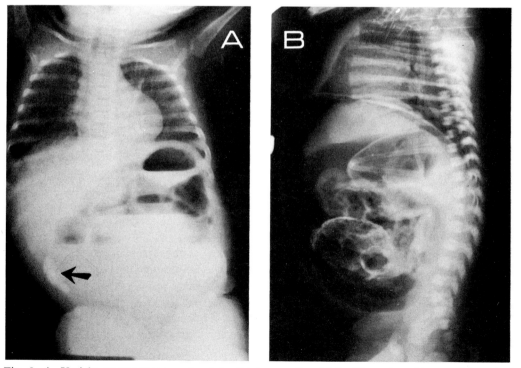

Fig. 8. A. Upright roentgenogram of a baby 24 hours after birth. There is evidence of intestinal obstruction with dilated loops and fluid levels. There is calcification in the right side of the abdomen. B. Twelve hours later, pneumoperitoneum has developed.

MECONIUM PERITONITIS

Meconium peritonitis should not be confused with meconium ileus. By definition, meconium peritonitis is the result of an abdominal catastrophe during fetal life which produced an intestinal perforation and peritonitis. The cause of the break in intestinal continuity may be some congenital band or other lesion that produced intestinal obstruction and perforation. The pouring out of meconium into the peritoneal cavity caused an inflammatory reaction which has subsided by birth, leaving adhesions and in many instances calcification (Fig. 7). Neuhauser (1946) was one of the first to call attention to the calcification which is often but not invariably found in this condition.

On rare occasions, a baby may develop a perforation and meconium peritonitis, yet have an intact, functioning intestinal tract at birth. The diagnosis in such situations is made from the multiple irregular abdominal masses and the calcification indicated in abdominal roentgenograms. The more common situation is intestinal obstruction either from adhesions or from destruction of a segment of intestine, and not infrequently the infant will accumulate air in the peritoneal cavity shortly after birth. These babies will have the signs of intestinal obstruction, they will vomit bile-stained fluid, and their abdomens will be distended. Masses may be detected on abdominal examination. Abdominal roentgenograms will outline calcification in addition to dilated intestine, fluid levels, and free air in the peritoneal cavity (Figs. 8 and 9).

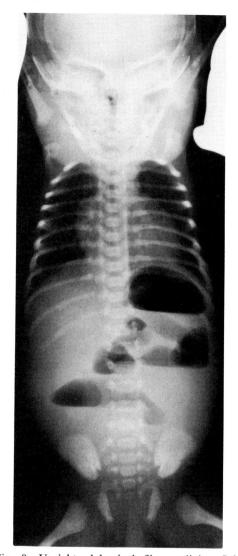

Fig. 9. Upright abdominal film outlining fluid levels and some calcification.

OPERATION

Preparation for operation is limited by the clear urgency with which an intestinal leak is associated. To postpone operation to prepare the child is not a wise course of action in infants with intestinal perforations. Often the neonate's condition will deteriorate despite parenteral fluids. Best results are obtained by starting a blood transfusion and promptly taking the infant to surgery. Each case is different; and, regardless of what is done, survivals are uncommon. A large cavity containing air and intestinal contents may be found. If the signs of intestinal obstruction are not definite, drainage of the cavity may be sufficient. Dissection of the intestine may be an almost impossible task, but when there is definite obstruction this approach offers the only hope of a cure. If the loops of intestine can be separated and the point of obstruction identified, freeing of adhesions is mandatory. When a perforation is identified, exteriorization is preferable to resection and primary anastomosis (Fig. 10). In some instances a limited amount of intestine may be involved, and resection of the entire mass is possible with end-to-end anastomosis to establish continuity. Generally, the postoperative course is complicated and prolonged. However, some recoveries do occur, and these patients thrive. For the technique of resection and anastomosis, see the section on atresia (Ch. 37).

Until the past 20 years survivors were virtually unknown. Some reports now indicate that a 50 percent survival rate is possible. Postoperatively, two entities must be eliminated by appropriate tests. About 20 to 40 percent of the infants will have pancreatic fibrocystic disease. The diagnosis can most readily be made with sweat tests, providing the examination is made 2 or 3 weeks after birth. Rectal biopsy will determine if aganglionosis is present.

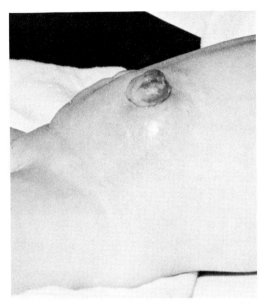

Fig. 10. A baby who had meconium peritonitis. The perforation was in the sigmoid. The sigmoid was exteriorized, and the baby did well. This photograph was taken three months later when the patient had closure of the colostomy.

OBSTRUCTIONS CAUSED BY CONGENITAL BANDS

Congenital bands of various sorts, such as from Meckel's diverticulum to the umbilicus, may be the cause of intestinal obstruction in the newborn. The history and physical signs are identical to those discussed under General Considerations, Chapter 34. Surgical treatment is simple, provided operation is performed before strangulation of the intestine has taken place. Simple division and excision of the band effects a cure. If there has been a delay in diagnosis, and necrosis of the intestine has taken place, resection with end-to-end anastomosis is the operation of choice. For this technique, see the section on atresia (Ch. 37).

MESENTERIC DEFECTS

In a large series of cases of all types of intestinal obstruction, mesenteric defects will be the cause in about 10 percent. The defects are most common in the mesentery of the terminal ileum, and the cause may be inadequate blood supply in the area between the last intestinal vessel and the ileocecal artery. A congenital defect in the blood supply seems more likely as a cause than does inflammation.

As intestine prolapses through a mesenteric defect and filling of the lumen occurs, the loop may become securely trapped, and necrosis of the intestine will occur early. Shock is an early finding, probably related to the closed-loop type of obstruction so frequently seen in these cases.

Early operation is most imperative. If the intestine is viable, the hernia is reduced and the mesenteric defect is carefully sutured with interrupted sutures. Frequently, the involved bowel is not viable, and resection with end-to-end anastomosis is then the procedure of choice. For details of an end-to-end anastomosis, see the section on atresia (Ch. 37).

Incarcerated hernia is another possible cause of intestinal obstruction. For a description of this condition, see the discussion of inguinal hernia (Ch. 33).

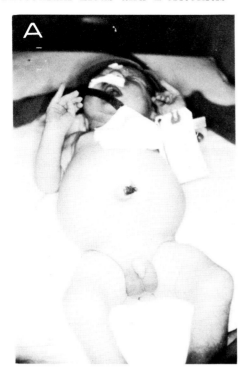

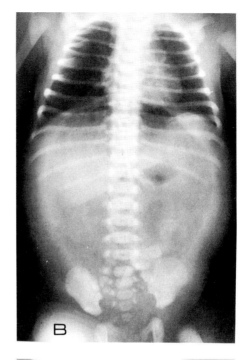

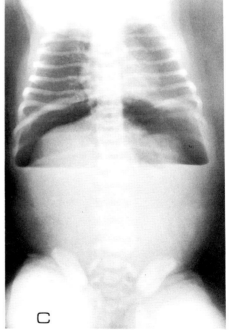

Fig. 11. A. Photograph of neonate with massive abdominal distension. B. Plain film outlining massive abdominal cavity free air. C. Upright film of same patient.

PNEUMOPERITONEUM IN THE NEWBORN

Intestinal perforations are frequently associated with some congenital malformation but in some instances are spontaneous, par-ticularly when the stomach is involved (Fig. 11). In patients with Hirschsprung's disease, there may be perforation of the large intestine with pneumoperitoneum in the early neonatal period. Bands causing intestinal obstruction necrose the intestine and are the cause of air in the peritoneal cavity. There may be congenital defects in the enteric wall to account for the perforation. Ulceration of the duodenum may produce perforations and pneumoperitoneum. Some of these perforations may occur just prior to birth, and as soon as the intestinal tract fills with air the pneumoperitoneum becomes evident. In an average situation, the lesion is associated with some degree of prematurity. At birth, the infant appears perfectly well, but in a few hours abdominal distension and respiratory distress develop. The degree of distension becomes grotesque, and a roentgenogram will identify the cause. It is known that gastric acidity rises during the first 24 hours of life and then subsides, following which there is a gradual rise to normal when the baby is several months of age. It is possible that the hormones in the mother may produce increased levels of circulating adrenal

cortical steroids, and this may be a factor in duodenal perforations. The gastric perforations seem to be unassociated with ulcer. They are clean-cut perforations which may be related to structural defects in the gastric wall.

Prompt recognition of this serious entity with effective therapy will lower the mortality rate. Initially, when the disease was described the mortality rate was near 100 percent. In the more recent reports, the mortality rate is less than 50 percent. These patients should not go through a lengthy preoperative preparation. Rather, prompt operation and closure of the defect if possible should be accomplished. Simultaneous with operation intravenous fluids and blood can be administered to help maintain the patient in reasonable condition.

ORVAR SWENSON

REFERENCES

AREY, L. B. Developmental Anatomy, 6th Ed. Philadelphia, W. B. Saunders Co., 1954.

BERNSTEIN, J., VAWTER, G., HARRIS, G. B. C., YOUNG, V., and HILLMAN, L. S. The occurrence of intestinal atresia in newborns with meconium ileus (the pathogenesis of an acquired anomaly). Amer. J. Dis. Child., 99: 804, 1960.

BISHOP, H. C., and KOOP, C. E. Management of meconium ileus: Resection, roux-en-Y anastomosis and ileostomy irrigation with pancreatic enzymes. Ann. Surg., 145: 410, 1957.

BIRD, C. E., LIMPER, M. A., and MAYER, J. M. Surgery in peptic ulceration of stomach and duodenum in children. Ann. Surg., 114: 526, 1941.

BOIKAN, W. S. Meconium peritonitis from spontaneous perforation of the ileum in utero. Arch. Path. (Chicago), 9: 1164, 1930.

BRAUNSTEIN, H. Congenital defect of gastric musculature with spontaneous perforation. J. Pediat., 4: 44, 1934.

BRYK, D. Meconium ileus (demonstration of the meconium mass on barium enema study). Amer. J. Roentgen., 95: 214, 1965.

BUCHANAN, D. J., and RAPOPORT, S. Chemical comparison of normal meconium and meconium from a patient with meconium ileus. Pediatrics, 9: 304, 1952.

CORDONNIER, J. K., and IZANT, R. J., Jr. Meconium ileus equivalent. Surgery, 54: 667, 1963.

ELLIS, D. G., and CLATWORTHY, H. W., Jr.

The meconium plug syndrome revisited. J. Pediat. Surg., 1: 54, 1966.

FARBER, S. Pancreatic function and disease in early life: 5. Pathologic changes associated with pancreatic insufficiency in early life. Arch. Path., 37: 238, 1944.

———— The relation of pancreatic achylia to meconium ileus. J. Pediat., 24: 387, 1944.

FONKALSRUD, E. W., ELLIS, D. G., and CLATWORTHY, H. W., Jr. Neonatal peritonitis. J. Pediat. Surg., 1: 227, 1966.

FOX, P. F., and POTTS, W. J. Meconium ileus and meconium peritonitis. Arch. Surg. (Chicago), 74: 733, 1957.

FRANKLIN, A. W., and HOSFORD, J. P. Meconium peritonitis due to a hole in the foetal intestinal wall and without obstruction. Brit. Med. J., 2: 257, 1952.

GLANZMANN, E. Dysporia entoro-broncho-pancreatica congenita familiaris. Ann. Pediat., 166: 289, 1946.

GROSS, R. E. The Surgery of Infancy and Childhood. Philadelphia, W. B. Saunders Co., 1953.

HILL, J. T., SNYDER, W. H. Jr., and POLLOCK, W. F. Uncomplicated meconium ileus. Arch. Surg. (Chicago), 88: 522, 1964.

————SNYDER, W. H., Jr., and POLLOCK, W. F. Management of complicated meconium ileus. Amer. J. Surg., 108: 233, 1964.

HOLSCLAW, D. S., ECKSTEIN, H. B., and

NIXON, H. H. Meconium ileus (a 20 year review of 109 cases). Amer. J. Dis. Child., 109: 101, 1965.

LANDSTEINER, K. Darmverschluss durch eingedicktes Meconium: Pankreatitis. Zbl. Allg. Path. 16: 903, 1905.

LYNN, H. B. Meconium ileus. Amer. Surgeon, 30: 597, 1964.

MEEKER, I. A., Jr., HILL, J. T., KINCANNON, W. N. Meconium ileus: Inspissated meconium with intestinal obstruction in the newborn. Surg. Clin. N. Amer., 44: 1483, 1964.

MOORE, T. C. Giant cystic meconium peritonitis. Ann. Surg., 157: 566, 1963.

NEUHAUSER, E. B. D. The roentgen diagnosis of fetal meconium peritonitis. Amer. J. Roentgenol., 51: 42, 1944.

———— Roentgen changes associated with pancreatic insufficiency in early life. Radiology, 46: 319, 1946.

OLNICK, H. M., and HATCHER, M. B. Meconium peritonitis. J.A.M.A., 152: 582, 1953.

RHODES, M. P., GELLER, M. J., and BECKER, J. M. Meconium peritonitis secondary to intestinal atresia. Surgery, 48: 812, 1960.

ROGERS, C. S. Pneumoperitoneum in the newborn. Surgery, 56: 842, 1964.

SCHWACHMAN, H., PRYLES, C. V., and GROSS, R. E. Meconium ileus (a clinical study of twenty surviving patients). Amer. J. Dis. Child., 91: 223, 1956.

SHURTLEFF, D. B. Meconium peritonitis presenting as an abdominal mass. J. Pediat., 58. 267, 1961.

SIMPSON, J. Y. Meconium peritonitis in the fetus in utero. Edinburgh Med. J., 15: 390, 1838.

SNYDER, W. H., Jr., GWINN, J. L., LANDING, B. H., and ASAY, L. D. Fecal retention in children with cystic fibrosis report on three cases. Pediatrics, 34: 72, 1964.

WRIGHT, L. T., and SCOTT, B. E. Perforated gastric ulcer in the newborn infant. J. Pediat., 37: 905, 1950.

ZUELZER, W. W., and NEWTON, W. A. The pathogenesis of fibrocystic disease of the pancreas. Pediatrics, 4: 53, 1949.

41

Duplications of the Intestine

In the past, this lesion has been referred to in the literature as "enteric cysts and giant cell diverticulum," or "reduplication of the intestine," the latter term being particularly inappropriate since it indicates redoubling. This is a fairly rare anomaly, with most large children's hospitals reporting two to five cases a year.

EMBRYOLOGY

Explanation of duplications from an embryological standpoint is difficult. The common explanation is based on the work of Johnson (1913) which primarily was a study of intestinal mucosa formation. He described a stage where the intestinal structure was a solid cord, and lumen was reconstituted by the formation and coalescence of vacuoles. Incomplete coalescence of the vacuoles might produce cystic duplication and possibly some of the tubular lesions of limited extent.

Serious doubt has been raised regarding the validity of this embryological explanation, due to the fact that Johnson could be positive in identifying this process only in the upper small intestine. Evidence that it occurred in the lower intestine was less convincing, and none was presented indicating that this was a normal course of events in the colon. On the other hand, there have been other observations, particularly in the human embryo, which do not entirely agree with the experimental material that Johnson

has published and indicate that on occasion the process has been identified below the duodenum. Long duplications would be more difficult to explain on the basis of the solid cord vacuolization phenomena. Bremer (1944) has suggested that these may be due to the adherence of adjacent walls of the lumen with coalescence and formation of long duplications.

To explain the duplication cysts which are not in the mesentery of the intestine is somewhat more difficult. Such cystic structures have been described in the retroperitoneal space, and because the lining of the structure was that of the gastrointestinal tract it is assumed that it is a form of duplication. It is also difficult to explain some of the thoracoabdominal duplications where there is a communication of the duplication with the upper small intestine and extension into the thoracic cavity.

The fact that there are associated anomalies is not surprising, and this has been noted particularly in the thoracic duplications where in a high percentage of patients there is hemivertebrae in the region of the duplication. Such vertebral anomalies are not as evident in the gastrointestinal form of duplication. However, atresia of the intestine has been associated with duplication, and this fact raises the possibility of intrauterine accidents being the cause of duplications. This may be the case particularly since there have been a number of reported cases of atresia associated with duplication. Duplication may

686

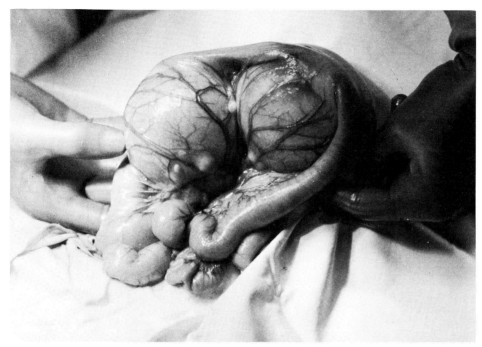

Fig. 1. Two adjacent noncommunicating duplications.

be multiple in a small percentage of cases (Fig. 1).

PATHOLOGY

In order to treat duplication surgically, it is appropriate to review the pathology and anatomy of duplication. In the course of the intestinal tract the duplication is invariably in the mesentery of the adjacent intestine. The exceptions to this are those related to the stomach where they may be separated, and there have been instances of retroperitoneal cysts being classified as duplications. These are rare and do not detract from the general anatomical arrangement of duplication. There is a thick muscular wall about the duplication, and it is interesting that in the area where the duplication is adjacent to the normal intestine there is a common muscular wall so that a normal cleavage plane is usually not present between the structures.

The feature about duplication which is a considerable factor in the symptomatology that this lesion produces is the peculiarity of the mucosa. Generally the lining of the duplication will mimic that of the adjacent bowel. However, there may in many instances be patches and in others large areas completely lined with gastric mucosa (Fig. 2). Production of acid fluid sets the stage for ulceration and bleeding which is one of the cardinal symptoms of duplication.

There is an almost infinite variety of types of duplication. Generally they can be classified in large groups. The first is the noncommunicating duplications which are usually spherical and of considerable size compared to the adjacent normal intestine (Fig. 3). These may be lined with some gastric mucosa and may contain a fluid which has a low pH indicating the acidity of the fluid produced by the gastric mucosa.

The tubular form is the second category of duplications. Here there is a considerable length to the lesion and not a great deal of dilatation beyond that of the adjacent bowel, providing there is a communication between the duplication in its distal portion and the normal bowel wall (Fig. 4). When the distal end of the tubular duplication ends blindly

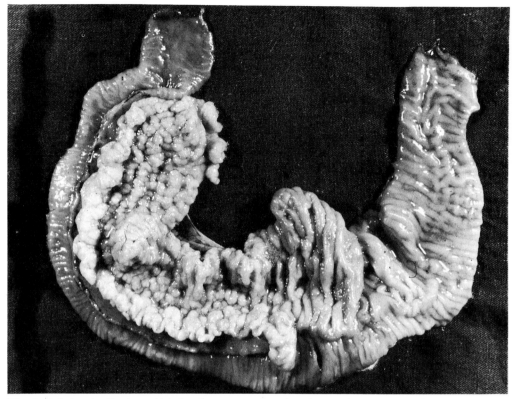

Fig. 2. Tubular duplication which has been opened so that the gastric mucosa can be compared to the adjacent intestinal mucosa.

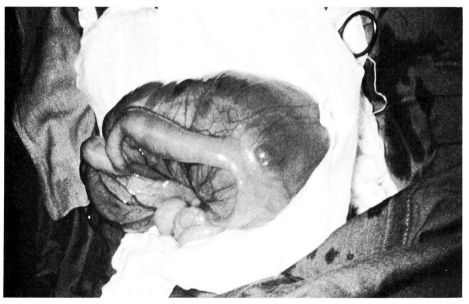

Fig. 3. Large noncommunicating duplication of intestine.

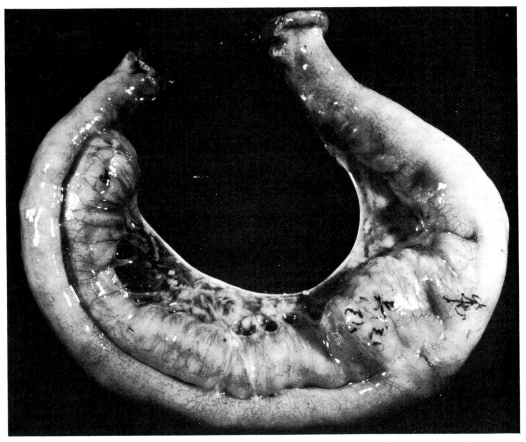

Fig. 4. Tubular duplication which had a proximal communication with adjacent bowel.

and communicates only with the bowel at its proximal end, there may be considerable dilatation of the duplication as normal peristaltic activity fills the dilated tubular duplication with intestinal contents. There may be communications at both ends of the duplication, and in such instances unless there are areas of stricture within there will be no dilatation of these duplications. In the tubular form of duplication, abdominal pain is limited to the situation in which the communication is proximal. This may lead to distension of the duplication with abdominal pain. Despite the absence of gastric mucosa in such a structure the fact that it is a blind pouch may make it become chronically infected and have a detrimental effect on the absorption of various materials required for normal hematopoiesis. Bleeding is evidence of gastric mucosa in the lining. The duplication which

communicates distally or at both ends, providing it has a sufficient area of gastric mucosa, will produce linear ulcerations where it empties into the normal intestine, and will cause intestinal hemorrhage. On the other hand, tubular duplications that communicate distally and do not contain gastric mucosa will be asymptomatic. There is the rare exception to this statement when the duplication is in the distal part of the gastrointestinal tract and communicates with the vagina or urinary system as a fistula (Fig. 5). In such instances, urinary tract infection or soiling through the vaginal fistula will require surgical attention to these lesions despite the fact that they may have no gastric mucosa in their lining (Fig. 6).

Special attention should be directed toward the rare duplication which may be present in the relation to the distal colon

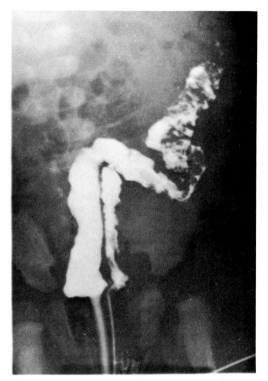

Fig. 5. Roentgenogram with contrast medium in the rectum and rectosigmoid. A small catheter was passed into the duplication by way of a vaginal fistula. The contrast medium filled the duplication and demonstrated a proximal communication with the rectosigmoid.

and appear as a pelvic mass or actually protrude posteriorly and be superficially similar to a sacrococcygeal teratoma.

SYMPTOMATOLOGY

The symptoms which may be produced by duplication can be classified under five general headings. In the various series that have been reported, there is considerable variation in the frequency with which these symptoms appear, and it is difficult to state which is the most common complaint.

ASYMPTOMATIC PALPABLE MASS

In small babies undergoing routine physical examination an asymptomatic palpable abdominal mass may be detected. The fact that it is freely movable and at times can be located in varying quadrants of the abdomen speaks strongly in favor of the mass being a duplication.

RECTAL BLEEDING

Where there is a communication of the duplication with the intestinal tract and there is sufficient area of gastric mucosa, the production of a highly acid fluid that produces ulceration and bleeding can be chronic or spasmodic and fairly massive in quantity. The color of the blood when it is passed per rectum depends on the location of the duplication within the gastrointestinal tract. High in the small intestine such bleeding may well produce a black stool, whereas lower in the gastrointestinal tract bleeding may produce brick-red or frank bloody stools.

INTESTINAL OBSTRUCTION

The mechanism of intestinal obstruction in relation to duplication is in two distinct entities. Where the duplication is small and located in the terminal ileum, it may become the leading point of what is clinically fairly routine ileocolic intussusception. With the current vogue of hydrostatic reduction of intussusception, it is advisable to have such examinations and treatments performed by skilled radiologists who are on the alert for the detection of a leading point. This has been possible in several instances and has led to surgical exploration and removal of a duplication or other abnormality serving as a leading point despite the fact that the duplication was reduced hydrostatically.

In another group of patients the duplication may be fairly large and may become fixed in one position and contribute to a segmental volvulus. Thus it may be the cause of intestinal obstruction. In other instances, there seems clearly to have been obstruction from the adjacent cystic duplication with pressure on the normal adjacent bowel wall. In our experience, this is rare; it is more likely to detect a volvulus factor in such obstructions.

ABDOMINAL PAIN

Abdominal pain has been listed as the leading symptom in patients with duplica-

tions. Mellish and Koop (1961) have felt that this is a fairly common symptom and relate it to contraction of the cystic duplication or ulceration of the lining. On the other hand,

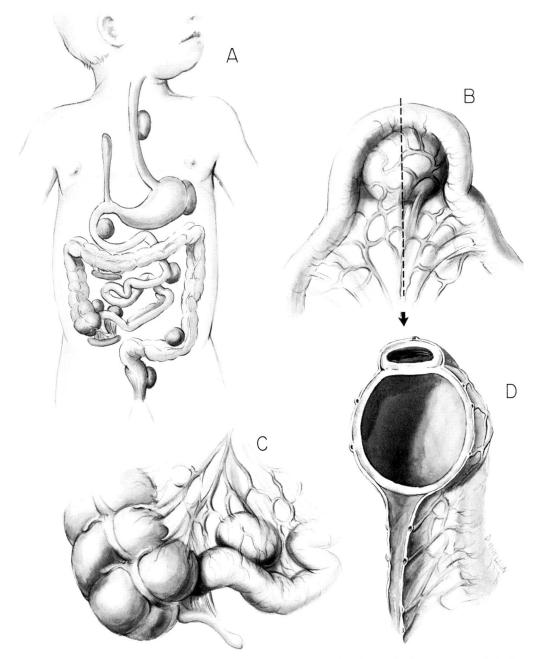

Fig. 6. Types of duplication of the intestine. A. Diagrammatic drawing indicating positions of duplication along the gastrointestinal tract. B. Cystic duplication of intestine which is noncommunicating. C. Small cystic duplication of terminal ileum. These may serve as a leading point for intussusception. D. Cross-section diagram through duplication and adjacent bowel. Note common adjacent muscular wall.

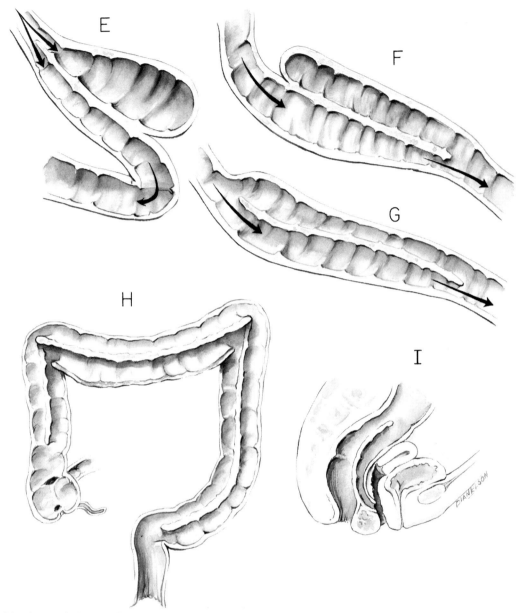

Fig. 6 (cont.). Types of duplication of the intestine. E. Diagram of tubular duplication which communicates proximally and hence becomes dilated. F. When the communication is distal, there is no dilatation. G. The tubular communication may communicate at both ends. H. An intensive duplication may be found which involves most of the colon. I. Rectal duplication with a communication with vagina.

it is well to caution that many children have chronic recurrent abdominal pain which may be quite incidental to the duplication. In other situations, the relationship seems to have been quite clear cut with cessation of all symptoms with removal of the duplication.

MISCELLANEOUS

The fifth category is the miscellaneous rare situations of a sacral cystic mass or an unusual rectovaginal fistula.

DIAGNOSIS

The lesion can rarely be identified with certainty preoperatively. The presence of a mass that is movable and negative results of other examinations, such as intravenous urograms, give some suggestion that a duplication is present. There is one situation where the diagnosis can be made with considerable accuracy radiographically. This is in patients with a dilated pouch duplication where the communication is at the proximal end of the tubular duplication (Fig. 7). In such patients there will be a pocketing and delay of barium which can be readily detected on serial roentgenograms of the abdomen. In such situations the diagnosis of a duplication can be made with considerable accuracy.

TREATMENT

Obviously, there may be duplications that are of no concern to the patient. These may be tubular in nature with communications at the distal end or at both ends, and with no acid-producing mucosa in their lining. Such lesions may be detected incidentally during surgical procedures and need not be given surgical attention. However, when the lesion is a cystic structure, when it has been bleeding into the gastrointestinal tract, when there is pain, the cause of which is unknown, or when the duplication is associated with intestinal obstruction, active surgical therapy is indicated. The ideal surgical procedure is resection with end-to-end aseptic anastomosis. This is possible in the cystic lesions and in the tubular lesions that have been the cause of bleeding or are dilated because of failure to have a communication distally, providing the lesions are not excessive in length.

Usually the lesion is unsuspected, and therefore bowel preparation has not been possible. Consequently we prefer an aseptic end-to-end anastomosis to restore intestinal continuity. The procedure utilizes small crushing Kocher clamps with division of the bowel with endothermy and placement of a

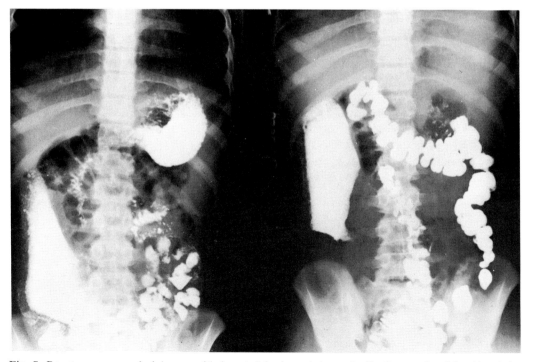

Fig. 7. Roentgenograms of abdomen with ingested barium. A large duplication on the right side of the abdomen is filled. Patient had a severe anemia from chronic blood loss. The duplication communicated with the proximal jejunum. It had no distal communication with the intestinal tract.

row of 6-0 interrupted black silk Halsted sutures. After all the sutures have been placed, the clamps are removed, the sutures tied, and the diaphragm broken. This has proved an extremely effective form of anastomosis and has yielded extremely good results with a paucity of complications. An open anastomosis is practiced by many surgeons. It would seem that complications would inevitably be greater in this group of patients and there would be a delay in restoration of gastrointestinal function.

In patients with long duplications (and these have been reported most often to be in the colon) and significant bleeding indicating the presence of gastric mucosa, surgeons have been reluctant to remove virtually the whole of the colon. Other procedures have been performed with success. It has been possible to open such duplications at intervals and to remove the mucosal lining, thus preventing further bleeding and leaving the patient's normal colon in place.

In the perisacral form of duplication, removal has been possible without sacrificing the adjacent rectum and rectosigmoid. There are longer duplications in this area with rectovaginal fistulas. The treatment of choice in one such case was dissection of the duplication fistula to free the vagina, closure of the vaginal defect, and then performance of a resection utilizing a pull-through technique such as is widely used in the treatment of Hirschsprung's disease to resect the rectum and rectosigmoid with the adjacent duplication and restore intestinal continuity with an anastomosis. This proved extremely satisfactory in that case.

POSTOPERATIVE CARE

Postoperative care is essentially that of a patient with intestinal anastomosis. When the aseptic one-layer technique has been used intestinal function returns within 24 to 48 hours. It is necessary to maintain the patients on nasogastric suction during this period. Passage of a stool and the return of audible peristalsis and a decrease in the amount of fluid produced by the nasogastric suction are indications for removal of the gastric suction. As soon as the nasogastric tube is removed a period of 6 or 8 hours is permitted to pass if the patient does not show signs of accumulation during this period of time. Feedings with glucose sweetened water are started. If this is tolerated for 8 hours a dilute formula is initiated and rapidly changed to full strength.

The results are extremely gratifying. Those patients that have had chronic anemias or acute episodes of bleeding are relieved of this troublesome problem in the future. The patient with the abdominal mass and those with intestinal obstruction are relieved, and since the patients with abdominal duplications are rather free of associated anomalies they tend to progress and be perfectly normal individuals.

ORVAR SWENSON

REFERENCES

BREWER, J. L. Diverticula and duplications of the intestinal tract. Arch. Path., 38: 132, 1944.
ELLIS, W. B. Duplications of the alimentary tract: Review of literature and report of case. Surgery, 34: 140, 1953.
FOSTER, R. L. Duplication of the stomach (case report). Amer. Surgeon, 31: 202, 1965.
GARDNER, C. E., Jr., and HART, D. Enter-ogenous cysts of the duodenum. J.A.M.A., 104: 1809, 1935.
GROSS, R. E., HOLCOMB, G. W., Jr., and FARBER, S. Duplications of the alimentary tract. Pediatrics, 9: 449, 1962.
HOLINGER, P. H., BROWN, W. T., and MAURIZI, D. G. Endoscopic aspects of post-surgical management of congenital esophageal atresia

and tracheo-esophageal fistula. J. Thorac. Cardiov. Surg., 49: 22, 1965.

JOHNS, B. A. E. Developmental changes in the esophageal epithelium in man. J. Anat., 86: 431, 1952.

JOHNSON, F. P. Development of the mucous membrane of the large intestine and vermiform process in the human embryo. Amer. J. Anat., 14: 187, 1913.

JOHNSTON, P. W., and SNYDER, W. H. Problems with the surgery of esophageal atresia and fistula. Amer. Surgeon, 30: 501, 1964.

MELLISH, R. W. P., and KOOP, E. E. Clinical manifestations of duplication of the bowel. Pediatrics, 27: 397, 1961.

SIEBER, W. K. Alimentary tract duplications. Arch. Surg., 73: 383, 1956.

42

Intussusception

Intussusception has been known in medical history for centuries. Hippocrates alluded to the possibility of reducing the intussusception with the injection of air into the colon. In many of the early writings, intussusception was mixed with other forms of intestinal obstruction. Consequently, many of the reports are not clear, and it is difficult to separate the true cases of intussusception from among the other diverse entities producing intestinal obstruction. Hutchinson (1874), who is known for his wide interest in medicine and surgery was the first to successfully treat an intussusception with operative reduction. This was accomplished in 1871. However, the mortality from surgical reduction of intussusception was so high that it is understandable that other methods of treatment were sought. Hirschsprung (1865) in Copenhagen used hydrostatic pressure for the reduction of intussusception and reported the results of his five years' experience with this method. He achieved a considerable improvement over the then current 90 percent mortality, reducing it to 35 percent. This indirect method of reduction had disadvantages, and consequently surgical therapy became more prevalent with improvement in anesthesia and surgical technique. Surgical treatment became prominent in the United States, and very early excellent results from surgical therapy were reported. For instance, in 1925 Taylor reported a series of 87 operative cases with a 3.7 percent mortality,

and Gross and Ware reduced the mortality to 2.7 percent in 1948.

Olsson and Pallin (1927) and Pouliquen and De La Marnierre (1927) suggested the possibility of achieving reduction with the use of radiographic control of the therapeutic enema, and this method treatment gained popularity in the Scandinavian countries. It was not until 1939 that Ravitch started to popularize this technique in the United States. In Australia, hydrostatic reduction of intussusception was an early method of treatment and remains so today.

ETIOLOGY

A great deal of speculation has centered on the etiology of intussusception. To date, no common clear-cut etiological agent has been described. The great majority of the patients are under two years of age, and over 50 percent are usually between three and nine months old. In this period the disease is idiopathic in that there are rarely gross associated abnormalities to account for the intussusception. It has been stated that a change in diet may be a factor, particularly in Europe. In investigations where diet has been given attention, no definite relationship can be established in the United States. The relationship with upper respiratory infection has been mentioned and seems probable. It may be that with upper respiratory infections there is hyperplasia of lymphoid tissue, and Peyer's patches may enlarge to the extent that they can become the leading point in intussusception. The seasonal variations of upper respiratory infection and intussusception coincide, and while this may be coincidental, it may indicate a relationship. Diarrhea is common in the first year of life, and this is given as a possible etiological agent. It is true that in over 10 percent of some series there has been an episode of gastroenteritis with hypermotility of the intestine within a reasonable period preceding the intussusception.

Recently, a group of investigators in Sheffield, England, have studied patients with in-

tussusception for the presence of virus and found that there might be some relationship. The evidence is suggestive but not conclusive. Patients with intussusception had a lower incidence of having had the specific viral infection preceding the intussusception than did the general population. After intussusception they developed evidence of having had the viral disease in the same proportion as in the normal population.

In children beyond two years of age, there is a definite instance of a leading point for the intussusception. The commonest associated lesion is a Meckel's diverticulum which tends to invaginate into the lumen of the

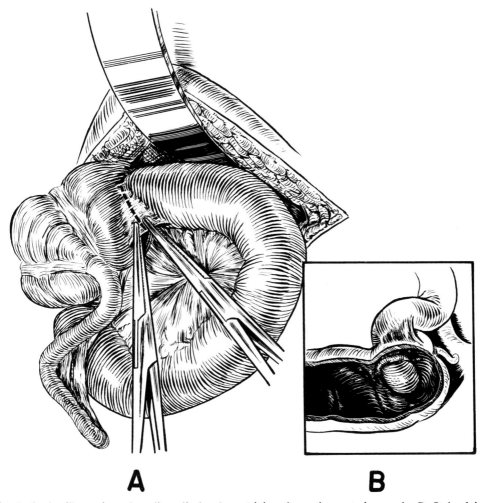

A   **B**

Fig. 1. A. An illustration of an ileocolic band containing the antimesenteric vessels. B. It is claimed that this band may hold the ileum partially prolapsed into the cecum, thus setting the stage for intussusception.

small intestine and thus become the leading point. The second most common is polyps of the small intestine, and less frequent is a duplication in the region of the ileocecal valve. Additional rare causes are tumors such as lymphosarcoma, aberrant pancreas, and hypertrophy of Peyer's patches.

Various bands have been described that may be related to intussusception, but none are so prominent and constant in their relationship to establish definitely such abnormal bands as a proven etiologic agent (Fig. 1). In the postoperative patient there is an unusual form of idiopathic small bowel intussusception which, while rare, can be quite baffling to the observing surgeon.

PATHOLOGY

It is now generally agreed that the leading point of an intussusception is stationary during the process of invagination. There are two major forms of intussusception—the ileocolic which is in all series the most common, and the ileoileocolic which is in effect a double intussusception. Rare coliccolic

forms have been described, and it is well for the surgeon to be aware of the possibility of small bowel intussusception in the postoperative patient. These can occur anywhere in the small intestine and are not of the variety that prolapses through the ileocecal valve.

The ileocolic form of intussusception is the simplest and is composed of three cylindrical layers. The ileoileocolic is a more complicated form and begins as a process of the small intestine and at the ileocecal valve produces a second invagination so that there are five cylinders or layers of intestinal wall. In 5 to 10 percent of the cases of intussusception the cause is an inverted Meckel's diverticulum, a small duplication at the ileocecal valve, a tumor, or polyp. A Meckel's diverticulum is the most common associated lesion. Polyps are the next commonest form of the cause of intussusception. We have seen patients with a local lymphosarcoma of the bowel which served as a leading point (Fig. 2). It is of some clinical value to note that these lesions are usually in older children beyond two or three years of age.

Intussusception is a form of intestinal ob-

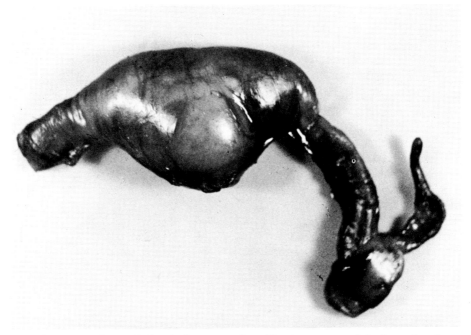

Fig. 2. A bisected specimen of chronic intussusception. The tumor proved to be a lymphosarcoma. The patient had had symptoms dating back three months.

struction. At first it is only a partial obstruction of the lumen, but as the lesion progresses and edema takes place, lumen obstruction may become more complete. The second aspect of the obstruction is constriction of the vascular supply, for the intussuscepted bowel must take with it its blood supply, drawing the mesentery into the space between the cylinders of the intussusception. The local swelling and edema can well be appreciated from the vascular occlusion which occurs fairly early due to the above-mentioned arrangement of the blood supply to the intussusception. The lymphatics become obstructed, and this situation accentuates the edema and contributes to the eventual complete lumen obstruction that may take place. Ulceration and necrosis are most likely to occur in the region of the leading point and trail off from this area. Because of the edema and swelling, damage to the permeability of vessels and barriers within the lumen wall takes place, and cultures of intussusceptions without perforations often yield bacterial growths. This may be related to the clinical experience that reduction of intussusception is associated with an increased instance of wound infection, when compared to the occurrence in clean laparotomies.

CLINICAL CHARACTERISTICS

This disease in the infant age groups is observed in otherwise perfectly normal, healthy babies. There is a preponderance of males over females in most reported series, the ratio being as high as three to one. There has been a question whether the disease is as common in the Negro race as in the Caucasian. As more clinical data have become available, it would appear to be equally common in the two races. Difference of instance in various parts of the world is well documented. It is interesting that most of the large children's hospitals in the United States see an average of about ten cases a year. In European hospitals, the instance is far greater than this. While a number of factors may influence this, such as the fact that treatment of this condition in adult hospitals may take place in the United States to a greater extent than in various European centers, nevertheless it appears that there is not a uniform instance in all parts of the world.

The initial symptom in most of the babies is vomiting. It is presumed that the small infants have abdominal pain when they cry, double up, and repeat this at a periodic interval. There may be paleness and sweating during the attacks which are undoubtedly related to increased intestinal activity. The vomiting at first appears to be on a reflex basis and consists of stomach contents. Later in the course of the disease, the small intestine begins to empty and the characteristic so-called fecal vomiting becomes evident. Some infants will appear to be quite depressed and may be suspected of having some form of drug intoxication. Patients have been admitted to the hospital with a diagnosis of central nervous system disease, and in the course of a careful work-up, abdominal examination has revealed a typical sausage-shaped mass of intussusception.

About 60 percent of the patients have gross blood in the stool. This is to be expected in view of the fact that there is such an early vascular component in this form of intestinal obstruction. Compression of the venous return probably occurs early and bleeding through the damaged mucosa accounts for the passage of blood. Initially, this is mixed with fecal material. Later it is mixed with mucus and has a characteristic currant jelly appearance. The incidence of blood in the stool can be increased if routine rectal examination is performed and the stool on the glove used in the examination tested for occult blood.

The mortality rate of this disease if left untreated is high. There are undoubtedly cases where an intussusception spontaneously reduces itself. This can be deduced from the fact that palpable masses have been clearly outlined and at operation some patients have no intussusception. There are also reported cases where sloughing of the intussusception has taken place. Presumably this must take place rather rapidly before the patient is overwhelmed by the prolonged intestinal obstruction. The reported cases have been in older children and the process takes from 15 to 21 days. Except for these unusual instances, the untreated disease results in intestinal obstruction and death.

UNUSUAL FORMS OF INTUSSUSCEPTION

There are variations from this clinical course. There may be a recurrent form of intussusception in patients who have as a leading point a small duplication or polyp in the terminal ileum. For some unknown reason, the intussusception does not progress far and spontaneously reduces itself. In rare instances, there may be chronic intussusception. We recently had a patient with a lymphosarcoma of the terminal ileum with symptoms of three month's duration. On the other hand, we have observed patients with chronic intussusception as determined by symptomatology which persisted for as long as six months without any associated pathology, such as a Meckel's diverticulum or tumor. Another rare form of intussusception should be mentioned. This occurs in the postoperative patient and is limited to the small intestine. Such patients will do well for two or three days after their abdominal operation and then begin to develop partial intestinal obstruction. These are hard to detect because the obstruction is partial. However, careful examination of the abdomen may reveal the presence of a mass, or the administration of Gastrografin may outline the partial obstruction.

PHYSICAL SIGNS

A great deal has been written about the diagnosis of intussusception from palpation of the abdomen. The pathognomonic sign is the finding of a sausagelike mass in the upper abdomen. The slightly crescent shape of the mass is probably related to the fact that the mesentery acts as a deterent on one side and tends to bow the intussusception to a certain extent. On rare occasions, the lesion may be felt in the right side of the abdomen. Usually the lesion is transverse in the midportion of the abdomen. The mass may be difficult to outline in an irritable crying child, and in such a situation it is perfectly acceptable to administer a small amount of barbiturate to the patient to provide satisfactory conditions for abdominal palpation. In a small percentage of the patients, the intussusception may progress and actually protrude through the anus. In some patients the leading point can be detected on rectal examination. When the intussusception protrudes through the anal canal, care must be taken to differentiate between a rectal prolapse and an intussusception. When an intussusception is present the examing finger can be passed between the anal canal and the intussusception well up into the rectum. On the other hand, when a prolapse has occurred, it is not possible to insert a finger beyond the pectinate line. There is a group of patients comprising probably 10 to 15 percent of the total group where the abdominal mass cannot be palpated. These are usually rather localized lesions and are tucked into the right upper quadrant below the protruding liver edge. In such patients the diagnosis can be established with a barium enema.

RADIOGRAPHIC EXAMINATION

Plain films of the abdomen are not too profitable in the early stages of intussusception before signs of intestinal obstruction have developed. Ladd (1913) was the first to publish a roentgenogram of a barium enema which was diagnostic of intussusception. The diagnosis can be made accurately, for as barium enters the colon in the area of intussusception, the leading point can be detected, and as the barium spreads between the bowel and intussusception, it may form a coil-spring appearance which is pathognomonic of intussusception (Fig. 3).

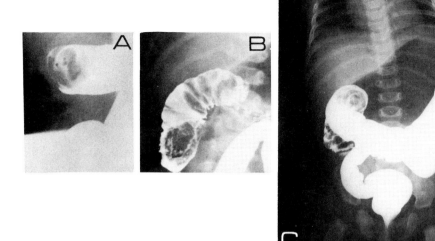

Fig. 3. A. A spot roentgenogram demonstrating the barium outlining the apex of the intussusception. B. The barium has flowed between the cylinders and the intussusception, forming the so-called coiled-spring sign which is pathognomonic of intussusception. C. Roentgenogram of the abdomen. The barium has filled the colon except for the right side where the intussusception is clearly outlined.

A considerable amount has been written about Dance's sign which is emptiness in the right lower quadrant on examination. This positive finding, at best vague, cannot be taken as conclusive evidence of intussusception. The seriousness of intussusception depends on the duration of the disease, a factor repeatedly demonstrated in publications. Providing the patient is presented for therapy within 24 hours of onset the results are excellent. It is in the patients with symptoms beyond 24 hour's duration that mortality occurs.

TREATMENT

In the past, considerable emphasis has been placed on the speed with which therapy is instituted. On the other hand, in analyzing reports of fatalities, it is clear that some are due to inadequate preparation of the patient. Consequently, the necessity for speed in therapy of this disease should not overshadow the importance of thorough preparation of the patient. In the infant with a short history of eight to ten hours, preparation need not be long. However, intravenous fluids are required, and in most instances administration can be accomplished most satisfactorily by exposing a small vein in the ankle and inserting a cannula or polyethylene tube for a route of infusion of fluid. It is wise to have blood crossmatching so that should reduction prove to be difficult or an unexpected resection become necessary, supportive therapy will be available. When the illness has lasted beyond 24 hours, it may require an additional 12 hours to prepare the patient adequately for operation. Preparation consists of careful decompression of the dilated upper intestinal tract with the use of nasogastric suction or a long tube for decompression of the small intestine. Replacement of fluids and electrolytes is imperative. Equally important is the use of transfusion. The patient with an intussusception has lost blood, and while the volume is not great, when it is added to the considerable loss of colloid material which has passed into the edematous tissue of the intussuscepting intestine, it becomes significant and can only be corrected with blood or plasma transfusions. Such severely ill patients probably have a reduced blood volume, and it is wise to insert a catheter for central venous pressure monitoring and to continue the repair with blood plasma and fluids until the venous pressure rises to 8 or 10 cm of water pressure.

CHOICE OF METHOD

In the past, there has been a tendency toward outlining therapy as surgical versus hydrostatic reduction. As evidence accumulates, it is clear that both of these forms of treatment have a definite place and that each patient must be carefully evaluated and the proper therapy instituted. It is now evident that with satisfactory safeguards, barium enema reduction can be safely performed, and approximately 30 percent or more of the patients can be saved from abdominal exploration. While the mortality does not differ and therefore this cannot be used as evidence to favor one method of therapy over the other, the fact that the incidence of postoperative adhesions is 3.5 percent in the surgical group and is virtually nonexistent in the other should be the deciding factor in the use of barium enema reduction of intussusception.

BARIUM ENEMA REDUCTION

Ravitch (1952) has established a series of conditions which are important to follow in order to provide safe hydrostatic reduction. When the diagnosis is made, the patient should be posted for operation, and the surgeon should accompany the patient to the department of radiology for an attempt at reduction. While Ravitch maintains that the duration of the disease has no relationship to whether this technique should be tried or not, most authors place a definite limitation in this regard. Patients with a history beyond 24 hours are usually relegated directly to surgical therapy. Patients beyond two or three years of age should be subjected directly to surgical therapy because of the relatively high instance of associated pathology. Where there is excessive evidence of abdominal distension, by physical examination and on plain films of the abdomen, hydrostatic reduction should not be attempted.

A number of rules and regulations must be followed carefully during the radiographically controlled reduction. Pressure should be limited by placing the enema can no higher than three feet above the table. Manipulation of the abdomen is to be discouraged. Ravitch forbids it, stating that this is a potential cause of perforations. The time limit that should be placed on indirect reduction varies from clinic to clinic. Ravitch states that it is permissible to proceed with hydrostatic methods as long as progress is evident. Other authors believe that three periods of 5 to 8 minutes each should limit the attempt at indirect reduction.

One of the criticisms of this form of treatment has been the absence of absolute criteria of complete reduction. As experiences accumulate, it becomes clear that there must be a free reflux of barium into the small intestine to attest to a complete reduction. This may be difficult to observe in some of the patients due to the large amount of barium in the distended colon. Postevacuation films usually permit a clear view of ileal reflux. All authorities agree that these patients should be hospitalized and carefully observed for a period after barium enema reduction. Most important of all is that if there should be a doubt about the completeness of the reduction either from the radiographic appearance or the behavior of the patient postreduction, exploration should be undertaken without hesitation. A word of caution should be given that at times a palpable mass may persist after complete reduction which may be edematous bowel. As an isolated finding it is not an indication for exploration. Passage of flatus and stool, disappearance of abdominal distension, and absence of pain are all clinical signs which are to be expected after successful therapy. Should these events fail to materialize serious consideration should be given to surgical exploration.

SURGICAL THERAPY

In the patient who comes to exploration to ascertain the completeness of a barium en-

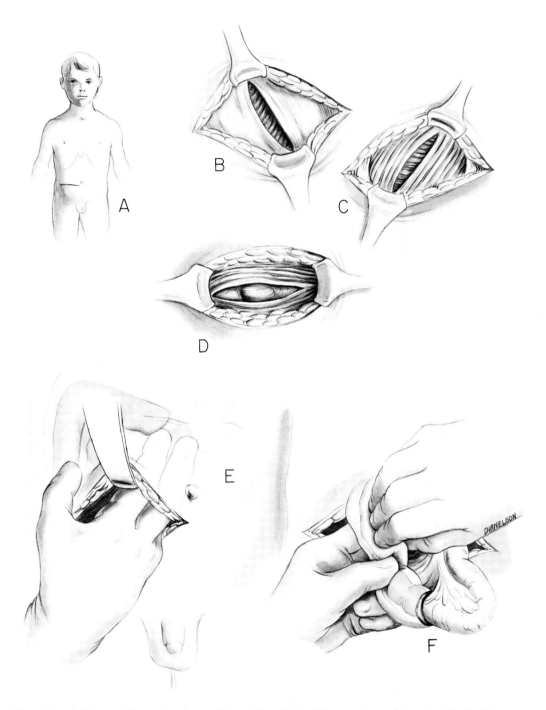

Fig. 4. A. A diagram illustrating the position of the skin incision. B., C., and D. The skin incision. The operator has inserted his index and third fingers through the incision, and the leading point of the intussusception is being pushed back toward the cecum. F. The reduction is completed after the ascending colon and terminal ileum have been delivered through the incision. This enables the operator to place more direct pressure on the leading point of the intussusception.

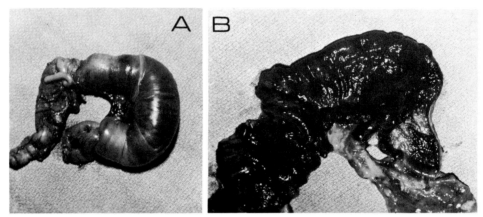

Fig. 5. A. Irreducible intussusception which requires resection with ileotransverse colostomy. B. The same specimen after it had been opened. There was extensive necrosis of the intestinal wall.

ema reduction, or who has been selected directly for surgical therapy, or who proves to have an intussusception which proved irreducible on barium enema, the exposure that is advocated in our hospital is a large McBurney incision (Fig. 4). The skin incision should be placed higher than the classical McBurney incision and should be transverse. The incision should be made slightly above the umbilicus with the lateral extension between the costal margin and the iliac crest. The value of this incision is that intussusception can be reduced and the patient safely discharged from the hospital two or three days after operation. This is possible because the McBurney type of incision is immune to dehiscence; consequently early discharge can be practiced safely. On the other hand, when a transverse muscle-cutting incision or a vertical muscle-retracting incision is used, the patient faces the possibility of evisceration for a period of five to eight days after operation, and discharge from the hospital before this time has unacceptable risks. When the peritoneal cavity is open, it is possible for the surgeon to insert his index and third fingers through the incision and to use the opposite hand for counter pressure on the abdominal wall. By this maneuver, he can readily trace the extent of the intussusception, place the fingers behind the leading point, and then gently push it backward. It is possible in most instances to reduce all but the terminal part of the duplication readily. When the cecal part of the intussusception remains, it can be delivered through the McBurney incision and given direct attention. In patients with considerable swelling, it may be possible to place general pressure over the whole intussusception before continuing the reduction. It is dangerous to use traction on the invaginated bowel in an attempt to dislodge it. Some traction can be placed at the same time the pressure is being applied to the leading point. This should be done with care. In the advanced intussusception it may take very little time to determine that it is irreducible or is composed of necrotic bowel (Fig. 5). However, in a number of patients it will be difficult to determine whether a resection is required. Usually the surgeon should err on the side of doing unnecessary resections rather than permitting the return of bowel into the peritoneal cavity which will perforate and cause a death. With the low mortality from resection and end-to-end anastomosis, it is wise to use this procedure a little more liberally than has been customary in the past. Resection may also be required after the reduction has been completed due to the poor appearance of the bowel and to obvious gangrene. Also there may be an associated large malformation, such as duplication, which requires resection.

A number of techniques are available to

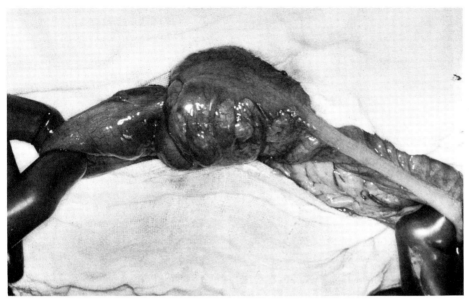

Fig. 6. A recurrent intussusception.

the surgeon in dealing with intussusception which must be resected. We have favored an aseptic resection with an end-to-end anastomosis using one row of interrupted fine silk sutures. This has a number of advantages. There is no gross contamination of the peritoneal cavity. There is a good stoma since only one layer of sutures is used. There are no occluding clamps placed on the bowel beyond the anastomosis to retard the return of intestinal function. On the other hand, resection with a two-layer anastomosis is commonly practiced, and good results are reported. We have been able to perform 15 resections consecutively with our technique without a mortality.

Gross and Ware (1948) have advocated the exteriorization of the intussusception with an obstructive type of resection. They add the additional step of sewing together the anti-mesenteric borders of the bowel adjacent to the resection or the colostomy so that a crushing clamp can be applied early in the postoperative period. It is their practice to have the colostomy closed within a relatively short period of time. Other authors advocate a Mikulicz type of resection with a formal closure of the colostomy with end-to-end

anastomosis of the intestine at a later date. More recently, Dennison (1948) has revived the older technique of doing an entero-enterostomy to form a short circuit proximal to the intussusception. This has had fairly good results in their hands. Apparently the intussusception reduces itself and is not the cause of long-term problems.

The problem of removing the appendix presents itself when the intussusception is reduced. Most surgeons follow the rule that

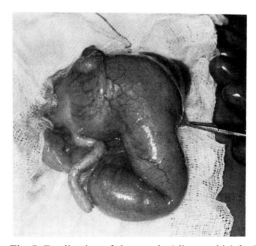

Fig. 7. Duplication of the terminal ileum which had produced recurrent intussusception.

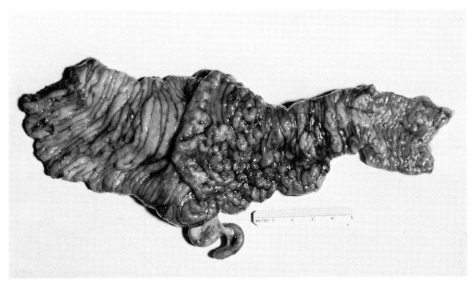

Fig. 8. Cecum and terminal ileum from a patient with a recurrent intussusception. The specimen was removed at a time when intussusception was present. No abnormal pathology except hypertrophy of the ileocecal valve was found.

if there is not excessive edema or abnormalities of the cecal wall, appendectomy may be performed with safety. On the other hand, when there is hemorrhage and edema in the cecal wall, it is unwise to perform appendectomy. With these guidelines about half the patients with surgical reduction of intussusception have an incidental appendectomy.

Another question arises as to the wisdom of removal of a Meckel's diverticulum when it is found as the leading point of a manually reduced intussusception. It is preferable to reduce the intussusception in such situations and to let the patient recover. Reoperation should be done in a month for definitive treatment of the Meckel's diverticulum. When there is little edema or other abnormalities of the intestinal wall, removal of the diverticulum can be accomplished when intussusception is reduced.

COMPLICATIONS

The recurrence rate of intussusception is 2 to 3 percent and seems to be the same whether hydrostatic reduction is achieved or direct manual reduction is practiced (Fig. 6). There is a difference of opinion on the treatment of recurrent intussusception; some

believe that it is wise to perform surgical resection, and others advocate hydrostatic pressure for the first recurrence. Certainly after the second recurrence, resection is mandatory (Fig. 7). The reason for this is that there is usually some local abnormality to account for the recurrence which can only be eliminated by a resection. Special atten-

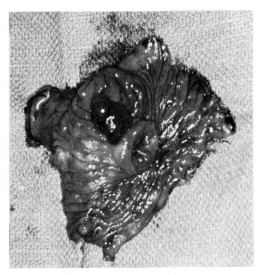

Fig. 9. A polyp in the cecum adjacent to the ileocecal valve. Patient had a history of several year's duration of recurrent bouts of abdominal pain and vomiting.

tion should be given to a rare form of recurrent intussusception which occurs in older children with recurrent bouts of abdominal pain (Fig. 8). These intussusceptions tend to be quite short and to reduce spontaneously. Consequently it is not possible in most instances to palpate the lesion and to establish the diagnosis in this way. Barium enemas are useless unless the examination is performed during an acute attack when the intussusception is taking place. In all of these patients, treatment should be surgical, and resection should regularly be practiced (Fig. 9).

The most common complication is wound infection. This is probably related to the fact that positive cultures can be secured in many instances of intussusception, before perforation of the bowel has taken place. These patients can be subjected to all of the other complications of intra-abdominal surgery. These should be sought for in the postoperative period and efforts made to combat them before they develop into major problems. It is well to maintain these patients on nasogastric suction until there is a good return of bowel function.

ORVAR SWENSON

REFERENCES

BENSON, C. D., LLOYD, J. R. and FISCHER, H. Intussusception in infants and children (an analysis of 300 cases). Arch. Surg. (Chicago), 86: 745, 1963.

CLUBBE, C. P. B. The Diagnosis and Treatment of Intussusception. London, Oxford University Press, 1921.

DENNIS, C. Resection and primary anastomosis in the treatment of gangrenous or nonreducible intussusception in children. Ann. Surg., 126: 788, 1947.

DENNISON, W. M. Acute intussusception in infancy and childhood. Glasgow Med. J. 29: 71, 1948.

FORSHALL, I. Intussusception of vermiform appendix with report of seven cases in children. Brit. J. Surg., 40: 305, 1953.

FOX, P. F. Intussusception: Surgical treatment. Surg. Clin. N. Amer., 36: 150, 1956.

GELLER, F. C., and HAYS, D. M. Subacute intussusception: A clinical entity in pediatric surgery. Amer. Surgeon, 28: 83, 1962.

GROSS, R. E., and WARE, P. F. Intussusception in childhood: Experiences from 610 cases New Eng. J. Med., 239: 645, 1948.

HAYS, D. M. Intussusception as a post operative complication in pediatric surgery. Surg. Gynec. Obstet., 112: 583, 1961.

———— GELLER, F. C., NORRIS, W. J., and SNYDER, W. H. A review of the management of intussusception in a pediatric center (1939–1958) 382 consecutive cases. Arch. Surg. (Chicago), 80: 788, 1960.

HIPSLEY, P. L. Intussusception and its treatment by hydrostatic pressure. Med. J. Aust., 2: 201, 1926.

HIRSCHSPRUNG, H. 107 Falle von Derminvagination dei Kindern, Behandelt in Konigen Louisen-Kinderhospital in Kopenhagen wahrend der Jahre 1871–1904. Mitt. a.d. Grenzeb. d. Med. u. Chir., 14: 555, 1865.

HUTCHINSON, J. A. A successful case of abdominal section for intussusception. Trans. Roy. Med. Chir. Soc. Glasgow, 57: 31, 1874.

IZANT, R. J., Jr., and CLATWORTHY, H. W., Jr. Surgical Treatment of Intussusception, In Mulholland, J. H., Ellison, E. H., and Friesen, S. R., eds. Current Surgical Management. Philadelphia, W. B. Saunders Co., 1957, pp. 349–357.

KELLOGG, H. B., Jr., and BILL, A. H., Jr. The treatment of intussusception (an evaluation of surgical and of barium enema reduction in a series of eighty cases). Amer. J. Surg., 101: 626, 1961.

LADD, W. E. Progress in the diagnosis and treatment of intussusception. Boston Med. Surg. J., 168: 542, 1913.

NELSON, T. Y. Place of hydrostatic pressure in treatment of intussusception. Med. J. Aust., 1: 825, 1949.

OLSSON, I., and PALLIN, G. Uber das bild der akuten Derminvagination bei Rontgenuntersuching und uber Desvagination mit Hilfe von Kontrastlavements. Acta Chir. Seand., 61: 371, 1927.

ORLOFF, M. J. Intussusception in children and adults. Inter. Abstr. Surg., 102: 313, 1956.

PACKARD, G. B., and ALLEN, R. P. Intussusception. Surgery, 45: 496, 1959.

PECK, D. A., LYNN, H. B., and DuSHANE, J. W. Intussusception in children. Surg. Gynec. Obstet., 116: 398, 1963.

POULIQUEN, E., and DE LA MARNIERRE. Indication du lavement bismuthe dans certaines formes d'invaginations intestinales. Bull. Mem. Soc. Nat. Chir., 53: 1016, 1927.

RAVITCH, M. M. Jonathan Hutchinson and intussusception. Bull. Hist. Med., 25: 342, 1951.

RAVITCH, M. M., and MORGAN, R. H. Reduction of intussusception by barium enema. Ann. Surg., 135: 596, 1952.

———— Intussusception in infancy and childhood. New Eng. J. Med., 259: 1058, 1958.

SANTULLI, T. V. Intussusception. Amer. J. Surg., 107: 443, 1964.

SNYDER, W. H., Jr., KRAUS, A. R., and CHAFFIN, L. Intussusception in infants and children (a report of 143 consecutive cases). Ann. Surg., 130: 200, 1949.

SOPER, R. T., and BROEN, M. J. Recurrent acute intussusception in children. Arch. Surg. (Chicago), 89: 188, 1964.

STRANG, R. Intussusception in infancy and childhood: A review of 400 cases. Brit. J. Surg., 46: 484, 1959.

SWENSON, O., and OECONOMOPOULOS, C. T. The operative treatment of acute intussusception in infants and young children (an analysis of ninety-seven consecutive case reports). Amer. J. Surg., 103: 599, 1962.

TAYLOR, W. Discussion of acute intestinal obstruction. Brit. Med. J., 2: 993, 1925.

WRIGHT, J. E. Intussusception (a survey of 107 cases). Aust. New Zeal. J. Surg., 32: 320, 1963.

ZACHARY, R. B., and POTTER, C. W. Aetiology of intussusception. Proc. Roy. Soc. Med., 54: 1018, 1961.

43

Gastrointestinal Bleeding in Infants and Children

Bleeding from the alimentary tract is a common occurrence during childhood. In most of the cases it is temporary and of little significance, requiring no more than reassurance of the parents, who have been taught to fear rectal bleeding as a sign of cancer. One or two follow-up visits usually suffice to confirm the permanent cessation of the bleeding. Occasionally, however, massive exsanguinating hemorrhage or serious chronic bleeding necessitate extensive diagnostic and therapeutic measures.

Hematemesis is the vomiting of blood, which may have been swallowed or produced by bleeding from the esophagus, stomach, or duodenum. When exposed to the hydrochloric acid of the gastric juice the blood becomes dark brown in color and develops an appearance similar to that of coffee grounds. *Melena* is the passage of dark tarry material from the rectum in association with bleeding from the upper gastrointestinal tract. The blood is altered by digestion as it passes distally, becoming a tarry black color through the action of the digestive enzymes. In general, it must come at least from above the ileocecal valve in order to undergo this transformation. Bright or dark red rectal bleeding with clots is given the somewhat inelegant name of *hematochezia*. In children unaltered blood may come even from the stomach, since peristalsis is often stimulated by the presence of intraluminal blood. Although the color of the blood as described

above is of some diagnostic value, the character of the rectal discharges may vary considerably during the course of severe gastrointestinal bleeding, and great reliance must not be placed upon it in attempting to localize the source of the bleeding.

Gastrointestinal bleeding is of widely varied etiology, and it occurs from many sites along the alimentary tract. At different ages during childhood there are characteristic causes which should first be considered before extensive and unnecessary diagnostic tests or operations are performed. In the neonatal period, for example, gastrointestinal bleeding is due to nonsurgical conditions in more than 95 out of 100 cases. Swallowed maternal blood and clotting abnormalities are the main causes in this age group. From one month to two years of age, the usual source of bleeding is the anal fissure, and surgical or serious medical conditions account for only about one third of the cases. It is not necessary to do extensive studies in most of the cases at this age. After the age of two, surgical causes of bleeding account for a higher proportion of the cases. In older children, therefore, serious disease should always be considered to be present whenever rectal bleeding is encountered and a careful diagnostic evaluation is always in order.

The following paragraphs deal briefly with the diagnosis of the usual sources of gastrointestinal bleeding in the various childhood age groups. Some of the more common lesions are discussed in some detail in this chapter, while the remainder are considered in other chapters.

The major surgical causes of bleeding are depicted in Figure 1. Systemic causes of intestinal bleeding which are of importance include leukemia, thrombocytopenic and allergic purpura, hemophilia, scurvy, and familial telangiectasia. These systemic disorders must be ruled out by appropriate physical and laboratory examinations before the purely surgical causes of intestinal bleeding are considered in the differential diagnosis.

GASTROINTESTINAL BLEEDING IN THE NEWBORN

ETIOLOGY

Several authors have assembled statistics on intestinal bleeding during the newborn period. In Table 1 are listed the causes responsible for 155 cases of neonatal gastrointestinal bleeding seen by Craig (1961) during an 11-year period.

DIAGNOSIS

The diagnosis of intestinal bleeding during the neonatal period can be very difficult. While infants may pass red blood per rectum from any portion of the gastrointestinal tract, and regurgitate it from below the ampulla of Vater, occasionally serious internal bleeding occurs without any obvious external sign. The infant may suddenly become limp, cold, and pale and be found to have cyanotic extremities and a rapid feeble pulse. When there is no obvious sepsis, and even slight hematemesis has occurred in such a baby, the diagnosis of duodenal ulcer should be seriously considered. No matter what the anticipated etiology, a catheter should be inserted into an arm vein and connected to a manometer to record the central venous pressure, and plasma should be adminis-

TABLE 1.   GASTROINTESTINAL
BLEEDING IN 155 NEWBORN INFANTS*

PRIMARY COAGULATION DEFECT		94
Melena	28	
Hematuria	12	
Melena and hematemesis	37	
Intestinal bleeding with other hemorrhage	17	
SWALLOWED BLOOD		54
Melena	17	
Hematemesis	19	
Melena and hematemesis	18	
GASTRO-DUODENAL ULCERS (HEMATEMESIS AND MELENA)		2
HIATUS HERNIA HEMATEMESIS		2
PYLOROSPASM HEMATEMESIS		1
HEMOLYTIC DISEASE: TERMINAL HEMATEMESIS		1
UNCERTAIN—? ASPHYXIA		1
Total		155 Cases

* Modified from Craig, W. S. On real and apparent external bleeding in the newborn. Arch. Dis. Child., 1961.

tered without delay. The temperature is recorded continuously and maintained within the normal range by incubation of the infant in a high-oxygen humidified environment. It is important to draw blood for crossmatching and also for prothrombin and clotting times, following which 1 mg of vitamin K analogue is given parenterally. These measures are essential to prepare for a possible exsanguination while the diagnosis is being made. If the bleeding seems severe, but the general condition of the infant remains stable, exsanguinating hemorrhage is not present. Nevertheless it is still safer to place a catheter into a vein, since it is impossible at first to predict which babies do and do not have serious intestinal bleeding.

Once the condition of the infant can safely be controlled, suitable investigations should be performed. It is of first importance to differentiate *secondary* from *primary* bleeding. The former term refers to swal-

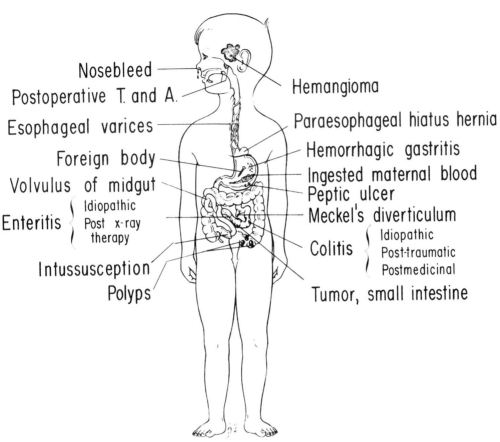

Nosebleed
Postoperative T. and A.
Esophageal varices
Foreign body
Volvulus of midgut
Enteritis { Idiopathic / Post x-ray / therapy
Intussusception
Polyps

Hemangioma
Paraesophageal hiatus hernia
Hemorrhagic gastritis
Ingested maternal blood
Peptic ulcer
Meckel's diverticulum
Colitis { Idiopathic / Post-traumatic / Postmedicinal
Tumor, small intestine

Fig. 1. Major causes of intestinal tract bleeding in children. (From Chisholm, Snyder, and McParland. Pediat. Clin. N. Amer., 9: 201, 1962.)

lowed maternal blood, which accounts for some 35 percent of the cases. The history of excessive hemorrhage or the presence of blood-stained amniotic fluid during the delivery is of significance. Fetal and maternal hemoglobin can be distinguished by the method of Apt and Downey (1955)—1 ml of the stool in question is dissolved in 10 ml of distilled water, and the mixture is filtered. Fetal hemoglobin remains pink and adult hemoglobin turns brown when 2 ml of 1 percent sodium hydroxide are added to the filtrate.

Primary bleeding due to coagulation defects accounts for most of the cases of newborn rectal bleeding. In the report of Craig, only 5 of 99 newborn infants with primary bleeding had an identifiable organic cause. Two had duodenal ulcers. As in most of the reported cases of gastroduodenal ulceration in the newborn, hematemesis had preceded the passage of blood per rectum by 10 to 30 hours. The symptoms of peptic ulceration begin on the first day of life in more than one half of the babies and within 48 hours in over 90 percent. The ulcers are probably due to excessive gastric acidity (which rises rapidly between 3 to 8 hours after birth) and to high pepsinogen activity, which is also increased during the first 5 days of life. There is undoubtedly an inborn tendency to the disorder, since occasionally fatal ulcerations have developed in identical twins (Fig. 2).

Other lesions causing acute neonatal he-

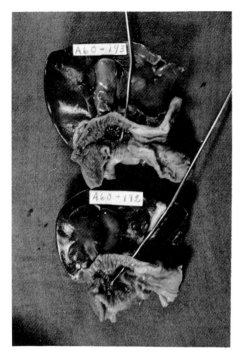

Fig. 2. Identical duodenal ulcers in newborn twins.

matemesis are peptic ulceration of the lower esophagus associated with free cardioesophageal reflux, and gastric mucosal irritation associated with gastric retention due to pylorospasm or pyloric stenosis. The bleeding from these conditions is only moderate in its severity, and the vomited blood is usually altered to a coffee-ground material. All

other surgical conditions leading to intestinal bleeding in the newborn are so rare as to be curiosities.

Upper gastrointestinal roentgen examination usually reveals the organic lesions which cause hematemesis in the newborn period. The duodenal ulcers are usually large. Although they may not produce the spasm of the bulb which is seen in older individuals, their craters are nearly always clearly visible (Fig. 3). Prior to the introduction of the barium it is essential to obtain supine and upright views of the abdomen to rule out the presence of free air in order to avoid the escape of barium into the peritoneal cavity through a perforated stomach or duodenum.

The reflux associated with hiatus hernia is easily demonstrable, and an irregular inflamed esophageal mucosal pattern or a small ulcer may be visible (Fig. 4). Significant pylorspasm with mucosal edema is also quite evident on upper gastrointestinal examination.

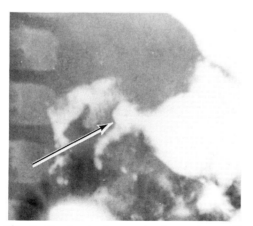

Fig. 3. Duodenal ulcer crater in newborn. The infant recovered after blood transfusions alone.

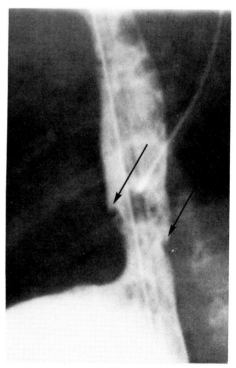

Fig. 4. Peptic esophagitis with hemorrhage in a premature infant with chalazia.

TREATMENT

PRIMARY RECTAL BLEEDING

Primary rectal bleeding is practically never fatal during the immediate newborn period. It may represent an inflammatory response of the colon to the invasion of the normal colonic flora, with the excessive bleeding being due to a clotting deficiency. This inflammation is soon controlled by the defense mechanisms which develop against the invading organisms, and the bleeding ceases. Proctoscopy is rarely indicated in newborns, and the treatment should be expectant. Bleeding of this nature is less active than is the bleeding of a duodenal ulcer. A transfusion of fresh whole blood, the administration of vitamin K, and specific chemotherapy for pathogenic organisms will usually effect a cure.

ESOPHAGEAL REFLUX

Esophageal reflux can be controlled by placing the infant in the upright position (Ch. 30). Elixir of Donnatal, 3 drops every 4 hours, may aid in controlling hyperacidity and in improving gastric emptying. Frequent small feedings thickened with rice cereal are also of value. Pylorospasm may be controlled by the same regimen. Operation for these conditions is rarely indicated.

DUODENAL ULCERS

The treatment of duodenal ulcers in the newborn is not a simple matter. Many of these will stop bleeding spontaneously within 4 to 5 days without later recurrence of hemorrhage, but others continue briskly until the baby has exsanguinated. It seems reasonable to place a Levin tube in the stomach, administer Elixir of Donnatal, and replace the blood as necessary to maintain an adequate venous pressure (9 to 10 cm H_2O) and pulse (120 to 160 per minute). Continuous aspiration of the gastric contents should be combined with half hourly instillations of 10 ml of a thinned suspension of magnesium carbonate which is immediately reaspirated, in order to raise the gastric pH and decrease the activity of the pepsin.

OPERATION FOR DUODENAL ULCER IN THE NEWBORN

If more than 50 ml of blood are required per hour to maintain the vital signs, or the loss of blood approaches 75 percent of the baby's blood volume, early operation through a right paramedian muscle-retracting incision is indicated. The ulcers are usually large and deep, extending to the serosa in the cases which have not perforated. There may be erosion of a discrete vessel, but the bleeding from the edges is just as often diffuse. It is extremely important to remove all clot from the ulcer bed and to cleanse the bed by brisk sponging. This maneuver opens up any clotted vessels so that they may be controlled by ligature. If this scrubbing of the ulcer is not done, a second exsanguinating hemorrhage may follow the operation as soon as the clot in a large vessel is softened by the digestive enzymes. Both gastrectomy and oversewing of the ulcer combined with a Finney pyloroplasty have been successful. We have used the latter procedure together with vagotomy in three infants, two of which survived. Section of the nerves does not appear to be necessary, since the tendency to ulceration passes off rapidly during the first week or two of life. Perforation is treated by utilization of the rent in the construction of a pyloroplasty, or, if the area has a good blood supply, by excision of the edges followed by a two-layer closure. Gastrectomy has been used successfully for both perforation and bleeding, but it seems rarely to be indicated.

Studies by Boley and his colleagues (1965) and others have revealed that vagotomy and pyloroplasty do not lead to any significant alteration of the growth pattern in puppies. Some impairment of growth did follow subtotal gastrectomy. Followup studies in our clinic lead us to believe that neither of these procedures alters the growth pattern of infants and children.

INTESTINAL HEMORRHAGE FROM ONE TO TWENTY-FOUR MONTHS OF AGE

By one month, swallowed blood is gone, the hyperacidity of the newborn period has regressed, and the important causes of intestinal bleeding after this age are more likely to be surgical in nature. On the other hand, a number of insignificant causes of bleeding bring these older infants to the attention of the physician. Among these the *anal fissure* is by all odds the most common lesion. Whenever rectal bleeding occurs, the history of the amount and the apparent source of the bleeding must be obtained very carefully. Most parents are alarmed by the discoloration produced by 10 ml of blood, even though the child continues to appear well. If bright red blood is noticed on the diaper on several occasions, and the child's hemoglobin remains within normal limits, treatment for an anal fissure should be instituted. This treatment includes the use of Desitin ointment to reduce the spasm associated with anal pain and to soothe the anal region. A suppository is given to ensure daily evacuations, and added fruit or excess sugar promote loose stools which do not cause stretching of the painful anal membrane. The bleeding usually clears on this program, and no further investigation is necessary.

If the rectal bleeding is dark in color, or if it is more massive, with clots, a careful study of the patient should be done at once. A measured fall in the hemoglobin or the presence of anemia are of the greatest importance in assessing the significance of the bleeding. The most common surgical lesions are an intussusception or a bleeding Meckel's diverticulum. Colonic polyps are not infrequent, but they do not usually produce acute gross bleeding leading to significant anemia, and they ordinarily do not require surgical removal. The important considerations in the treatment of massive intestinal bleeding in older infants are to establish an intravenous route for the maintenance of the blood

TABLE 2.   CAUSES OF MASSIVE GASTROINTESTINAL HEMORRHAGE FROM 1–24 MONTHS OF AGE

MAIN CAUSES
Meckel's diverticulum
Polyps
Intussusception

OTHER CAUSES
Peptic esophagitis due to achalasia
Volvulus
Hemorrhagic gastritis
Esophageal varices
Stress ulcers
Duplications
Colitis—Infectious and non-specific
Foreign body
Trauma, especially liver and duodenum

volume, to type and crossmatch one or two units of blood, and then to proceed with an orderly investigation. Time is usually available to permit a thorough work-up. The diagnosis and treatment of the most important causes, which are listed in Table 2, are discussed elsewhere in this volume.

BLEEDING IN CHILDREN OVER THE AGE OF TWO YEARS

Intestinal bleeding in older children is rarely exsanguinating in nature. Time is available to make a thorough investigation, unless associated bowel obstruction is present. There are many causes for rectal bleeding in this age group (Table 3). Henoch-Schönlein purpura, ulcerative colitis of infectious or nonspecific origin, a hemorrhagic diathesis, and several other purely medical conditions should be excluded. A proctoscopy, coagulation studies, and upper and lower intestinal roentgenograms must be done before a child is subjected to laparotomy for diagnostic purposes. Rare causes of bleeding in older children are the duplications, intestinal telangiectasia (often associated with Turner's syndrome in girls), regional enteritis and idiopathic ulcerative colitis, mulitple polyposis, the Peutz-Jeghers syndrome, paraesophageal hiatus hernias, chronic duodenal ulcer, and acute hypertrophic gastritis. Large hemangiomas may occasionally be present in the rectum or higher in the intestinal tract. Occasionally a significant bleeding episode may be produced by a small localized hemangioma or telangiectasia which is not apparent either on x-ray examination or on external inspection of the bowel. Aside from the intestinal telangiectasias, which are impossible to identify radiographically, the remaining lesions can almost always be diagnosed by appropriate preoperative studies.

In addition to the usual gastrointestinal lesions producing hemorrhage, other sources of bleeding must be considered. A tarry stool after tonsillectomy is not unusual, particularly if a definite bleeding complication has occurred. Epistaxis may lead to the swallowing of blood which is followed by melena. The juvenile nasopharyngeal angiofibroma may uncommonly present in this way. Trauma to the buccal mucosa occasionally leads to excessive bleeding with hematemesis. When the bleeding is from esophageal varices, the signs of portal hypertension are often discernible. It is important, therefore, to begin one's consideration of the source of bleeding from the top (or the bottom) of the alimentary tract, excluding those diagnoses which do not fit the clinical picture and physical findings which are present.

LAPAROTOMY FOR UNDIAGNOSED BLEEDING

Shandling (1965) has detailed the findings in 61 infants and children (from a group of 801 patients) with intestinal bleeding who were subjected to laparotomy when no diagnosis could be made from preoperative investigations. Thirty of these patients had positive findings, and 31 did not (Fig. 5). Twenty-four patients had a Meckel's diverticulum; only 3 of these patients had a hemoglobin level above 8 g percent. A colloid carcinoma of the jejunum and a jejunojejunal intussusception were the most important of the other 6 cases. In 31 patients no correctable lesion was found to explain the bleeding episode. Sixteen of these latter patients were contacted for follow-up examinations. Eleven of them had no further bleeding, and in only 1 of the remaining 5 who bled once again was the cause (a rectal polyp) discovered.

The rare condition of generalized intestinal telangiectasis may account for some of the obscure cases of rectal bleeding. This interesting condition is associated with Turner's syndrome in a number of the cases (Fig. 6). In a girl with chronic anemia and stools positive for blood, a buccal smear may reveal absence of or a decrease in the number of the Barr bodies, an indication of the chromosomal abnormality (the XO genotype) which is present in this syndrome. When the bleeding has been localized in this condition to a particular area of the bowel by a careful investigation at operation, removal of that portion of the bowel may result in cure of the anemia. In most of the cases, however, the condition is more gen-

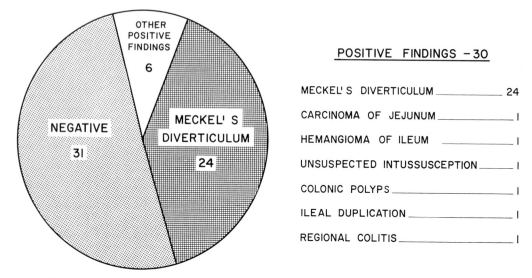

POSITIVE FINDINGS - 30

MECKEL' S DIVERTICULUM _____ 24

CARCINOMA OF JEJUNUM _____ I

HEMANGIOMA OF ILEUM _____ I

UNSUSPECTED INTUSSUSCEPTION _____ I

COLONIC POLYPS _____ I

ILEAL DUPLICATION _____ I

REGIONAL COLITIS _____ I

Fig. 5. Exploratory laparotomy for rectal bleeding in 61 children. (From Shandling. Pediatrics, 35:787, 1965.)

eralized, and the best that can be hoped for from subtotal removal of the affected bowel is a reduction in the need for repeated transfusions.

Small intestinal hemangiomas of the colon may bleed repeatedly, giving rise to anemia and debilitation. While the larger ones may be visible on radiographic examination, the smaller ones are not. Even more difficult to find are the rare localized telangiectasias of the colon or small bowel which are sometimes the source of serious bleeding. The only finding at operation in these cases may be slight dilatation of veins in the mesentery of the affected part. If no bleeding lesion in the intestinal tract is found at laparotomy for rectal bleeding, the entire mesentery should be inspected carefully by transillumination for evidence of dilated veins. If such dilated mesenteric veins are seen, removal of that portion of the intestine is indicated, as described in a recent clinical pathologic conference discussion of this difficult problem (Farber and Vawter, 1962).

TECHNIQUE OF SIGMOIDOSCOPY

A clear liquid diet is given the night before, and in the morning preparation of the lower colon is readily accomplished with a Dulcolax suppository. Unless continued bleeding obscures the field from above, the child clears the colon and a clean lumen is obtained about 45 minutes after introduction of the suppository. For infants, a 1-cm sigmoidoscope, 12 cm in length, is available. The rectum is approximately 5 cm in length and up to 3 cm in diameter in the infant age group. In older children, a sigmoidoscope 1.5 by 15 cm is perfectly adequate both for viewing the mucosa and for taking specimens with the rectal biopsy forceps (Fig. 7).

With the infant or child held in the knee-chest position, the *warmed* and lubricated sigmoidoscope is gently introduced after a digital exploration of the rectum has been accomplished. The sigmoidoscope will proceed several centimeters by its own weight, and then it should be advanced under direct vision (Fig. 8). We prefer the knee-chest to the Sims position because it is easier to hold the children in this manner, and a certain amount of straightening and dilatation of the rectosigmoid occurs as the result of gravitation of the intestinal mass to the upper abdomen.

It should be remembered that 6 cm in the infant rectum and sigmoid is equivalent to 25 cm in the adult. It should also be remembered that the rectosigmoid colon of infants

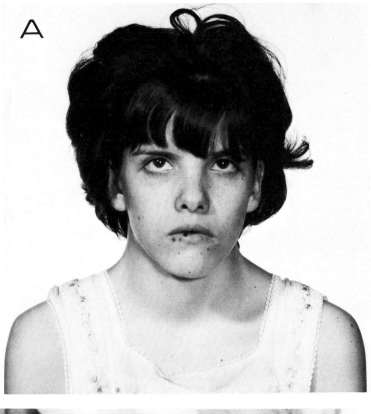

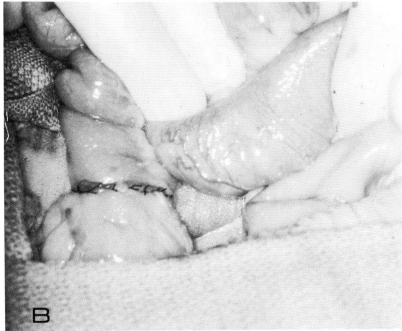

Fig. 6. A. Webbed neck of Turner's syndrome. Multiple cutaneous angiomas are also present. B. Residual angiomatosis of small bowel after subtotal colectomy and ileosigmoidostomy.

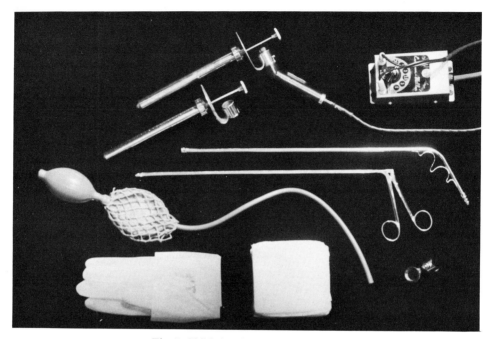

Fig. 7. Child-size sigmoidoscope outfit.

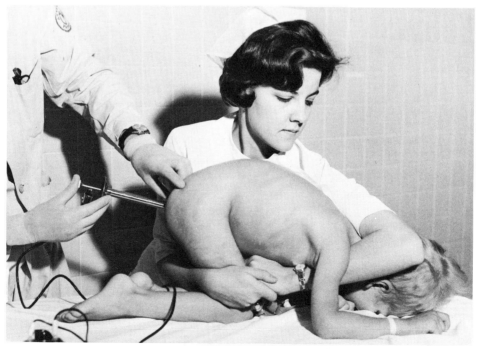

Fig. 8. Knee-chest position for sigmoidoscopy. The nurse holds the child firmly behind the neck and across the popliteal space.

is thin and friable. A perforation is very easily produced by rough manipulation or deep biopsy. Aside from these considerations, the procedure is rapid and atraumatic. General anesthesia is not necessary for proctosigmoidoscopy in infants and children.

PREPARATION FOR EMERGENCY BARIUM ENEMA

Cathartics are contraindicated in preparation for a lower gastrointestinal series when bleeding is present. Excellent preparations can be achieved by the use of a Dulcolax suppository followed by a thin barium mixture as a cleansing enema. If the preparation is not adequate, this preliminary mixture should be evacuated. A second study is then performed with a thicker mixture in conjunction with air-contrast studies to reveal mucosal detail.

SUMMARY

Many abnormalities may lead to gastrointestinal bleeding in children. The specific lesions are considered in other chapters of this book. An attempt has been made in the present chapter to give an overall view of the problem and to suggest measures for the immediate management of the bleeding patient.

In one's approach to the diagnosis and treatment of intestinal bleeding, it is best to begin with the age of the patient and the probable level of the bleeding. Most newborn infants with intestinal bleeding do not have surgical lesions and recover spontaneously. The incidence of exsanguinating disorders is high enough, however, that an intravenous route for the administration of fluids should be established immediately on the baby's admission to the hospital. Vitamin K, normal feedings, and occasionally a blood transfusion result in cessation of the bleeding in 95 percent of the cases during the neonatal period. If upper gastrointestinal hemorrhage continues despite constant gastric drainage and the administration of antacid agents

through an indwelling nasogastric tube, an acute bleeding duodenal ulcer is probably present. It can usually be diagnosed by roentgen examination, which should also include an investigation of the lower esophagus. Operative treatment is indicated if more than 75 percent of the infant's total blood volume has had to be replaced.

In the 1- to 24-month age group, intussusception, Meckel's diverticulum, and duplications are the usual surgical causes of bleeding, but sepsis with stress ulceration and infectious colitis are important alternative diagnoses. Acute anal fissure is the condition which brings most children of this age to the physician. After two years of age, idiopathic ulcerative colitis, Meckel's diverticulum, a variety of polyps and tumors, esophageal varices, regional enteritis. duplications, intussusceptions, a peptic ulcer, or Henoch-Schönlein purpura will usually be discovered.

The immediate management of the individual patient with significant rectal bleeding requires the physician to distinguish the surgical from the medical problems associated with bleeding, and to determine whether or not operation is indicated. Quite obviously urgent treatment is required for intussusception, segmental volvulus, esophageal varices which continue to bleed, and other strangulating or exsanguinating gastrointestinal lesions. The situation is not so clear cut when a bleeding Meckel's diverticulum is suspected, for the diagnostic features of this disorder are not definite, and truly massive hemorrhage leading to death is a rare event (Ch. 38). The patient with a bleeding Meckel's diverticulum can usually be observed safely under hospital conditions until appropriate diagnostic studies are completed.

A workable therapeutic plan in the management of severe gastrointestinal bleeding in older infants and children is to establish a route for the administration of blood and to follow the vital signs, the venous pressure, and the hematocrit while diagnostic studies are being done. If the hemorrhage ceases and the hemoglobin remains above 7 g percent, repeated diagnostic investigations should include complete coagulation studies, upper and lower intestinal roentgenograms, proctosigmoidoscopy, and occasionally esophagoscopy.

If no diagnosis can be made and the stools continue markedly positive for blood, or if a second massive hemorrhage occurs which reduces the hemoglobin below 6 g percent, the patient should be transfused to a level of 12 g of hemoglobin before an exploratory operation is performed. This program will identify the responsible lesion in more than 90 percent of the cases.

If the stools become negative for occult blood during the period of observation, followup investigations should be performed at 1, 3, 6, and 12 months. The physical examination, hemoglobin level, and stool guaiac examinations are usually sufficient for this purpose. Of those children in whom an exploratory operation fails to locate any responsible lesion, about 70 percent continue well without further intestinal tract bleeding. The remainder are usually subjected to reoperation for another episode of bleeding, and an abnormality is eventually uncovered in the great majority of the cases.

WILLIAM L. DONNELLAN
ORVAR SWENSON

REFERENCES

ABRAMS, B., and LYNN, H. B. Rectal bleeding in children. Amer. J. Surg., 104: 831, 1962.

ALWAY, R. H. Gross bleeding from the alimentary tract in infants and children. Amer. Surgeon, 20: 216, 1954.

AMES, M. D. Gastric acidity in the first ten days of life of the prematurely born baby. Amer. J. Dis. Child., 100: 252, 1960.

APT, L., and DOWNEY, W. S., Jr. "Melena" neonatorum; the swallowed blood syndrome. J. Pediat., 47: 6, 1955.

BOLEY, S. J. et al. The effect of operations for peptic ulcer on growth and nutrition of puppies. Surgery, 57: 441, 1965.

BRAYTON, D., and NORRIS, W. J. Gastrointestinal hemorrhage in infancy and childhood. J.A.M.A., 150: 668, 1952.

CHISHOLM, T. C., SPENCER, B. J., and McPARLAND, F. A. Acute massive gastrointestinal hemorrhage. Pediat. Clin. N. Amer., 9: 201, 1962.

COLE, A. R. C. Gastric ulcer of the pylorus simulating hypertrophic pyloric stenosis; report of a case in an infant nine weeks old. Pediatrics, 6: 897, 1950.

CRAIG, W. S. On real and apparent external bleeding in the newborn. Arch. Dis. Child., 36: 575, 1961.

FARBER, S., and VAWTER, G. F. Clinical pathological conference, The Children's Hospital Medical Center, Boston. J. Pediat., 61: 638, 1962.

FISHER, J. H. Duodenal ulcers in infants. Amer. J. Dis. Child., 79: 50, 1950.

GROSS, R. E., HOLCOMB, G. W., Jr., and FARBER, S. Duplications of the alimentary tract. Pediatrics, 9: 449, 1952.

HODGSON, J. R., and KENNEDY, R. L. J. Bleeding lesions of the gastrointestinal tract in infants and children. Radiology, 63: 535, 1954.

HOFFERT, P. W., and HURWITT, E. S. The significance of rectal bleeding. Surg. Clin. N. Amer., 35: 1221, 1955.

HOLLANDER, M. H., and STARK, M. W. Duodenal ulcer in infancy, with presentation of a case. Pediatrics, 6: 676, 1950.

KIESEWETTER, W. B., CANCELMO, R., and KOOP, C. E. Rectal bleeding in infants and children: With a hitherto unreported etiological factor. J. Pediat., 47: 660, 1955.

KOOP, C. E. Rectal bleeding in infants and children. Pediat. Clin. N. Amer., 3: 207, 1956.

LADD, W. E. Surgical significance of melena in childhood. New Eng. J. Med., 217: 649, 1937.

LAWRENCE, B. A., and BLOXSOM, A. Pneumonia complicated by acute hemorrhage and ulcerative gastroenteritis in a child. Amer. J. Dis. Child., 58: 1265, 1939.

LEIX, F., and GREANY, E. M., Jr. Surgical experience with peptic ulcer in infancy and childhood. Amer. J. Surg., 106: 173, 1963.

MACBETH, R. A. Rectal bleeding in infancy and childhood. Canad. Med. Ass. J., 85: 1040, 1961.

McPARLAND, F. A., and KIESEWETTER, W. B. Meckel's diverticulum in childhood. Surg. Gynec. Obstet., 106: 11, 1958.

MILLER, R. A. Observations on the gastric acidity during the first month of life. Arch. Dis. Child., 16: 22, 1941.

OECONOMOPOULOS, C. T. Low intestinal hemorrhage in children. Amer. J. Proctol., 2: 379, 1960.

RAFFENSBERGER, J. G., CONDON, J. B., and GREENGARD, J. Complications of gastric and duodenal ulcers in infancy and childhood. Surg. Gynec. Obstet., 123: 1269, 1966.

SCHUSTER, S. R., and GROSS, R. E. Peptic ulcer disease in childhood. Amer. J. Surg., 105: 324, 1963.

SHANDLING, B. Laparotomy for rectal bleeding. Pediatrics, 35: 787, 1965.

SPENCER, R. Gastrointestinal hemorrhage in infancy and childhood: 476 cases. Surgery, 55: 718, 1964.

STOTTS, C. S., and FRIESEN, S. R. Perforation of duodenal ulcer in the newborn with operation and survival. Surgery, 41: 863, 1957.

THOMPSON, N. W., TUBERGEN, D. G., and YULL, A. B. Duodenal ulcer in the newborn infant. Arch. Surg., 90: 233, 1965.

44

Polyps and Other Tumors of the Gastrointestinal Tract

BENIGN POLYPS

THE JUVENILE OR INFLAMMATORY POLYP

Benign polyps in the childhood age group differ from adult intestinal polyps both in their histology and their behavior. The juvenile polyp is often called an "inflammatory" polyp since it is composed mainly of connective tissue elements containing large numbers of lymphocytes, plasma cells, polymorphonuclear leukocytes, and some eosinophils. Granulation tissue covers the surface of the polyp. Obstruction of the orifices of the remaining intestinal glands by overgrowth of this tissue results in the formation of large cystic spaces (Fig. 1). By contrast, adult or "adenomatous" polyps are true epithelial growths with a frondlike development of myriads of mucous glands of approximately the same size.

About 75 percent of juvenile polyps are pedunculated, and 25 percent are sessile. It is the presence of a large pedicle of normal mucosa which often permits spontaneous amputation of the polyp during the passage of stools (Fig. 2) or prolapse of the polyp through the rectum. Juvenile polyps are usually located in the colon, but they may occur anywhere along the course of the intestinal tract. Seventy to 85 percent are found to be

within the reach of proctosigmoidostomy, with lesser numbers lying more proximally. In 75 percent of the cases the polyp is solitary, and in over 90 percent no more than three polyps are discovered. Malignancy is rare in juvenile polyps. Although Gordon and his colleagues (1957) found 8.5 percent of 104 childhood polyps to harbor potential malignancy, no case of invasion of epithelial elements beneath the muscularis mucosae

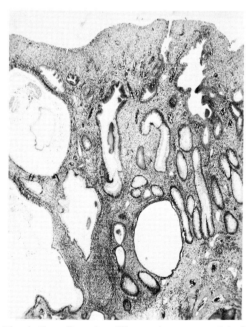

Fig. 1. Juvenile polyp. The cystic spaces and lack of surface epithelium are characteristic.

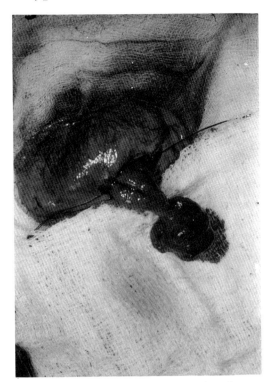

Fig. 2. Colonic polyp drawn through colotomy incision to show long pedicle.

was present in 58 polyps which could be extensively examined. In any case, it is generally accepted that carcinoma in association with intestinal polyposis is not a problem under the age of 11 years (discussed elsewhere) and that it occurs not with juvenile polyps, but with the truly neoplastic adenomatous variety.

SIGNS AND SYMPTOMS

The usual time of discovery of a colonic polyp is between the ages of 2 and 6 years. It appears that the lesions may regress, since they are rare after 11 years of age. The cardinal symptom is *bright red rectal bleeding*. In some series significant bleeding occurred in over 99 percent of the cases. The bleeding is rarely severe. It consists usually of oozing from the inflamed surface, and when only one or two polyps are present anemia does not develop. Occasionally the avulsion of a large polyp exposes a good-

sized vessel in the base, and a bout of sharp bleeding requiring transfusion may then occur.

Prolapse of the polyp through the anus is the next most frequent complication, resulting in the diagnosis of about one fifth of the cases (Fig. 3). Such prolapse is often associated with severe pain. It may be followed by avulsion of the polyp with subsequent bleeding. When such spontaneous amputation occurs, the mother is likely to bring the polyp when the child arrives for the examination.

Abdominal pain was present in only 5.5 percent of the cases reported by Mallam and Thomson (1959). In other series it has occurred in up to 20 percent. The pain is cramping in nature and very probably results from traction on the polyp during peristaltic activity or from partial intussusception which can be demonstrated by barium enema examination.

When many polyps are present, *diarrhea* may be a prominent complaint. Excessive mucus and watery stools probably result from irritation of the normal mucosa about the polyps and from bouts of partial bowel obstruction. This symptom occurs in from 3 to 10 percent of the cases.

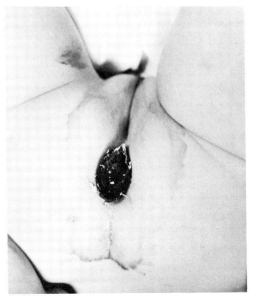

Fig. 3. Prolapse of polyp through the rectum in small child.

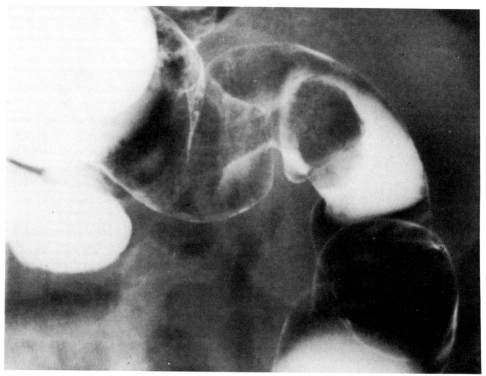

Fig. 4. Polyp of the sigmoid colon. The stalk is clearly visible.

DIAGNOSIS

The majority of polyps of the colon and rectum can be palpated at rectal examination. From 50 to 70 percent can be diagnosed in this way. At the same time the more common *anal fissure* can be eliminated as a cause of mild rectal bleeding. If no polyp is felt, and there is no anal spasticity or other evidence of a fissure, proctosigmoidoscopy should be performed.

We have found Dulcolax to be a satisfactory preparation for sigmoidoscopy. If the bleeding is not severe, a clear liquid diet is given the night before the examination together with two Dulcolax tablets. One hour before the sigmoidoscopy a Dulcolax suppository is inserted, and the child is allowed to evacuate any remaining stool. This preparation produces a clear and dry mucosa which is not hidden by excessive mucus production.

Sometimes a hemorrhagic area on the wall of the rectum testifies to the previous avulsion of a polyp. If no other lesions are seen nothing further need be done. Most of the polyps are single, and it is probable that any others will remain asymptomatic. A stool should be examined for occult blood one month later. If blood is present, a barium enema with air-contrast studies must be performed.

A careful preparation of the colon must be done prior to barium enema examination. If the colon is not cleared of feces a round fecalith may erroneously be mistaken for a polyp. A filling defect which persists as a round barium-covered protrusion into the colonic lumen is almost certainly a polyp (Fig. 4). Postevacuation films may reveal other smaller polyps, but usually only one or two are present at any single examination.

DIFFERENTIAL DIAGNOSIS

Rectal bleeding is a prominent symptom of many lesions of the small bowel and colon. The major causes in the 2- to 6-year-old age group are polyps, colitis, an anal fissure, and a Meckel's diverticulum. When no lesion is discovered by proctosigmoidoscopy and barium enema examination, an orderly investigation for the cause of bleeding should be performed in the manner outlined in Chapter 43.

TREATMENT

If a single polyp is present in the rectum it can be removed by a sigmoidoscopic snare and electrocautery technique, or occasionally by prolapsing the polyp through the rectum for ligation of its base. About 25 percent of colonic polyps cannot be reached from below, however, and laparatomy must be considered.

It is our opinion that single polyps, or even two or three polyps, do not necessarily require removal by abdominal section. Many authors believe that spontaneous regression may occur, and certainly a number will be avulsed by peristaltic activity. Unless the bleeding is troublesome or a serious anemia develops, colotomy or colectomy are not indicated for the removal of juvenile polyps, since the one important problem—the possibility of malignant change—does not exist. This is particularly true in the smaller children. On the other hand, large polyps which persist and cause repeated episodes of abdominal pain, or those which are found after the age of ten are more likely to produce serious complications, and they may harbor invasive malignancy. We believe that these should be removed surgically when they are discovered. In addition, the discovery on microscopic examination that the polyp is adenomatous rather than juvenile in type indicates that more careful followup studies will be necessary, since a potentially dangerous condition, that of malignant change, is present. According to Kottmeier and Clatworthy (1965), children have either juvenile inflammatory or adenomatous polyps, never both together. For that reason, the finding of a juvenile polyp in one location implies that other polyps which may be present are of the same histological type, and that their subsequent excision by abdominal section is not necessary.

PROGNOSIS

The removal of a single juvenile polyp from the rectum will be followed by recurrence in only about 5 percent of the cases. Adenomatous polyps and particularly the polyps associated with familial polyposis are almost certainly more likely to recur. When more than ten polyps, whether juvenile or adenomatous are present, recurrence is the rule after colotomy with local excision. It is recommended by several authors that subtotal colectomy to remove the polyp area be accomplished in this situation, in order to avoid the hazards of repeated abdominal operations.

In summary, about 15 to 20 percent of all rectal bleeding during childhood is due to the presence of colonic polyps. The bleeding is usually mild, but it may on occasion be massive. Over two thirds of colonic polyps can be felt per rectum, and if one rectal polyp is present, others will be discovered on further examination in about 25 percent of the cases. If the histological diagnosis of juvenile rather than adenomatous polyps is confirmed, those polyps which cannot be reached sigmoidoscopically do not usually require abdominal section for their removal.

ADENOMATOUS POLYPS

Adenomatous polyps are true neoplasms. They develop through alteration of the columnar cells at the base of the crypts. Taller groups of cells which contain increased numbers of mitotic figures are seen to develop in the deeper portions of the crypts. As the proliferation of these cells increases, a sessile nodule develops which in the course of time is drawn into the lumen of the bowel and becomes pedunculated. The usual adenomatous polyp is rarely larger than 2 to 3 cm in diameter. Microscopically the appearance is that of rather regular proliferating glands supported on a thin vascular connective tissue stroma. The base of the polyp is made up of normal mucosa and submucosa, and its surface is lined, not by inflammatory granulation tissue as is the case with the juvenile polyps, but with a regular orderly columnar surface epithelium punctuated by the openings of the glands.

Adenomatous polyps are rare in children. Kottmeier and Clatworthy found only 3 patients with this type in a group of 50 children who were found to have intestinal polyps. In two of the adenoma cases the polyps were multiple. Carcinoma developed in one of the patients at the age of 12.

TREATMENT

It is recommended that adenomatous polyps be removed whenever they are dis-

covered. If a rectal polyp is found to be of this variety, extensive studies of the rest of the colon are indicated, and resection should be done if any more polyps are found by sigmoidoscopy or radiographic study. Multiple polyps are often clustered in one area of the colon. If this is found to be the case, they should be removed by a segmental colon resection which includes all of the affected area. Followup studies are indicated at yearly intervals to determine if other polyps are forming.

FAMILIAL MULTIPLE POLYPOSIS OF THE COLON

Multiple polyposis may be familial or sporadic. The distinction between polyposis and multiple scattered polyps is a difficult one to make. True familial multiple polyposis is an uncommon condition which is transmit-

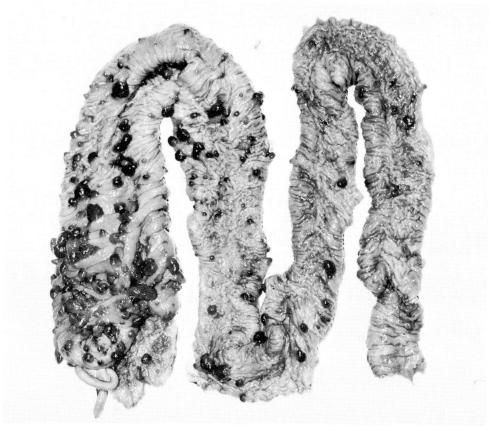

Fig. 5. Multiple polyposis in a six-year-old boy.

ted as a mendelian autosomal dominant, that is, it occurs in one half of the children of either sex when one parent has the disease. The entire colon is studded with large numbers of small sessile or pea-sized polyps (Fig. 5). The stomach and small bowel are almost never affected. The condition makes itself known by bleeding or recurrent diarrhea during later childhood and early adolescence. Small polyps are undoubtedly present and in many cases can be demonstrated before puberty in known polyposis families, but symptoms of the disease rarely occur before the age of 11 and are usually delayed until about the twenty-first year. Malignant degeneration is so common as to be the rule, and carcinoma, often multiple, has been reported in patients with this condition as young as 12 years of age. For this reason total colectomy with ileorectostomy is the procedure of

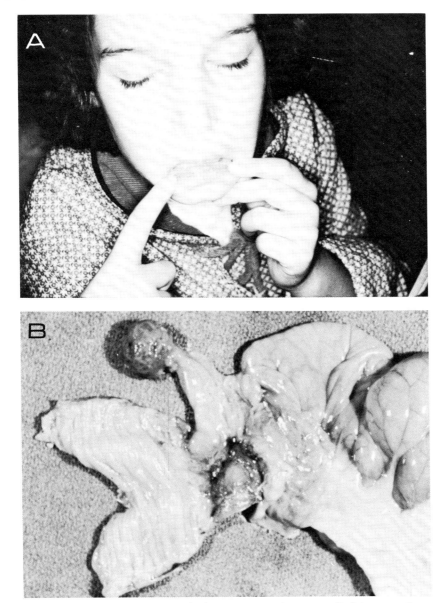

Fig. 6. The Peutz-Jeghers syndrome. A. Melanin spots on oral mucosa. B. Intussusception was caused by the polyp shown.

choice. Some surgeons prefer to resect the entire colon and rectum, with anastomosis of the ileum by the pull-through technique to the terminal 2 cm of the anal canal. The stools vary from 6 to 10 in number per day in different patients after the initial recovery period, and good fecal control is achieved. Because perineal excoriation may follow low ileorectostomy, however, we prefer to do an ileosigmoid anastomosis and to follow the patients by sigmoidoscopy for the treatment of recurrent polyps. At operation the well-prepared bowel is opened from above and the residual polyps are excised and fulgurated. A similar procedure is also done from below prior to the discharge of the patient from the hospital.

Frequent follow-up examinations at six-month intervals are required for the duration of the patient's lifetime. Recurrent polyps must be fulgurated as they appear. According to Localio (1962) and several other authors, spontaneous regression of the rectal polyps may occur after high ileoproctostomy. On the other hand, carcinoma will develop under observation in 5.2 percent of patients in whom the rectum is left in place. If carcinoma does develop while the patient is under observation, it can still be treated and cured by more radical surgical therapy. For this reason we believe that ileosigmoidostomy or high ileoproctostomy is the treatment of choice, since the patients are comfortable and their eventual cure rate is excellent. Total proctocolectomy with permanent ileostomy, as has been recommended by some authorities, does not seem to be warranted in an effort to eliminate the relatively small number of patients who return with carcinoma in the retained rectum.

THE PEUTZ-JEGHERS SYNDROME

A fourth type of intestinal polyposis is that associated with mucocutaneous pigmentation. First noted by Peutz in 1921, this association was reviewed by Jeghers and his colleagues in 1949. The condition appears to be ge-

netically determined, since a positive family history is present in about 50 percent of the cases.

Pigmentation of the lips and oral mucosa does not necessarily imply that intestinal polyps are present. Nevertheless Peutz-Jeghers polyposis should be suspected whenever this type of unusual spotty pigmentation is discovered (Fig. 6). Other sites include the palms and digits, the umbilicus, and the anorectal mucosa. The pigmentation is noted during early childhood as a rule and tends to fade after puberty.

The most common symptom of this type of intestinal polyposis is recurrent *cramping abdominal pain* accompanied by borborygmi, which results apparently from transient intussusceptions. It usually occurs shortly after meals or upon arising, and rarely when the patient is at rest. Next in frequency are rectal bleeding, anemia, rectal prolapse, and bouts of vomiting. When these symptoms are noted in conjunction with mucocutaneous pigmentation, the demonstration of polyps by gastrointestinal radiography confirms the diagnosis of the Peutz-Jeghers syndrome.

PATHOLOGY

The polyps occur anywhere from the esophagocardiac junction to the anus. They are usually multiple. The small intestine is always involved, with affection of the colon, rectum, stomach, and duodenum occurring in that order of frequency. Many small micropolyps may be present in addition to the larger lesions. According to Dormandy (1957) "crops" of polyps are produced which mature together. Recurrence of the polyps is the rule after excisional treatment, but several months or years may elapse before further symptomatic polyps develop. The microscopic appearance is characteristic and quite different from both the juvenile and adenomatous varieties. The glands are relatively normal in appearance, but they are unusually long and markedly branched. Their epithelial cells are those of the mucous membrane of that portion of the gastrointestinal tract which is involved. Bands of smooth muscle coursing through the polyp are characteristic of the growth, which is generally considered to be hamartomatous in nature.

TREATMENT

Since intestinal polyps of the Peutz-Jeghers type apparently do not become malignant, and since they are continually forming in the intestinal tract, conservatism in their surgical management is the best course to follow. Multiple intussusceptions occur, but for some reason they only very rarely progress to complete obstruction or devitalization of the bowel. The intussusceptions usually can be reduced manually by pressure on the abdomen or by the giving of an enema, and these methods of relief have often been discovered by the patient or his parents before the diagnosis is made.

A rare complication which requires operative treatment is chronic anemia. If chronic rectal bleeding develops and the hemoglobin level cannot be maintained, the largest polyps should be removed. Continued bouts of severe pain may also require operation. In distinction to the treatment of multiple colonic polyps, which are best managed by resection of the offending portion of the bowel, Peutz-Jeghers polyps require that only local removal be done, since it is difficult to predict how much bowel will eventually be affected by the development of further areas of polyposis. At operation many intussusceptions may be discovered. These are reduced manually, and the lead polyps are removed through small enterotomies. Other large polyps should also be removed at the same sitting. Further operations may be required by the recurrence of pain or bleeding, but again a conservative approach should be the rule.

PROGNOSIS

The prognosis for a normal life span is good. Affected patients must expect to experience further symptoms even after most of the polyps are removed at operation. These recurrent symptoms may occur a few months or several years after the initial treatment. Untreated intussusception has occasionally led to the death of a patient with the Peutz-Jeghers disorder, but this need not occur. The best service which can be rendered to these patients is to acquaint them fully with the nature of the disease and to reassure them that while the complications of the polyposis are distressing, they are not dangerous to life, and that if the complications of strangulating intussusception or serious bleeding occur they can be managed in a straightforward manner.

UNUSUAL POLYPS OF THE COLON

Two unusual types of polyps of the colon should be mentioned. Occasionally an overgrowth of lymphoid tissue occurs in the mucosa and submucosa of the colon, giving rise to a polypoid mass which may partially occlude the bowel lumen or may ulcerate to cause rectal bleeding. These masses are usually circumscribed and single. They can be dealt with by a segmental resection. The histology of the lesion is not that of lymphosarcoma, for there are germinal centers and few mitotic figures. Furthermore, recurrence or generalization of the disease to leukemia does not occur.

A second unusual polyp is that formed by granulation tissue. These masses occur in the rectum, and may cause rectal bleeding or diarrhea. The etiology is unknown. It is possible that the lesion arises from a traumatic ulceration of the rectal mucosa which has failed to epithelialize in the normal manner. There is no indication of specific bacterial or viral etiology. When the lesions are small electrocautery may suffice for cure, but larger lesions require segmental resection either by the posterior operation of Kraske or, if they are higher toward the pelvic brim, by means of an anterior resection with anastomosis. A margin of 1 cm is sufficient for good healing

TABLE 1.   MALIGNANT GASTROINTESTINAL NEOPLASMS*

SARCOMAS (76 CASES)

Tumor Type		Distribution	
Lymphosarcomas	71 (93.4%)	Duodenum	2
Reticulum cell sarcoma	2	Jejunum	2
Angiosarcoma	1	Ileum	59
Spindle cell sarcoma	1	Ileocecal	2
Unspecified	1	Cecum	3
		Colon	4
		Rectum	4
	76		76

CARCINOMAS (142 CASES)

Rectum	70 ⎫	
Rectosigmoid	12 ⎬ 71.7%	
Sigmoid	20 ⎭	
Duodenum	6	
Jejunum	6	
Cecum	7	
Colon	20	
Unclassified	1	
	142	

* From Bonelli. Clin. Proc. Child. Hosp. Wash., 3:151, 1947.

of the anastomosis, and permanent control of the problem is usually achieved.

MALIGNANT NEOPLASMS OF THE GASTROIN-TESTINAL TRACT

In a collective review of 218 patients under the age of 20 with malignancy of the small and large intestines, Bonelli lists the types of tumors in Table 1.

In this large collected series of cases sarcomas occurred at a much earlier age than carcinomas (Table 2). In those reports in which the age of the patient is given there were 17 cases of sarcoma in the 0- to 5-year-age group, with a decreasing incidence with increasing age. By contrast, all the carcinomas were found beyond the age of 11 years. A little more than one half developed in the 11- to 15-year-age group and the rest in the 15- to 20-year-age group.

In our experience lymphosarcoma has been the most common malignancy, followed (at great distance) by reticulum cell sarcoma, leiomyosarcoma, malignant carcinoids, and adenocarcinomas. Our youngest patient with lymphosarcoma was 2 years of age. We have encountered three carcinomas of the rectum or sigmoid, one in a 12-year-old girl with multiple polyposis, one at 13 years in association with ulcerative colitis, and a third in a 12-year-old boy without other disease. Mayo and Madding (1940)

TABLE 2.   CLASSIFICATION OF TYPES OF TUMOR BY AGE*

SARCOMAS		CARCINOMAS	
0–5 years	17	11–15 years	79
6–10 years	11	15–20 years	63
11–15 years	7		
16–18 years	3		

* From Bonelli. Clin. Proc. Child. Hosp. Wash., 3:151, 1947.

mention a rectosigmoid carcinoma in a 4-year-old boy, but the tumor was described as a polyp of "grade I malignancy," and was without metastatic spread.

The *symptoms* of gastrointestinal malignancy in children are vague. There may be moderate recurrent abdominal pain or a soreness over the lesion. Weight loss is uncommon and occurs only late in the course of the disease, but anemia may develop from chronic blood loss. Occasionally obvious rectal bleeding is the first symptom of a malignant tumor. Obstruction with vomiting may occur, particularly when the tumor is located in the upper bowel or ileocecal region, since intussusception leads to the diagnosis in about 24 percent of the cases. Tumors in the free portion of the intestine, however, may attain a relatively gigantic size before producing enough symptoms to bring the patient to the attention of a physician (Fig. 7).

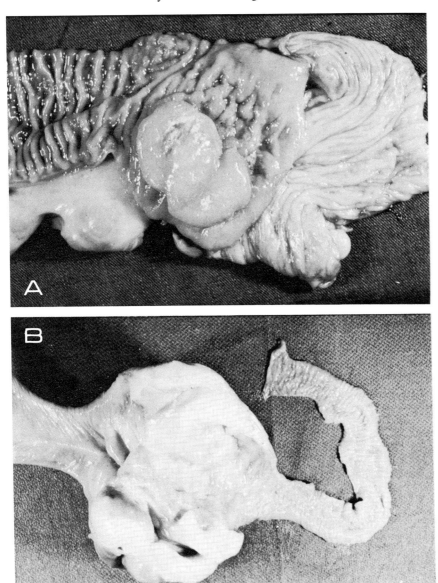

Fig. 7. A. Small reticulum cell sarcomas of the type which produce intussusception. B. Very large lymphosarcoma which produced only moderate symptoms of obstruction.

When a lymphosarcoma develops in the region of the cecum its ulceration may result in infection and pain in the right lower quadrant. It is not surprising, therefore, that children are not infrequently referred for further treatment after an exploration for appendicitis has led to the discovery of a large cecal or terminal ileum lymphosarcoma. In such cases the mass is usually easily palpable, the pain is more diffuse than that of appendicitis, and the tenderness is less marked than in the case when an appendiceal abscess is present. The finding of a mass in the right lower quadrant should at least lead to the suspicion that a tumor rather than appendicitis is the cause of symptoms, particularly when a good history for perforation of the appendix cannot be obtained. Abdominal pain is common during childhood. While it is usually temporary and of little importance, it is more likely to be significant if it is recurrent or if it is associated with weight loss, a change in the bowel habits, regurgitation of food materials, or intestinal bleeding. When these symptoms are present a complete investigation of the gastrointestinal tract must be performed at once.

TREATMENT

Most gastrointestinal malignancies during childhood lead to the death of the patient. The tumors are highly invasive, and because of their late discovery they have usually spread before they are discovered. The local removal of a lymphosarcoma which has not spread to the local nodes is occasionally followed by cure, with or without radiation therapy. Most such successes are incidental to appendectomy or to cases in which the tumor has produced an intussusception early in its growth.

The removal of the portion of the intestine which contains the tumor should always include wide resection of its mesentery and the draining lymph nodes. Radiation therapy to the abdomen is begun on the day of operation and is carried out to 2,000 to 2,500 rads through multiple parts for a total of 20 days. Although some unresectable tumors have disappeared with radiation therapy, it is still doubtful whether this adjunct to treatment is of real value. Adequate removal of the tumor and its drainage areas will be followed by cure if no residual malignant cells remain behind. If local or distant metastases have occurred they usually lie outside the field of irradiation.

Generalization of the lymphosarcoma is the most usual outcome of treatment. A leukemic blood picture develops, and multiple enlargements of the lymph nodes and invasion of the bone marrow make their appearance. This is the common sequel to the surgical removal of an intestinal lymphosarcoma, and it is therefore the opinion of some observers that antileukemia chemotherapy is preferable to local irradiation. One treatment with intravenous or intra-arterial alkylating agents should be given on the day of operation. Subsequent treatments are given after the seventh postoperative day, in view of the findings of Mrazek and his associates (1959), and of Newcombe (1966), that healing is delayed if antimetabolites are given during the time of tissue mobilization for wound repair.

PROGNOSIS

The cure of an intestinal lymphosarcoma is unlikely. At The Children's Memorial Hospital we have encountered 13 of these tumors in the past 15 years. Three of the children were transferred after previous operations, and 10 were treated primarily. Two patients survived beyond 2 years and appear to be cured. The third has been asymptomatic for 8 months postoperatively. Two of these surviving patients had intussusceptions which led to early diagnosis; the third, who has now survived 5 years, had an ulcerating lesion associated with large mesenteric nodes. The tumor in this patient was only partially resected. It was treated by a combination of irradiation, prednisone and prolonged Cytoxan therapy, with the result that the residual tumor appears to have been ablated. In the large series of Simpson-Smith (1938), 60 percent of children with intestinal sarcoma died within six months, and 92 percent were dead within one year.

Adenocarcinomas of the colon in children have an equally gloomy prognosis. Their treatment should be exactly the same as in the adult. Prophylactic surgical attention to polypoid masses or to prolonged ulcerative colitis in children over the age of ten years would seem to be the best way to improve the prognosis for the rare carcinomas of the intestinal tract which occur during childhood.

WILLIAM L. DONNELLAN
ORVAR SWENSON

REFERENCES

ABRAMS, B., and LYNN, H. B. Rectal bleeding in children. Amer. J. Surg., 104: 831, 1962.

BONELLI, W. R. Malignant tumors of the small and large intestines in infants and children. Clin. Proc. Child. Hosp. Wash., 3: 151, 1947.

DORMANDY, T. L. Gastrointestinal polyposis with mucocutaneous pigmentation (Peutz-Jeghers syndrome). New Eng. J. Med., 256: 1093, 1957.

GORDON, D. L. et al. Polyps of the colon in children. Arch. Surg., 75: 90, 1957.

HORRILENO, E. G., ECKERT, C., and ACKERMAN, L. V. Polyps of the rectum and colon in children. Cancer, 10: 1210, 1957.

HUBBARD, T. B., Jr. Familial polyposis of the colon: The fate of the retained rectum after colectomy in children. Amer. Surgeon, 23: 577, 1957.

JEGHERS, H., McKUSICK, V. A., and KATZ, K. H. Generalized intestinal polyposis and melanin spots of oral mucosa, lips and digits: Syndrome of diagnostic significance. New Eng. J. Med., 241: 993, 1949.

KOTTMEIER, P. K., and CLATWORTHY, H. W., Jr. Intestinal polyps and associated carcinoma in childhood. Amer. J. Surg., 110: 709, 1965.

LOCALIO, S. A. Spontaneous disappearance of rectal polyps following subtotal colectomy and ileoproctostomy for polyposis of the colon. Amer. J. Surg., 103: 81, 1962.

MALLAM, A. S., and THOMSON, S. A. Polyps of rectum and colon in children. Canad. J. Surg., 3: 17, 1959.

MAYO, C. W., and MADDING, G. F. Carcinoma of the rectum and rectosigmoid in the young. Arch. Surg., 40: 83, 1940.

MESTEL, A. L. Lymphosarcoma of the small intestine in infancy and childhood. Ann. Surg., 149: 87, 1959.

MIDDELKAMP, J. N., and HAFFNER, H. Carcinoma of the colon in children. Pediatrics, 32: 558, 1963.

MRAZEK, R. et al. Prophylactic and adjuvant use of nitrogen mustard in the surgical treatment of cancer. Ann. Surg., 150: 745, 1959.

NEWCOMBE, J. F. Effect of intraarterial nitrogen mustard infusion on wound healing in rabbits. Ann. Surg., 163: 319, 1966.

SIMPSON-SMITH, A. Sarcoma of the intestine in children. Brit. J. Surg., 26: 429, 1938.

SNYDER, W. H., Jr., CHAFFIN, L., and SNYDER, M. H. Neoplasms of the colon and rectum in infants and children. Pediat. Clin. N. Amer., 3: 93, 1956.

WAUGH, J. M., HARP, R. A., and SPENCER, R. J. The surgical management of multiple polyposis. Ann. Surg., 159: 149, 1964.

WILLIAMS, C., Jr. Carcinoma of the colon in childhood. Ann. Surg., 139: 816, 1954.

WILLIAMS, R. D., and FISH, J. C. Multiple polyposis, polyp regression, and carcinoma of the colon. Amer. J. Surg., 112: 846, 1966.

45

Aganglionic Megacolon or Hirschsprung's Disease

There are references to a disease in the literature that resemble congenital megacolon which antedate Hirschsprung's paper of 1868. His report was limited to two patients. However, it was unusual in that the clinical description followed these patients' life course and ended with a description of their postmortem examinations. The narrow distal segment of colon was described as well as the massive proximal colon, making it certain that Hirschsprung was describing the lesion which we now know as aganglionic megacolon.

The instance of Hirschsprung's disease has been found to be 1 in 5,000 births. Others have estimated it to be 1 in 2,000 to 1 in 20,000. As experience accumulates it would appear that it is more common than the earlier estimates had anticipated. In reported series of neonatal obstruction it is not unusual for aganglionic megacolon to stand as the most common cause.

ETIOLOGY

The etiology of the lesion is unknown. Why there is an absence of ganglion cells in the distal part of the colon is only surmised. It is known that the neural elements grow in after the bowel has begun to form into a viscus. Why the defect is common in the distal colon supplied normally by the pelvic parasympathetic system is undetermined. Present studies indicate that perhaps the rigid division between the parasympathetic and the sympathetic autonomic system is not as clear as originally considered by the neuroanatomist. Nevertheless, this lesion appears to be a defect of the pelvic parasympathetic system. It is generally agreed that the gastrointestinal tract up to the midpoint of the transverse colon is supplied by the autonomic fibers from the vagus. Beyond this, the colon is supplied by the pelvic parasympathetic system, and in the majority of the patients this is the part of the autonomic system which is defective in aganglionic megacolon.

About 4 percent of the patients have siblings with the lesion. We have seen the lesion in identical twins, and it has also occurred in children with one parent having had the disease. Passarge has found that a female having the disease has a 7.2 percent chance of having an offspring with the disease, while a male under the same conditions has a 2.6 percent chance. In the general population it is .02 percent. As more information accumulates there may well be an established genetic factor in the etiology of this disease.

One other interesting fact is that there is now a known association of mongolism and aganglionic megacolon. In a group of patients with aganglionosis this association is seen in 2 percent. That two such relatively rare lesions should occur together indicates that there may be some relationship in causation. So far chromosomal studies indicate

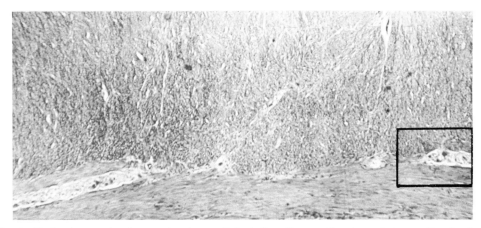

Fig. 1. Photomicrograph of normal colon wall including the ganglion layer between the circular and longitudinal muscular coats. Ganglion cells are present in two areas. (Hematoxylin and eosin stain.)

that trisomy 21 is the common abnormality found in the few cases where studies have found alterations from normal.

PROGNOSIS

A patient with Hirschsprung's disease faces a grave risk in the first few weeks of life. It has been stated that untreated neonatal Hirschsprung's disease is associated with a mortality of about 80 percent in the first month of life. Rarely does the patient with this untreated disease survive beyond the age of 12. That occasionally patients survive beyond this age is well known. Our oldest patient was 45 years of age at the time of resection. Some of the patients that survive for long periods of time have had surgical therapy of some sort which may have contributed to their survival. This disease is in-

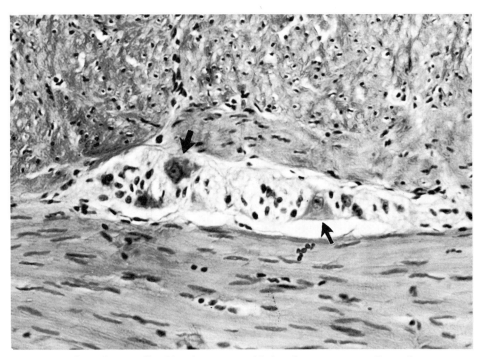

Fig. 2. Area outlined in Figure 1 magnified to demonstrate ganglion cells.

capacitating and considerably reduces lon-
gevity.

PATHOPHYSIOLOGY

It is interesting that the defect in ganglion
cells was described many years before any
surgical therapy was based upon this pathological finding. The earliest reports are probably from Germany in 1907. At a later date,
DeValle (1924) in Italy reported absent
ganglion cells in megacolon. In the more recent medical literature, there are publications
by Zuelzer and Wilson (1948) and Whitehouse (1948) describing absence of ganglion
cells in the terminal portion of the colon
(Figs. 1 and 2).

The absence of ganglion cells is complete
(Fig. 3). There is a transition zone of 1.5

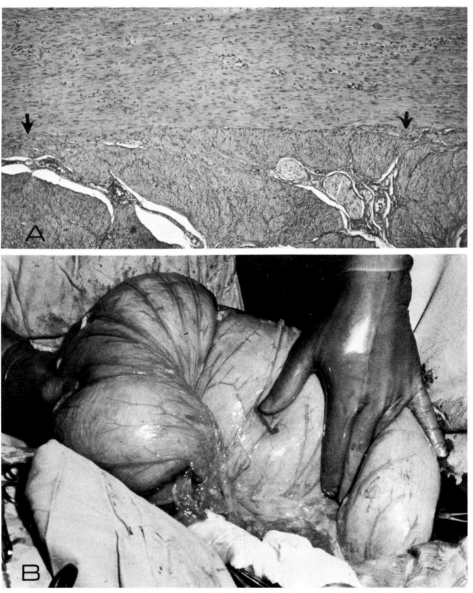

Fig. 3. A. Photomicrograph of colon from a patient with Hirschsprung's disease. The section was taken
from the aganglionic rectosigmoid. Arrows indicate sandwich area between circular and longitudinal
muscular layers. There are no ganglion cells. B. Photograph of colon with Hirschsprung's disease.

to 2 cm in length where there may be diminished ganglion cells; then a normal concentration prevails. The absence of ganglion cells always extends to the distal end of the colon and includes the internal sphincter. The proximal extension is variable. Eighty-five percent of the patients have the lesion limited to the left side of the colon. It is important to realize that 10 percent of the aganglionosis extends across the colon, and this should be in the surgeon's mind when he is performing transverse colostomy. Blind placement of colostomies in the colon may end in a poor result or a fatality unless biopsies are taken to assure that the colostomy is placed in normal colon.

There is considerable discussion about skipped areas, that is, an area of absence of ganglion cells in a segment of intestine well above the rectum with normal innervation above and below. We have not encountered such skipped areas in about 400 specimens that we have had an opportunity to examine. A similar experience in over 200 cases is reported from Great Ormand Street Hospital for Sick Children in London. There has been a published case where a skipped area was claimed. Nevertheless, if the skipped area does exist, it must be extremely rare.

The changes in intestinal function with ganglionic defects have not been studied widely. Over 20 years ago we recorded the colonic function in a group of normal patients and compared these tracings with those secured from children with aganglionosis. Patients with transverse colostomies were selected so that recording balloons could be positioned at the splenic flexure, the descending colon, and the rectosigmoid. In normal patients the peristaltic waves could be recorded from all three positions, while in patients with aganglionosis the peristaltic waves were limited to the normal colon, there being no peristalsis in the aganglionic portion (Figs. 4 and 5). This explains the partial obstruction which is a common part of these patients' history. We postulated that removal of this aganglionic segment would restore intestinal function.

As experience has accumulated it is clear that the internal sphincter which is also aganglionic has a role in this disease. The rectal wall receives inhibiting fibers from the sympathetic system and motor innervation from the parasympathetic fibers. The internal sphincter receives motor innervation from the sympathetic system and inhibition from the parasympathetic system. Therefore a defect in parasympathetic fibers, as is the case with Hirschsprung's disease, would prevent

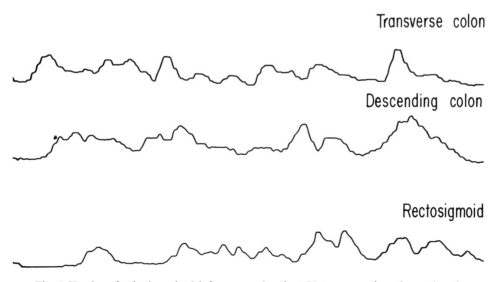

Fig. 4. Tracing of colonic peristalsis in a normal patient. Note progression of wave in colon.

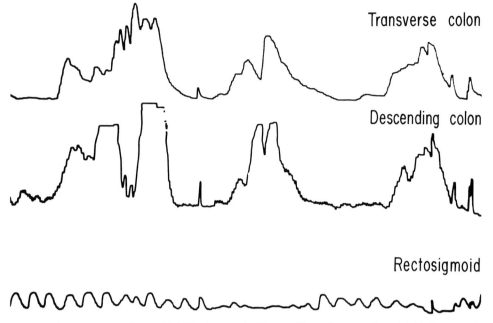

Transverse colon

Descending colon

Rectosigmoid

Fig. 5. Tracing from a patient with Hirschsprung's disease. Note absence of peristalsis in rectosigmoid which was aganglionic when the resected specimen was examined.

relaxation of the internal sphincter. In addition there would be unapposed motor function which would produce the tight internal sphincter which is common in congenital megacolon. Recently direct measurements have been taken which demonstrate that with distension of the rectum, there is contraction of the internal sphincter. In normal subjects, there is relaxation with distension of the rectum.

Grossly the internal sphincter is hypertrophied especially in patients with short aganglionic lesions. It is a common observation that the poorest results from surgical treatment are the children with short aganglionic segments. We have overcome this with a partial resection of the internal sphincter. Rehbein (1960) has used forceful anal dilatation with the purpose of destroying the internal sphincter.

The question of autonomic lesions of the bladder has been widely discussed. Some years ago we had an opportunity to examine a number of patients with enlarged bladders that were not associated with any mechanical obstruction. It was found in such situations that ganglion cells were difficult to find.

They were not completely absent but certainly were diminished from the concentration in normal bladders. It is to be recalled that ganglion cells in the bladder are concentrated in the periureteral areas, and consequently biopsy to determine this concentration is difficult to achieve. The studies were done by dividing the entire bladder into serial sections and evaluating a group of patients with enlarged bladders without obstruction against a series of patients with normal bladders. We could identify the enlarged bladders histologically by the paucity of ganglion cells. In the fixed state the megalobladders were shrunken and no larger than normal bladders. This concept has been challenged by Liebowitz (1963). Clinically megalobladders with megaloureters continue to be found in about 2 to 3 percent of the patients with colonic aganglionosis. The defect in bladder function is not incontinence; rather there is difficulty of emptying despite a high intravesical pressure. The megaloureters develop as a result of the increased intravesical pressure (Fig. 6). To have two lesions as rare as these in the same patient suggests a common etiological agent. It is

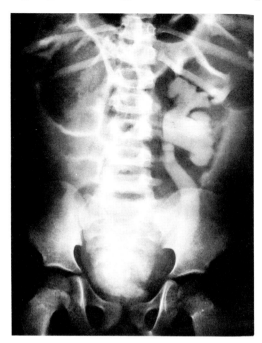

Fig. 6. Excretory urogram of a patient with megacolon and megaloureters.

argued by some that the large fecal impaction causes the megaloureters and enlargement of the bladder. However, we have observed these changes in patients who have had a colostomy shortly after birth and therefore have had no impaction to account for the lesion. While the etiology is not entirely clear, the clinician should be aware of the fact that the two lesions are found occasionally in the same patient. From a probability standpoint it would seem reasonable that a defect in the pelvic parasympathetic system with a colonic defect may well be associated with a similar lesion in the bladder.

CLINICAL SYNDROME

In the past, attention was directed toward the older child with Hirschsprung's disease. As experience has grown it has become evident that the patient with aganglionosis presents a typical syndrome at birth. Considering the high mortality in the first few weeks of life, salvaging a majority of the patients with Hirschsprung's disease requires detecting the lesion early and providing effective

treatment before the lethal complication of gastroenteritis becomes established.

For simplicity and clarity we will divide characteristics of this disease and its diagnosis in the neonate, the infant, and the older child.

NEONATAL HIRSCH-SPRUNG'S DISEASE

It would appear at the present time that the first clue that is extremely valuable in detecting Hirschsprung's disease is delay in passage of meconium. The vast majority of normal babies will pass meconium within 24 hours. Delay in passage should be taken seriously. Recently, there has not been much interest in nurseries in the time of passing meconium. Consequently, accurate records are frequently not maintained. With the possibility of detecting Hirschsprung's disease by delay in passage of the meconium, there has been a revival of interest in the time of passage and the establishment of rules in all nurseries that delay in passage of meconium is a warning symptom which requires investigation. Not only is there a delay in passage of meconium, but a majority of these patients develop all the signs and symptoms of intestinal obstruction. In a series that we studied some years ago, 75 percent presented with mechanical intestinal obstruction. They had vomiting of bile-stained material, failure to pass meconium, and generalized abdominal distension (Fig. 7). In view of the fact that the patient with Hirschsprung's disease faces a mortality rate of 80 percent, needless exploration with a mistaken diagnosis of small bowel intestinal obstruction should be avoided. This unfortunate train of events can be prevented providing the physician and surgeon are alert to the possibilities of Hirschsprung's disease. It is imperative in all patients with signs and symptoms of small bowel obstruction that abdominal roentgenograms be obtained. These will reveal dilated loops of intestine. However, in the neonate it is impossible to identify the dilated intestine as small or large. This distinction can

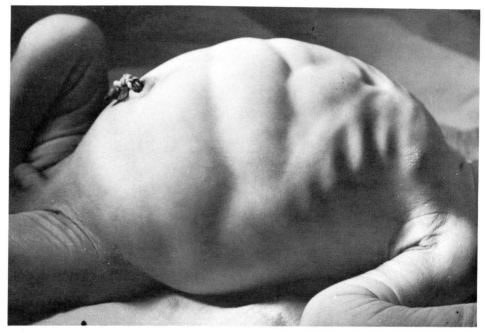

Fig. 7. Neonate with congenital megacolon. He had signs and symptoms of intestinal obstruction.

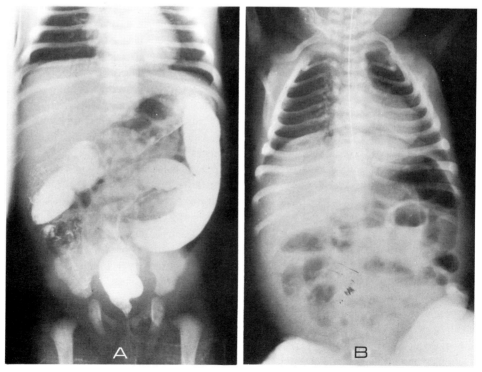

Fig. 8. A. Barium enema of newborn with Hirschsprung's disease. B. Plain upright film of same patient.

be made by having a barium enema performed. If this reveals a normal or dilated colon, the possibility of there being a small bowel mechanical obstruction is nil, and surgical exploration is contraindicated (Fig. 8). On the other hand, when the barium enema outlines a small unused colon, the diagnosis of mechanical intestinal obstruction or meconium ileus is established and abdominal exploration is imperative (Fig. 9).

Unfortunately, the diagnosis of Hirschsprung's disease cannot be established with certainty in the neonate with the barium enema. In the child beyond six weeks of age the barium enema performed and evaluated by an experienced radiologist will be as accurate as rectal biopsy in diagnosing aganglionosis. In rare instances of short lesions the roentgen examination may fail to detect the lesion, but a false positive diagnosis should not be made. This is not true in patients under six weeks of age. We have seen patients with hypothyroidism who have had all the signs and symptoms of neonatal Hirschsprung's disease and whose barium enema examination has revealed the characteristic

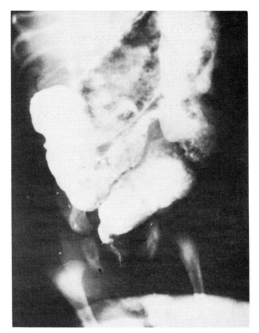

Fig. 10. Barium enema in patient with hypothyroidism.

narrowed distal colon with proximal dilatation (Fig. 10). This same situation can be found in patients with the so-called meconium plug syndrome (Fig. 11). Conse-

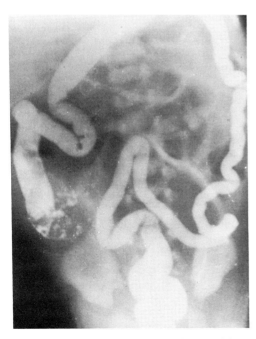

Fig. 9. Barium enema of patient with small bowel intestinal obstruction.

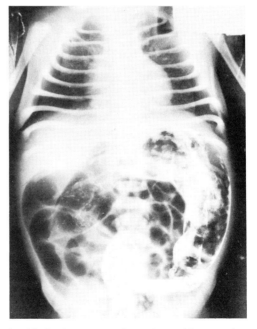

Fig. 11. Barium enema in patient with meconium plug syndrome.

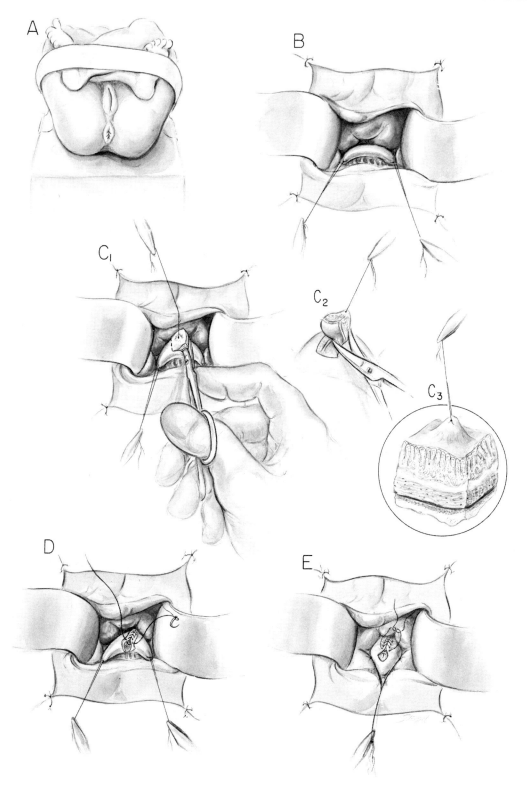

quently, surgical therapy should not be undertaken unless the diagnosis of aganglionosis is established by rectal biopsy.

RECTAL BIOPSY

This is a difficult biopsy to perform because of the small space which the rectum affords, particularly in infants. A vigorous dilatation is advantageous, since it provides better exposure for the procedure. The perianal skin is prepared with soap and Zephiran, and drapes are secured. To facilitate the subsequent resection, we have recently used the posterior wall as the site for biopsy (Fig. 12A).

The anal canal is cleaned with three Zephiran sponges, and one is left in place to prevent gross contamination from the colon. Small retractors are placed on each side to expose the posterior rectal wall (Fig. 12B). Two traction sutures are placed 2 cm above the mucocutaneous line. Traction brings the appropriate portion of the posterior wall into view, and a fine silk suture is placed between and above the traction sutures. A full-thickness biopsy is taken, and the specimen is removed with the fine silk suture (Fig. 12C). One can actually see the layer between the circular and longitudinal muscular coats as a white line. When there is doubt about the adequacy of the biopsy a frozen section can be made to prove the proper tissue has been removed. The defect in the rectal wall is closed with fine silk sutures to the muscular coats and with chromic catgut to the mucosa (Figs. 12D and E). Complications are extremely rare.

To secure accurate interpretation of biopsy requires the services of an experienced pediatric pathologist who has constant experience with this disease (Figs. 13A and B). Such an individual gains his skill by having frequent opportunities to examine histological sections for ganglion cells. Through experience he can determine whether a biopsy is adequate or not (Fig. 14). Up to the present time we have used full-thickness rectal biopsy to establish the diagnosis. This has some disadvantage in that the subsequent resection is more difficult. Consequently we are now tending to use mucosal biopsy. However, it has not proven as yet in our experience to be 100 percent satisfactory. The difficulty with mucosal biopsy is that diverting colostomy cannot be done at the time rectal biopsy is accomplished because frozen section diagnoses are unreliable on histological sections from mucosa alone. Full-thickness biopsy in the hands of a competent experienced pediatric pathologist enables a positive diagnosis of aganglionosis to be made from frozen sections. When mucosal biopsies are used, it is necessary for permanent sections to be made and serial sections of the entire biopsy prepared to be sure that there are no ganglion cells in Meisner's plexus. Our practice is to take the neonate who has had failure to pass meconium beyond 24 hours and has decompressed spontaneously or as the result of rectal irrigations, and to perform a mucosal biopsy. On the other hand, with infants, particularly where decompression has been incomplete and there is urgent need for a colostomy, we recommend full-thickness rectal biopsy in order that a frozen section diagnosis can be made and colostomy performed with one anesthetic. Should the frozen section reveal no ganglion cells, a colostomy is immediately undertaken.

COLOSTOMY

A blindly placed transverse colostomy should be avoided at all cost to prevent a

---

Fig. 12 (opposite page). Rectal biopsy. A. Position of infant for rectal biopsy. B. Two small retractors expose the posterior rectal wall. Traction sutures pull the rectal wall downward. C_1. A full-thickness biopsy is taken of the rectal wall. C_2 The biopsy is removed with a suture of fine silk previously placed. C_3. One can see the sandwich layer between the circular and longitudinal coats of muscle. D. The muscular coat is closed with interrupted fine silk sutures. E. The mucosa is closed with chromic catgut sutures.

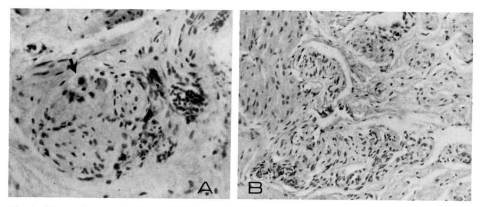

Fig. 13. A. Photomicrograph of rectal biopsy containing ganglion cells. B. Photomicrograph of rectal biopsy from patient with Hirschsprung's disease.

number of complications. The first difficulty is that in about 10 percent of cases, the aganglionosis extends across the transverse colon. We have had a number of patients sent to us with blindly placed transverse colostomies who have shown failure to improve after this procedure. What has happened is that the patient has more extensive aganglionosis than thought, and the colostomy has been placed in the aganglionic segment and is of no value to the patient.

The second difficulty with a blindly placed colostomy is that when there is a long aganglionic lesion extending into the descending colon, there is a considerable problem in reconstruction. This is so simply because the colon is attached to the abdominal wall in the transverse portion at the site of colostomy, and there is inadequate length of bowel to extend to the perineum for the reconstructive procedure. What has to be done in such situations is either to close the colostomy and make a new one or to discard a lot of normal colon, take down the colostomy, and use the right side of the colon for the reconstruction. This does not give the patient as good a result as in those instances where a more adequate length of colon is left in place.

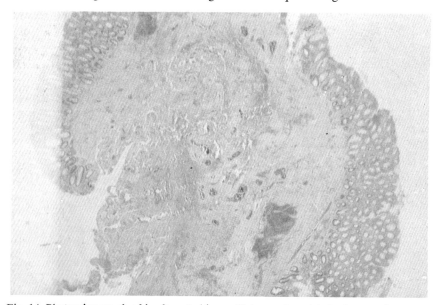

Fig. 14. Photomicrograph of inadequate biopsy. It does not contain both muscular coats.

The third reason for avoiding transverse colostomy is that the patient then has a defunctionalized segment of normal colon which becomes quite small in caliber. At the time of anastomosis there will be a postoperative stricture simply because of the diminished caliber of the colon that one has for the reconstruction.

The fourth reason one should not do a blind transverse colostomy is that a small baby needs as long a segment of colon above the colostomy as possible for good growth and nutrition.

Last, and probably least important, is that when one does a blind transverse colostomy, he subjects the patient to a three-stage procedure—colostomy, resection of the aganglionic segment, and closure of the colostomy.

When the colostomy is placed at the junction of the normal and abnormal colons, treatment can be accomplished with two operations—colostomy and resection of colostomy and aganglionic segment with reconstruction of intestinal continuity.

We place the colostomy at the junction of normal and abnormal colon. This area is discrete in the older child but is indefinite and consequently unreliable in the neonate. Therefore extramucosal biopsies of the colonic wall are made, frozen sections are taken, and a diagnosis of presence or absence of ganglion cells is made. These biopsies are done at the level where the junction of disease and normal bowel is anticipated from gross examination of the colon. If the first biopsy contains no ganglion cells, additional higher biopsies are taken until normal ganglionated bowel is encountered. The advantage of doing these biopsies without entering

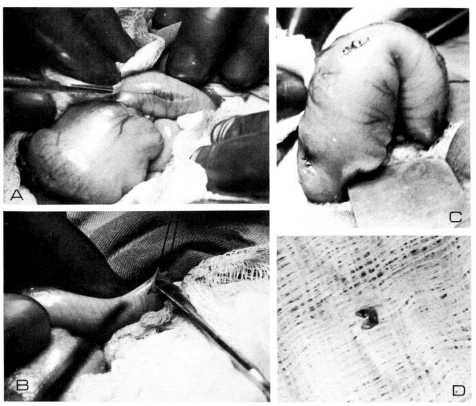

Fig. 15. Biopsy procedure. A. An incision has been made down to the mucosa of the colon. B. The mucosa is pulled from the muscular coat with a blunt dissector. C. Colon. Three biopsies were required to identify normal colon. D. Biopsy material; note how it curls.

the colonic lumen is obvious. This can be accomplished by placing two 6-0 silk traction sutures and then making parallel incisions about $\frac{1}{8}$ inch apart through the muscular coats down to the mucosa. Thus a strip of colonic muscular wall about 1 cm in length can be excised readily. An alternate method is an incision down to the mucosa and then the freeing of the muscular coats from the mucosa with blunt dissection until an edge

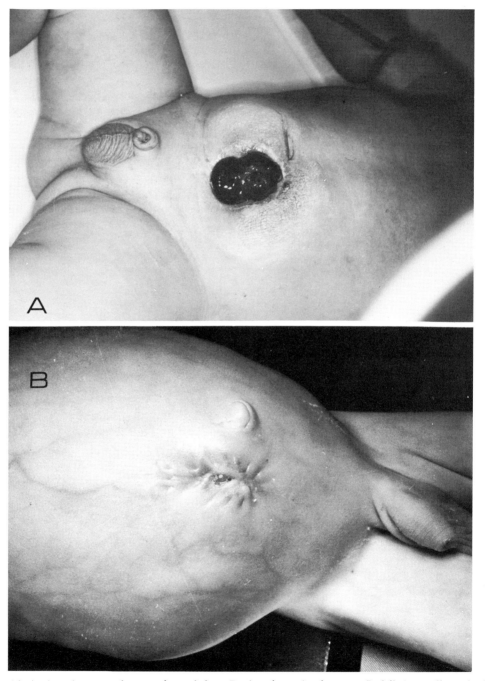

Fig. 16. A. An adequate colostomy in an infant. B. A strictured colostomy. It failed to relieve the infant's partial intestinal obstruction.

can be excised with scissors. The defect is closed with 6-0 interrupted silk (Fig. 15). The specimen curls naturally and when placed on the freezing plate presents a cross-cut surface where ganglion cells can readily be identified in the sandwich area between the circular and longitudinal fibers. A colostomy is then performed. It is important to realize that evisceration of small intestine around the colostomy in the neonate is a constant hazard. Consequently the peritoneum must be sutured to the colon where the colostomy is made with a series of interrupted 6-0 silk sutures. It is also wise to suture the fascia to the colon as an additional safeguard against evisceration. A glass rod through the mesentery under the bowel is left in place to keep the colon well exteriorized and to prevent retraction. Postoperatively the colostomy is opened about twelve hours after operation. The rod is left in place for seven days. At the time it is removed, clamps are placed across the colon, and it is completely divided. This is extremely important in fashioning a good functioning colostomy. The bridge of fibrous tissue which forms across the colostomy as a result of bowel division is a great deterrent to prolapse (Fig. 16). This technique is simpler than dividing the colon, closing the distal end, and leaving it in the abdominal cavity, with immediate maturation of the colostomy.

INFANTS' HIRSCH-SPRUNG'S DISEASE

The infant with Hirschsprung's disease often presents an unexpected clinical syndrome. He may be admitted to the hospital because of gastroenteritis, and when this is severe, prolonged, or recurrent, the possibility of Hirschsprung's disease should be given serious consideration. Normally infants suffering from enteritis will not have abdominal distension, while infants with aganglionosis will have pronounced distension despite the diarrhea. In situations with the patient beyond six weeks of age, the diagnosis can be established by a barium enema. On the other hand, in patients below this age who have gastroenteritis and suspected Hirschsprung's disease, rectal biopsy offers the only sure method of establishing the diagnosis. Once the diagnosis is made, it is a question of proper therapy. We are convinced that immediate colostomy is not indicated in all the patients. In the very sick child with severe infection, it is well to delay colostomy until the patient is brought into more suitable condition for surgical therapy. This is accomplished by the administration of broad-spectrum antibiotics. Before these are administered, it is imperative that a blood culture be secured, as well as stool cultures. However, the instance of septicemia is so high in these patients that it may be lifesaving to administer broad-spectrum antibiotics until their need is disproved by negative blood cultures and stool cultures. Cultures have the additional advantage of guiding chemotherapy when the organism's sensitivities are established.

The second part of the therapy is related to the abdominal distension which is present in patients with acute enterocolitis. One can gently insert a large rectal 24 to 28 F tube. The tube is then gently irrigated with 10 ml aliquots of warm saline. In most instances, one can decompress the babies and thus avoid an emergency colostomy, for the intestine is full of gas and liquid feces. By repeating these irrigations three or four times a day, decompression of the intestine can be maintained. When the child is in good condition colostomy is performed.

POSTOPERATIVE CARE

The postoperative care of the patient with a colostomy who has had severe gastroenteritis is extremely difficult. Many of these cases have an appallingly rapid transit time and consequently pour fluid from their colostomy, due to the severe intestinal infection which involves small intestine as well as the colon. It may be that the intestinal absorption mechanism is so permanently altered that return of normal alimentation is delayed or impossible. Consequently, oral feeding may have to be delayed a considerable length of time simply because of the fact that feeding them when the intestinal transit time is rapid is of no avail and actually is disadvantageous since it increases the loss of intestinal fluids through the colostomy. Gradual feeding with formulas composed of monosaccharides and medium length glycerides rather than the usual fat may be helpful. Supplementation with intravenous fluids may have to be continued for days or even weeks before alimentation becomes effective in maintaining the youngster. We have had situations where supplementation with intravenous fluids has been required for a 30-day period after colostomy in order to have the patient survive. Once the baby is able to maintain himself on oral feedings, there is usually a most gratifying improvement. These infants will become plump and healthy in a matter of two or three months. We have delayed resection until the babies weigh about 15 pounds and are in excellent health.

HIRSCHSPRUNG'S DISEASE IN THE OLDER CHILD

In the older child, the classical picture of Hirschsprung's disease is observed. These children have a great deal of constipation. An important clinical fact to keep in mind when seeing children with severe constipation is that when there is associated soiling, the likelihood of aganglionosis is nil. The patient with aganglionosis also has a history of bowel trouble dating back to early infancy. Another feature that is of importance to the clinician when he is considering a diagnosis is the presence of intermittent abdominal distension, a condition rarely found in patients with chronic constipation and almost inevitably present in the patient with Hirschsprung's disease (Fig. 17). These cases tend to have small thin extremities with a massive abdomen. There is increase in the antero-posterior diameter of the chest due to the chronic abdominal distension. Large intra-

abdominal impactions are common and tend to be in the right lower quadrant, due to the fact that the massive sigmoid usually exhibits the distal portion on the right side. These impactions are not in the pelvic cavity and consequently are movable and not fixed. On the other hand, the patient with chronic constipation usually has a large impaction right down to the external sphincter. It is often said that the patient with Hirschsprung's disease has an empty rectum. While this is generally true, there may be small amounts of hard fecal material in the rectum detectable on digital examination. However, the presence of a large impaction in this location is unknown in Hirschsprung's disease, for in these patients the impactions are above the aganglionic segment.

Individuals with this disease tend to have chronic anemia which is probably due to both blood loss and infection. There may be a number of minute colonic ulcera-

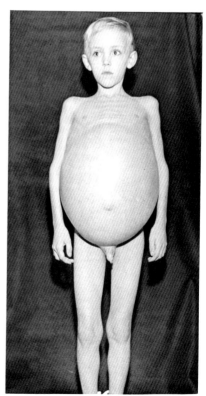

Fig. 17. A boy with advanced Hirschsprung's disease.

tions with blood loss which contribute to the anemia. The general state of debilitation may be an additional factor in the anemia. The diagnosis can be established in a majority of children with a barium enema. In the occasional short lesion, the barium enema examination may be negative, and a diagnosis can be established with a rectal biopsy.

DIAGNOSIS

The differential diagnosis between chronic habit constipation and Hirschsprung's disease can be made in most instances from the patient's history. In Hirschsprung's disease, the symptoms date from birth; in habit constipation, the child's intestinal inertia begins at two or three years of age. Furthermore, abdominal distension is rarely present in habit constipation. Although the parents often insist that distension does occur, it will rarely be found on examination. Additional clinical help in differentiating Hirschsprung's disease from chronic constipation is the fact that the child with habit constipation will be well developed and well nourished, and normal or above normal in height and weight. Often in advanced habit constipation the child has a tendency to pass enormous-sized

stools which frequently block toilet facilities, and there is constant or intermittent soiling. Neither of these symptoms is present in Hirschsprung's disease.

RADIOGRAPHIC DIAGNOSIS

While a presumptive diagnosis of Hirschsprung's disease can be made from the data secured from the history and physical examination of the patient, the diagnosis is not established without demonstrating the pathognomonic lesion by barium enema or by rectal biopsy. The roentgen examination is difficult to perform. The task of the radiologist will be simplified if the colon is fairly well cleaned out by a series of enemas prior to examination. There are several points to be mentioned in connection with the proper roentgen examination of the patient. First, only a small amount of barium should be used so that the narrow segment will be filled completely and the dilated portion incompletely. If a large amount of barium is used, the dilated portion becomes filled and overlaps the rectosigmoid and rectum, obscuring the lesion; it becomes impossible for an accurate radiographic diagnosis to be made. Second, considerable maneuvering of the pa-

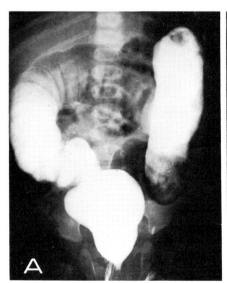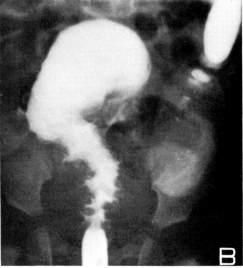

Fig. 18. A. Barium enema failed to outline a narrow segment of colon because an excess of contrast material was used. B. Same patient reexamined with a small amount of barium which outlined the lesion.

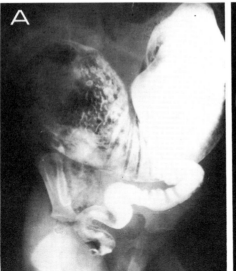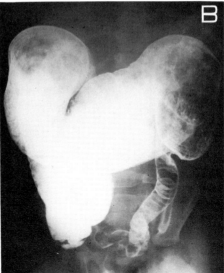

Fig. 19. A. Barium enema outlining a long narrow segment. B. Postevacuation film of same patient.

tient is necessary to obtain adequate fluoro-scopic views of the rectosigmoid and rectum, such as the placing of the patient in the Trendelenburg position and manipulating the sigmoid into the upper part of the abdomen by manual pressure on the abdominal wall. An unobstructed view of the lesion is most

likely to be obtained with the patient in the lateral or oblique position.

Narrowing of the distal colon and dilata-tion of the proximal colon are the pathogno-monic radiographic findings in Hirsch-sprung's disease (Fig. 18). The longer the segment of narrowing, the more readily the diagnosis is made (Fig. 19). In some situa-tions a superior view of the rectosigmoid may be obtained by placing the patient in the Chassard-Lapine position (Fig. 20). A lo-calized indentation of the colon in the sig-moid may be mistaken for Hirschsprung's disease. It is tempting to postulate a so-called skip area, that is, a short aganglionic segment with normal ganglion cells distally, a condi-tion which is extremely rare. We have not observed a patient with such a lesion in whom the diagnosis was established beyond reasonable doubt. It is advisable to secure a postevacuation film, for incomplete empty-ing is a constant feature of Hirschsprung's disease.

In a small number of patients it may be impossible to establish an absolute diagnosis of Hirschsprung's disease from radiographic examination of the colon. This is particu-larly true of those patients with a short lesion in whom the area of narrowing does not ex-tend above the rectum (Fig. 21). It is also

Fig. 20. Roentgenogram of rectosigmoid outlining pathognomonic lesion of Hirschsprung's disease. This is a Chessard-Lapine projection.

difficult at times to diagnose the condition when all of the colon is aganglionic, for in this condition the entire colon may be narrow, and characteristic dilatation of the proximal colon may be absent. The diagnosis is also difficult to make in patients who have had a functioning transverse colostomy for a period of a year or more (Fig. 22). In such situations, the colon beyond the colostomy becomes surprisingly narrow, and the usual changes in contour which are pathognomonic of Hirschsprung's disease may not be demonstrated on barium enema examination.

MANAGEMENT

The treatment of patients with Hirschsprung's disease in the older age group depends on their general health. If they are in fairly good health, a primary resection can be performed after adequate correction of the anemia and hypovolemia. In our experience, in only 10 or 15 percent of the older

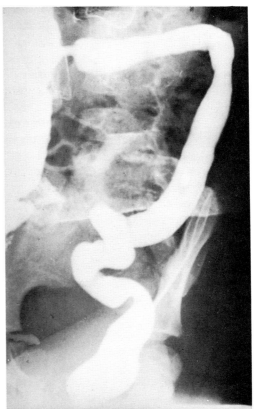

Fig. 22. Roentgenogram of barium enema made two years after transverse colostomy. The aganglionic lesion extended into the sigmoid. Two years of disuse had made the entire distal colon narrow.

patients is a colostomy necessary in order to prepare the patient for resection. Once a colostomy is made, and it should be made at the junction of the normal and aganglionic bowel, the child should be permitted to make a full recovery before resection is undertaken. Attention to anemia and hypovolemia is important, and correction with blood transfusion will provide a better operative risk.

TOTAL AGANGLIONOSIS OF THE COLON

In a recent study of 50 cases of proven aganglionosis 31, or 62 percent, had aganglionosis limited to the rectosigmoid. The lesion included the sigmoid in 4 and the descending colon in 3. The splenic flexure was involved in 4 instances, the transverse

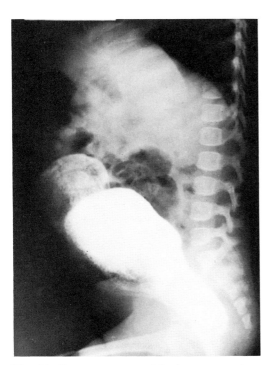

Fig. 21. Roentgenogram of barium enema in a patient with a short aganglionic lesion. The diagnosis could not be established from the radiographic studies. It was established by rectal biopsy.

colon in 3, and the hepatic flexure in 1. The entire colon was involved in 3, which is 6 percent of the patients having total aganglionosis of the colon. This is a little higher than has been reported previously. A recent patient had aganglionosis extending into the midileum. A preoperative diagnosis of meconium ileus was made, and gross finding of a dilated proximal ileum containing thick meconium and a narrow distal segment containing dried bits of meconium seemed to confirm this diagnosis. However, a segment of bowel just proximal to the point of narrowing examined histologically contained no ganglion cells. Undoubtedly, this is a rare form of Hirschsprung's disease. Nevertheless the possibility should be considered in all evident cases of meconium ileus.

All patients with total colonic aganglionosis will present as newborns with signs and symptoms of intestinal obstruction. Barium enema is not diagnostic, for it will outline a normal or slightly smaller than normal colon (Fig. 23). The dilatation will be in the small intestine, indicating small bowel obstruction. At the indicated laparotomy the absence of mechanical obstruction and the finding of a dilated ileum terminating in a narrow segment should alert the surgeon to the possibility of aganglionosis and prompt him to secure a muscular biopsy which will establish the diagnosis of Hirschsprung's disease.

We have had an opportunity to treat a number of such children with resection of the colon and reconstruction of the gastrointestinal tract, anastomosing the terminal ileum to the rectal cuff as we have practiced in all of our patients with megacolon. The management of these patients is extremely important. When such a lesion is encountered in a neonate it is our practice to perform an ileostomy. There will be a satisfactory gain of weight and growth despite the ileostomy. It has been stated by some workers that ileostomy is incompatible with normal growth and development in the newborn baby. This opinion has probably been based on experience where the patient has had severe infection, particularly severe enterocolitis, before ileostomy is performed. It is our conviction that severe enterocolitis not only involves the colon but also produces changes throughout the intestinal tract. The result is that such patients have extremely rapid transit time with poor absorption of both fluids and nutrient substances. It may take many days, even weeks, for the intestinal mucosa to acquire normal function. During

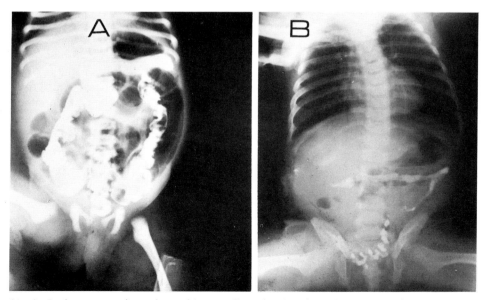

Fig. 23. A. Barium enema in patient with aganglionosis of entire colon. B. A plain film of the same patient two months after ileostomy was performed. Note retention of barium in colon.

this period it is essential to supplement findings with intravenous fluids, including blood and plasma, in an attempt to support the baby. It has recently been suggested that monosaccharides rather than the disaccharides in the formulas have a distinct advantage in this type of situation. It has also been thought that the medium-chain triglycerides should be used as fats in the formula since these are more readily absorbed. Such formulas should be tried. As yet it is impossible to state the exact value they will have in treating these patients. On the other hand, when an ileostomy is performed on a neonate who has not had preceding enterocolitis or infection, there will be little problem in the patient's maintaining his weight with this anatomic arrangement. There may be an adjustment period of several days when it will be necessary to supplement oral feeding with intravenous fluids. However, this should not be a prolonged necessity.

After the patient has made a good adjustment to the ileostomy and is gaining weight satisfactorily, a process which usually takes six to eight months, our policy is to resect the ileostomy and colon, anastomosing the ileum to the rectum. It is advisable not to delay the second stage too long. The infant can be more readily cared for than the older child during the immediate postoperative period which can be quite troublesome due to frequent loose bowel movements. These may number as many as 10 and 12 a day. However, within two or three months the frequency subsides, and the child has 3 or 4 bowel movements a day. During this period the child is a constant nursing problem. The mother must have her household so arranged that she can spend considerable time with the infant. Unless such precautions are taken, the child will develop deep excoriations of the skin of the perineum which greatly complicate the problem. We have followed some of these patients almost 20 years. Growth and development have been normal. They have 2 to 3 bowel movements a day and are in good health (Fig. 24).

It has been suggested that a Duhamel type

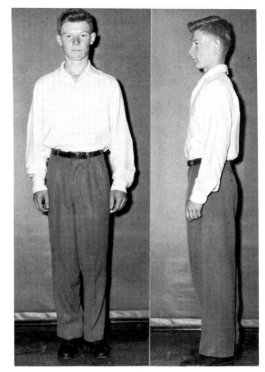

Fig. 24. Two views of a boy who had colostomy and anastomosis of ileum to lower rectum 2 cm above mucocutaneous line. He is healthy 19 years after operation.

of operation be performed on these patients, leaving their entire colon in place. Time will determine whether this long inert colonic segment, left in place, will not distend and become a large diverticulum filled with fecal impactions which will eventually be a great source of trouble. In view of the satisfactory results we have observed by resection of the entire colon, we believe that this additional risk of future trouble should be eliminated by colectomy.

OPERATIVE TREATMENT

A number of operations have been suggested in the last few years for the treatment of Hirschsprung's disease. The concept of the aganglionic defunctioned segment in the distal colon, published by us in 1948, is the basis upon which all of these operations are based. About ten years ago, Duhamel (1960)

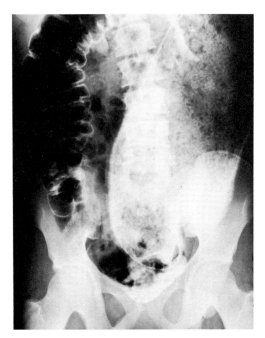

Fig. 25. Plain roentgenogram of abdomen in a patient with Hirschsprung's disease taken eight years after a State type of resection. The film was made after a number of enemas had been used to empty the colon. The patient had severe symptoms.

suggested a modification of the established resection for Hirschsprung's disease. This was to leave the rectum in place, to dissect behind it, to bring the proximal bowel through the posterior rectal wall, and then

to crush with clamps the adjacent bowel walls to form a communication between the rectum and the colon. This operation violates the basic concept of the pathophysiology of Hirschsprung's disease which is that the aganglionic segment is the cause of the disease, by leaving abnormally innervated rectum and rectosigmoid in place. This accounts for the complication of the rectal stump's dilating and becoming the site of large fecalomas. Furthermore, it must be remembered that in order to evaluate these operations, a considerable length of time is necessary. We have observed, for instance, that patients with segmental resections of the type advocated by State (1952) do fairly well for several years (Fig. 25). One patient did well for ten years before the bowel decompensated and a full recurrence of symptoms took place. Consequently, one must be careful in evaluating the results of Duhamel's procedure due to the fact that at the present time there are no reports of long-term results. Complications with this type of operation have also been numerous and should be taken into consideration by the surgeon who elects to use it. Ravitch (1968) has stated that complications are more frequent than anticipated when this technique is used. That this method is not altogether satisfactory is attested to by the fact that numerous modifi-

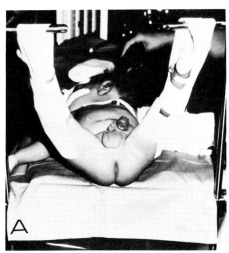
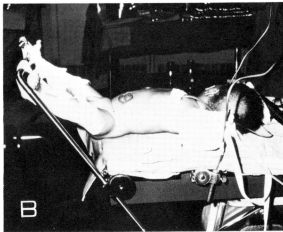

Fig. 26. A. Photograph of infant with legs suspended from bar to provide exposure of abdomen and perineum. B. Side view of same patient.

cations of the original Duhamel procedure had been made, including those suggested by Duhamel himself. Some workers who have used this operation and tested it thoroughly, such as Grob (1964) in Switzerland, have abandoned it because it was inadequate and because the incidence of fecal incontinence was unacceptable.

Anterior resection has had some popularity and is being used by Rehbein in Germany. Rehbein acknowledges the fact that aggressive dilatations are needed in all of the patients after this type of operation for two reasons—stricture at the anastomosis and an abnormal internal sphincter which is left undisturbed by this operation. We have observed recurrence after anterior resection as long as ten years postoperatively. It would seem to be sensible to use an operative procedure which would not require unpleasant rectal dilatations postoperatively and did not have a record of delayed recurrences.

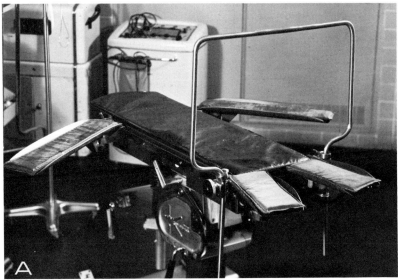

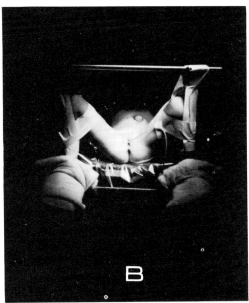

Fig. 27. A. Photograph of table used in operation. Here the foot supports are in place. Children have their knees flexed and strapped to the bar. B. A patient in position.

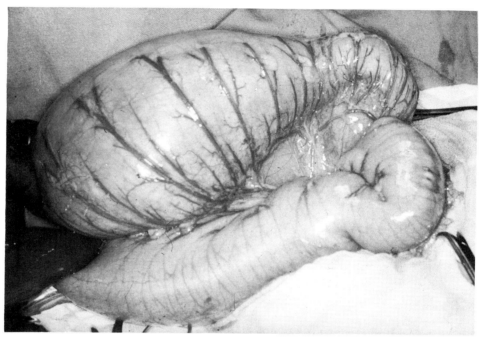

Fig. 28. A typical lesion of Hirschsprung's disease.

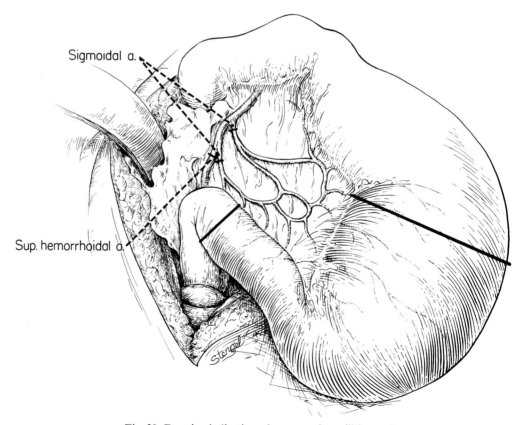

Fig. 29. Drawing indicating where resection will be made.

More recently, Soave (1964) in Italy has revived the Hochenegg type of resection for Hirschsprung's disease. He has removed the mucosa from the rectum and part of the rectosigmoid and passed the bowel down through the remaining muscular tube. This has a number of theoretical objections. In the first place it leaves aganglionic rectum in place and most important leaves the entire abnormal internal sphincter undisturbed. We have used this operation on four occasions, in attempts to resect stricture, and the complications of infection between the pulled-through bowel and the rectal muscular wall were a problem. In the second place we have also observed the internal sphincter and external sphincter cut through the prolapsed rectum permitting the bowel to retract with stricture reformation. In contemplating the use of this operation the surgeon should give considerable thought to the fact that the hypertrophied abnormal muscular coats of the rectosigmoid and rectum are left in place and that, most important, the internal hypertrophied internal sphincter is undisturbed.

TECHNIQUE OF OPERATION

On the basis of our studies of the abnormal pathophysiology in Hirschsprung's disease published in 1948, we proposed removal of the aganglionic segment. This could only be accomplished by a pull-through technique since an anterior resection would leave several centimeters of aganglionic rectum in place. Consequently, the operation that we have performed now for twenty years seems best suited to accomplish a cure on the basis of the known pathophysiology of the disease. In our experience it is the most difficult operation that we encounter in pediatric surgery. Where the surgeon has not had training in its use and an opportunity to perform it under supervision, it is recommended that he perform the operation on a number of animals in the laboratory before undertaking its use on patients. The operation is

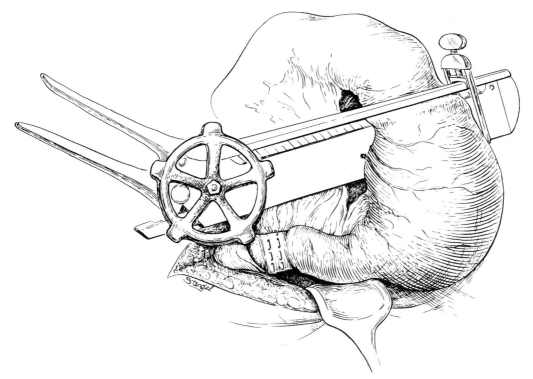

Fig. 30. The Von Petz clamp is used to facilitate the resection.

a tedious one and consumes four to five hours. That the patients tolerate it well is attested to by the fact we have never had shock during operation or postoperatively. We attribute this to thorough preoperative preparation and adequate replacement of blood during operation. To quantitate blood loss, we weigh sponges and replace blood on this basis meticulously. The preparation of the patient is not prolonged. We do not attempt to do more than irrigate the colon for two or three days preceding operation. It is usually impossible to remove large impactions in the sigmoid loop by any method,

and fortunately it is unnecessary to do so before operation.

No attempt is made to reduce the bacterial flora in the colon by administration of antibiotics. This was attempted in a series of patients some years ago, and our complication rate increased, particularly the instance of severe gastroenteritis. In the chronically ill patient the correction of anemia and hypovolemia is important. We insist upon the existence of a good avenue for injection of blood before the operation is undertaken. We also place a catheter through the urethra into the bladder. It is important to position the

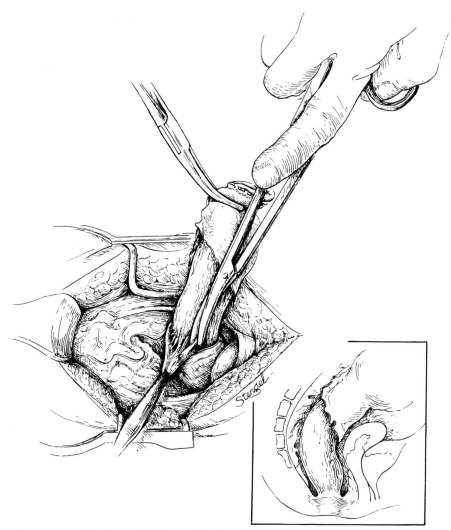

Fig. 31. The dissection is kept on the bowel wall to prevent damage to the autonomic system.

patient in such a way that both the abdomen and the perineum can be exposed simultaneously. In small babies under two years of age, we attach the legs to an overhead bar with adhesive strapping (Fig. 26). This can be lowered so that during the abdominal part of the operation, there is no hindrance from the lithotomy position of the child. Older children are handled in a different way, the feet being placed on small holders at the end of the table with the legs flexed at the knees and strapped with adhesive tape to an overhead bar (Fig. 27). Other types of supports should be used with caution to prevent damage to the perineal nerve. By using the technique illustrated in Figure 27, we have never had any damage to this nerve despite operations lasting 8 hours. The abdomen is prepared and draped with a large sterile drape, and the abdominal part of the operation

undertaken. A left rectus muscle-retracting incision is advantageous particularly when the splenic flexure unexpectedly needs to be detached, for the incision can be extended upward to facilitate this maneuver. If a transverse incision is used, there may be difficulty should the need arise for detaching the splenic flexure. Once the abdomen is opened, the sigmoid is delivered. Usually the lesion is in the distal sigmoid or rectosigmoid, and there may be a large impaction in the sigmoid. We select a proximal line of resection 10 to 12 cm above the narrow colon and divide the bowel using a von Petz stapling clamp to accomplish rapid and effective closure of the bowel ends (Figs. 28, 29, and 30). No infection has been observed with the use of this clamp. We divide the bowel with endothermy. The next task is to divide one or more sigmoidal arteries to provide ade-

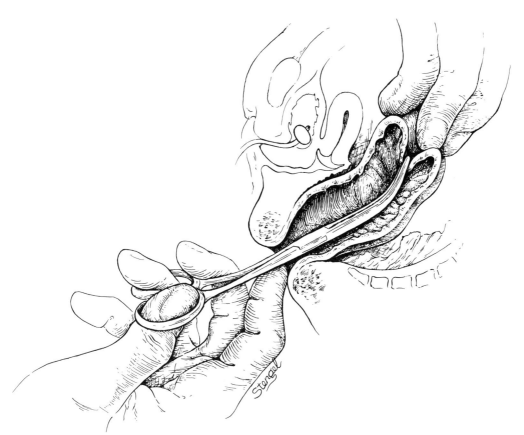

Fig. 32. A long curved clamp is inserted through the anus, grasping the closed rectosigmoid so that it can be everted.

quate length of bowel to reach to the perineum without tension (Fig. 31). Rather than take a chance with inadequate length of bowel it is wise when necessary to divide the left colic artery and to detach the splenic flexure, thus providing an adequate length. Not only must there be sufficient length, but a vigorous blood supply must be present in the most distal part of the colon. When the lesion is in the transverse colon there is insufficient length of colon for the conventional reconstruction. Ligation and division of the middle colic artery is required, and the right side of the colon is turned down to the perineum, precautions being taken that the terminal ileum is not obstructed or the right ileocolic vessel compromised. The peritoneum is then divided down along the rectosigmoid and rectum, and the incisions from the sides are united in the cul-de-sac anterior to the rectum. In the male it is important to identify both vasa and both ureters before proceeding with the peritoneal incision. The bowel is then detached down to the rectosigmoid where it is again transected with the use of the von Petz stapling clamp and diathermy. Thus the large impaction is removed

with the specimen. The resected bowel is given to the pathologist so that a frozen section can be made and the state of ganglion cells determined at the proximal line of resection. If ganglion cells are absent, 2 or 3 inches more of bowel is resected proximally, and this is repeated until cells are encountered. It is important not to ligate the superior hemorrhoidal vein but to ligate the superior hemorrhoidal artery to reduce bleeding during the pelvic dissection. At a point well above the superior hemorrhoidal vessels, the pelvic dissection is brought to the bowel wall. This is an important precaution to prevent damage to urinary bladder innervation and to guard against any subsequent defect in ejaculation (Fig. 32). At this point, we free the peritoneum on each side in the pelvis for a short distance and suture it to the anterior peritoneum adjacent to the abdominal incision. This effectively walls off the small intestine from the field and obviates the necessity of large packs to keep the small intestine out of the pelvic cavity during the dissection. The dissection is made right on the bowel wall, a tedious procedure which necessitates that a large number of small

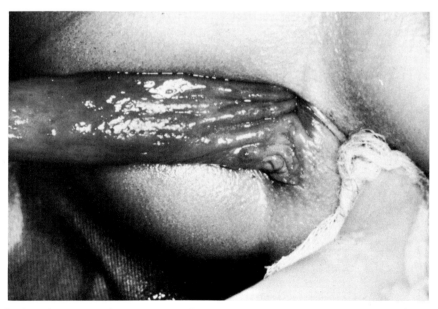

Fig. 33. Prolapsed rectum. With traction on the rectum and countertraction on the perianal skin the mucocutaneous line is clearly visible. The pelvic dissection must be deep enough to permit this amount of prolapse.

vessels be ligated. We ligate the vessels on the pelvic side with fine silk and use endothermy to cauterize the vessels on the specimen side. It is impossible to determine definitely from the intra-abdominal part of the dissection when the bowel has been freed sufficiently for proper resection. We dissect a reasonable depth into the pelvis and then prolapse the distal segment to be sure that it has been freed sufficiently. This is determined when one can, by placing traction on the prolapsed rectum and countertraction on the perianal skin, actually see the junction of mucosa and the perineal skin (Fig. 33). This is important posteriorly and laterally, but not superiorly. Unless the bowel has been freed so that this can be accomplished it is returned to the pelvic cavity and the dissection extended for a centimeter or two further. It may be necessary to return the rectal stump two to three times into the pelvic cavity in order to have the dissection at exactly the precise distance.

The alternative technique of prolapsing the colon has many disadvantages despite its theoretical appeal of preventing infection. First, the resection method permits testing of the adequacy of the dissection by prolapsing the rectal stump, a simple maneuver compared to the situation when the intussuscepting technique has been used. Furthermore, the pathologist has ample material to determine the ganglion cell situation. An additional advantage is that the fecalith is in the segment of colon removed during the abdominal phase of the operation.

Most important, the adequacy of the distal resection is difficult to determine with the massive colon pulled through the rectum when the intussuscepting technique is used. Palpation may erroneously indicate that an adequate resection is being performed, when 6 to 8 cm of rectum may actually be left in place, a situation we have proved in some patients sent to us postoperatively by other surgeons.

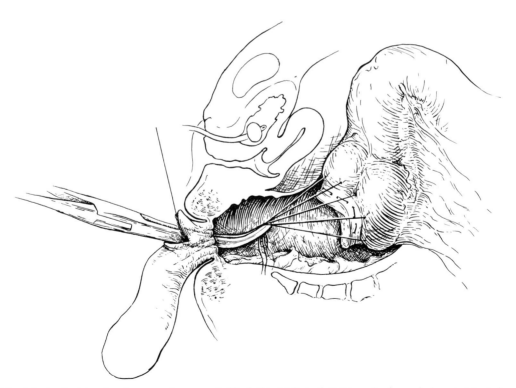

Fig. 34. An incision has been made across half of the prolapsed rectum. A clamp is inserted to bring the proximal segment to the perineum.

Our only change in the technique of the operation, since it was published 20 years ago, is that we excise part of the internal sphincter. This is accomplished by cutting back diagonally across the prolapsed rectum so that we are virtually at the mucocutaneous margin posteriorly. Not more than 0.5 cm of mucosa should be left. If the patient has a low lesion, it is well to cut it to the skin margin. It is important to make the cut anteriorly and halfway across the bowel and then to pull the proximal bowel through. Before this is done, the bowel should be prepared for the anastomosis by excising the mesentery for a distance of at least 1 cm to provide a clean area. It may be necessary to cut one

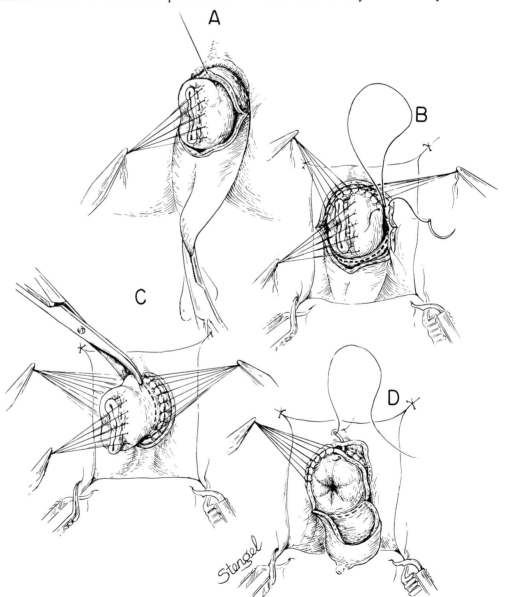

Fig. 35. Anastomosis. A. The anastomosis is begun anteriorly. A single suture has been placed on the muscular layer of the everted rectum. B. The muscular coats are approximated with interrupted silk sutures. C. When this row is completed, the proximal segment is opened along the row of silk sutures. D. The anastomosis is completed with interrupted sutures of catgut to the mucosal layers.

or two sigmoidal vessels in order to have sufficient length. After these are cut, it is important to be sure that there is a vigorous blood supply to the end which is to be used in the anastomosis. The anastomosis is not commenced until the pathologist has reported on a frozen section which he has taken from the proximal end of the resected colon. Unless ganglion cells are present at this point, additional bowel is resected until normal colonic wall is encountered. A cut is made anteriorly 2 to 3 cm from the mucocutaneous line on the prolapsed rectum, and a clamp is inserted to pull the prepared proximal segment through (Fig. 34).

The anastomosis must not be attempted unless 2 or 3 cm of colon can be brought through without tension, particularly at the mesenteric border. The anastomosis is one of the most difficult to make in intestinal surgery. It must be absolutely watertight and able to withstand the extreme high pressure which the colon is capable of developing, higher than any other region of the gastrointestinal tract. We make the anastomosis in children with 5-0 silk; in small infants under two years of age with interrupted 6-0 silk sutures. These are placed close together so that we will have an absolutely watertight suture line (Figs. 35A and B). The difficult part of the anastomosis is posteriorly, and precautions must be taken to provide for discrepancies of bowel size of the two segments. This is accomplished by taking sutures across the large segment and parallel to the long axis of the smaller segment. As the last part of the anastomosis is made posteriorly, it is well to work from both sides and to place the patient in the Trendelenburg position so that a clear view can be had. It is in the posterior aspect of the anastomosis that most difficulties arise, and the surgeon should guard against them with careful placement of sutures. He must prevent folding of the large bowel that has been pulled through. If he allows such a fold to exist without proper suturing, there will be a catastrophe from a leak.

The anastomosis is then completed by excising the cap of the proximal bowel and approximating the mucosa of the two segments with 4-0 chromic catgut sutures in the older child and 5-0 chromic catgut sutures in the younger child (Figs. 35C and D).

While the anastomosis is being made, the abdominal incision is closed with interrupted silk sutures with a continuous 5-0 plain catgut suture to the skin with a collodion dressing. In children under one year of age, a suprapubic cystotomy is made. We have had poor drainage from penile catheters in small children. In older children, the catheter is left in place five or six days postoperatively.

POSTOPERATIVE CARE

The patients have a surprisingly benign postoperative course providing they have been well prepared and the operation properly executed. The average hospital stay postoperatively is less than 12 days. Recently, it has been possible to discharge some of the patients within 8 days after operation. The danger from perforation of the suture line should be small providing adequate blood supply has been provided in the proximal segment of bowel and a careful, tight anastomosis has been accomplished. Unless this has been achieved at the time of operation, a colostomy should be instituted before the abdomen is closed. The critical postoperative period is the first 4 days. During this time perforation of the suture lines, should it occur, will take place. When the patient has an unexplained elevation of temperature or abdominal distension which cannot be readily relieved by the insertion of a large rectal tube, a perforation of the suture line should be ruled out with a contrast enema. To prevent overlooking a small leak, it is important to use Diodrast as contrast material rather than barium. Should a patient become distended postoperatively and an upright abdominal film reveal free air under the diaphragm, the diagnosis of a leak is established and a contrast study is unnecessary. Should a leak be detected postoperatively, immediate colostomy is imperative. Providing this precaution is promptly taken, the development of a stricture is unknown. On the other hand, we have had patients referred to us who have had a leak at the suture line where there has been a delay of weeks or months in performing a colostomy. It is in such situations that chronic infection becomes so well established in the pelvis that an impermeable stricture is inevitable. Furthermore, early detection of a leak may be lifesaving.

We administer a broad-spectrum antibiotic postoperatively since operation involves a potentially contaminated field. Such administration of antibiotics is not prophylactic. The antibiotics are continued for four or five days, and then Gantrisin is substituted for the rest of the hospital stay and for a week after the patient leaves the hospital. This is done to guard against urinary tract infections which may result from the use of an inlying bladder catheter.

Should any abdominal distension develop after operation, the insertion of a large, soft, open-ended rubber catheter is required. Gentle irrigation through the tube should be limited to maintain patency of the tube. The complication of mild or severe enterocolitis postoperatively has been all but eliminated by a more radical resection which includes part of the internal sphincter. The role of the greatly hypertrophied aganglionic internal sphincter has not been fully appreciated in the therapy of this disease. If left undisturbed, it continues to be a considerable physiological obstruction to colonic emptying. Prior to our partial resection of the internal sphincter, we had occasional bouts of enterocolitis postoperatively. Should these occur, it is important to insert a large rectal tube to irrigate the colon gently with small aliquots of saline to completely decompress the abdominal distension. In no instance have we encountered in the immediate or delayed postoperative period enterocolitis of a severity that would require a colostomy. Rather we have performed a medical colostomy, that is, the use of a large rectal tube

with irrigations. Prior to our use of partial resection of the internal sphincter, small infants, particularly, returned occasionally with severe enterocolitis associated with excessive abdominal distension and retention of liquid fecal material. There was soon such severe intestinal wall inflammation that ileus supervened and prevented passage of any intestinal contents. Unless this possibility is promptly recognized, and drainage of the colon instituted by the insertion of a large rectal tube, a fatality may result or the condition may develop into a chronic ulcerative colitis that is extremely difficult to treat. Irrigations two or three times a day may be required for several days to help the baby through an attack of enteritis. Fortunately, this complication has been largely eliminated by an extension of the operation to include partial resection of the internal sphincter.

FOLLOW-UP

The care of these patients after they leave the hospital is extremely important. In the first place, the surgeon must realize that the family, particularly of the older children, are so concerned about bowel function that their anxiety will continue postoperatively and may disturb intestinal function in the postoperative patient. To guard against this, the surgeon must have adequate talks with the parents to allay their anxiety for the patient postoperatively. Our rule is that no parent may give the child a laxative, enema, or suppository postoperatively without consulting us by telephone. Any technique that will build up the patient's and the parents' confidence postoperatively should be used by the surgeon, according to his own preferences.

The patients can be on a normal diet with the exception that some will experience diarrhea with certain foods, particularly green corn. The parents should observe this and quickly eliminate such items from the patient's diet.

Postoperatively, the patient will tend to have loose stools, and as long as this state persists there will be some soiling during passage of intestinal gas (which is profuse in many cases). This is often misinterpreted as true incontinence. Actually, one can talk this over with older children, and observant parents will relate that the soiling occurs with the passage of flatus. The older child can be warned to go to the bathroom if he is to pass flatus and thus not soil himself. As the stool becomes more firm passage of flatus is accomplished without soiling. Usually this takes place about six months after operation although it can be variable.

It is also important to impress upon parents of infants the necessity of delaying vigorous attempts at bowel training. Too vigorous attempts may give the patient a common variety of constipation due to holding back. The parents are urged to be lenient in train-

Fig. 36. A. Photograph of patient before operation. B. Same patient several years after operation.

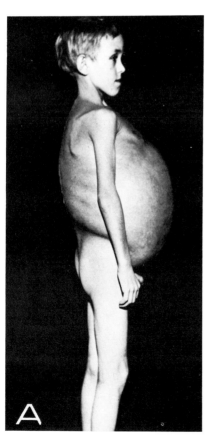

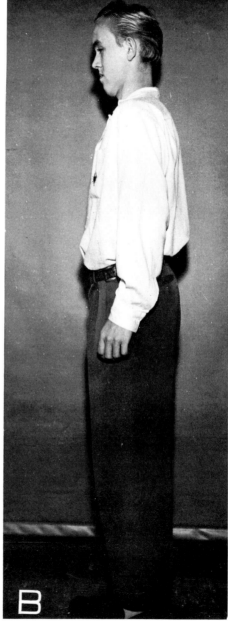

ing, their efforts being limited to making sure that the child has a chance to observe normal behavior in older children and to make suitable equipment available.

COMPLICATIONS

With the use of the new technique of partial internal sphincter resection we have reported a series of 32 patients without a significant complication. Two patients had slight urinary tract infection postoperatively. No intra-abdominal infection, difficulty with suture line, or stricture developed in these patients. To be sure, some of the infants had bouts of enteritis postoperatively, usually in conjunction with siblings affected with this

same disease. They were able in most instances to handle enteritis without the development of the abdominal distension and ileus which was a postoperative complication in some of our patients prior to the use of this technique. The mortality from the operation of resection has remained in the vicinity of 2.5 percent. The instance of leak at the anastomosis is about 5 percent. In none of these patients has stricture developed. We attribute this to the fact that prompt colostomy has been made. A variety of usual and unusual complications has occurred, such as acute appendicitis in the postoperative patient, jejunoileal intussusception, and intestinal obstruction from postoperative adhesive bands. Persistent fecal incontinence has not been present in our postoperative patients, and we

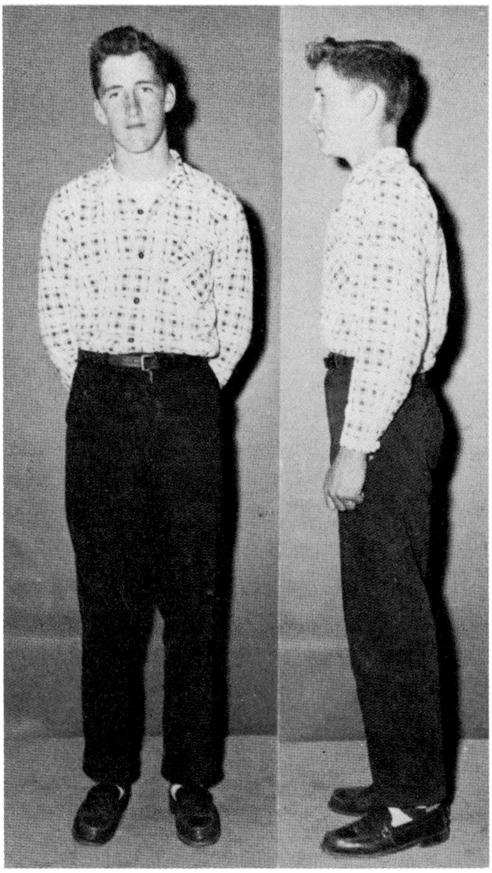

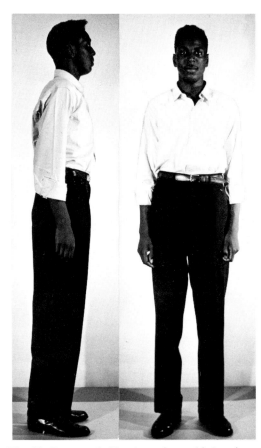

Fig. 37. Front and side views of our first male patient who was resected. The followup has been for 20 years.

Fig. 38. Front and side view of our third patient, who is well 20 years after operation.

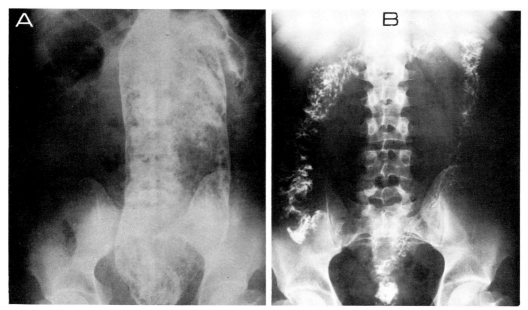

Fig. 39. A. Preoperative barium enema. B. Barium enema one year following resection.

have now had an opportunity to observe some of them for twenty years. Urinary incontinence has never occurred. We have had two instances where there has been difficulty to complete emptying of the bladder. In these situations, the use of a tidal irrigator for two or three weeks postoperatively has completely corrected the situation. The bowel habits vary. Most patients settle to one or two bowel movements a day and later may occasionally miss a day. Constipation as observed in normal children has rarely been encountered in our postoperative patients. In two or three instances we have observed the patient develop a holding back syndrome, particularly during the age of two or three when the child tends to be extremely negative. Mild impactions have occurred in these patients. The use of enemas and suppositories for short periods of time, plus the elimination of milk, breads, and ice cream from the diet have proved entirely effective.

Disturbance of ejaculation was thought to be a complication of this type of resection. We can now state that a number of patients, some who were resected in their teens and others at a younger age, are now married,

and there is no reported instance of inability to have children. One mother who was resected has had four children, one with aganglionosis. We have had another interesting family in which the mother had five children, all with aganglionosis. Her husband was killed, and following remarriage she has had three normal children. The danger of this disease being passed on to subsequent generations from affected mothers and fathers seems to be very small as far as we can tell from our experience at the present time. There has been no recurrence of the disease in our patients, even those who have been followed for as long as twenty years. We are quite confident that once provision of an adequate resection is done, particularly with partial resection of the internal sphincter, permanent cures are achieved. Resection of part of the internal sphincter is probably less necessary in the older child who can overcome the defect by a more forceful contraction of the abdominal musculature during defecation. While the operation is a long and tedious one, it pays off handsomely in having a low mortality rate, few complications, and permanent cure.

The results improve as time passes after operation. We have a number of patients who 10 to 19 years after the operation are perfectly well (Figs. 36–38). The colon may take several years to return to normal. However, it empties completely. Some return to normal in one year (Fig. 39).

ORVAR SWENSON

REFERENCES

BERMAN, C. Z. Roentgenographic manifestations of congenital megacolon (Hirschsprung's disease) in early infancy. Pediatrics, 18: 227, 1956.

BOGGS, J. D., and KIDD, J. M. Congenital abnormalities of intestinal innervation: absence of innervation of jejunum, ileum and colon in siblings. Pediatrics, 21: 261, 1958.

DALLA VALLE, A. Contributo alla conoscenza della forma famigliare del megacolon congenio. Pediatrics, 32: 569, 1924.

DUHAMEL, B. A new operation for the treatment of Hirschsprung's disease. Arch. Dis. Child., 35: 38, 1960.

EHRENPREIS, T. Megacolon in the newborn; a clinical and roentgenological study with special regard to the pathogenesis. Acta Chir. Scand., 94: 1, 1946.

EMANUEL, B., PADORR, M. P., and SWENSON, O. Familial absence of myenteric plexus (congenital megacolon). J. Pediat., 67: 381, 1965.

——— PADORR, M. P., and SWENSON, O. Mongolism associated with Hirschsprung's disease. J. Pediat., 66: 437, 1965.

GROB, M. Personal communication.

LAWSON, J. O. N., and NIXON, H. H. Anal canal pressures in the diagnosis of Hirschsprung's disease. J. Pediat. Surg., 2: 544, 1967.

LIEBOWITZ, S., and BODIAN, M. A study of the vesical ganglia in children and the relationship to the megaureter megacystitis syndrome and Hirschsprung's disease. J. Clin. Path., 16: 342, 1963.

MADSEN, C. M. Hirschsprung's disease. Copenhagen, Munksgaard, 1964.

McDONALD, R. G., and EVANS, W. A., Jr. Hirschsprung's disease. Roentgen diagnosis in infants. Amer. J. Dis. Child., 87: 575, 1954.

POTTS, W. J., BOGGS, J. D., and WHITE, H. Intestinal obstruction in the newborn infant due to agenesis of the myenteric plexus (congenital megacolon). Pediatrics, 10: 253, 1952.

RAVITCH, M. Emergency surgery in the newborn. Surg. Gynec. Obstet., 126: 597, 1968.

REHBEIN, F., and VON ZIMMERMANN, H. Results with abdominal resection in Hirschsprung's disease. Arch. Dis. Child., 35: 29, 1960.

SHIM, W. K. T., and SWENSON, O. Treatment of congenital megacolon in 50 infants. Pediatrics, 38: 185, 1966.

SOAVE, F. A new surgical technique for treatment of Hirschsprung's disease. Surgery, 56: 1007, 1964.

STATE, D. Physiological operation for idiopathic congenital megacolon (Hirschsprung's disease). J.A.M.A., 149: 350, 1952.

SWENSON, O. Partial internal sphincterectomy in the treatment of Hirschsprung's disease. Ann. Surg., 160: 540, 1964.

——— Follow-up on 200 patients treated for Hirschsprung's disease during a 10 year period. Ann. Surg., 146: 706, 1957.

——— and IDRISS, F. Excision of rectal stricture with end-to-end anastomosis. Arch. Surg. (Chicago), 93: 54, 1966.

——— and FISHER, J. H. Hirschsprung's disease during infancy. Surg. Clin. N. Amer., 36: 1511, 1956.

WHITEHOUSE, F. R., and KERNOHAN, J. W. The myoenteric plexus in congenital megacolon. Arch. Intern. Med., 82: 75, 1948.

ZUELZER, W. W., and WILSON, J. L. Functional intestinal obstruction on congenital neurogenic basis in infancy. Amer. J. Dis. Child., 75: 40, 1948.

INDEX

1